42⁵⁰

VENOUS PROBLEMS

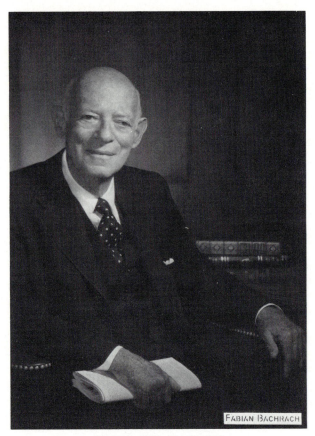

FABIAN BACHRACH

GEZA DE TAKATS

Scientist, Raconteur, Clinical Investigator, Surgeon Extraordinaire, Respected Intellectual.

Past President, Society for Vascular Surgery; Past President, North American Chapter, International Cardiovascular Society; Past International President, International Cardiovascular Society; Past President, Chicago Surgical Society; Past President, Chicago Heart Association.

Recipient of Many Honorary Awards.

Author of 270 Medical Articles and Countless Short Stories.

VENOUS PROBLEMS

Edited by
JOHN J. BERGAN, M.D.
AND
JAMES S. T. YAO, M.D., PH.D.

Blood Flow Laboratory, Division of Vascular Surgery,
Department of Surgery,
Northwestern University Medical School,
Chicago, Illinois

YEAR BOOK MEDICAL PUBLISHERS, INC.
CHICAGO • LONDON

This Symposium was supported by a generous grant from Scholl, Inc. whose continued interest in this field is well known worldwide.

Library of Congress Catalog Card Number: 77-81529

International Standard Book Number: 0-8151-0686-6

Foreword

THE SYMPOSIUM ON VENOUS PROBLEMS to honor Dr. Geza de Takats has served at least two important purposes. First, the meeting was a fitting tribute to a remarkable man and a long-standing contributor to the understanding of vascular disease. Second, the Symposium provided an opportunity to gather a large number of scientists and clinical investigators in a single conference to discuss the complex problems of venous disease. I cannot recall a similar symposium that has provided comparable comprehensive review of the pathophysiology of venous circulation and of venous disease.

This book is a tribute to Doctor de Takats and to those who participated in the Symposium. In addition, Drs. John J. Bergan and James S. T. Yao and their associates deserve commendation for publication of the material that made this conference successful. Even a cursory review of this book will provide evidence of the depth of coverage of venous problems, and a study of each chapter will reward the reader with detailed information on each aspect of venous circulation and disease.

So often medical symposia suffer from presentation of familiar findings and repetition of data that are available in journals. It is to the credit of the contributors to this Symposium that the papers present current concepts and new data to challenge the reader.

The contributions from international participants from England and from Sweden enhance the value of this volume as a source of reference material. I consider this book to be a timely publication that should be of interest to surgeons in general, as well as those who are specifically interested in vascular disease.

JOHN M. BEAL, M.D.

Professor and Chairman, Department of Surgery
Northwestern University Medical School
Chicago

RICHARD J. DALEY
MAYOR

CITY OF CHICAGO

PROCLAMATION

WHEREAS, Dr. Geza de Takats was the founder of vascular surgery in Chicago and has had a long career of leadership in the development of vascular surgery throughout the world;

WHEREAS, Dr. de Takats no longer practices surgery, but is continually consulted for his opinions and ideas about vascular surgery and vascular disorders; and

WHEREAS, at the age of 84, Dr. de Takats has been an inspiration to others seeking careers in vascular surgery and vascular disorders; and

WHEREAS, great dedication and devotion to the health of his fellow men and women is evident from the assignments he has accepted in medicine—Director of the Vascular Clinic at Northwestern University; Professor of Surgery (now Emeritus) at the University of Illinois College of Medicine, and Professor of Surgery Emeritus at Rush Medical College; and

WHEREAS, despite the demands of his medical career, he still found time to devote to the presidencies of the Chicago Heart Association, Chicago Surgical Society, Society of Vascular Surgery, North American Chapter of the International Cardiovascular Society, and other; and

WHEREAS, Northwestern University Medical School has honored Dr. de Takats by holding a symposium in his name;

NOW, THEREFORE, I, RICHARD J. DALEY, Mayor of Chicago, do hereby proclaim Thursday, December 2, 1976, to be DR. GEZA de TAKATS DAY IN CHICAGO, AND CALL UPON ALL CITIZENS TO HONOR AND SALUTE THIS GREAT DOCTOR.

Dated this 2nd Day of December, 1976.

MAYOR

Contributors

FREDERICK A. ANDERSON, JR., M.S.

Department of Surgery,
University of Massachusetts
Medical School,
Worcester, Massachusetts

RICHARD J. ARMENIA, B.S.

Research Technologist,
Research Service,
Veterans Administration
Hospital,
West Roxbury, Massachusetts

WILEY F. BARKER, M.D.

Chief, Division of General
Surgery and Professor of
Surgery,
University of California
School of Medicine,
Los Angeles

JOHN S. BELKO, M.S.

Biochemist-in-Charge Research
Service,
Veterans Administration
Hospital,
West Roxbury, Massachusetts

JOHN J. BERGAN, M.D.

Magerstadt Professor of Surgery,
Chief, Division of Vascular
Surgery,
Northwestern University
Medical School,
Chicago, Illinois

SVEN-ERIK BERGENTZ, M.D.

Professor of Surgery,
University of Lund,
Malmö General Hospital,
Malmö, Sweden

NORMAN L. BROWSE, M.D., F.R.C.S.

Professor of Vascular Surgery,
St. Thomas' Hospital Medical
School,
London, England

K. G. BURNAND, F.R.C.S.

Lecturer in Surgery,
St. Thomas' Hospital Medical
School,
London, England

ARTHUR J. CANOS, M.D.

*Kachelmacher Memorial
  Laboratory for Peripheral
  Venous Diseases and
Department of Surgery,
Good Samaritan Hospital,
Cincinnati, Ohio*

JULIUS CONN, JR., M.D.

*Professor of Surgery,
Northwestern University
  Medical School,
Chicago, Illinois*

LEONARD T. COTTON, M.CH.,
  F.R.C.S.

*Dean-Elect, King's College
  Hospital Medical School,
London, England*

JOHN J. CRANLEY, M.D.

*Director, Kachelmacher
  Memorial Laboratory for
  Peripheral Venous Diseases
  and
Director, Surgery Medical
  Education,
Good Samaritan Hospital,
Cincinnati, Ohio*

JAMES K. CREASY, M.D.

*Fellow in Peripheral Vascular
  Surgery,
Department of Surgery,
Northwestern University
  Medical School,
Chicago, Illinois*

W. ANDREW DALE, M.D.

Professor of Clinical Surgery,

*Vanderbilt University School of
  Medicine,
Nashville, Tennessee*

RICHARD H. DEAN, M.D.

*Associate Professor of Surgery,
Vanderbilt University School of
  Medicine,
Nashville, Tennessee*

JAMES A. DeWEESE, M.D.

*Professor of Surgery and
  Chairman, Division of
  Cardiothoracic Surgery,
University of Rochester School
  of Medicine,
Rochester, New York*

LAZAR J. GREENFIELD, M.D.

*Professor and Chairman,
Department of Surgery,
Medical College of Virginia,
Virginia Commonwealth
  University,
Richmond, Virginia*

WILLIAM S. GROSS, M.D.

*Assistant Professor of Surgery,
University of Michigan School
  of Medicine,
Ann Arbor, Michigan*

JOHN T. HOBBS, M.D.,
  F.R.C.S.

*Consultant Surgeon and Senior
  Lecturer in Surgery,
St. Mary's Hospital Medical
  School,
London, England*

ROBERT W. HOBSON, II, M.D.

Associate Professor of Surgery,
College of Medicine and
*   Dentistry of New Jersey and*
Chief, Surgical Service,
Veterans Administration
*   Hospital,*
East Orange, New Jersey

MICHAEL HUME, M.D.

Professor of Surgery,
Tufts University School of
*   Medicine and Chief of the*
*   Surgical Services,*
Lemuel Shattuck Hospital,
Boston, Massachusetts

E. A. HUSNI, M.D.

Department of Surgery,
Huron Road Hospital,
Cleveland, Ohio

ROBERT L. KISTNER, M.D.

Department of Peripheral
*   Vascular Surgery,*
Straub Clinic and Hospital, Inc.
*   and Associate Professor of*
*   Surgery,*
John A. Burns School of
*   Medicine,*
University of Hawaii,
Honolulu, Hawaii

HAU C. KWAAN, M.D.,

Professor of Medicine,
Northwestern University
*   Medical School and*
Chief, Hematology Section,
Veterans Administration

Lakeside Hospital,
Chicago, Illinois

KARL A. LOFGREN, M.D.

Head, Section of Peripheral
*   Vein Surgery,*
Mayo Clinic and Mayo
*   Foundation and*
Associate Professor of
*   Surgery,*
Mayo Medical School,
Rochester, Minnesota

JERE W. LORD, JR., M.D.

Professor of Clinical Surgery,
New York University School of
*   Medicine and*
Chief, Vascular Surgery,
Cabrini Health Care Center,
Columbus Hospital Division,
New York, New York

MARIAN F. McNAMARA, M.D.

Coon Fellow in Peripheral
*   Vascular Surgery,*
Northwestern University
*   Medical School,*
Chicago, Illinois

KRISHNAMURTHI MAHALINGAM, M.D.

Kachelmacher Memorial
*   Laboratory for Peripheral*
*   Venous Diseases and*
Department of Surgery,
Good Samaritan Hospital,
Cincinnati, Ohio

KAZI MOBIN-UDDIN, M.B., B.S.

Department of Surgery,
The Frederick C. Smith Clinic,
Marion, Ohio

HARVEY L. NEIMAN, M.D.

Associate Professor of
  Radiology,
Northwestern University
  Medical School
Chicago, Illinois

A. N. NICOLAIDES, M.S.,
  F.R.C.S., F.R.C.S.E.

Senior Lecturer and Honorary
  Consultant Surgeon to the
  Cardiovascular Unit and
Director of the Vascular
  Laboratory,
St. Mary's Hospital Medical
  School,
London, England

JOHN H. OLWIN, M.D.

Clinical Professor of Surgery,
  Emeritus
Rush Medical College and
Attending Surgeon, Emeritus
Rush-Presbyterian-St. Luke's
  Medical Center,
Chicago, Illinois

J. CUTHBERT OWENS, M.D.

Professor of Surgery,
University of Colorado Medical
  Center,
Denver, Colorado

NILIMA A. PATWARDHAN, M.D.

Department of Surgery,
University of Massachusetts
  Medical School,
Worcester, Massachusetts

GEORGE P. POLLOCK, PH.D.

Assistant Professor of
  Physiology,
Loyola University,
Stritch School of Medicine,
Maywood, Illinois

WALTER C. RANDALL, PH.D.

Professor of Physiology,
Loyola University,
Stritch School of Medicine,
Maywood, Illinois

NORMAN M. RICH, M.D., COL.,
  M.C., U.S. ARMY

Chief, Peripheral Vascular
  Surgery Service,
Walter Reed Army Medical
  Center and
Professor and Chairman
  Department of Surgery,
Uniformed Services University
  of the Health Sciences,
Washington, D. C.

V. C. ROBERTS, PH.D., M.I.E.E.

Deputy Director,
Department of Biomedical
  Engineering,
King's College Hospital
  Medical School,
London, England

EDWIN W. SALZMAN, M.D.

Professor of Surgery,
Harvard Medical School and
Associate Director of Surgery,
Beth Israel Hospital,
Boston, Massachusetts

ARTHUR A. SASAHARA, M.D.

Chief, Medical Service,
Veterans Administration
* Hospital,*
West Roxbury, Massachusetts
* and*
Professor of Medicine,
Harvard Medical School,
Boston, Massachusetts

SIMON SEVITT, M.D.,
  F.R.C.P.I., F.R.C.PATH.

Consultant Pathologist,
Birmingham Accident Hospital,
Birmingham, England

G. V. R. K. SHARMA, M.D.

Director, MICU-CCU,
Veterans Administration
* Hospital,*
West Roxbury, Massachusetts
* and*
Instructor in Medicine,
Harvard Medical School,
Boston, Massachusetts

JOHN T. SHEPHERD, M.D.

Director of Research,

Mayo Clinic and Mayo
* Foundation,*
Rochester, Minnesota

D. E. STRANDNESS, JR., M.D.

Professor of Surgery,
University of Washington School
* of Medicine,*
Seattle, Washington

DAVID S. SUMNER, M.D.

Professor and Chief,
Section of Peripheral Vascular
* Surgery,*
Southern Illinois University
* School of Medicine,*
Springfield, Illinois

KENNETH G. SWAN, M.D.

Chief, Division of General and
* Vascular Surgery and*
Professor of Surgery,
College of Medicine and
* Dentistry of New Jersey,*
Newark, New Jersey

HARVEY TAKAKI, M.D.

Fellow in Peripheral Vascular
* Surgery,*
Northwestern University
* Medical School,*
Chicago, Illinois

DONALD E. TOW, M.D.

Chairman, Nuclear Medicine
* Service,*
Veterans Administration
* Hospital,*
West Roxbury, Massachusetts
* and*

Assistant Professor of
  Radiology,
Harvard Medical School,
Boston, Massachusetts

Bonno van Bellen, M.D.

Assistant Professor of Surgery,
Santo Amaro Medical School,
São Paulo, Brazil

H. Brownell Wheeler, M.D.

Professor and Chairman,
Department of Surgery,
University of Massachusetts
  Medical School,
Worcester, Massachusetts

Creighton B. Wright, M.D.

Associate Professor of Surgery,
Division of Thoracic and
  Cardiovascular Surgery,
University of Iowa and
Veterans Administration
  Hospital,
Iowa City, Iowa

James S. T. Yao, M.D., Ph.D.

Associate Professor of Surgery
  and Director,
Blood Flow Laboratory,
Northwestern University
  Medical School,
Chicago, Illinois

Table of Contents

Symposium on Venous Problems: Introductory Remarks

MAY I EXPRESS my sheer delight, great pride and deep gratitude to Northwestern University Medical School, and primarily to John Bergan and to Jim Yao, for having organized this meeting. It was just 50 years ago when Allen B. Kanavel generously offered me a half-time surgical fellowship at this institution which enabled me to combine teaching and research with patient care.

A curious sequence of events led me to establish a Vein Clinic. I had 7 years of surgical residency abroad which included neurologic and orthopedic surgery, but found that in the climate of the mid-1920s I would hardly be able to survive unless I selected a subspecialty. With the encouragement of Allen Kanavel, to whom I really owe all I have ever accomplished, I started an elective course in Local Anesthesia and taught a course in Surgical Physiology, both of which were new additions to the curriculum. I was also struck with the plight of the patient suffering from varicose veins and even more with those having postphlebitic ulcers, since they wandered from one clinic to another, getting varied and highly indifferent treatment. I read the report of a Danish surgeon named Meisen, who injected a hypertonic dextrose solution into the veins of horses and obtained firm thrombi. We started the injection treatment of veins and combined it with ambulatory saphenous vein ligation. Later more and more attention was paid to incompetent valves in the perforators. We became aware of deep venous insufficiency. The flood of leg ulcers was treated with glycerin-gelatin boots and many an old Northwestern alumnus still grumbles about the Unna's paste he had to apply in the clinic. Later we widely excised and grafted these ulcers. It soon became obvious, however, that many patients had arterial, arteriolar or lymphatic involvement. Because we were operating in a vacuum, with no internists, cardiologists, coagulationists or plastic surgeons exhibiting the slightest interest in this material, a Peripheral Circulatory Clinic was

1

born around 1930. By the time I transferred to the University of Illinois in 1935, a fully developed program had been established. In addition to venous problems, the lymphatics were studied and also the peripheral arterial tree, which was found to react in the brain, heart, kidney and mesentery not unlike the vascular tree in the extremities. I also became entranced with the autonomic nervous system.

This obviously called for a team approach. During my traveling fellowship supported by the Rockefeller Foundation in 1924–1925, I had the privilege of being assigned to Allen O. Whipple at Columbia who established a spleen clinic, a thyroid clinic and later a hypertension clinic, with a great deal of success. I managed to gather a group of aggressive and talented physiologists, internists and neurologists and later a coagulationist, who all converged on the patients two afternoons a week, instead of the patient—frequently from downstate—limping from one clinic to another. The entire team attended the clinic and were not just on call by the house staff. In addition, with small grants from here and there, which would seem minuscule today, we had a technician and a nurse attached to the Vascular Clinic; they studied the clotting mechanism and gave treatments with suction boots and rhythmic constrictors. Plethysmographs and ergographs became available. Skin temperature and galvanic resistance measurement were used.

All this seems terribly far away and superannuated. Certainly the cardiothoracic surgeon today will seldom study histamine flares in the skin or bother with venous pressure measurements when the patient is walking or standing still. Most of them still doubt the importance of vascular reflexes in pulmonary embolism and venous hypertension. And yet in a few institutions, of which the Division of Vascular Surgery at Northwestern is an outstanding example, this specialty managed to survive and flourish. Excellent patient care backed by clinical research in hemodynamics, in the clotting-fibrinolytic balance and in the autonomic nervous system continue here. To all the participants of this Symposium, some of whom came from a great distance, and to its efficient organizers, John Bergan and Jim Yao, my very best wishes and deep gratitude.

GEZA DE TAKATS

BASIC PHYSIOLOGY IN VENOUS CIRCULATION

Introduction

THE AUTHORS of the following papers concerning basic physiology of the venous circulation have condensed a tremendous amount of complex, highly pertinent information into their presentations. It is appropriate that the conference on venous problems began in this way since, ultimately, the accurate diagnosis and effective treatment of any disease rests on a complete understanding of the pathophysiology.

Despite an almost mystical fear of pulmonary embolism, most surgeons, internists and medical students are strangely apathetic toward venous disease. It never seems to excite the imagination in the same way that cardiac or arterial problems do. For this reason, many of us have a scattered, fragmentary knowledge of venous physiology.

Awareness of our ignorance is easily expanded to the feeling that little is known. In fact, as the following papers demonstrate, there is a great body of solid information applicable to the understanding of venous pathophysiology.

The work of Doctor Shepherd and his colleagues has greatly expanded our knowledge of venous control mechanisms. As clinicians, we are often aware of the effects of change in arterial diameter. Yet changes in venomotor tone may make a greater contribution to the total circulatory response to stress than changes in arterial tone.

Doctor Strandness has capably reviewed the literature on venous hemodynamics in both normal and diseased states. His implication that venous disorders represent a continuum is apropos. Classification of each patient's disease demands careful documentation of the type and magnitude of existing hemodynamic aberration.

Although techniques for recognizing venous obstruction and valvular incompetence have been available for some time, ability to quantitate the degree of disturbance has been lacking. Perhaps the plethysmographic methods mentioned will fill this need. With these or similar objective methods, a longitudinal study of chronic venous insufficiency could be undertaken. Such a study would further our understanding of the natural history of these diseases and allow them to be treated more rationally.

Doctors Pollock and Randall have summarized the complex anatomy and function of the pulmonary vasculature as it is currently understood. The importance of the numerical approach is emphasized by their review of the function of the lung as a reservoir.

Certainly, there are many challenging problems to be solved and many questions to be asked. For example, what is the possible therapeutic role of pharmacologic agents in controlling venous capacity? What is the role of reflex pulmonary arterial constriction in patients with pulmonary embolism, a question raised long ago by Doctor de Takats.

1 / Reflex Control of the Venous System

JOHN T. SHEPHERD, M.D., M.CH., D.SC.

Mayo Clinic and Mayo Foundation, Rochester, Minnesota

THE GREATER PART of the blood volume is contained in the low pressure side of the circulation. This includes the postcapillary systemic vessels, the right heart, the pulmonary vessels and the left atrium. Thus, these channels function as the capacitance part of the circulatory system. While the total blood volume is maintained relatively constant by appropriate reflex adjustments of renal hemodynamics and hormonal effects on the renal tubules, shifts of blood do occur between different parts of the cardiovascular system, especially between the cardiopulmonary vessels and the systemic veins. This is especially important in humans because of the shift of blood from the heart and lungs to the systemic veins which occurs as the subject moves from the horizontal to the upright position. As a consequence, the filling pressure of the ventricles is reduced and the cardiac output decreases. The major function of the systemic venous system is to counteract this shift in order to maintain an adequate intrathoracic blood volume and filling pressure for the heart in response to any stress imposed upon it.

The role of the systemic venous system is best understood by an analysis of its three major components: the splanchnic veins, the veins within the skeletal muscles and the cutaneous veins (Fig 1-1). The splanchnic and cutaneous veins are richly supplied with sympathetic nerves, whereas the muscle veins have little or no sympathetic innervation (Fig 1-2).

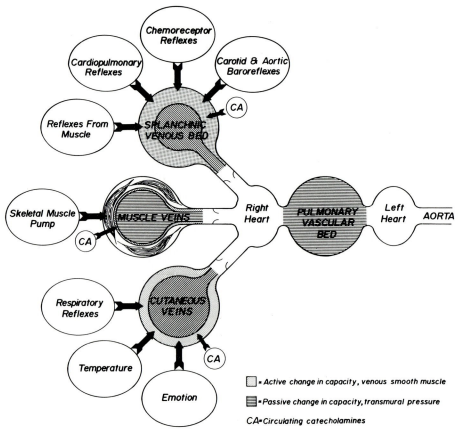

Fig 1–1.—Schematic representation of the regulation of the intrathoracic blood volume (*right heart, pulmonary vascular bed* and *left heart*) by the three major components of the systemic venous system (*splanchnic venous bed, muscle* and *cutaneous veins*). These three components adjust the intrathoracic blood volume and hence the filling pressure of the heart by active expulsion of blood due to contraction of the venous smooth muscle and by passive expulsion due to a decrease in venous distending pressure resulting from constriction of the precapillary resistance vessels. The latter will occur in the systemic venous bed with any stimulus that causes an increase in sympathetic outflow to the systemic resistance vessel or an increase in circulating catecholamines. In the skeletal muscles the compression of the veins by the contracting muscles is an additional but important means for their passive emptying. While the active expulsion of blood from the splanchnic venous bed is controlled primarily by mechanoreflexes and chemoreflexes from the carotid sinus region, the aortic arch, the heart and lungs and the skeletal muscles, that from the cutaneous veins is governed mainly by local and central changes in temperature, by respiratory reflexes and by emotion. The veins of the skeletal muscles have little or no sympathetic innervation, but like the splanchnic venous bed and the cutaneous veins they can be constricted by circulating catecholamines.

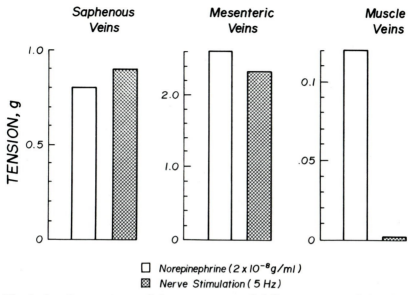

Fig 1–2.—Comparison of the responses of different veins of the dog to electric field stimulation and norepinephrine. The response to norepinephrine is an indication of the density of the smooth muscle population, while that to electric stimulation is an indication of the density of adrenergic innervation. Note the differences in scale. Mean data for six strips of different dogs in each group. (Modified from Shepherd, J. T., and Vanhoutte, P. M.: *Veins and Their Control* [London: W. B. Saunders Company, Ltd., 1975]. Used by permission.)

The Splanchnic Venous Bed

In resting conditions, the splanchnic vascular bed contains about one fifth of the total blood volume and receives a similar proportion of the cardiac output. Because of its capacity to take up and release blood, and the influence of the gut in counteracting gravitational changes in venous transmural pressure, the splanchnic venous bed plays a major role in the regulation of cardiac filling pressure. The potential contribution of the different components of this bed can be demonstrated by their response to electric stimulation of the splanchnic nerves. In the dog, the spleen seems to be an ideal blood reservoir because it has the capability of releasing 6–14% of the total blood volume with a hematocrit value of more than 80%.[1] In the cat and the dog, the small intestine can mobilize an amount of blood that corresponds to 30–60% of its blood content; in comparison with the spleen the actual volume of blood released is small. For example, in dogs with an average weight of 10 kg, stimulation of the sympathetic nerves at outflow pressures of 10 cm H_2O expels 5 or 6 times more blood from the spleen than from the small intestine.[1,2] In the cat, stimulation of the hepatic nerves can result in expulsion of more than 50% of the blood in the liver, thus making the latter potentially an important blood reservoir.[3]

The release of blood from the splanchnic bed with activation of the sympathetic nerves is a result of active and passive expulsion of blood from the veins. When the nerves are stimulated, the precapillary vessels constrict. As a result there is a decrease in the venous distending pressure because of the increased resistance to flow through the precapillary resistance vessels and the resultant loss of energy. Hence, there will be a passive expulsion of blood from the veins as the trans-

Fig 1–3.—Active and passive expulsion of blood from splanchnic region in dog. Total splanchnic inflow and outflow are continuously recorded with electromagnetic flowmeters. Alteration of blood volume is computed as the difference between inflow and outflow. Control flow is set equal to zero, and increases and decreases from this level are shown. *Left panel,* arterial and venous blood flow changes are plotted during an 18-sec thoracic splanchnic nerve stimulation (15 v, 15 Hz, 3 msec). Active plus passive emptying amounts to 112 ml. *Middle panel,* blood flow changes during an 18-sec mechanical arterial inflow occlusion to the same flow level causes passive emptying of 55 ml. *Right panel,* computed change in splanchnic blood volume (57 ml) represents active emptying during previous electric stimulation. (Data from Brooksby, G. A., and Donald, D. E.: Circ. Res. 31:105, 1972. By permission of the American Heart Association, Inc.)

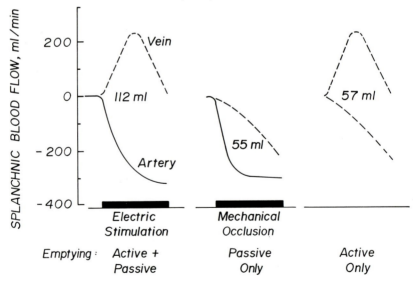

mural pressure within them decreases. At the same time the increased activity of the sympathetic nerves to the veins causes them to constrict and actively expel blood; thus, the active and passive components reinforce each other in supplying blood to the heart (Fig 1–3).

The various components of the splanchnic circulation make different contributions to the active and passive release of blood. For example, in the dog, the spleen expels blood in an almost wholly active manner while the small intestine has a large passive component.[1]

The changes in capacity of the splanchnic bed are mediated mainly by the sympathetic nerves whose activity is altered in response to reflexes from the carotid and aortic baroreceptors, the cardiopulmonary receptors, the carotid and aortic chemoreceptors and receptors activated by contraction of the skeletal muscles.

A decrease in carotid sinus pressure causes contraction of the spleen and constriction of the ileal and colic veins. In the total splanchnic bed, blood flow and blood volume change in proportion to the carotid sinus pressure (Fig 1–4). The greatest changes are seen when this pressure fluctuates within 30 mm Hg of the normal blood pressure. Over the full range of carotid sinus activity, the amount of blood mobilized corresponds to 60% of that expressed by maximal electric stimulation of the splanchnic nerves.[4]

The cardiopulmonary receptors are strategically located to signal changes in central blood volume. When this volume is reduced by gravitational forces or blood loss, the resulting decreased activity of

Fig 1–4.—Increases and decreases in splanchnic blood volume and flow in response to graded changes in pressure in the isolated carotid sinus in five dogs. (From Brooksby, G. A., and Donald, D. E.: Circ. Res. 29:227, 1971. By permission of American Heart Association, Inc.)

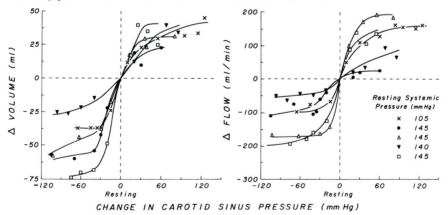

CHANGE IN CAROTID SINUS PRESSURE (mm Hg)

these receptors causes constriction of the splanchnic resistance and capacitance vessels and an active and passive mobilization of blood. By contrast, when the central reservoir is overfilled and the activity of the receptors is increased, the splanchnic bed accommodates more blood. The influence of the cardiopulmonary receptors on splanchnic blood volume is maximal when the inhibitory input to the vasomotor centers from the carotid baroreceptors is absent or minimal.[5] In dogs, the effect on hepatic blood volume of withdrawal of inhibitory traffic from the carotid sinus and the cardiopulmonary receptors was compared by reducing carotid sinus pressure from 220 to 40 mm Hg and then cold-blocking the vagi. Combined withdrawal of carotid sinus

Fig 1–5.—Constriction of the splanchnic veins and muscle resistance vessels and dilatation of the cutaneous veins in response to hypoxic stimulation of carotid chemoreceptors in dog. The vagi are cut. The carotid sinuses are vascularly isolated and perfused at constant pressure; the latter is maintained at 40 mm Hg to eliminate the inhibitory influence of carotid baroreceptors. Stimulation is caused by perfusion with autologous blood collected in a reservoir and equilibrated at PO_2 37 mm Hg; PCO_2 and pH normal. Systemic PO_2, PCO_2 and pH were normal. Muscle resistance vessels and cutaneous vein were perfused at constant flow with autologous blood; thus, changes in perfusion pressure were caused by constriction or dilatation of the respective vessels. Response of the splanchnic veins was estimated from changes in pressure in the spleen, whose circulation was temporarily arrested. (From Shepherd, J. T.: Circulation 50:418, 1974. By permission of American Heart Association, Inc.; data from Pelletier, 1972 and Pelletier and Shepherd, 1972.)

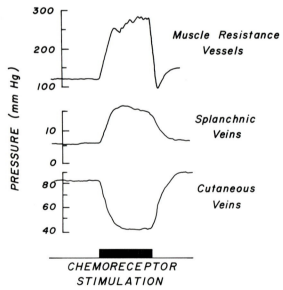

and cardiopulmonary inhibitory traffic reduced hepatic blood volume by a mean of 13 ml/100 gm. The carotid sinus was responsible for 63% of this total change and the cardiopulmonary receptors for 37%.[4a] Activation of the carotid chemoreceptors causes the splanchnic veins to constrict (Fig 1-5).

Direct electric stimulation of afferent nerves from the muscles causes pressor or depressor responses, depending on the intensity and frequency of stimulation. Similar responses can be obtained when the muscles are made to contract. Electric stimulation of brachial plexus afferents in the cat causes constriction of the splanchnic capacitance vessels. In the dog, similar responses are obtained in the spleen with high frequency stimulation of the afferent nerves from muscle or with sustained tetanic contraction induced by electric stimulation of the gastrocnemius and quadriceps muscles. The constriction of the spleen is reflexly induced by the contraction of the skeletal muscles; after neuromuscular blockade, stimulation at the same voltage and frequency causes relaxation. By contrast, low intensity stimulation of the afferent nerves from muscle or rhythmic muscle contractions causes a relaxation of the spleen. Since this persists after neuromuscular blockade, it may be due to direct stimulation of nociceptive fibers. The reflex constriction of the splanchnic veins which results from tetanic contraction of the skeletal muscles is mediated by small myelinated (group III) and nonmyelinated (group IV) afferent fibers; the nature of the receptors in the skeletal muscles activated in this way remains to be determined.[6, 7]

Muscle Veins

These veins have little or no sympathetic innervation.[8, 9] Active venoconstriction may occur in response to catecholamines either released from the adrenal medulla overflowing into the bloodstream at the precapillary level or liberated by the few adrenergic nerve fibers in the vein wall. However, the precapillary resistance vessels in muscle are densely innervated and play an important role in blood pressure control through the carotid and aortic baroreflexes and the chemoreflexes. Hence, if the precapillary resistance vessels are constricted this will lead to a passive decrease in volume of the muscle veins. However, the major factor involved in the emptying of these veins is the muscle pump, especially of the leg veins in man in the upright position.

During contraction of the leg muscles, the resulting increase in intraluminal pressure in the deep veins causes them to empty. When the muscles relax, the intraluminal pressure in these veins decreases abruptly below that in the cutaneous veins so that the blood flows from the latter to the former. The emptying of the veins during and after the contraction restores the competence of the valves, so that the long hydrostatic column is broken into shorter segments; thus the pressure of the cutaneous veins is decreased.[10] As the blood flows into the veins, the partially collapsed deep and superficial veins refill and the pressure within them increases at a rate that is determined by the blood flow through the leg. The venous pressure remains low if successive contractions occur before the veins become overdistended and the valves become incompetent.

A similar venous pump mechanism also operates for the foot. The deep veins of the sole are compressed either by the weight of the body or by contraction of the plantar muscles or both; the blood is pumped along perforating veins into the superficial veins on the dorsum of the foot, reflux being prevented by valves.[11]

Cutaneous Veins

The hypothalamic thermoregulatory centers dominate the neurogenic control of the cutaneous veins. Thus, if the temperature of the body core is varied over the range of 40–33 C, the cutaneous veins constrict progressively (Fig 1–6). The neurogenic thermoregulatory control is reinforced by the local effects of temperature. Local cooling augments and local warming depresses the cutaneous venomotor reactions to adrenergic nerve stimulation (Fig 1–7). While cooling augments the contraction of isolated venous strips, it decreases the efflux of neurotransmitter (Fig 1–8) One explanation is that cooling results in a greater affinity of the membrane for the released norepinephrine.

The modulation of cutaneous venomotor reactions by temperature, together with the changes in adrenergic venomotor outflow, operate to restrict or increase heat loss from the skin according to the thermal requirements of the organism. The cutaneous venoconstriction with body cooling not only decreases heat loss by decreasing the venous surface area but it also directs venous flow through the venae comitantes where transfer of heat from the accompanying artery takes place. Such a countercurrent exchange creates a thermal short circuit that carries some of the arterial heat back into the body.[12, 13] Because the deep limb veins do not participate in venomotor reflexes and because they dilate when perfused with colder blood,[14] this facilitates

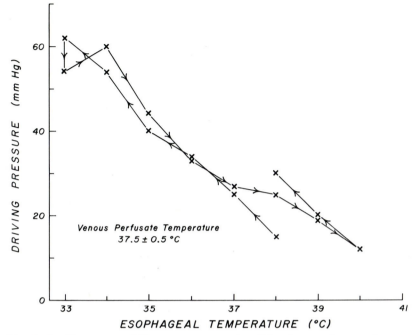

Fig 1–6.—Response of the cutaneous vein of the dog to changes in central temperature, with local temperature constant. The lateral saphenous vein was perfused at constant flow so that changes in driving pressure were caused by constriction or dilatation of the vein. Note that venous responses to esophageal temperature change appear to be linear over the range 33–40 C. (From Webb-Peploe, M. M., and Shepherd, J. T.: Circ. Res. 23:693, 1968. By permission of American Heart Association, Inc.)

both the shift of blood from the superficial to the deep veins and the countercurrent exchange with the arterial blood.

While stimulation of the carotid chemoreceptors causes the splanchnic venous bed to constrict together with the resistance vessels in the splanchnic bed, the muscle bed and the skin due to an increase in sympathetic outflow, the cutaneous veins dilate due to a decrease (see Fig 1–5).[15, 16]

The stress of mental arithmetic or unpleasant thoughts is enough to activate the adrenergic nerves to the cutaneous veins. The venoconstriction is accompanied by a dilatation of the resistance vessels in the skeletal muscles, due probably to both activation of cholinergic fibers and circulating catecholamines (Fig 1–9).

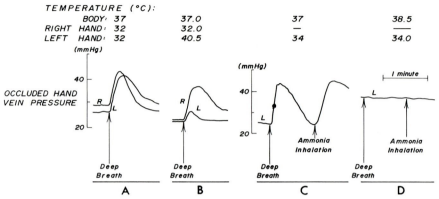

Fig 1−7.—Experiment showing that in man the cutaneous veins are governed by both local and central thermoregulatory mechanisms. **A,** voluntary deep breath with body temperature at 37 C and both hands at 32 C produced marked increase in venous pressure (occluded limb technique) in both hands. **B,** warming left hand to 40.5 C greatly attenuated the response in that hand. **C,** returning hand temperature to 34 C restored response to deep breath and ammonia inhalation. **D,** increasing body temperature to 38.5 C abolished response to same stimuli when hand temperature was maintained at 34 C. (From Shepherd, J. T., and Webb-Peploe, M. M.: Cardiac Output and Blood Flow Distribution During Work in Heat, in Hardy, J. D., Gagge, A. P., and Stolwijk, J. A. J., (eds.): *Physiological and Behavioral Temperature Regulation* [Springfield, Ill.: Charles C Thomas, Publisher, 1970], p. 237. Used by permission. The original data were kindly supplied by R. S. Zitnik).

During sleep, the veins of the hand became more distensible, possibly because emotional influences are absent or because the pattern of respiration is changed. Transient increases in venous tone during sleep could be associated with dreaming.[17]

The cutaneous veins also react to unpleasant or painful stimuli. For example, the application of ice to the forehead or the sudden immersion of one hand in cold water activates the sympathetic nerves to the cutaneous veins and causes their constriction.

Taking a deep breath causes a transient reflex constriction of the cutaneous veins. The response usually begins within 2−4 sec, reaches its maximum in 20−60 sec and returns to control value within about 2 min. With repeated deep breaths at rapid intervals, the constriction is not sustained.[18] It is caused by a spinal reflex because it is present in tetraplegics with complete spinal cord transection; in this regard it is similar to the reflex constriction of the skin resistance vessels in response to the same stimulus. Obstruction of the airways during either

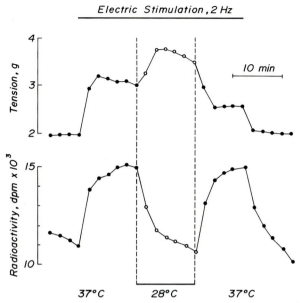

Fig 1–8. — Effect of cooling from 37 to 28 C on tension and ³H efflux in a helical strip of dog's saphenous vein previously incubated with (³H) norepinephrine and contracted by electric field stimulation. Cooling augments the contraction but decreases the efflux of tritiated compounds. (From Shepherd, J. T., and Vanhoutte, P. M.: *Veins and Their Control* [London: W. B. Saunders Company, Ltd., 1975]. Used by permission.)

inspiration or expiration causes an increase in tone of the cutaneous veins, but this only occurs occasionally with passive inflation of the lungs. Hence, stretch receptors in the latter are not responsible, and the afferent source of this spinal reflex probably is in the chest wall or diaphragm.[19]

As with a single deep breath, hyperventilation of brief duration causes constriction of the cutaneous veins.[18] This response is little altered during overbreathing of carbon dioxide, indicating that it is not due to hypocapnia. Cutaneous venoconstriction also occurs in the anesthetized subject breathing 8% carbon dioxide but not if active respiratory movements are prevented by muscle relaxants. Thus, the venoconstriction is not due to emotion but, like the response to a single deep breath, is reflexly induced by the expansion of the thoracic structures.

Other respiratory maneuvers such as the Valsalva also evoke a venoconstriction, presumably by activating the same reflex.

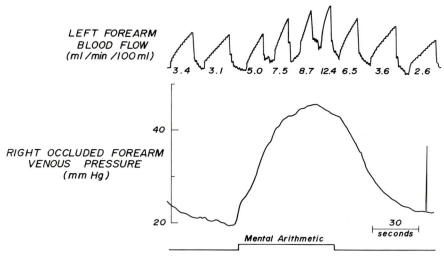

LEFT FOREARM
BLOOD FLOW
(ml/min /100 ml)

3.4   3.1   5.0 7.5 8.7 12.4 6.5   3.6   2.6

RIGHT OCCLUDED FOREARM
VENOUS   PRESSURE
(mm Hg)

40

20

30
seconds

Mental Arithmetic

Fig 1–9.—Constriction of cutaneous veins and dilatation of resistance vessels in skeletal muscle during mental stress. (From Marshall, R. J., and Shepherd, J. T. : *Cardiac Function in Health and Disease* [Philadelphia: W. B. Saunders Company, 1968]. Used by permission.)

Unlike the resistance vessels and the splanchnic veins the cutaneous veins show no consistent immediate response to arterial baroreceptor activity.[20] If, as a result of a decrease in arterial baroreceptor activity, the blood levels of catecholamines increase this may cause their constriction. The cutaneous veins also are unaffected by changes in the activity of the cardiopulmonary receptors when the blood volume is normal. During hypervolemia, however, interruption of afferent vagal traffic causes them to dilate in contrast to the increase in tone in the splanchnic capacitance bed.[5]

Exercise

The major stress on the cardiovascular system is caused by muscular exercise. The upper limit of exercise is determined by the ability of this system to meet the demands for oxygen of the active muscles and at the same time provide adequate circulation to the coronary vessels, the brain and the skin for thermoregulation. An analysis of the cardiovascular responses to rhythmic exercise in man demonstrates the important role of the systemic veins in meeting this demand.

Almost simultaneously with the onset of muscular contractions there is a dilatation of the resistance vessels in the exercising muscles.

This dilatation, mediated through a local mechanism whose precise nature is as yet unknown, permits an increase in blood flow proportional to the increase in metabolic rate of the active muscles. In spite of the rapid decrease in systemic vascular resistance caused by this dilatation there is little change in systemic arterial blood pressure because of rapidly adaptive changes in the circulation. The adrenergic outflow is augmented to the systemic vessels. As a consequence the blood flow to the splanchnic region, the kidney and the nonworking muscles is progressively decreased as exercise increases in severity so that the arterial blood pressure is maintained and the increase in left ventricular output is directed to the working muscles. Simultaneously there is a reflex decrease in splanchnic blood volume. Of the reflexes which might be responsible for the increase in sympathetic outflow during exercise, those most frequently discussed are the arterial baroreflexes, reflexes originating in the contracting muscles and central "irradiations."[21] As respiration increases the increase in intra-abdominal pressure through the action of the abdominothoracic pump forces blood into the thorax. With the onset of exercise the pumping action of the muscles reduces the volume of blood in the limb veins. This is especially important when exercise is carried out in the standing position. In changing from supine to quiet standing the cardiac output and the volume of blood in the heart and lungs decreases by 20% and the stroke volume may decrease by 40% or more; even mild leg exercise is sufficient to restore these values to normal. In addition the decrease of the pressure in the leg veins during upright exercise increases the pressure difference between the arteries and veins of the lower limbs and thus augments the blood flow through them.[22]

Thus, the combination of the reflex decrease in splanchnic blood volume together with the action of the muscle and abdominothoracic pump aids venous return and thereby maintains or increases the filling pressure of the right ventricle, augments the cardiopulmonary blood volume, pulmonary capillary filling and pulmonary diffusing capacity and contributes to the filling pressure of the left ventricle.

At the start of rhythmic exercise there is a generalized constriction of the cutaneous veins that is proportional to the severity of the exercise (Fig 1–10). As exercise continues and body heat production increases, the thermoregulatory mechanisms dominate and the cutaneous veins relax simultaneously with the skin resistance vessels. If the severity of the exercise is increased, both sets of vessels constrict again, but this too is transient (Fig 1–11). Local cooling of the skin causes a marked increase in venous tone of the resting limb and enhances the cutaneous venomotor response to exercise. At high work

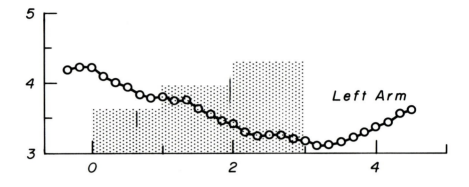

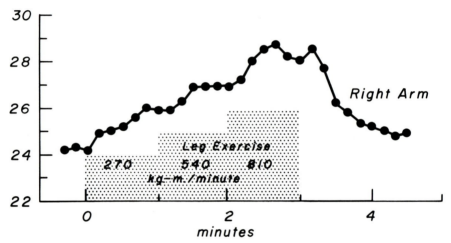

Fig 1–10.—Proportional constriction of forearm veins with increasing severity of leg exercise. Changes in capacity of forearm vessels (**top**) and pressure in an isolated venous segment (**bottom**) as shown by simultaneous measurements in both upper limbs. (From Bevegård, B. S., and Shepherd, J. T.: J. Appl. Physiol. 20:1, 1965. By permission of American Physiological Society.)

loads, if the skin is kept cool, cutaneous venous tone may be maintained for as long as 10 min despite an increase in body temperature.[23] This is due to the effect of cold increasing the reactivity of the cutaneous venous smooth muscle. When exercise is carried out in a hot environment, the cardiovascular system is stressed severely in simultaneously providing for the oxygen requirements of the contracting muscles and the need for heat transport to the skin. The maximal heart

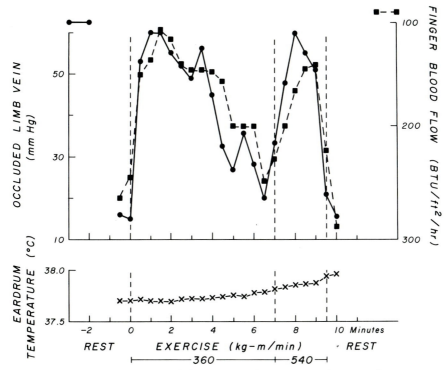

Fig 1–11.—Relationship of duration and intensity of supine leg exercise and of central body temperature *(eardrum temperature)* to skin blood flow (measured by heat elimination from finger) and tone in hand veins (measured by "occluded limb" technique). The hand veins constrict at the start of exercise, as demonstrated by the increase in venous pressure. As the body temperature begins to increase, the veins relax. They constrict again when exercise is increased in severity, but this too is transitory and the veins relax again as the body temperature continues to increase. The pattern for finger blood flow is identical. (From Zitnik, R. S., and Shepherd, J. T.: Prog. Cardiol. 1:185, 1972. By permission of Lea & Febiger.)

rate is reached at a lower oxygen consumption in the heat than in a cool environment. The stroke volume is less, with a resultant decrease in maximal cardiac output. The decrease in stroke volume may be due to a lower filling pressure of the heart as a consequence of the decrease in intrathoracic blood volume that may result from the displacement of blood into the capacious skin veins. The increased capacity of these veins is due to both the withdrawal of sympathetic activity and the increased distending pressure caused by the large increase in skin blood flow. With total skin blood flow well in excess of 5 L/min, the increased cutaneous circulation to the legs will contribute to the rapid filling of the leg veins between muscular contractions; in these circumstances the muscle pump is less effective in maintaining the intrathoracic blood volume. The decrease in this volume cannot be compensated for by the blood released from the splanchnic capacitance vessels; although the extent of the active venoconstriction is unknown, an important passive mobilization must occur because the splanchnic resistance vessels are maximally constricted.[24]

Veins in Clinical States

As in normal subjects, studies of the veins in patients with various diseases have been confined to those in the limbs. Before attributing any alteration in function of the cutaneous veins to a particular disease, evidence must be presented that the changes are not due to psychic stimuli or to local or central changes in temperature.

When the valves in the leg veins are congenitally absent or damaged by thrombosis, there is exaggerated pooling of blood in the upright position; during exercise the ability to displace blood from the legs is impaired so that the stroke volume and hence the cardiac output do not increase normally.[25]

In vasovagal syncope two of the major mechanisms responsible for the blood pressure decrease are bradycardia and dilatation of the resistance vessel in skeletal muscles.[26] Despite suggestion that reflex dilatation of the limb veins might contribute to the syncope by causing peripheral pooling of blood, these veins in fact constrict during syncope induced either by head-up tilt or lower body negative pressure. This together with the observation that central venous pressure did not fall immediately prior to or during syncope suggests that the capacitance vessels by constricting help to maintain the filling pressure of the heart and thereby the cardiac output.[27]

Regarding primary varicose veins, the cause is uncertain. Isolated segments from these veins are more distensible than are similar preparations from normal subjects.[28] The sensitivity of the smooth muscle to vasoactive agents seems unchanged and the defect is probably due to the presence of abnormal or immature connective tissue in the vein wall. The activity of lysosomal enzymes that interfere with the metabolism of mucopolysaccharides is significantly higher in varicose than in normal human saphenous veins and this could be the origin of the abnormal physical properties of the vein wall.[29]

Summary

The greater part of the blood volume is contained in the low pressure side of the circulation, including the postcapillary systemic vessels, right heart, pulmonary vessels and left atrium. Since in man a shift of blood from the heart and lungs to the systemic veins occurs as the subject moves from the horizontal to the upright position, the major function of the systemic venous system is to counteract this shift in order to maintain an adequate intrathoracic blood volume.

The role of the venous system is best understood by an analysis of its three major components, the splanchnic veins, the veins within the skeletal muscles and the cutaneous veins. The splanchnic and cutaneous veins are richly supplied with sympathetic nerves whereas muscle veins have little or no sympathetic innervation. In man, the major factor involved in emptying of muscle veins is the muscle pump, which operates in the leg and the foot. During exercise, there is a reflex decrease in splanchnic blood volume and an augmentation of cardiopulmonary blood volume due to the actions of the muscle pump and the abdominothoracic pump, which aids venous return.

When leg vein valves are destroyed by thrombosis or are congenitally absent, there is exaggerated pooling of venous blood in the upright position. The inability to displace blood from the legs to the heart decreases stroke volume and cardiac output. In primary varicose veins, abnormal physical properties of the vein wall may be due to abnormal or immature connective tissue, or the activity of lysosomal enzymes might interfere with metabolism of mucopolysaccharides since these enzymes are known to be significantly greater in concentration in varicose than in normal human saphenous veins.

Acknowledgments

My thanks are due to Mr. Robert Lorenz for assistance with the manuscript and for the preparation of the figures, and to Mrs. Joan Y. Troxell for the typing.

REFERENCES

1. Donald, D. E., and Aarhus, L. L.: Active and passive release of blood from canine spleen and small intestine, Am. J. Physiol. 227:1166, 1974.
2. Folkow, B., Lewis, D. H., Lundgren, O., Mellander, S., and Wallentin, I.: The effect of graded vasoconstrictor fibre stimulation on the intestinal resistance and capacitance vessels, Acta Physiol. Scand. 61:445, 1964.
3. Greenway, C. V., Stark, R. D., and Lautt, W. W.: Capacitance responses and fluid

exchange in the cat liver during stimulation of the hepatic nerves, Circ. Res. 25:277, 1969.

4. Brooksby, G. A., and Donald, D. E.: Dynamic changes in splanchnic blood flow and blood volume in dogs during activation of sympathetic nerves, Circ. Res. 29:227, 1971.

4a. Carnerio, J. J., and Donald, D. E.: Personal communication.

5. Shepherd, J. T., and Vanhoutte, P. M.: *Veins and Their Control* (Philadelphia: W. B. Saunders, Co., 1975), p. 269.

6. Clement, D. L., Pelletier, C. L., and Shepherd, J. T.: Role of muscular contraction in the reflex vascular responses to stimulation of muscle afferents in the dog, Circ. Res. 33:386, 1973.

7. Clement, D. L., and Shepherd, J. T.: Influence of muscle afferents on cutaneous and muscle vessels in the dog, Circ. Res. 35:177, 1974.

8. Fuxe, K., and Sedvall, G.: The distribution of adrenergic nerve fibres to the blood vessels in skeletal muscle, Acta Physiol. Scand. 64:75, 1965.

9. Ehinger, B., Falck, B., and Sporrong, B.: Adrenergic fibres to the heart and to peripheral vessels, Bibl. Anat. 8:35, 1966.

10. Ludbrook, J.: *Aspects of Venous Function in the Lower Limbs* (Springfield, Ill.: Charles C Thomas, Publisher, 1966).

11. Pegum, J. M., and Fegan, W. G.: Physiology of venous return from the foot, Cardiovasc. Res. 1:249, 1967.

12. Webb-Peploe, M. M., and Shepherd, J. T.: Response to the superficial limb veins of the dog to changes in temperature, Circ. Res. 22:737, 1968.

13. Vanhoutte, P. M., and Shepherd, J. T.: Thermosensitivity in veins, J. Physiol. (Paris) 63:449, 1971.

14. Abdel-Sayed, W. A., Abboud, F. M., and Calvelo, M. G.: Effect of local cooling on responsiveness of muscular cutaneous arteries and veins, Am. J. Physiol. 219:1772, 1970.

15. Pelletier, C. L.: Circulatory responses to graded stimulation of the carotid chemoreceptors in the dog, Circ. Res. 31:431, 1972.

16. Pelletier, C. L., and Shepherd, J. T.: Venous responses to stimulation of carotid chemoreceptors by hypoxia and hypercapnia, Am. J. Physiol. 223:97, 1972.

17. Watson, W. E.: Distensibility of the capacity blood vessels of the human hand during sleep, J. Physiol. (Lond.) 161:392, 1962.

18. Samueloff, S. L., Bevegård, B. S., and Shepherd, J. T.: Temporary arrest of circulation to a limb for the study of venomotor reactions in man, J. Appl. Physiol. 21:341, 1966.

19. Browse, N. L., and Hardwick, P. J.: The deep breath-venoconstriction reflex, Clin. Sci. 37:125, 1969.

20. Brender, D., and Webb-Peploe, M. M.: Influence of carotid baroreceptors on different components of the vascular system, J. Physiol. (Lond.) 205:275, 1969.

21. Goodwin, G. M., McCloskey, D. I., and Mitchell, J. H.: Cardiovascular and respiratory responses to changes in central command during isometric exercise at constant muscle tension, J. Physiol. (Lond.) 226:173, 1972.

22. Marshall, R. J., and Shepherd, J. T.: *Cardiac Function in Health and Disease* (Philadelphia: W. B. Saunders Co., 1968) p. 409.

23. Hanke, D., Schlepper, M., Westermann, K., and Witzleb, E.: Venetonus, Haut- and Muskel-durchtlutung an Unterarm und Hand bei Beinarbeit, Pfluegers Arch. 309: 115, 1969.

24. Rowell, L. B.: Human cardiovascular adjustments to exercise and thermal stress, Physiol. Rev. 54:75, 1974.

25. Bevegård, B. S., and Lodin, A.: Postural circulatory changes at rest and during exercise in five patients with congenital absence of valves in the deep veins of the legs, Acta Med. Scand. 172:21, 1962.

26. Barcroft, H., and Edholm, O. G.: On the vasodilatation in human skeletal muscle during post haemorrhagic fainting, J. Physiol. (Lond.) 104:161, 1945.

27. Epstein, S. E., Stampfer, M., and Beiser, G. D.: Role of the capacitance and resistance vessels in vasovagal syncope, Circulation 37:524, 1968.
28. Bocking, J. K., and Roach, M. R.: The elastic properties of the human great saphenous vein in relation to primary varicose veins, Can. J. Physiol. Pharmacol. 52:153, 1974.
29. Přerovský, I., Linhart, J., Dejdar, R., Svejcar, J., Kruml, J., and Vavrejn, B.: Research on the primary varicose veins and chronic venous insufficiency, Rev. Czech. Med. 8:171, 1962.

2 / Applied Venous Physiology in Normal Subjects and Venous Insufficiency

D. E. STRANDNESS, JR., M.D.

Professor of Surgery, University of Washington School of Medicine, Seattle, Washington

THE PHYSICS AND PHYSIOLOGY of venous blood flow is in many respects much more complex than on the arterial side of the circulation. Venous dynamics are complicated by some of the following factors: (1) the collapsibility of veins; (2) the presence of valves; (3) the relatively low intravenous pressure; (4) the effect of gravity; and (5) the occurrence of retrograde pulse transmission from the right side of the heart.

In clinical terms, there is no doubt that the venous circulation is considered a poor second cousin to the arterial side. This is probably due to the fact that arterial surgery is the most dramatic representation of the direct approach in correcting the anatomic abnormalities created by disease. In contrast, diseases of the venous system are often lumped into broad diagnostic categories such as thrombophlebitis, the postphlebitic syndrome and the lowly varicose vein without giving serious consideration to the pathophysiology of the condition. Physicians recognize that valves are important, but, beyond this, there is considerable ignorance. In fact, many of the operations designed to correct venous problems could have been predicted to fail if the basic physiology of venous flow had been clearly understood.

Now the situation is changing somewhat as physicians and surgeons have become aware of not only the need but the availability of methods for studying venous physiology. It is possible that this interest has been in large part stimulated by the realization that the most common serious venous disease, acute venous thrombosis, can be prevented, resulting in not only the saving of lives but the prevention of chronic venous insufficiency. In the case of the author, it has become clear that the general and vascular surgeon must understand the physiology of the venous system at least as well as the arterial circulation to approach and treat patients with venous disorders.

From a practical standpoint, most diseases of the venous system produce problems by two mechanisms—venous thrombosis, producing complete occlusion of the involved segment, and incompetence of the venous valve. It is apparent that one or both of these mechanisms can be present, particularly in the patient with chronic venous insufficiency. If this simple fact is kept in mind many of the symptoms, signs and physical changes observed in patients can be readily understood.

The valves are primarily responsible for protecting the tissues distal to their location. As will be shown, this implies that not any one single valve is critical but that a whole system of valves is normally necessary to protect both the superficial and deep veins and their surrounding tissue. It must also be remembered that the perforating veins, those that provide a communication between the superficial and deep veins, are often the vital link. Their anatomic distribution in large part explains the localization of the soft tissue changes that accompany chronic venous insufficiency.

For the discussion which follows, it is necessary to review venous pressure, flow and the role of the muscular pump separately. These considerations are followed by a brief presentation of the state of the art with regard to assessment of venous physiology in the clinical setting.

Venous Pressure—Normal

The recording of venous pressure presents special problems because of the low magnitude of the pressures that are present. Brecher[1] has indicated that the development of the mercury manometer may in fact have hindered the progress in measurement of venous pressure. The great density and inertia of the mercury column makes it impossible to follow not only small pressure changes but also the rapid phasic changes that occur in veins in proximity to the right side of the heart as influenced by not only the myocardial contractile events but respiration as well.

To measure mean pressure, it is only necessary to have a vertical column of saline and an accurate ruler. A common reference point must be used if the values are to be compared from patient to patient. Winsor and Burch[2] described the phlebostatic axis which is a point which lies midway between the anterior and posterior surface of the thorax at the level of the fourth intercostal space. The phlebostatic level is a horizontal plane at the level of the axis. Venous pressures are generally expressed as the height of the fluid column above this level.

Theoretically, the pressure at the foot level in the erect 6-foot "dead man" would be 140 mm Hg and a pressure of zero (atmospheric at the top of the head). In fact, the pressure at the foot would be equal to the distance from the foot to the right atrium or about 100 mm Hg. The basis for this and its explanation which would appear to deviate from hydrostatic theory is shown in Fig 2–1. When the volume in the system is inadequate to distend the entire vascular tree, there will be a point at which the veins will collapse. The point at which the vein collapses is at atmospheric or zero pressure.

When the "dead man" model is related to the horizontal plane, the hydrostatic pressures will be equal at all points (Fig 2–2). There is a point just below the diaphragm where the pressure is the same regardless of whether the subject is horizontal or vertical. This has been called the hydrostatic indifferent point (HIP).[3, 4] It must be emphasized that the presence of the pump in the circuit does not change the

Fig 2–1.—The hydrostatic pressures measured in an upright "dead man." The *middle tube* represents the pressure levels in a rigid tube of similar height. On the *right* is depicted the pressures present in a continuous fluid system of parallel columns. (From Strandness, D. E., Jr., and Sumner, D. S.: *Hemodynamics for Surgeons* [New York: Grune & Stratton, 1975]. Used by permission.)

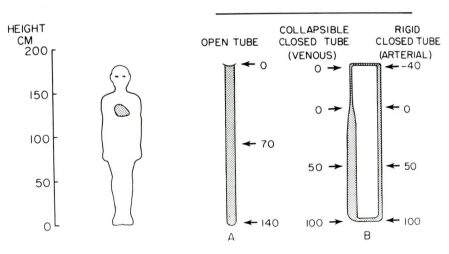

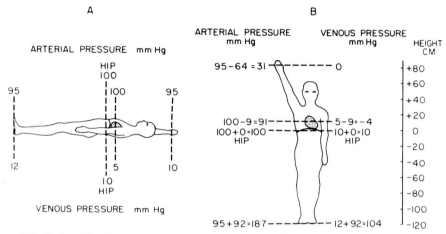

Fig 2–2.—Total pressures present at various levels of the venous system. *HIP* represents the hydrostatic indifferent point which is located just below the diaphragm. (From Strandness, D. E., Jr., and Sumner, D. S.: *Hemodynamics for Surgeons* [New York: Grune & Stratton, 1975.] Used by permission.)

hydrostatic pressure relations even though it has a marked effect upon intravascular pressure.

VENOUS PRESSURE AT REST

The pressures measured in the veins of the lower limb at rest will be equal to the height of the column of blood at the point of estimation to the third interspace at the sternum. Pollack and Wood[5] carried out some measurements and found the following values at the level of the ankle: (1) recumbent, 11.7 mm Hg (7–16.0 mm Hg); (2) sitting, 56.0 mm Hg (45–67 mm Hg); and (3) standing, 86.8 mm Hg (78.5–92.6 mm Hg). Ludbrook[6] found the pressures to be equal in the deep and superficial venous system. Arnoldi[7] noted the pressure in the posterior tibial vein to be about 1 mm Hg higher than in the greater saphenous at the same level. It was his contention that this higher pressure would keep the valves in the perforating veins in the closed position.

The situation with regard to the arm veins is more complex. Sitting upright with the arm dependent, the reference level is not the right atrium but rather at the level of the subclavian vein where it enters the thorax. With a negative intrathoracic pressure, the subclavian vein will collapse at the point where it passes into the chest.

The perfusion pressure at the capillary level is the same in the leg, whether the subject is upright or recumbent, approximately 83 mm Hg. However, it is important to consider the transmural pressure changes that occur with different positions since these are very important. It is this pressure which is acting either to distend or collapse the vein.

There are striking changes in the transmural pressures in the legs in going from the recumbent to standing position. Intramuscular pressure is usually on the order of 5 mm Hg in recumbent subjects. Thus, the pressure across the vein wall may increase from levels of 5–15 mm Hg to greater than 80 mm Hg. With the intracapillary pressure normally being 25 mm Hg, this is usually balanced by an interstitial colloid osmotic pressure of 20 mm Hg and the tissue pressure of 5 mm Hg. The normal transcapillary exchange from the proximal capillary end where the pressure is higher is equal to that resorbed at the distal end where the colloid osmotic pressure exceeds the intracapillary pressure. Nevertheless, assuming the upright position adds approximately 80 mm Hg on both sides of the capillary, which must result in fluid loss into the tissues. While some of this fluid will be picked up by the lymphatics, other mechanisms must be operative if edema is not to develop.

During the assumption of the upright position, approximately 500 ml of blood will be accumulated in the veins of the leg.[8] The volume increase occurs in part due to reflux and arterial inflow. With prolonged standing there will be a gradual increase in leg volume which is due to the fluid extravasation that occurs. While there is a rise in tissue pressure, this is not enough to prevent the accumulation of fluid in the tissues. The extent to which the edema may occur is evident in the blood volume reduction which may be as much as 15% by quiet standing.[3]

VENOUS PRESSURE WITH EXERCISE

The most dramatic changes which occur in lower limb venous pressure take place with exercise. Indeed, it is these changes which have been studied most extensively in distinguishing the normal venous system from that which is the site of acute and chronic venous disease.

The so-called "muscle pump" serves three useful functions: (1) to lower venous pressure in the dependent limb; (2) to reduce venous volume in the exercising area; and (3) to facilitate venous return (Fig 2–3).

During exercise, the muscle pump reduces hydrostatic pressure on the venular side of the capillary. Since the pressure on the arteriolar

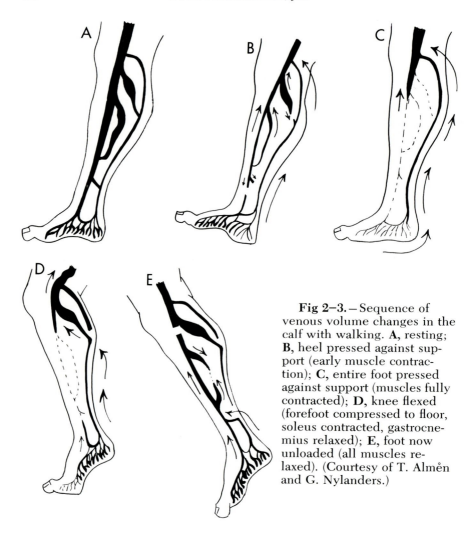

Fig 2–3.—Sequence of venous volume changes in the calf with walking. **A,** resting; **B,** heel pressed against support (early muscle contraction); **C,** entire foot pressed against support (muscles fully contracted); **D,** knee flexed (forefoot compressed to floor, soleus contracted, gastrocnemius relaxed); **E,** foot now unloaded (all muscles relaxed). (Courtesy of T. Almén and G. Nylanders.)

side is not reduced, the transcapillary pressure gradient goes up. This increased gradient assures a greater blood flow during exercise. It is important to briefly review these pressure changes. As shown in Figure 2–4 from the classic work of Pollock and Wood,[5] there is a dramatic fall in pressure at the ankle with a single step. The mean venous pressure decreases about 60 mm Hg during the first three to 12 steps of walking. The fall in pressure is also accompanied by a fall in calf volume but this is not sustained (Fig 2–5). A steady state mean pressure is finally reached which will remain unchanged. When walking is

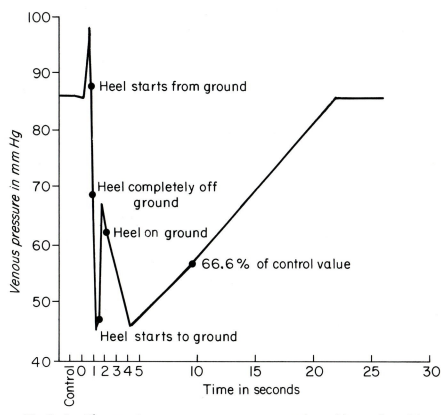

Fig 2–4.—Changes in mean venous pressure at the ankle produced by a single step. (From Pollack, A. A., and Wood, E. H.[5])

stopped, the pressure requires about 30 sec to return to the resting level.

The extent to which the intramuscular pressure rises with contraction has been studied by Ludbrook.[9] By means of a plastic catheter inserted into the soleus and gastrocnemius muscles, he found pressures above 200 mm Hg. These muscle groups constitute the major components of the muscle pump. The pressures in the thigh rose to a much less degree (Table 2–1).

Venous Flow—Normal

Under resting conditions in the recumbent position, venous flow is phasic and in large part dominated by respiratory movements. In the

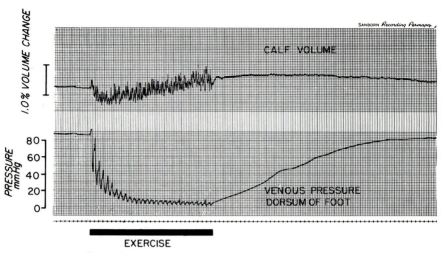

Fig 2–5. — Effect of exercise on venous pressure and calf volume. Note that the decrease in calf volume is not sustained during the exercise period. (From Strandness, D. E., Jr., and Sumner, D. S.: *Hemodynamics for Surgeons,* [New York: Grune & Stratton, 1975]. Used by permission.)

lower limb at the level of the common femoral vein, flow is decreased during inspiration and increased with expiration (Fig 2–6). This same pattern is observed as far peripherally as the posterior tibial vein. If the intra-abdominal pressure changes are accentuated by a Valsalva maneuver, flow normally stops completely without reversal of flow.

The venous flow patterns and direction during exercise are dependent upon the competence of the valves. Stegall[10] showed that venous flow was accelerated in both the deep and superficial veins simultaneously with the onset of calf contraction. This is in contrast to an older view which held that flow in superficial veins decreased or ceased with exercise. Stegall felt that the superficial veins are also com-

TABLE 2–1. — INTRAMUSCULAR PRESSURES (mm Hg)*

MUSCLE	RELAXED	QUIET STANDING	MAXIMAL CONTRACTION	
			SINGLE	SUSTAINED
Soleus	15	48	250	250
Gastrocnemius	9	22	230	215
Vastus lateralis	9	16	140	115
Adductor longus	7	12	60	55

*Derived from Ludbrook, J.[9]

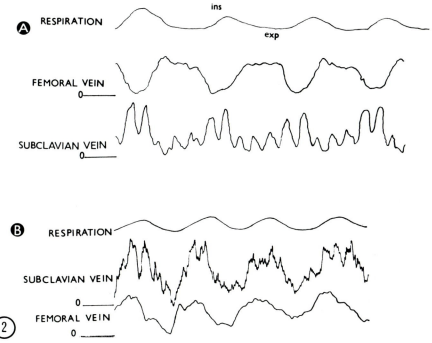

Fig 2–6. — Simultaneous recordings of subclavian and femoral vein velocity and respiration. When the patient position is changed from the horizontal (**A**) to the vertical (**B**), there is a phase shift in the femoral vein velocity. (From Lewis, J., Hobbs, J., and Yao, J.: Normal and Abnormal Femoral Vein Velocities, in Roberts, V. C. (ed.): *Blood Flow Measurement* [Baltimore: Williams & Wilkins, 1972].)

pressed by muscular activity which is transmitted through the investing deep fascia.

The direction of flow between the superficial and deeper compartments depends entirely upon the valves in the communicating or perforating veins. In the foot, flow is normally directed from the deep to the superficial system.[11, 12] This is in contrast to the lower leg where the direction of flow is in the opposite direction — superficial to deep.

Summary of Normal Pressure-Flow Relations with Exercise

With the onset of calf muscle contraction, the increased intramuscular pressure essentially empties the capacious veins within the soleus and gastrocnemius muscles. The more proximal end of the posterior tibial vein is partially compressed by this external muscular force. On the other hand, the distal posterior tibial vein increases in diameter. The pressure in the distal posterior tibial vein rises secondary to the increase in flow from the muscles and the external compressing force and by the narrowing of the proximal vein.[7, 13] The pressure in the popliteal vein will rise to a degree as the blood displaced by the calf pump fills this segment. The very steep pressure gradient that results, plus the competent valves, insures unidirectional flow during exercise.

Obviously, during the normal exercise pattern, flow is maintained within the deep system alone without egress of blood via the perforating veins which are protected by valves. However, during the relaxation phase, flow will be from superficial to deep veins as the pressure gradient becomes reversed.

Acute and Chronic Venous Disease

The two major changes that take place and lead to problems on the venous side of the circulation involve obstruction, valvular incompetence or both. Obviously, it is important to localize not only the site of involvement but to estimate, if at all possible, whether the disease is confined to the superficial or deep veins or both because the pathophysiology that follows may vary greatly. While it is not common to speak of venous collaterals, it must be kept in mind that these channels are equally important as their counterpart on the arterial side of the circulation.

Venous Pressure

Acute Venous Thrombosis

Acute obstruction of the arterial system results in regional hypotension, the magnitude of which is dependent upon the collateral artery resistance. On the venous side, acute thrombosis will produce regional hypertension, the magnitude of which is dependent again upon the extent of the collateral venous resistance. As might be expected, the degree to which the venous pressure rises is extremely variable.

Husni et al.[14] found the mean venous pressure in the foot of 22.5 ± 9.3 cm in 25 subjects with acute venous thrombosis. This was approximately 2.5 times normal pressures. These were all measured in the supine position. The reflection of the high collateral venous resistance was also exemplified by the fact that with ambulation, there was no fall in the venous pressure in patients with acute thrombosis as compared to normals.

DeWeese and Rogoff[15] related the extent of the pressure rise to the location of the occluding process. The supine pressures as related to level of disease were as follows: (1) popliteal or veins distal to knee, 11.5–25.0 cm saline; (2) superficial femoral vein (three subjects), 27, 33 and 70 cm saline; and (3) ileofemoral venous thrombosis (ten patients), 44–113 cm saline, average 68 cm saline. These pressures coincide with the effectiveness of venous collaterals and the extent to which they are capable of "decompressing" the areas distal to the occlusion. The degree of swelling also correlated with the level of the occlusion and, in turn, with the degree of pressure elevation. Thus, the more proximal disease, such as ileofemoral venous thrombosis, is associated with the greatest pressure increases and edema. The pressure measurements are rarely necessary for diagnosis of acute venous thrombosis but do correlate well with some of the clinical impressions relating the extent of disease and the degree of edema that occurs.

Chronic Venous Insufficiency

When there is residual venous obstruction with loss of valvular competence in the remaining segments, the pressure changes, particularly with walking, are distinctive. Data as summarized from the work of Hjelmstedt[16, 17] are shown in Table 2–2. The degree to which the pressure falls appears to be roughly related to the extent of the occlusive process. The venous pressure fluctuation between calf contraction (systolic phase) and relaxation (diastolic phase) are greater than seen in normals often by a factor of two or greater. As mentioned earlier, the rate of return to preexercise levels in normal subjects is quite slow but is very rapid (within 1 or 2 sec) in the postphlebitic limbs.

Most of the pressure measurements have been from superficial veins which only partly answers the questions. Arnoldi et al.[13] have, in part, resolved the problems with regard to the pressures in the deep and superficial venous systems in patients who were placed 78 degrees from horizontal. These investigators found little difference between the pressure in the superficial and deep venous circuits with the subjects motionless. Pressure in the midposterior tibial vein rises to a very high level (approximately 80 mm Hg above right atrial pressure). Pressure in the distal posterior tibial vein rises very high because of the absence of functioning valves.

With regard to the energy differential between the deep and super-

TABLE 2–2.—VENOUS PRESSURE CHANGES IN SUBJECTS WALKING AT 40 STEPS PER MINUTE
(DORSUM OF FOOT)

CONDITION	NO. PATIENTS	MEAN	AVERAGE FALL IN VENOUS PRESSURE (MM HG)		AMPLITUDE OF PRESSURE FLUCTUATION (MM HG)*
			DURING RELAXATION	DURING CONTRACTION	
Normal	45	61.5	80.6	46.0	34.6
Varicose veins	12	52.3	74.3	31.1	43.2
Postphlebitic degree of thrombosis					
1–2 of main trunks of lower leg†	15	48.3	70.4	28.1	42.3
4–6 of main trunks of lower leg†	4	52.3	83.3	23.3	60.0
Deep veins of lower leg and femoral vein	4	27.3	68.0	+22.0‡	90.0

*Maximum pressure swing between period of relaxation and contraction
†Refers to venae comitantes of the trifurcation arteries
‡This indicates a rise in pressure, not a fall.

ficial systems, Arnoldi et al.[13] found large differences. The distal posterior tibial vein pressure was 24 ± 15 mm Hg greater than in the saphenous vein. Because of this pressure differential, flow will occur from deep to superficial via the incompetent perforating veins. In fact, the maximum pressure level reached in the superficial veins was 71% of the deep system in the postphlebitic limb and 73% in patients with varicose veins. In normals, this value was only 32% of the pressure in the deep system. This venous hypertension will occur only with both deep venous insufficiency plus incompetent perforating veins. During relaxation, the pressure gradients are essentially reversed.

VENOUS FLOW

Because of the difficulty in directly measuring venous flow from any specific segment, information pertaining to flow is relatively sparse. However, Bjordal[18] has successfully used the electromagnetic flowmeter to evaluate flow in the saphenous veins and incompetent perforators.

When the deep valves are competent but the perforators are incom-

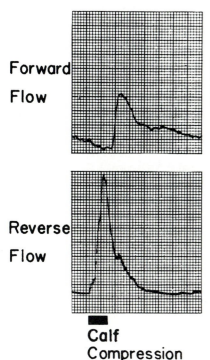

Forward Flow

Reverse Flow

Calf Compression

Fig 2–7.—Bidirectional flow in the incompetent perforating vein produced by rhythmic contraction of the calf. (From Folse, R., and Alexander, R. H.: Surg 67:144, 1970.)

petent, flow in the saphenous vein is retrograde into the deep system (circus motion). When the deep valves are incompetent but those in the superficial are intact, blood flow is cephalad in the saphenous system. When both systems are incompetent, blood simply surges up and down without any net upward flow in the saphenous vein.

The development of a directional, continuous wave velocity detector has permitted a qualitative assessment of the directional flow changes that accompany diseases of the superficial and deep venous system. It is clear from these studies that flow in the normal venous system is unidirectional. To demonstrate valvular incompetence, i.e., reverse flow, it is simply necessary to perform a Valsalva maneuver or suddenly compress the venous segment being studied proximal to the position of the Doppler probe. Likewise, if the probe is placed over the perforating vein, limb compression will demonstrate to and fro flow through this short incompetent segment (Fig 2–7).

"VENOUS VOLUME"

In an attempt to quantify further some of the changes that occur in response to both acute and chronic venous disease, a variety of plethysmographic methods have been employed to examine this problem.[19-26] While it would be more appropriate to use the term limb volume, the major changes which do occur with most methods are indirect indices of venous function. In practice, the techniques are quite similar and employ a pneumatic tourniquet(s) on the thigh with the volume sensor, often a mercury strain gauge, on the calf (Fig 2–8). The techniques are used to examine two aspects of venous function. The first is the rate of maximal venous outflow. This refers to the peak rate of venous emptying when the pressure in the thigh cuff is suddenly released. The cuff pressure is 50 mm Hg which is sufficient to produce venous congestion and a relatively stable calf volume increase within 1–3 min. A typical slope is shown in Fig 2–9. The initial slope can be used to calculate peak outflow based upon the following equation:

$$\text{MVO} = -\left[\frac{2}{C} \cdot \frac{dc}{dt} \cdot 60.1000\right]$$

where MVO = maximal venous outflow in cc/min/100 cc tissue
C = circumference
$\dfrac{dc}{dt}$ = rate of change in circumference

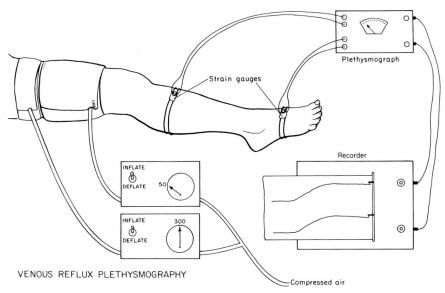

VENOUS REFLUX PLETHYSMOGRAPHY

Fig 2–8.—Using the two cuff system with the mercury strain gauge on the calf, it is possible to measure maximal venous outflow, maximal venous reflux flow and volume. (See text for explanation.) (From Barnes, R. W., Collicott, P. E., Mozersky, D. J., Sumner, D. S., and Strandness, D. E., Jr.[20])

Left Popliteal Thrombosis

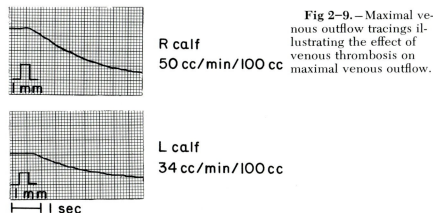

R calf

50 cc/min/l00 cc

L calf

34 cc/min/l00cc

Fig 2–9.—Maximal venous outflow tracings illustrating the effect of venous thrombosis on maximal venous outflow.

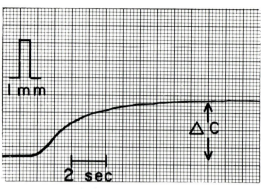

Fig 2–10. — Method of calculating maximal venous reflux volume. C, limb circumference. (From Barnes, R. W., Collicott, P. E., Mozersky, D. J., Sumner, D. S., and Strandness, D. E., Jr.[20])

Max. venous reflux volume

$$(cc/100cc) = \frac{2}{C} \cdot \Delta C \cdot 100$$

The technique also measures venous reflux. By using two cuffs on the thigh, a small proximal and larger distal one, it is possible to assess venous reflux. The principle is simple. Arterial inflow to the limb is occluded by inflating the proximal cuff to over 300 mm Hg. With the entire blood volume in the limb trapped, it is possible to measure the calf volume change when the second cuff is inflated to 50 mm Hg. If

Fig 2–11. — Method of calculating maximal venous reflux flow. The value of ΔC is determined at 10 seconds after inflation of the distal thigh cuff with complete arterial inflow occlusion. (From Barnes, R. W., Collicott, P. E., Mozersky, D. J., Sumner, D. S., and Strandness, D. E., Jr.[20])

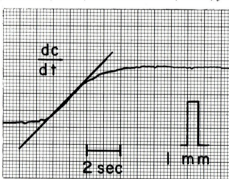

Max. venous reflux flow

$$(cc/min/100cc) = \frac{2}{C} \cdot \frac{dc}{dt} \cdot 60 \cdot 100$$

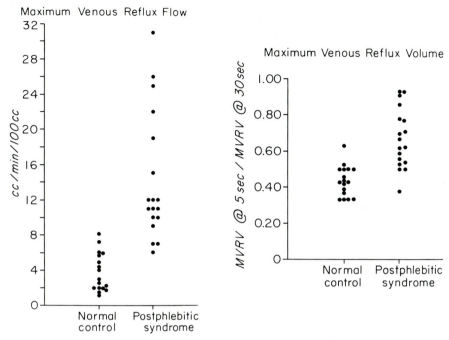

Fig 2–12.—Comparisons of maximal venous reflux flow and volume as compared to normals. (From Barnes, R. W., Collicott, P. E., Mozersky, D. J., Sumner, D. S., and Strandness, D. E., Jr.[20])

the valves are incompetent, blood will be translocated distally. It is then possible to calculate both the maximal venous reflux volume (Fig 2–10) and maximal venous reflux flow (Fig 2–11) at the calf level. As Barnes et al.[20] have shown, there are distinct differences between normals and patients with the postphlebitic syndrome (Fig 2–12).

Pathophysiology of the Postphlebitic Syndrome

It is fitting to conclude this chapter with a brief review of the pathogenesis of the changes noted with far-advanced venous disease. There is considerable confusion in this area and it is still not uncommon to hear physicians refer to varicose ulcers implying that varicose veins are the underlying cause. The fact that varicose veins alone are rarely the cause of ulcers has been known since the classic studies by Bauer in 1942.[27]

The terminology used—postphlebitic—implies that patients with the induration, pigmentation and ulcers had at some point in time acute venous thrombosis as the principle factor leading to the venous damage of the deep venous system. In the series reported by Cockett and Jones,[28] only 27 of 80 cases with venous ulceration could be definitely related to previous deep venous thrombosis.

Since there have not been any prospective studies of the fate of patients with established acute venous thrombosis, the basis for the ulceration has largely rested upon the findings relative to the state of the deep, superficial and perforating veins. The known facts include the following. (1) The location of the areas of induration and pigmentation are characteristic. By far, the most common site is in the region of the medial malleolus which coincides with the initial portion of the greater saphenous vein. The second most common site is laterally in the area drained by the lesser saphenous vein. (2) The perforator veins have their greatest concentration in the areas of induration. (3) It is nearly always possible to find an incompetent perforating vein in the vicinity of the ulcer. Indeed, Arnoldi et al.[13] in studying 493 cases of venous leg ulcers concluded that ulcers occur only where perforating veins are incompetent. The incompetence of the deep and superficial systems can easily be documented at the bedside by the use of a directional velocity detector (Fig 2–13).

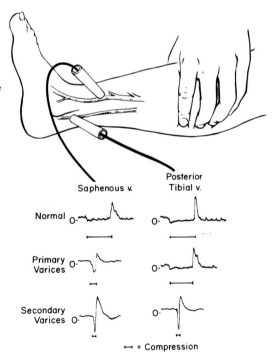

Fig 2–13.—Comparison of the directional flow changes in normals, patients with primary varicose veins and the postphlebitic syndrome. (From Barnes, R. W., Ross, E. A., and Strandness, D. E., Jr.: Surg. Gynecol. Obstet. 141:207, 1975.)

However, even accepting this fact does not explain mechanistically the changes that lead to the tissue damage which occurs. The current theories which relate the known level of incompetence are as follows.

1. The perforators constitute the conduits for the so-called high pressure leak or "ankle blow-out syndrome." This implies that the high pressures generated with walking are transmitted via the incompetent perforating veins to the subcutaneous tissues leading to a reduction in capillary flow and relative hypoxia. As a result, there would be an increased leakage of protein and possibly red cells into the interstitium.[29] Presumably these changes with time lead to progressive tissue fibrosis and damage. Cockett and Jones[28] postulate that the high venous pressure leads to dilatation and tortuosity of the smaller veins in the vicinity, stagnation with thrombosis, localized fibrosis and eventual ulceration.

2. Decreased capillary blood flow has been discussed. It has been noted by Cockett and Jones[28] that the number and size of perforating arteries in the region where ulcers commonly occur are less than in the foot. Thus, occlusion of the smaller arteries in this area may have a more serious effect than in other areas of the leg. While this is theoretically possible, there is little evidence to support it.

3. Venous hypertension has also been implicated. Disregarding for a moment the known changes in the venous anatomy, there appears to be one factor common to patients with chronic venous insufficiency and that is the presence of ambulatory venous hypertension. Ludbrook[30] found that skin changes were present only in those extremities in which the mean pressure in the saphenous vein remained above 80 mm Hg with exercise. Arnoldi and Linderholm[29] concluded it was the peak level of the "systolic" pressure during exercise which was important. Ulcers were present in those limbs where the venous pressure reached 40–60 mm Hg above the resting level during repeated calf muscle contraction. Bjordal[31] did not have similar findings, yet in all but three of 33 limbs the "systolic" pressure did rise above the resting level. The implication is that the high pressure levels reached are possible because of incompetent perforating veins. Certainly in the author's experience, it is rare indeed to have an ulcer without combined incompetence of both the deep and perforating veins.

Summary

The physics and physiology of venous blood flow are in many respects much more complex than on the arterial side of the circulation.

In clinical terms, the venous circulation is considered a poor second cousin to the arterial circulation. Now the situation is changing somewhat as physicians and surgeons become aware of the need and the availability of methods for studying the venous physiology.

REFERENCES

1. Brecher, G. A.: History of venous research, IEEE Trans. Biomed. Eng. 6:236, 1969.
2. Winsor, T., and Burch, G. E.: Phlebostatic axis and phlebostatic level, reference levels for venous pressure measurements in man, Proc. So. Exp. Biol. 58:165, 1945.
3. Gauer, O. H., and Thron, H. L.: Postural Changes in the Circulation, in Hamilton, W. F., and Dow, P. (eds.): *Handbook of Physiology,* sect. 2, Circulation, vol. III. (Washington, D.C.: American Physiological Society, 1965), pp. 2409–2439.
4. Rushmer, R. F.: Effects of Posture, in *Cardiovascular Dynamics* (3d ed.; Philadelphia: W. B. Saunders Co., 1970), pp. 192–219.
5. Pollack, A. A., and Wood, E. H.: Venous pressure in the saphenous vein at the ankle in man during exercise and changes in posture, J. Appl. Physiol. 1:649, 1949.
6. Ludbrook, J.: Functional aspects of the veins of the leg, Am. Heart J. 64:796, 1962.
7. Arnoldi, C. C.: Venous pressures in the leg of healthy human subjects at rest and during muscular exercise in the nearly erect position, Acta Chir. Scand. 30:510, 1965.
8. Henry, J. P., Slaughter, O. L., and Greiner, T.: A medical massage suit for continuous wear, Angiology 6:482, 1955.
9. Ludbrook, J.: The musculovenous pumps of the human lower limb, Am. Heart J. 71:635, 1966.
10. Stegall, H. F.: Muscle pumping in the dependent leg, Circ. Res. 19:180, 1966.
11. Kuster, G., Lofgren G. P., and Hollinshead, W. H.: Anatomy of the veins of the foot, Surg. Gynecol. Obstet. 127:817, 1968.
12. Pegum, J. M., and Fegan, W. G.: Physiology of venous return from the foot, Cardiovasc. Res. 1:249, 1967.
13. Arnoldi, C. C., Greitz, T., and Linderholm, H.: Variation in cross-sectional area and pressure in the veins of normal human leg during rhythmic muscular exercise, Acta Chir. Scand. 132:507, 1966.
14. Husni, E. A., Ximenis, J. O. C., and Goyette, E. M.: Elastic support of the lower limbs in hospital patients—a critical study, JAMA 214:1456, 1970.
15. DeWeese, J. A., and Rogoff, S. M.: Phlebographic patterns of acute deep venous thrombosis of the leg, Surgery 53:99, 1963.
16. Hjelmstedt, A.: Pressure decrease in the dorsal pedal veins on walking in persons with and without thrombosis, Acta Chir. Scand. 134:531, 1968.
17. Hjelmstedt, A.: The pressure in the veins of the dorsum of the foot in quiet standing and during exercise in limbs without signs of venous disorder, Acta Chir. Scand. 134:335, 1968.
18. Bjordal, R. I.: Circulation patterns in incompetent veins in the calf and in the saphenous system in primary varicose veins, Acta Chir. Scand. 138:251, 1972.
19. Barnes, R. W., Collicott, P. E., Mozersky, D. I., Sumner, D. S., and Strandness, D. E. Jr.: Noninvasive quantitation of maximum venous outflow in acute thrombophlebitis, Surgery 72:971, 1972.
20. Barnes, R. W., Collicott, P. E., Mozersky, D. J., Sumner, D. S., and Strandness, D. E. Jr.: Noninvasive quantitation of venous hemodynamics in postphlebitic syndrome, Arch. Surg. 107:807, 1973.
21. Cranley, J. J., Gray, A. Y., Grass, A. M., and Simeone, F. A.: A plethysmographic technique for the diagnosis of deep venous thrombosis of the lower extremities, Surg. Gynecol. Obstet. 136:385, 1973.
22. Dahn, I., and Eiriksson, E.: Plethysmographic diagnosis of deep venous thrombosis of the leg, Acta Chir. Scand. (Suppl.) 398:33, 1968.

23. Dohn, R.: Plethysmography during functional states for investigation of the peripheral circulation. Proc. Second Intern. Cong. Phys. Med., Copenhagen, Dansk Fijsurgisk Selskab, 1956.
24. Hallböök, T. and Gothlin, J.: Strain gauge plethysmography and phlebography in diagnosis of venous thrombosis, Acta Chir. Scand. 137:37, 1971.
25. Hallböök, T. and Ling, L.: Pitfalls in plethysmographic diagnosis of acute deep venous thrombosis, J Cardiovasc. Surg. 14:427, 1973.
26. Wheeler, H. B., Pearson, D., O'Connell, D., and Mullick, S. C.: Impedance phlebography, technique, interpretation and results, Arch. Surg. 104:164, 1972.
27. Bauer, G.: A roentgenological and clinical study of the sequels of thrombosis, Acta Chir. Scand. 86 (Suppl. 74):1, 1942.
28. Cockett, F. B., and Jones, D. E. E.: The ankle blow-out syndrome, a new approach to the varicose ulcer problem, Lancet 1:17, 1953.
29. Arnoldi, C. C., and Linderholm, H.: On the pathogenesis of the venous leg ulcer, Acta Chir. Scand. 134:427, 1968.
30. Ludbrook, J.: Valvular defect in primary varicose veins, cause or effect? Lancet 2: 1289, 1963.
31. Bjordal, R. I.: Pressure patterns in the saphenous system in patients with venous ulcers, Acta Chir. Scand. 136:309, 1971.

3 / The Pulmonary Vasculature

George P. Pollock and Walter C. Randall

Department of Physiology, Loyola University, Stritch School of Medicine, Maywood, Illinois

The pulmonary vasculature is unique because it functions in such a low and variable pressure environment. It is subjected intravascularly to the rhythmic distending pressures generated by myocardial contraction. It is also exposed transmurally to the fluctuating pressures, on both sides of atmospheric pressure, which originate from external respiratory mechanics. It is, therefore, interesting to consider what the structure of the pulmonary vasculature is like, and how it differs from counterpart components in the systemic circulation. Furthermore, it is important to consider what functions are performed by the pulmonary vasculature, and how the structural design facilitates these functions. Therefore, this paper will be divided into two major sections: (1) structure of the pulmonary vasculature, and (2) functions of the pulmonary vasculature.

Structure of the Pulmonary Vasculature

In the adult human lung, blood vessels and airways have a characteristic relationship to each other. The pulmonary arteries accompany the airways quite closely, while pulmonary veins are situated between the airways (Fig 3–1). This arrangement is maintained throughout the lung, extending from the hilum to the periphery. Functionally, of course, the airways terminate in the alveoli where they come into intimate relationship with the capillary network which lies between the arteries and veins, this system making up what may

Supported by grant HL 08682 from the National Institutes of Health.

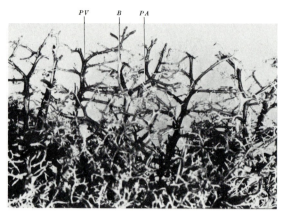

Fig 3–1. — Distal portion of a plastic cast of the bronchi *(B)*, pulmonary artery *(PA)*, and pulmonary vein *(PV)* of a mature human lung showing topographic relationships between these structures. (From Weibel, R. R.[41] Used by permission.)

be termed the "lung unit" (Fig 3–2). The entire organ is thus composed of millions of such units arranged in parallel.[41]

Surprisingly few data are available on the morphometry of the pulmonary vasculature as a whole. Cumming et al.[6] prepared resin casts from the pulmonary artery down to branches having a diameter of 800 μ, and counted (3,468 branches) and measured each component. Lengths and diameters of vascular branches in an intermediate zone were also measured from photographic prints made from different angles. The latter permitted measurement of branching angles, and accurate plots were drawn of the "generations" of divisions in each of the primary branches of the pulmonary artery. The individual blood vessels show progressive diminution from the center toward the periphery of the lung. Cumming et al. concluded from these measurements that the pulmonary circulation is markedly asymmetrical, and that the diameters decrease from branch order to branch order in an orderly fashion. He also determined that the volume of blood between the pulmonary valve and where the pulmonary veins enter into the left atrium is approximately 450 ml. In his calculation, total volume was roughly equally distributed in the arterial (150 ml), capillary (150 ml) and venous (150 ml) systems. The distribution of blood volume within the pulmonary artery was also defined by Cumming et al.[6] There were 634 vessels down to a diameter of 1.7 mm, which contained 90% of the blood. The remaining 10% was distributed between 450 million vessels down to a diameter of 8.5 μ. Thus, in the view of

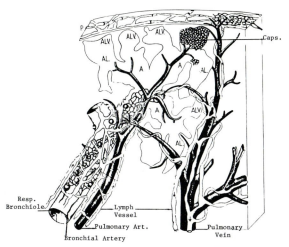

Fig 3–2. — General scheme of a primary lobule showing divisions of bronchial tree, pulmonary artery, pulmonary vein and the lymphatics. The bronchial arterial system is also represented on the surface of the bronchiole. The capillary bed enveloping several alveolar sacs is illustrated between the pulmonary artery and vein. Alveolar sacs are shown schematically, and the pleura *(P)* is related to the vein. *A, AL* and *ALV* refer to components of the pulmonary alveoli. (Modified from Miller, W. S.[32])

Cumming, the great bulk of blood volume within the pulmonary artery is located centrally.[7]

The *main pulmonary artery* extends only about 4 cm beyond the right ventricle before dividing into right and left branches. These branches supply blood to the right and left lungs, respectively. The pulmonary branches are all very short, but generally have much larger diameters than their systemic counterparts. The large pulmonary arteries have remarkably thin walls which are composed primarily of elastic tissue. Relatively small amounts of smooth muscle become apparent as the artery penetrates into the lung substance. The arteries accompany the airways down to the region of the terminal bronchioles. Those arteries ranging in diameter from 1.0 to 0.1 mm have a fairly prominent media of circularly arranged smooth muscle between the internal and external elastic laminas. Thus, while being similar to systemic muscular arteries in having a muscular media, the muscular pulmonary arteries are dissimilar in being extremely thin-walled.[17] They lie close to the bronchioles, respiratory bronchioles and alveolar ducts and branch with the bronchial tree. The anatomical structure of these arteries, with a thin media and relatively wide lumen, is associated with a low resistance to flow. However, the mere presence of muscle suggests the potential for constriction.

The walls of arterial branches smaller than 0.1 mm in diameter consist essentially of supporting endothelial tubes which abruptly break up into profusely anastomotic capillary networks. The precapillary vessels are sometimes called arterioles, although there is nothing which resembles muscular arteriolar sphincters which characterize the skeletal muscle circulation. There is, therefore, no functional mechanism comparable to a "stopcock action" familiarly attributed to systemic precapillary sphincters.

The *pulmonary capillaries* form a dense network of tiny vessels over the walls of the alveoli (Fig 3–3).[29] Weibel described a geometric model of the pulmonary capillary bed which consists of short, wedged, tubular segments which form interconnecting hexagonal units that almost totally cover the surface of the alveolus.[41] The length of each individual segment was considered to approximate its width, and be slightly greater than the diameter of a red blood cell. From morphometric analysis, the number of individual segments in the entire human lung has been estimated to be about 30×10^{10}, regardless of the overall size of the lung. Since each capillary segment is imbedded between two alveoli, Weibel calculated the number per alveolus to be between 1,800 and 2,000.[42] Thus, a concept of the pulmonary capillary system has arisen which is markedly different from that taught for systemic vascular beds. In Weibel's model, each vascular

Fig 3–3.—Photomicrograph of a capillary network in the frog lung following injection of "chromopaque" into the vasculature. A precapillary vessel is seen at top and two collecting venules appear at the bottom of the picture. A calibration line (100 μ) is shown at lower right. (From Maloney, J. E. and Castle, B. L.[29] Used by permission.)

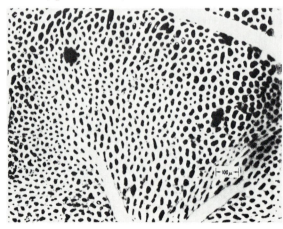

segment consists of wedged cylinders, while the overall network is a series of interconnected cylindrical tubes.

Sobin et al.[37] found a much closer mesh in the alveolar bed of the cat. This meshwork may be described as a sheet in which two parallel vascular endothelial surfaces are essentially held together by cells of connective tissue which act as posts. The difference between these two models may be clarified by considering the space "seen" by the red blood cell as it enters the interalveolar septum; the capillaries of the tube model would be seen as cylindrical tunnels which branch repeatedly. On the other hand, the space in the sheet model would appear as a parking garage with a floor, ceiling and intervening support posts. Flow through this latter system is conceived to be a continuous sheet of blood over the alveolar wall, presenting an extremely efficient mechanism for gaseous exchange.[14] Employing either of these models, it is evident that each red blood cell spends no longer than 1 sec in the capillary network, during which time it traverses two or three alveoli before it is collected in a small vein. This brief time is sufficient for nearly complete equilibration of oxygen and carbon dioxide between alveolar gas and capillary blood.[31]

The *pulmonary venules*, defined as vessels with diameters of less than 100 μ leading away from the capillary bed, appear microscopically to be identical in structure with the precapillary or arteriolar vessels (see Fig 3–3). The wall consists of endothelium with only a single elastic lamina and virtually no adventitia. Formed near bronchioles, they pass into the connective tissue septa between the secondary lobules to enter pulmonary veins.[17]

In contrast to the pulmonary arterial vessels, the veins are situated away from the bronchial tree, and the larger veins lie in the interlobular septa. Bundles of oblique and circularly arranged smooth muscle fibers are intermingled with collagen. The adventitia is distinct and fibrous and contains longitudinal elastic fibers. Occasionally, muscle is discernible. Like the pulmonary arteries, the veins are short in length, but their distensibility characteristics are similar to those in the systemic circuit. Cardiac muscle is continuous from the left atrium for varying distances along the pulmonary veins, and the adventitia contains numerous small vessels and nerves.

BRONCHIAL CIRCULATION

An accessory arterial circulation branches directly from the aorta through bronchial arteries to both lungs. Blood flowing in these vessels is oxygenated, in contrast to the partially deoxygenated blood in the pulmonary arteries. It supplies the supporting tissue of the lungs, including connective tissues, the septa and the bronchial system. Most of the bronchial venous blood returns to the heart by way of the left rather than the right atrium. Only 1–2% of the total cardiac output flows through the bronchial circulation, the majority of lung tissue receiving its oxygen supply directly from the pulmonary system.

LYMPHATICS

The lymphatic vessels extend from all of the supportive lung tissues, beginning in the perivascular and peribronchial spaces of the junctional regions between the alveoli. These smaller vessels coalesce along the venules and veins which course to the hilum of the lung and then mainly into the right lymphatic duct. Particulate matter which enters the alveolus can be removed rapidly by way of these channels. Protein is also normally eliminated, thereby preventing edema.

NERVE SUPPLY

The blood vessels of the lung potentially receive a generous nerve supply from both sympathetic and parasympathetic origins.[18] Adrenergic nerves are more abundant, in general, although species differences appear to be prominent. Both afferent and efferent fibers are present, presumably accompanying both systems.[33] On reaching the root of the lung, each vagus nerve divides into smaller branches which pass both in front of and behind the hilum to form the esophageal plexus. Branches arise from the anterior and posterior divisions of the vagus to form a small anterior and a larger posterior pulmonary plexus on each side. These plexuses communicate with the cardiac, aortic and esophageal plexuses. The left anterior pulmonary plexus communicates with the phrenic nerve. However, there is no convincing evidence to show that the parasympathetics exert a tonic effect on pulmonary blood vessels.[8] The sympathetic supply to the lungs originates from the second to the sixth thoracic segments of the spinal cord. Preganglionic fibers arise from cells in the lateral horns of these segments. They synapse with cell bodies of postganglionic fibers in the second to sixth thoracic ganglia and the stellate ganglion. Afferent sympathetic fibers have their cell bodies in the posterior root ganglia. The branches from the sympathetic chain, which carry fibers to and from the lung, are intimately intermingled with cardiac, aortic and esophageal branches. Most of these branches pass through the posterior pulmonary plexuses. From the pulmonary plexuses branches accompany the main bronchi and the pulmonary vessels into the lung.

At the third order branching of the bronchi, peripheral plexuses begin to develop. Nerve fibers pass even to the smallest muscular pulmonary arteries. Aggregates of nerve cells are found close to, or within, the adventitia of the muscular vessels, presumably representing parasympathetic postganglionic cells. Some of the cells undoubtedly supply the bronchial arteries as well.

The nerve supply to the pulmonary veins is probably closely associated with that to the left atrium, a fact which becomes evident as the veins approach the heart. The supply to the small intrapulmonary veins and the capillary bed is very scanty or absent. Thus, the lung appears to be rather extensively innervated in anatomical terms. However, the function of the neural structure remains poorly understood. Certainly a major portion consists of effector control of the bronchiolar system, and many afferent fibers pass from the lung substance to the central nervous system along these neural trunks.

Functions of the Pulmonary Vasculature

FUNCTION OF GASEOUS EXCHANGE

The primary function of the pulmonary vasculature is to serve as a system of conduits through which oxygen-deficient, carbon dioxide-laden blood is transported to the region of gaseous exchange. Hemodynamically,[32] the entire cardiac output (6.1 L/min) flows through the pulmonary artery (radius, 1.35 cm) at an average flow velocity of 17.8 cm/sec, with a mean pressure of 15 mm Hg and a mean vascular resistance of 105 dyne sec/cm.[5] The mean transit time through the lung is 4.33 sec with a mean pulmonary blood volume of approximately 440 ml. Pulmonary capillary transit time, however, is less than 1 sec and carbon dioxide and oxygen exchange normally occurs in less than one third of that time. The cardiovascular demands of exercise can increase the pulmonary capillary blood volume almost threefold, from approximately 70 to 200 ml.[4, 35, 41] Concomitantly, a threefold reduction in capillary transit time occurs. This, however, does not markedly impair the total gas transport process because of the rapidity of gaseous exchange.

FUNCTION AS A BLOOD RESERVOIR

Classically, the lung is considered to serve as a mobilizable reservoir of blood.[16] This concept implies that the pulmonary vasculature is more compliant than the systemic vasculature. However, literature values of systemic vascular compliance range from 1 to 4 ml/kg/mm Hg.[10, 16] These values are far greater than the reported values of 0.217 ml/kg/mm Hg for the rabbit pulmonary vascular compliance.[11] Permutt and colleagues measured pulmonary vascular compliance over two pulmonary arterial pressure ranges, approximating 15–22 mm Hg and 26–32 mm Hg, respectively.[34] They obtained values for pulmonary vascular compliance between 0.627 and 0.366 ml/kg/mm Hg. These data indicate that pulmonary vascular compliance varies as a function of the initial mean pulmonary vascular pressure.[16] It is evident from the above data that the systemic vasculature, as a unit, is 2–6 times more compliant than the entire pulmonary vasculature. This raises a serious question about the validity of the concept of the pulmonary circulation functioning as an effective blood reservoir.

The impression is frequently expressed that pulmonary blood volume can vary from as much as 200% greater than normal to 50% less than normal.[16] Using the above-stated value for pulmonary vascular compliance of 0.627 ml/kg/mm Hg, which is possibly high, and an initial volume of 440 ml of blood in the lung, let us consider what change in *mean pulmonary pressure* would be required to achieve a pulmonary blood volume of 1,320 ml in the average 70 kg man. A value close to 30 mm Hg is obtained from such a calculation. It is important to realize that this does not mean a 30 mm Hg change in mean pulmonary arterial pressure, but represents a pressure increase that, when the pulmonary bed is occluded, would result in an equilibrium pressure of 30 mm Hg in the entire pulmonary vasculature. Conversely, while assuming the same values, mean pulmonary pressure would have to be reduced by 5 mm Hg to realize a 50% reduction in pulmonary blood volume.

It is difficult to extrapolate to normal pulmonary vascular function from calculations derived from data acquired from static experimental conditions. However, in view of the low compliance of the pulmonary vasculature relative to the systemic vasculature, it is difficult to consider that the lungs serve as a blood reservoir of consequence.

FUNCTION OF PROTECTIVE SHUNTING INDUCED BY HYPOXIA

Since von Euler and Liljestrand proposed in 1946 that acute hypoxia elicited pulmonary vasoconstriction,[40] literally hundreds of papers have reported upon experimental probes into the fundamental basis for this phenomenon. A detailed review of the literature is beyond the scope of this paper, but the interested reader is directed to an excellent recent review of the subject by Fishman.[12] Therein is found documentation which supports the concept that hypoxic hypertension develops through pulmonary vasoconstriction. However, two key questions remain unanswered: (1) by what mechanism does hypoxia elicit vasoconstriction, and (2) what segment(s) of the pulmonary vasculature constricts? Two alternate hypotheses were presented by Fishman for consideration (Fig 3–4).

By this model, there may be an *indirect* effect of hypoxia which operates via an intrapulmonary chemical mediator which is released by nonmuscle cells of the lung. It is presumed that such a substance would diffuse to smooth muscle cellular receptors and activate the contractile process. Alternatively, a *direct* effect on pulmonary vascular smooth muscle is also possible. This mechanism might involve one or more stages in the contractile process, including excitation, contraction or a coupling of the two.

When pulmonary vascular volume changes do occur, it appears that the small vessel segment is the region which accommodates the change.[30] Two theories exist about how small pulmonary vessels accommodate changes in pulmonary blood volume: (1) the theory of recruitment, and (2) the theory of distention of patent vessels.[34] Analysis of the questions involved requires consideration of the model by West et al. for distribution of blood flow in the pulmonary capillaries.[43] In simplest terms, the capillaries of the lung may be exposed to different transmural pressures depending upon their position relative to the pulmonary artery. In apical zones of the upright lung, alveolar pressure may be greater than either pulmonary arterial pressure or pulmonary venous pressure. In a middle portion (zone) of the lung, blood flow is influenced by the fact that pulmonary arterial pressure may exceed alveolar pressure. In basilar zones of the lung, blood flow is primarily determined by classical arterial-venous pressure differences.

Fig 3–4. — Hypothesis presented by Fishman[12] to explain the development of hypoxic hypertension through pulmonary vasoconstriction.

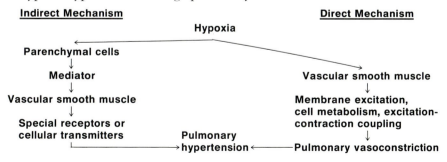

Following this theory, Glazier et al.[15] determined that capillary diameters increased as a function of capillary hydrostatic pressure when alveolar pressure was held constant. They, therefore, suggested that both recruitment and distention play roles in accommodating pulmonary blood volume changes. Thus, when pulmonary venous pressure exceeds alveolar pressure, capillary distention occurs. Also, when pulmonary venous pressure is less than alveolar pressure, capillary distention will provide for the increased volume. Maseri et al.[30] and Permutt et al.[34] used similar logic to interpret their flow reversal observations. They reasoned that distention would be indicated by a volume increase following an outflow pressure elevation sufficient to reduce flow. Since this did not occur, they suggested that capillary recruitment accounted for pulmonary blood volume changes.

From our conceptual point of view, hypoxic vasoconstriction would appear to function to actively shunt blood to ventilated regions of the lung. We do not consider the pulmonary vascular hypoxic response to be simply fortuitous. The response was clearly demonstrated to occur in dogs and cats.[3] Blood flow was demonstrated to be shunted away from the basilar portion of human lungs ventilated with argon gas.[2] It appears, then, that the shunting mechanism is a safety measure designed to maintain arterial oxygen tension.

FUNCTION OF THE LYMPHATICS

The lung possesses an extensive lymphatic system which functions to keep the lung fairly dry.[25] Failure in this function results in pulmonary edema.[36] Lung lymphatics exist in those regions of the lung where loose connective tissue is abundant, and, accordingly, the basilar portion of the lung possesses more lymphatics than the less dependent areas.[25] This arrangement is beneficial for accommodating the more extensive transcapillary filtration which results from the greater hydrostatic filtration forces extant in the basilar lung. The hypertrophy of pulmonary lymphatics which occurs in instances of chronic pulmonary edema gives credence to this concept.[39] The pulmonary lymphatic ultrastructure reveals large separations between adjacent endothelial cells.[25] The width of these separations may be variable because of guy wire-like filamentous attachments from the lymphatic endothelium to the surrounding connective tissue. Therefore, when pulmonary edema expands the interstitial space, the intercellular gaps may widen. It is conceivable that the lymphatics also are dilated by this mechanism.

That the lymphatic capillaries extend into the alveolar-capillary septum is questionable, the primary limitation being the narrow width (0.2 – 1 μ) of this barrier.[41] It is known, however, that lymphatic capillaries do exist adjacent to alveoli, but that they are embedded in substantially thick parenchymal tissue.[24] Valves are present in pulmonary lymphatic vessels whose diameters exceed 50 μ.[26] The structural design of these valves was resolved to be monocuspid, and their function assures unidirectional lymphatic flow.

Vascular Responses to Neural Excitation

It is difficult to demonstrate pulmonary vasoconstriction in the laboratory. It is also clear that neurogenic influences on pulmonary flow resistance are quite weak. Even maximum discharge rates in the sympathetic fibers seldom increase resistance more than 30 – 50%.[8, 9] Indeed, it may be argued that selective changes in the resistance of pulmonary vessels, which would produce regional differences in blood flow, could not have the same value for the lungs that they may have for the systemic circulation, since in the lungs all the tissues subserve the same function. It is conceivable that the vasoconstrictor nerves, while not markedly influencing pulmonary flow resistance, may actively expel considerable blood from the pulmonary blood reservoir into the left side of the heart.[13] However, the importance of this function would appear to be minimized by the arguments presented above.

The fact that the capacitance of the arterial side virtually matches that of the venous side has a potentially great advantage. If the increase in resistance accompanying neural discharge to the capacitance vessels is approximately matched by constriction on the precapillary side, there would be no secondary decrease in pre-/postcapillary resistance ratio, and hence no increase in pulmonary capillary pressure as a result of such a capacitance change. Kadowitz et al.[20-23] conclude that increase in resistance to flow in the lung results from activation of alpha-adrenergic receptors in venous segments and small arteries. These observations support evidence that strong sympathetic stimulation acts upon the pulmonary venous system to reduce blood volume,[1] to be mediated by an alpha-receptor mechanism. Ingram et al.[19] and Szidon et al.[38] reported that stellate ganglion stimulation did not increase pulmonary vascular resistance, but rather induced a rise in pulmonary systolic pressure, increased pulse wave velocity, decreased arterial compliance and rapid arterial runoff, while diastolic pressures remained essentially unchanged. These changes suggested diminished distensibility of the arterial tree rather than a diffuse constriction of small pulmonary vessels. These investigators concluded that the overall response was an altered vascular distensibility, affecting the entire pulmonary vasculature, rather than a selective increment in vascular resistance which characterizes the systemic responses to sympathetic stimulation. Employing the same experimental preparation, these authors also reported that sympathetic nerves to the bed can be engaged reflexly, and that this system may play a functional role in regulation of pulmonary vascular tone.

Another possible function of a vasomotor innervation was suggested by Hebb,[18] who reported a greater density of innervation at the branching points from the parent arterial system. She suggested that selective vasoconstriction would prevent engorgement of the blood vessels of the dependent portions of the lung and so act to keep flow more evenly distributed through all parts of the lung. On the other hand, employing anesthetized, open-chest canine models, Lloyd[28] reported that widespread sympathetic activation associated with elevated intracranial pressure does not significantly alter pulmonary vascular perfusion, and that the pulmonary hypertension arises passively with increased left atrial pressure and increased blood volume. Baroreceptor stimulation induces reflex dilatation of the pulmonary vessels, whereas chemoreceptor stimulation provokes reflex pulmonary vasoconstriction.[13] There is a suggestion that sympathetic nerves provide slight tonic vasoconstriction, and these reflex effects are abolished by stellatectomy.

The pulmonary trunk and the right and left pulmonary arteries are the sites of adventitially placed vagal mechanoreceptors,[5] similar in appearance to those in the carotid sinus and aortic arch. An increase in pressure in the pulmonary artery elicits bradycardia and hypotension, reflex responses generally similar to those induced by the sinoaortic baroreceptor mechanisms. Stimulation of the mechanoreceptors, situated at the junction of the pulmonary veins and the left atrium, on the other hand, induces tachycardia involving primarily, and perhaps only, the sympathetic nerves and is accompanied by significantly increased urine flow.[27] The full implication of these functional observations is not clearly understood, but they may be of considerable consequence in finally delineating comprehensive cardiopulmonary reflex mechanisms.

Summary

The pulmonary vasculature is unique because it functions in such a low and variable pressure environment. In the adult human lung, blood vessels and the airways have a characteristic relationship to one another, with pulmonary veins situated between the airways and the arteries accompanying them quite closely. This arrangement is maintained throughout the lung and extends from the hilum to the periphery. The anatomical structure of pulmonary arteries, with thin media and relatively wide lumen, indicates a very low resistance to flow. The mere presence of muscle suggests, however, the potential for constriction. The pulmonary capillaries form a dense network of tiny vessels over the walls of the alveoli. Since each capillary segment is imbedded between two alveoli, it has been calculated that the number per alveolus is between 1,800 and 2,000. The primary function of the pulmonary vasculature is to serve as a system of conduits through which oxygen-deficient, carbon dioxide-laden blood is transferred to the region of gaseous exchange. The pulmonary trunk and right and left pulmonary arteries are the site of adventitially placed vagal mechanoreceptors. An increase in pressure in the pulmonary artery elicits bradycardia and hypotension. On the other hand, stimulation of the mechanoreceptors situated at the junction of the pulmonary veins and left atrium induces tachycardia. The full implication of these functional observations is not clearly understood.

REFERENCES

1. Aarseth, P., Nicolaysen, G., and Waaler, B. A.: The effect of sympathetic nerve stimulation on pulmonary blood volume in isolated perfused lungs, Acta Physiol. Scand. 81:448, 1971.
2. Abraham, A. S., Cumming, G., Horsfield, K., and Prowse, K.: Regional hypoxia and distribution of pulmonary blood flow, Scand. J. Resp. Dis. 51:33, 1970.
3. Barer, G. R., Howard P., McCurrie, J. R., and Shaw, J. W.: Changes in pulmonary circulation after bronchial occlusion in anesthetized dogs and cats, Circ. Res. 25: 747, 1969.
4. Bates, D. V., Varvis, C. J., Donovan, R. E., and Christie, R. V.: Variations in the pulmonary capillary blood volume and membrane diffusion component in health and disease, J. Clin. Invest. 39:1401, 1960.
5. Coleridge, J. C. C., and Kidd, C.: Electrophysiologic evidence of baroreceptors in the pulmonary artery of the dog, J. Physiol. 150:319, 1960.
6. Cumming, G., Henderson, R., Horsfield, K., and Singhal, S. S.: The Functional Morphology of the Pulmonary Circulation, in Fishman, A. P., and Hecht, H. H. (eds.): *The Pulmonary Circulation and Interstitial Space* (Chicago: University of Chicago Press, 1969).
7. Cumming, G.: The Pulmonary Circulation, in Guyton, A. (ed.): MTP Int. Rev. Sci., *Cardiovascular Physiology*, Vol. 1, No. 1 (Baltimore: University Park Press, 1974).
8. Daly, I. deB., and Hebb, C. C.: *Pulmonary and Bronchial Vascular System* (Baltimore: Williams and Wilkins, 1966).
9. Daly, I. deB., and Daly, M. deB.: Sympathetic nerve control of pulmonary vascular resistance and impedance in isolated perfused lungs of the dog, J. Physiol. 234: 106P, 1973.
10. Drees, J. A., and Rothe, C. F.: A neurogenic component in the capacitance vessel pressure-volume response of the dog, Fed. Proc. 30:399, 1971.

11. Engelberg, J., and Dubois, A. B.: Mechanics of pulmonary circulation in isolated rabbit lungs, Am. J. Physiol. 196:401, 1959.
12. Fishman, A. P.: Hypoxia on the pulmonary circulation. How and where it acts, Circ. Res. 38:221, 1976.
13. Folkow, B., and Neil, E.: *Circulation* (New York: Oxford University Press, 1971).
14. Fung, Y. C., and Sobin, S. S.: Theory of sheet flow in the lung alveoli, J. Appl. Physiol. 26:472, 1969.
15. Glazier, J. B., Hughes, J. M. B., Maloney, J. E., and West, J. B.: Measurements of capillary dimensions and blood volume in rapidly frozen lungs, J. Appl. Physiol. 26: 65, 1969.
16. Guyton, A. C.: *Circulatory Physiology: Cardiac Output and Its Regulation* (Philadelphia: W. B. Saunders & Co., 1963).
17. Harris, P., and Heath, D.: *The Human Pulmonary Circulation* (Baltimore: Williams and Wilkins, 1962).
18. Hebb, C. C.: Motor Innervation of the Pulmonary Blood Vessels of Mammals, in Fishman, A. P., and Hecht, H. H. (eds.): *The Pulmonary Circulation and Interstitial Space* (Chicago: University of Chicago Press, 1969).
19. Ingram, R. H., Szidon, J. P., Skalak, R., and Fishman, A. P.: Effects of sympathetic nerve stimulation on pulmonary arterial tree of isolated lobe perfused in situ, Circ. Res. 22:801, 1968.
20. Kadowitz, P. J., Joiner, P. D., and Hyman, A. L.: Effect of sympathetic nerve stimulation on pulmonary vascular resistance in the intact spontaneously breathing dog, Proc. Soc. Exp. Biol. Med. 147:68, 1974.
21. Kadowitz, P. J., Sweet, C. S., and Brody, M. J.: Influence of prostaglandins on adrenergic transmission to vascular smooth muscle, Circ. Res. 31:36, 1972.
22. Kadowitz, P. J., Joiner, P. D., and Hyman, A. L.: Influence of prostaglandins E and F_2 on pulmonary vascular resistance in the sheep, Proc. Soc. Exp. Biol. Med. 145: 1258, 1974.
23. Kadowitz, P. J., Joiner, P. D., and Hyman, A. L.: Influence of sympathetic stimulation and vasoactive substances on the canine pulmonary veins, J. Clin. Invest. 56: 354, 1975.
24. Lauweryns, J. M.: The juxta-alveolar lymphatics in the human adult lung, Am. Rev. Resp. Dis. 102:877, 1970.
25. Lauweryns, J. M.: The Blood and Lymphatic Microcirculation of the Lung, in Lockhart, A., and Evans, P. (eds.): *Pathology Annual* (New York: Appleton-Century-Crofts, 1971).
26. Lauweryns, J. M.: Stereomicroscopic funnel-like architecture of pulmonary lymphatic valves, Lymphology 4:125, 1971.
27. Linden, R. J.: Function of cardiac receptors, Circulation 43:463, 1973.
28. Lloyd, T. C.: Effect of increased intracranial pressure on pulmonary vascular resistance, J. Appl. Physiol. 35:332, 1973.
29. Maloney, J. E., and Castle, B. L.: Pressure-diameter relations of capillaries and small blood vessels in frog lung, Resp. Physiol. 7:150, 1969.
30. Maseri, A., Caldini, P., Howard, P., Joshi, R. C., Permutt, S., and Zierler, K. L.: Determinants of pulmonary vascular volume—recruitment versus distensibility, Circ. Res. 31:218, 1972.
31. Milhorn, H. T., and Pulley, P. E.: A theoretical study of pulmonary capillary gas exchange and venous admixture, Biophys. J. 8:337, 1968.
32. Miller, W. S.: *The Lung* (Springfield, Ill.: Charles C Thomas, 1947).
33. Mitchell, G. A. G.: *Cardiovascular Innervation* (Edinburgh: Livingstone, 1956).
34. Permutt, S., Caldini, P., Maseri, A., Palmer, W. H., Sasamori, T., and Zierler, K.: Recruitment Versus Distensibility in the Pulmonary Vascular Bed, in Fishman, A. P., and Hecht, H. H. (eds.): *The Pulmonary Circulation and Interstitial Space* (Chicago: University of Chicago Press, 1969).
35. Roughton, F. J. W., and Forster, R. E.: Relative importance of diffusion and chemical reaction rates in determining rate of exchange of gases in the human lung, with

special reference to true diffusing capacity of pulmonary membrane and volume of blood in lung capillaries, J. Appl. Physiol. 11:290, 1957.

36. Rusznyak, J., Foldi, M., and Szabo, G.: in Youlton, Z. (ed.): *Lymphatics and Lymph Circulation; Physiology and Pathology* (Oxford: Pergamon Press, 1967).

37. Sobin, S. S., Tremer, H. M., and Fung, Y. C.: Morphometric basis of the sheet-flow concept of the pulmonary alveolar microcirculation in the cat, Circ. Res. 26:397, 1970.

38. Szidon, J. P., and Fishman, A. P.: Autonomic Control of the Pulmonary Circulation, in Fishman, A. P., and Hecht, H. H. (eds.): *The Pulmonary Circulation and Interstitial Space* (Chicago: University of Chicago Press, 1969).

39. Uhley, H. N., Leeds, S. E., Sampson, J. J., and Friedman, M.: Right duct lymph flow in experimental heart failure following acute elevation of left atrial pressure, Circ. Res. 20:306, 1967.

40. von Euler, U. S., and Liljestrand, G.: Observations on the pulmonary arterial blood pressure in the cat, Acta Physiol. Scand. 12:301, 1946.

41. Weibel, E. R.: *Morphometry of the Human Lung* (New York: Academic Press, 1963).

42. Weibel, E. R.: The Ultrastructure of the Alveolar-Capillary Membrane or Barrier, in Fishman, A. P., and Hecht, H. H. (eds.): *The Pulmonary Circulation and Interstitial Space* (Chicago: University of Chicago Press, 1969).

43. West, J. B., Dollery, C. T., and Naimark, A.: Distribution of blood flow in isolated lung; relation to vascular and alveolar pressures, J. Appl. Physiol. 19:713, 1964.

Discussion: Chapters 1 through 3

DR. ALTON OCHSNER, JR.: We have heard lucid discussions of venous physiology and pathophysiology, but with the exception of the paper on pulmonary vasculature, there was no emphasis on the role of the lymphatics.

The problems of venous insufficiency dealt with clinically, in chronic form, are basically problems of venolymphatic insufficiency. I hope that Doctor Shepherd and Doctor Strandness might give us their opinions of the role of lymphatics in the venous hemodynamics.

DR. EUGENE STRANDNESS: I was afraid somebody was going to ask about the role of the lymphatics in venous disease. I don't know of any good way of evaluating the two simultaneously in terms of their basic roles in the development of the stasis changes that we see. Undoubtedly, in the advanced stages of chronic venous insufficiency, lymphatic abnormalities will be found. However, I don't understand the role of the lymphatics in this whole problem, Doctor Ochsner, and if I did, I would have said something in my presentation.

DR. JOHN BERGAN: That is typically forthright.

DR. JOHN SHEPHERD: We are learning more about lymphatics. Clearly, they are important. They play an important role in every venous bed in the body, including the lung. It has been shown that the lymphatics have sympathetic innervation. Not only do they work through local mechanisms, but they also primarily play some role in coordinated function within the body.

62

CHRONIC VENOUS INSUFFICIENCY

Introduction

ALTHOUGH VARICOSE VEINS are common and their treatment is an ordinary surgical task, little hard data guide the conscientious surgeon who works in this field. As Professor Browse indicated in discussing these presentations, ". . . if you are keen, energetic and enthusiastic, you get good results." But, unfortunately, descriptions of treatment of varicose veins give little factual information about the cause of the varicosities themselves. This is important because if one is to tailor treatment to the primary abnormality, it is necessary to define that abnormality accurately.

The following three papers summarize a wide experience in treating varicose veins and, as such, present the state of the art as it existed in the mid-1970s.

A certain dissatisfaction with current treatment of varicosities seemed to underlie the discussion of these presentations, with Dr. John Olwin finally concluding that, once the actual etiology of varicose veins was uncovered, the surgeon's services eventually might be eliminated.

4 / The Surgical Management of Primary Venous Insufficiency: Varicose Veins

JOHN H. OLWIN, M.D.

Clinical Professor of Surgery, Emeritus, Rush Medical College; Attending Surgeon, Emeritus, Rush-Presbyterian-St. Luke's Medical Center, Chicago, Illinois

IN A SYMPOSIUM as comprehensive as this, involving contributors with varying experiences and interests, a certain amount of overlapping is unavoidable. In this presentation I shall attempt to limit my remarks to my assigned subject but shall allow myself a few liberties, since my experience may suggest contributions that bear on the subject under discussion.

Etiologic Factors

Factors involved in the development of primary varicose veins are no doubt multiple and are still only partially understood. Heredity has, for many years, been considered the most important factor. As techniques for studying venous flow and valvular competency have become more sophisticated, congenital absence of iliofemoral valves has assumed importance. An hereditary factor would appear to be involved in this congenital development as suggested by the finding of a significant incidence of absence of iliofemoral valves in children of patients with documented history of varices.[1, 2] Trauma, undoubtedly, is a factor in some cases. Most of us have seen a varicose segment of a greater saphenous vein in a young person who may have suffered trauma to a particular site, such as a kick, a blow or a gouge to the thigh or groin. Often there is no recalled history of trauma in such cases. A history of thrombophlebitis usually is not obtainable in a patient with primary varicose veins. A history of such, if reliable, is considered to exclude the varicosities from the primary category. Some clinicians will question this position. In this connection, the question arises of how much inflammation is necessary to produce scarring and insufficiency and how often such inflammation is subclinical. Some years ago a chemist in our laboratory discovered a thrombin-like enzyme activity which was present in the blood of "normal" persons and was significantly elevated in those with acute thrombophlebitis. It dropped to normal levels within 2 weeks and again became elevated in weeks to months after the acute episode. It was found to be elevated in patients with a history of thromboembolism. It was particularly high in women in the third trimester of pregnancy though not before, except in those patients with a history of thromboembolism or in those who developed thrombophlebitis prior to the third trimester.[3-5] It was unaffected by heparin but was lowered to normal or below normal levels by oral anticoagulant drugs. Of interest was its elevation in patients with varicose veins, primary or secondary, and in three generations of women with histories of thromboembolism and/or varicose veins.[6] These findings suggest that low-grade subclinical inflammation of veins may be a factor in the hereditary feature of primary varicose veins.

Objectives of Treatment

Most authorities agree that locating the various sites of valvular incompetency in the superficial venous systems and communicating veins, eliminating these sites of incompetency and the resulting dilated veins and, hopefully, preventing their recurrence, are the main objectives in the treatment of primary varicose veins. It is about the methods for achieving these objectives that the disagreement occurs. There is no foolproof method or combination of methods for any of these. The clinical methods of inspection, palpation, percussion and various tourniquet applications aid in locating perhaps 50% of the sites of incompetency. The use of fluorescin dye and phlebography is of further aid and apparently the most reliable means for locating incompetent communicating veins is by infrared techniques.[7] An added and important advantage of the latter is that it is noninvasive. The ultrasound technique, also noninvasive, has the additional advantages of relative economy and adaptability to office use. No one method or combination of methods is completely accurate and all may give false positive indications.

Another factor which plagues the varicose vein therapist is the anatomical variability of veins, particularly those of the superficial systems. Communications of these veins with one another and with the deep system (perforating veins) vary widely with the individual. Common sites of incompetent "perforators" are the middle and lower thirds of the thigh medially, upper third of the lower leg medially and the lower third of the lower leg laterally and medially. As Dodd and Cockett have emphasized in their classic volume,[8] there are often three sites in the so-called ulcer-bearing area occurring in the course of the posterior arch vein. In my own experience, I have found at least one of these more uniformly than any of the other sites mentioned above, possibly because (since they are in the ulcer-bearing area) I have sought them routinely, even when they have not been apparent clinically.

The surgeon must always bear in mind that any superficial vein may unexpectedly terminate in a deep vein. This is particularly true of the lesser saphenous vein which instead of its expected popliteal termination may progress to the greater saphenous vein or a tributary in the lower thigh and occasionally it will end in the posterior tibial vein in the midcalf region. It also may be found in a combination of these variations. The surgeon must always beware of injury to the sural nerve when attacking this vein directly. He must also be aware of the possibility of overlooking it since it is usually concealed, in its upper portion, by being invested within the aponeurosis of the gastrocnemius muscle.

Varicosities of the upper thigh and genital areas are usually a result of incompetency or congenital absence of valves in the internal iliac veins and subsequent incompetency of sciatic, gluteal, internal pudendal and/or obturator veins.

Techniques of Surgical Treatment

As indicated above, the first step in the surgical management of primary venous insufficiency is the identification of the sites of insufficiency. Since 100% identification of these sites has not as yet been possible, a certain recurrence rate is inevitable. Two recent papers have reported a 15 and 7% overall recurrence rate, respectively, on 10 and 6 – 10 year follow-up.[9, 10]

Whatever surgical technique is used, a careful marking of all veins and perforators is essential. I have relied on clinical methods for this procedure. It goes without saying that complete ligation of all tributaries at the saphenofemoral junction is imperative. This requires adequate exposure and clear visualization of the femoral vein for a minimum of 2 cm above and below the junction. I use a 6- to 10-cm incision parallel to and just below the inguinal crease, two thirds of the incision being medial and one third lateral to the femoral pulse. The two layers of the superficial fascia are incised and the saphenofemoral junction usually is readily identified. The greater saphenous vein must be ligated at its termination. Occasionally an "accessory" saphenous vein will enter a large saphenous vein near its termination and mimic a saphenofemoral junction. Thus, the femoral artery must always be identified. I use 3-0 chromic catgut for tie with a transfixion ligature just distal to the flush tie. Care must be taken to ligate all tributaries to the femoral vein lying above the fascia lata. The greater saphenous vein is isolated at the level of the medial malleolus and a Myers stripper is passed to the groin. At this point, I usually search for an accessory saphenous vein, a fair size tributary entering the greater saphenous near its termination. It is more often lateral but may be medial. If a stripper is introduced retrogradely into this, it often can be pushed to midthigh or further and pulled out through a small incision, thus removing a segment of vein which is easily overlooked and may be a site of recurrence later on. In some cases, the stripper, in being passed from the ankle to the groin, is obstructed in the lower leg or thigh by a sacculation, previous ligation or occasionally a scar of an injection. In such instances, it is brought out through an incision at the point of obstruction and is reinserted into the vein proximally. A 4- or 6-inch Tensor elastic bandage is applied to the leg from the ankle to upper thigh as the vein is stripped from its bed. This is left in place as the groin wound is closed in layers. All marked veins are then excised through individual incisions, segments being stripped where possible, but more often subcutaneous tunneling between incisions is necessary. Usually 1.5 to 2-cm transverse incisions are used at intervals of 4–6 cm. This provides not only complete eradication of the visible veins, but leads to other varicosities that were not apparent at the time of marking. It also turns up "perforators" that were not discovered by preoperative examination. Large plexuses, at whatever site, are excised through adequate incisions over the long axis of the plexus. A perforator is often found as a part of, and is an important causative factor in, such a plexus.

If the lesser saphenous vein is involved, it is picked up behind the lateral malleolus and a small stripper is passed to the termination of the vein, usually at the popliteal vein. With the patient prone or on his side, an incision is made over the leading head of the stripper just above and parallel to the popliteal crease, and the vein is ligated at its termination. It is then stripped as a Tensor bandage is applied. The wound is closed in layers, care being taken to approximate the popliteal fascia accurately. If the vein terminates in the greater saphenous vein, it is ligated at this point. Stripping of the former may have left the end of the lesser saphenous vein free, in which case it is readily stripped through a small incision. If the stripper meets an obstruction distal to the popliteal fossa, extreme care must be exercised in any incision between the ankle and the knee posteriorly to avoid injuring the sural nerve. In such cases, I usually settle for ligature at the saphenopopliteal junction and leave the vein in place. Some authorities advise against stripping of the lesser saphenous vein.[10]

Varicosities of the upper thigh are treated as veins elsewhere, being followed with multiple incisions and tunneling. The consideration of varicosities of the vulva is not within the scope of this paper but the reader is referred to the excellent report on this subject by Dixon and Mitchell.[11]

All wounds are closed with interrupted sutures of 4-0 silk or 5-0 nylon, 3-0 chromic catgut being used for the fascial layers. A fluffy gauze bandage (Kerlex) is applied directly to the skin from toes to upper thigh covered by several layers of sheet-wadding rolled on over this and Tensor bandages applied with gentle pressure (4-inch for the lower leg and 6-inch for the thigh). The distance from the top of the bandage to the groin is compressed with soft dressings held in place with elastic tape. The entire dressing is held in place with firm-fitting stockinette from toes to just below the groin. This prevents edema, allows immediate ambulation and in most patients prevents pain completely. Fifteen hundred units of heparin in 1,000 ml of lactated Ringer's or 5% dextrose solution are infused over 12-hr periods for the first 24 hr following surgery. The anticoagulant, antiphlogistic and diuretic properties of heparin contribute to the patient's comfort, promote healing and, hopefully, are factors in preventing thrombophlebitis. The patient is ambulant 3–5 min of each hour as soon as the anesthetic wears off and is discharged on the 1st to 3d postoperative day depending on his disposition and fortitude. The original dressing is left in place until the 8th postoperative day when alternate sutures are removed, and the remaining ones are taken out 5–7 days later. A Tensor elastic bandage to the knee is worn for 6 weeks after surgery and the patient is urged to elevate the leg when he is not actually walking. If his work allows frequent elevation, he may return after 2 weeks of convalescence. Patients who must stand continuously are advised to remain away from work for 6 weeks.

I have no statistics on recurrence rate with this routine but it has not been appreciable. I have occasionally missed a varicosity or a perforator and this is taken care of under local anesthesia at the patient's convenience.

Summary

The causes, pathology and principles of surgical treatment of primary varicose veins are discussed and the technique of treatment is described in some detail.

Factors involved in development of primary varicose veins are still only partially understood. An hereditary factor appears to be important and a low grade subclinical inflammation may be a factor. Objectives of treatment include elimination of sites of valvular incompetency in the superficial venous system and communicating veins. The first step in surgical management is identification of the sites of venous insufficiency. Careful marking of varicose veins and perforators is essential, and subsequently, complete ligation of all tributaries at the saphenofemoral junction is imperative. The operation requires meticulous technique and aftercare.

REFERENCES

1. Ludbrook, J., and Beale, G.: Femoral venous valves in relation to varicose veins, Lancet 1:79, 1962.
2. Reagan, B., and Folse, R.: Lower limb venous dynamics on normal persons and children of patients with varicose veins, Surg. Gynecol. Obstet. 132:15, 1971.
3. Koppel, J. L., Hough, D. M., and Olwin, J. H.: Possible relation of a plasma enzyme activity to thromboembolism, Surg. Gynecol. Obstet. 112:315, 1961.
4. Koppel, J. L., Lycette, R. S., and Olwin, J. H.: Generation of a plasma enzyme activity and its relation to thromboembolism, Surg. Gynecol. Obstet. 125:502, 1967.
5. Olwin, J. H., and Koppel, J. L.: Anticoagulant therapy during pregnancy. A new approach, Obstet. Gynecol. 34:847, 1969.
6. Koppel, J. L., Hough, D. M., and Olwin, J. H.: Unpublished data.
7. Patil, K. D., Williams, J. R., and Williams, K. L.: Localization of incompetent perforating veins by thermography, Br. J. Surg. 56:620, 1969.
8. Dodd, H., and Cockett, F. B.: *The Pathology and Surgery of Veins of the Lower Limb* (London: E. & S. Livingstone Ltd., 1956).
9. Larson, R. H., Lofgren, E. P., Myers, T. T., and Lofgren, K. A.: Long term results after vein surgery. Study of 1000 cases after 10 years, Mayo Clin. Proc. 49:114, 1974.
10. Rivlin, S.: The surgical cure of primary varicose veins, Br. J. Surg. 62:913, 1975.
11. Dixon, J. A., and Mitchell, W. A.: Venographic and surgical observations in vulvar varicose veins, Surg. Gynecol. Obstet. 131:458, 1970.

5 / Management of Varicose Veins: Mayo Clinic Experience

KARL A. LOFGREN, M.D.

Head, Section of Peripheral Vein Surgery, Mayo Clinic and Mayo Foundation; Associate Professor of Surgery, Mayo Medical School, Rochester, Minnesota

The Early Mayo Operation

THE MAYO CLINIC experience with the management of varicose veins began before the turn of the present century. Several years before the Mayo Clinic was formally organized, Dr. Charles H. Mayo performed his first operation on a patient with varicose veins, at St. Mary's Hospital in Rochester, Minnesota. This operation, performed in 1888, was mentioned in his report before the 32d annual meeting of the Minnesota State Medical Association in 1900.[9] The great saphenous vein was excised through a long incision extending from the upper region of the thigh to below the knee. Fifty-three more patients had been operated on by him for varicose veins up to the time of that report, and Mayo noted that many older operations, previously in disrepute because of high mortality and sepsis, had been revived with the advent of aseptic surgery resulting from Lister's discovery. He also advised the use of rubber gloves by the surgeon and his assistants to provide greater safety for the patient.

In a subsequent report, presented in 1904 before the 36th annual meeting of the Minnesota Medical Association,[10] Mayo stated that 125 patients had been operated on for varicose veins and that he still favored an extensive excision of the great saphenous vein in preference to the then popular surgical procedures described by Trendelenburg and by Schede.[15, 18] Trendelenburg ligated and resected the saphenous vein in the upper inner third of the thigh. Schede employed circumferential incisions around the leg, down to the muscular layer;

this often left residual numbness and swelling from interruption of sensory nerves and lymphatics. During Mayo's earlier operations, considerable time was required to close the long incision that extended all the way from the upper part of the thigh to below the knee. Now he described the use of a special pair of forceps and the more recent development of a special extraluminal stripper. With these newly devised instruments, shorter incisions replaced the longer one, and the saphenous vein was freed and removed in uncut areas between incisions. He described his new stripper as a "ring vein enucleator which consists of a one-fourth inch ring of steel with a long handle, the whole instrument being not unlike a blunt uterine curet, which would possibly serve the purpose with the ring bent at a more acute angle" (Fig 5–1).[10] After the incision was made over the saphenous vein in the upper third of the thigh, the vein was transected and its lower end was passed through the ring of the enucleator. With a gentle pushing force, the ring was pushed down the vein (which was held under tension) for a distance of 6–8 inches, where another incision was made and the vein segment was removed. The process was repeated to a lower point until a large segment of the saphenous vein had been removed. Three

Fig 5–1.—The early Mayo operation, using the extraluminal vein stripper.

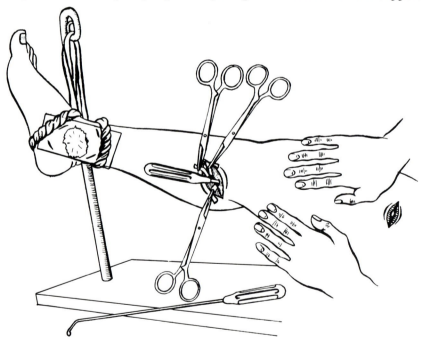

to five incisions of 1 inch in length, from the upper third of the thigh to the proximal third of the leg 6–8 inches below the knee, ordinarily were made. Hemorrhage was avoided by keeping the leg elevated on a gynecologic standard, and bleeding was controlled with a pressure pad held against the skin or a small pack placed into the incision. The Mayo operation with the extraluminal stripper was feasible for nearly all patients except in the very few instances where the varicose veins were enormously and irregularly dilated or their walls were extremely weak so that direct excision was required instead.

In a paper presented before the meeting of the Western Surgical and Gynecological Association in 1906, Mayo described his extraluminal stripper in more detail and included a sketch.[11] Stripping as well as local excision was employed, although the operation never extended up to the groin or down to the ankle or foot. Local excision was sometimes done for varicosities over the posterior aspect of the thigh or leg. Mayo mentioned that follow-up results in 51 patients 1–11 years after surgery were satisfactory in 84% and poor in 16% by examination. Recurrence was attributed to "a widening of the collateral veins, formation of new veins, and, it is claimed, from regeneration of the saphenous itself." The early Mayo operation was not as extensive as the complete stripping operation we now employ, for it left behind a considerable segment of the saphenous system in the groin and upper third of the thigh as well as in the lower half of the leg. Recurrence from residual varicosities was not uncommon.

Sclerotherapy

The Mayo operation for varicose veins was employed by the general surgeons of the Mayo Clinic staff for more than two decades, or until about 1927, when sclerotherapy replaced surgery as the treatment of choice. Hopes were initially high for improving the long-term results and avoiding the morbidity with sepsis and pulmonary embolism which had occasionally complicated the older surgical procedure. Sclerotherapy had begun in Europe, soon after Pravaz devised the hypodermic syringe in 1851.[14] After Linser, of the Tübingen Clinic, discovered in 1911 a sclerosing agent, bichloride of mercury, that was less toxic than those in use before,[5] injection therapy became widely accepted in most European countries as the best treatment for varicose veins. Dixon introduced sclerotherapy at the Mayo Clinic in 1928 and at first used a solution of quinine hydrochloride and urethane. He mentioned in an early report that recurrence after sclerotherapy was low, about 5%.[3] Sodium morrhuate (a fatty acid of cod liver oil, developed in England in 1930) was used at the Mayo Clinic by 1931. Still later, monolate solution (monoethanolamine oleate) became the favored sclerosing agent because of its very low incidence of side reactions. Smith, who carried out most of the sclerotherapy during that period, reported a low incidence of complications, with pulmonary embolism of nonfatal type occurring in one out of 692 patients.[17] Before long, however, it became evident that the recurrence rate was very high after sclerotherapy, particularly when the varicosities were also incompetent and would not remain occluded in the face of nature's efforts to recanalize thrombosed veins.

Ligation Combined with Sclerotherapy

Ligation combined with sclerotherapy was introduced at the Mayo Clinic in 1937 to improve the treatment for incompetent saphenous

Fig 5–2.—Comparison of follow-up results after ligation and injection (1940 group) and complete stripping (1950 group). (Courtesy of Lofgren, K. A., Ribisi, A. P., and Myers, T. T.[8]; copyright 1958, American Medical Association.)

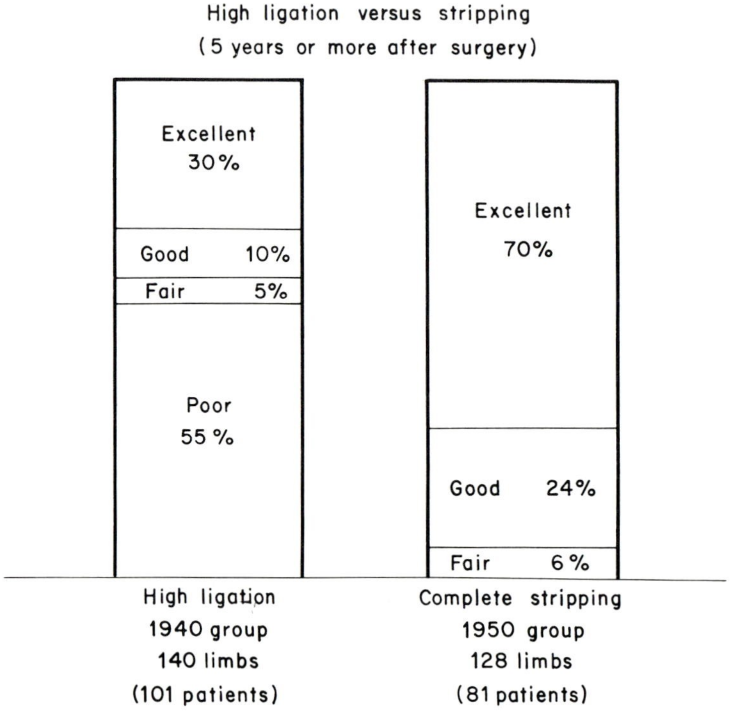

High ligation versus stripping
(5 years or more after surgery)

High ligation
1940 group
140 limbs
(101 patients)

Complete stripping
1950 group
128 limbs
(81 patients)

veins, with Waugh as an early, strong proponent. This procedure had originally been mentioned by Schiassi in 1908.[16] More recent reports especially by de Takats[1] and also by McPheeters and Anderson[12] in the early thirties, had greatly influenced the medical profession in this country to adopt this combined method of treatment. A paper published in the *Archives of Surgery* by de Takats and Quillin in 1933 stimulated additional enthusiasm for ambulatory ligation followed by injection.[2]

With the patient under local anesthesia, the great saphenous vein was ligated at its juncture with the common femoral vein, a short segment of the vein was resected, and the distal end of the vein was injected with 5% sodium morrhuate. Any remaining varicosities in the thigh or leg subsequently were injected during the immediate postoperative period. Initially, the follow-up results appeared to be very good, considerably better than with the sclerotherapy alone. Waugh at first believed that the recurrence rate would be less than 5% in 5 years, as compared with nearly 50% recurrences after injection alone.[19] However, the recurrence rate proved to be much higher with more time, as a later follow-up study revealed. When 101 patients were reviewed several years after original ligation and injection, only 40% were classified as having had excellent or good results, 60% having had poor or fair results; 36% of the entire group had needed subsequent additional surgery (Fig 5–2).

Complete Stripping

The present section of peripheral vein surgery was established at the Mayo Clinic in 1947, with Dr. Thomas T. Myers in charge. A more systematic approach to the diagnosis and treatment of varicose veins and peripheral venous disorders became possible. Surgical and medical management and a follow-up program for venous problems of the extremity were assigned to this special "vein clinic" within the larger Mayo Clinic, and soon two full-time surgeons were needed. The surgical treatment of varicose veins with stripping represented a radical departure from the older method of ligation (see Fig 5–2). Myers designed a new flexible intraluminal stripper, a much improved version of the short, rodlike intraluminal stripper described by Babcock in 1907. The intraluminal strippers were soon available in different lengths, acorns and tips so that veins of various dimensions could be easily removed. Unstrippable, tortuous varicosities and plexuses were removed by direct dissection. The stripping operation produced much better long-term results when performed completely rather than par-

TABLE 5-1.—FOLLOW-UP RESULTS AFTER VEIN SURGERY,
MAYO CLINIC EXPERIENCE

OPERATION (FOLLOW-UP)	NO. OF PATIENTS	RESULTS (%)			
		EXCELLENT	GOOD	FAIR	POOR
1906: Early Mayo operation	51	84 "satisfactory"		16 "un-	
(1-11 yr)				satisfactory"	
1954: Partial stripping	156	25	32	30	13
Complete stripping	555	64	30	5	1
(avg. 25 mo)					
1958: Ligation and injection	101	30	10	5	55°
Complete stripping	81	70	24	6	0
(5+ yr)					
1974: Complete stripping	278	44	41	15	0
(10+ yr)					

°Required further surgery.

tially (from foot to groin instead of from knee to groin) (Table 5-1).[13] The complete stripping operation, including meticulous dissection and excision of all varicose tributaries and incompetent perforating veins, became the standard operation for all patients needing vein surgery. It has remained the exclusive treatment of choice since 1950, and to the present time we have employed this method for more than 11,000 patients, or nearly 21,000 stripping operations.

Present Day Management of Varicose Veins

On the premise that a removed malfunctioning varix cannot recur, we believe that surgical treatment with stripping and excision offers the patient the best long-term prognosis. For patients in poor general health or those burdened with other more serious medical problems or for patients with trivial or cosmetic problems, alternatives to surgery are often employed. Among these, sclerotherapy has a leading place, along with elastic support, periodic elevation of legs and exercise. Sclerotherapy became an ancillary form of treatment after stripping began in the late 1940s and it is now used mainly for minor varicosities sometimes found at follow-up examinations or for spiderbursts and cutaneous venules that are of cosmetic concern to the patient. Sclerotherapy is not used for primary varicosities or for larger recurrent varicosities, for which we regard surgical excision as so much more effective. Elastic support with bandages or stockings provides symptomatic relief and protection for patients with larger varicosities or venous insufficiency when surgery is contraindicated for other medical reasons. Periodic elevation of legs and appropriate exercises help to promote better venous return flow and therefore are useful as adjunctive and alternative therapy in certain instances.

SURGICAL APPROACH

During the past quarter of a century, there has been no basic change in surgical technique, although the operation has gradually been extended to include a wider area of the saphenous system, from the dorsomedial aspect of the foot to the saphenofemoral juncture of the great saphenous system, and from the lateral aspect of the foot to the saphenopopliteal juncture of the small saphenous system. Each patient is selected critically for this elective, but extensive, vein operation. There must be valid indications for surgery, and clinical evidence for incompetence must be demonstrated. In our experience, the basic steps for successful surgical management of varicose veins include: (1) accurate preoperative diagnosis, (2) meticulous preoperative marking of the varicose pattern, including tributaries and perforating veins, (3) thorough surgical removal of the involved saphenous system by stripping, dissection and excision and (4) periodic follow-up of patients.

Preoperative Diagnosis

While the patient stands on a platform before the examining physician, facing adequate lights, varicose veins and signs of chronic venous insufficiency are looked for, from the groin and lower abdominal area downward to the ankles and feet. Past history of venous disorder and treatment should have been elicited before this examination. Attention is paid to any operative scars, unusual configuration of superficial veins or clinical signs of a postphlebitic condition such as edema, stasis cyanosis of skin, induration or ulceration. Pigmentation, dermatitis, induration and cellulitis are further signs of chronic venous stasis.

After inspection and palpation of superficial veins and subcutaneous tissue, the state of competence of the saphenous system is determined by two simple clinical tests that demonstrate reflux of venous blood flow if this is present. The first is the *compression test*, which is performed by compressing the great saphenous vein in the thigh with fingers of one hand and feeling for the transmitted downward impulse of venous blood with fingers of the other hand at a lower level in the leg. Compressing the small saphenous vein behind the knee (slightly flexed) transmits a similar impulse downward to the lower calf and ankle level. The compression test is also very useful in tracing the course and pattern of superficial veins.

The second test is the *retrograde filling test* (Brodie-Trendelenburg) which is done with the use of a rubber tourniquet around the lower thigh to test the competence of the great saphenous vein, or with the thumb applying pressure behind the knee to test the competence of the small saphenous vein. The superficial veins first are emptied by elevating the legs while the patient reclines before pressure is applied to the indicated saphenous vein and the patient resumes the standing position. After about 15 sec, pressure from the tourniquet (or thumb) is released and sudden retrograde filling or reflux of venous blood flow (incompetence) is looked for closely. This test is most important in establishing incompetence or reflux of either the great or the small saphenous vein, and the need for surgery is based on the existence of such incompetence. With incompetent perforating veins of large size, reflux usually can be demonstrated with release of finger pressure over the bulging vein, which normally overlies a palpable opening in the deep fascial layer. These veins more commonly are present over the inner lower third of the leg, where they not infrequently contribute to stasis changes of the tissues, especially in postphlebitic conditions. Incompetence of the great or small saphenous system must be diagnosed accurately and carefully differentiated by the surgeon, and normal or competent saphenous veins must be spared for possible future benefit to the patient. Crossover patterns with tributaries filling portions of the other saphenous system not infrequently are seen and should not be overlooked later during surgery.

Preoperative Marking

Meticulous marking of varicosities is the most important step in the surgical procedure, next to a thorough operation. All visible and palpable varicosities, including the saphenous main channel, tributaries, plexuses and perforating veins, are clearly marked with a special staining solution that does not rub or wash off (made by dissolving 5 gm of pyrogallic acid in ethyl alcohol, and adding 50 ml acetone, 40 ml of solution of ferric chloride and sufficient ethyl alcohol to make 100 ml). This is best done before hospital admission, while the patient stands on the examining platform before good lighting. Only the surgeon himself can perform adequate marking that provides the all-important guidelines during the long surgical procedure and calls his attention to many varicosities that otherwise could be missed easily.

Surgical Technique

Because of its extensive nature, the operation is best done with general anesthesia. In recent years, a split-leg operating table has been used very effectively because it permits easy access to the medial and posterior aspects of the patient's lower extremities by the surgical team (Fig 5–3). The lower limbs also can be elevated by flexing the operating table during the operation. With the *great* saphenous vein, the groin dissection is the first step. The saphenous vein is divided and all attached tributaries are followed out widely and ligated before the saphenofemoral juncture is ligated with simple and transfixion ligatures of chromic catgut. The medial and lateral femoral cutaneous tributaries, coursing down the thigh, are ligated or they are stripped out if they are large enough to admit a short stripper (38 cm).

Inserting the long flexible stripper (100 cm) into the saphenous vein on the dorsomedial aspect of the foot is the next step. The stripper is threaded upward under visual and palpable observation until it reaches the groin incision. In the foot incision, the vein is tied around the stripper, just ahead of the acorn, with a heavy silk tie. Before the long stripper is pulled out, several incisions are made to expose previously marked tributaries, which are freed and removed with the small stripper or with direct dissection. Any marked perforating vein is exposed

Fig 5–3.—Patient on split-leg operating table with all varicosities marked with staining solution before surgery.

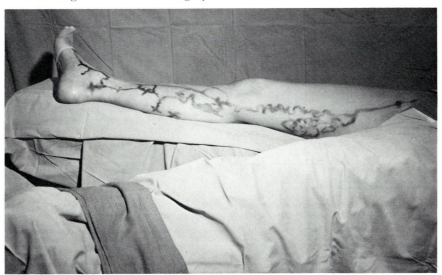

by individual incisions, followed down and ligated at the aperture of the deep fascial layer; joining superficial veins are excised. By flexing the operating table, the lower extremities are kept elevated from 12 to 15 degrees throughout the entire operation. The long stripper is then slowly pulled upward and out of the groin with the saphenous vein telescoped upon it. However, if resistance is met while the stripper is being pulled, additional incisions are made to expose and remove any joining, unmarked tributary. Alternative methods include stripping from the groin downward to the knee, although we prefer upward stripping from foot to knee-level with the use of the smallest acorn (¼-inch diameter) to avoid injury to the saphenous nerve.

With the *small* saphenous vein, a small transverse incision just above the popliteal fold, or a longitudinal incision just below the fold, is employed to expose the saphenous vein, while the leg is held up by an assistant. After the popliteal fascia has been incised longitudinally, the saphenous vein (which lies between the middle and lateral thirds of the popliteal fossa) is divided and followed upward to the close proximity of the saphenopopliteal juncture, where it is ligated with simple and transfixion ligature of chromic catgut. The intraluminal stripper is introduced into the small saphenous vein on the lateral ankle, threaded upward to the popliteal incision and pulled out after all attached tributaries over the calf region have been divided and removed through additional incisions. Again we favor stripping upward and using the smallest acorn (¼-inch diameter) on the medium length stripper (63 cm) to avoid injury to the sural nerve, which accompanies the saphenous vein from the ankle up to the midcalf level.

Small longitudinal incisions are used because they inflict less damage on superficial sensory nerves and lymphatic vessels. Dexon 3-0 sutures are used to close Scarpa's fascia in the groin or the popliteal fascia; 4-0 silk is used as interrupted vertical mattress sutures to close all skin incisions. Blood loss is controlled by elevating the lower extremities on the operating table, by applying external pressure or packing the wounds and by ligating larger vessels. Blood transfusions should not be necessary when the proper precautions have been observed.

During the postoperative period, the foot of the patient's bed is elevated 10–15 degrees. Higher elevation is not desirable because it impedes the arterial flow into the lower limb. In addition to surgical dressings and cotton padding, elastic bandages are applied and kept in place during the hospital stay. Bathroom privileges and short periods of ambulation are allowed on the morning after surgery. Skin sutures are removed 1 week after operation. Antibiotic or anticoagulant

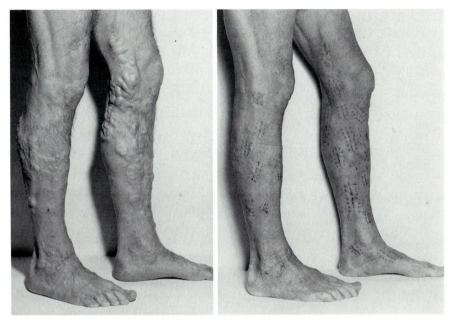

Fig 5–4.—Complete stripping operation. Preoperative (**left**) and postoperative (**right**) views of patient with extensive varicosities.

therapy is not prescribed. Elastic bandages are used daily for about 6 weeks after surgery, and longer or indefinitely if chronic deep venous insufficiency also exists. Sclerotherapy is ordinarily not necessary during the postoperative period if the varicosities have been removed thoroughly (Fig 5–4).

Postoperative complications have consisted of small hematomas, delayed wound healing and minor, nonfatal pulmonary emboli. The percentage of these complications has been extremely low. There have been no hospital deaths during the past 10 years, in which time we have operated on approximately 4,000 patients. As for pulmonary embolism, there were 16 patients during a recent 10-year period who had clinically suspected minor pulmonary emboli after vein stripping, a frequency of 0.39%.

Follow-Up Program

Follow-up is important for the best care of the patient, and it also helps the surgeon to evaluate the effectiveness of his operation. We routinely advise our patients to return in 1 year for a follow-up examination, after which they may wait 2 or 3 years for their next visit unless unexpected problems arise. Sometimes a smaller varicosity has developed which can be occluded with sclerotherapy. Sometimes the patient has special need for elastic support and should be seen more often, as during pregnancy or when there is a coexisting postphlebitic condition. At times other medical problems have developed for which the patient needs help and referral for adequate care. By and large, although a periodic follow-up program is time-consuming, it is well compensated by the service provided to the patient and by the information it provides the physician with regard to long-term control and results achieved.

LONG-TERM FOLLOW-UP RESULTS

In our experience, long-term follow-up results have been generally good (see Table 5–1). An early report in 1954 showed that the complete stripping operation (from foot to groin) produced much better results than did the partial operation (from knee level to groin).[13] Another report, in 1958, confirmed that the stripping operation was much superior to the older ligation and injection procedure.[8] A more recent follow-up study, published in 1974, involving a larger group of patients, revealed that 85% maintained excellent or good results, as noted by direct examination 10 years or more after vein surgery.[4]

Recurrence of varicosities after the stripping operation—enough to warrant further surgery—cannot always be prevented in spite of a thorough and complete surgical procedure. Pregnancy subsequent to the stripping operation is a strong predisposing factor for recurrence in many patients. In a separate 2-year review of surgical recurrence after stripping, we noted that pregnancy had occurred from one to four times subsequent to the original operation in 8 of the 11 patients who were operated on again by us (from 2 to 17 years later). In other patients, inherent constitutional weaknesses as well as the effects of time are undoubtedly important contributing factors for recurrence.

The number of our own patients needing further surgery after the complete stripping operation has been low, but this does not necessarily reflect the true incidence of surgical recurrence because many patients never return for follow-up examination and still others decline any reoperation because they are well pleased with their results from a symptomatic standpoint. In our follow-up study wherein 43 patients, 15% of the examined group (see Table 5–1), were classified as having had only fair results 10 years or more after the stripping operation, 34 still thought that their results had been either good or excellent because of subjective improvement, and many declined further surgery.

Summary

The Mayo Clinic experience with the management of varicose veins goes back to the turn of the present century. The early Mayo operation was a fairly effective, radical operation for its time, even though incomplete by present standards. It was used by our general surgeons for another two decades or more before being replaced by sclerotherapy for a decade and by ligation and sclerotherapy for still another decade. The stripping operation became the treatment of choice in the late 1940s and with continued emphasis on completeness it has offered promising long-term results, objectively and symptomatically. A permanent surgical cure cannot be guaranteed for all patients. Over the past quarter of a century, we have learned that a thorough operation combined with periodic follow-up will provide the best management of varicose veins for the lifetime of most patients.

REFERENCES

1. de Takats, G.: Ambulatory ligation of the saphenous vein, JAMA 94:1194, 1930.
2. de Takats, G., and Quillin, L.: Ligation of the saphenous vein: A report on two hundred ambulatory operations, Arch. Surg. 26:72, 1933.
3. Dixon, C. F.: The results of injection treatment of varicose veins, Proc. Staff Meet. Mayo Clin. 5:42, 1930.
4. Larson, R. H., Lofgren, E. P., Myers, T. T., and Lofgren, K. A.: Long-term results after vein surgery: Study of 1,000 cases after 10 years, Mayo Clin. Proc. 49:114, 1974.
5. Linser, P.: Die Behandlung der Krampfadern mit Sublimateinspritzungen und ihre Erfolge, Med. Klin. 17:1445, 1921.
6. Lofgren, E. P., and Lofgren, K. A.: Recurrence of varicose veins after the stripping operation, Arch. Surg. 102:111, 1971.
7. Lofgren, E. P., and Lofgren, K. A.: Alternatives in the management of varices, Geriatrics 30:111, 1975.
8. Lofgren, K. A., Ribisi, A. P., and Myers, T. T.: An evaluation of stripping versus ligation for varicose veins, Arch. Surg. 76:310, 1958.
9. Mayo, C. H.: Varicose veins of the lower extremity, St. Paul Med. J. 2:595, 1900.
10. Mayo C. H.: The surgical treatment of varicose veins, St. Paul Med. J. 6:695, 1904.
11. Mayo, C. H.: Treatment of varicose veins, Surg. Gynecol. Obstet. 2:385, 1906.
12. McPheeters, H. O., and Anderson, J. K.: *Injection Treatment of Varicose Veins and Hemorrhoids* (2d ed.; Philadelphia: F. A. Davis Company, 1939).
13. Myers, T. T., and Smith, L. R.: Results of the stripping operation in the treatment of varicose veins, Proc. Staff Meet. Mayo Clin. 29:583, 1954.
14. Pravaz, C. G.: Cited by McPheeters and Anderson.[12]
15. Schede, M.: Ueber die operative Behandlung der Unterschenkelvaricen, Berl. Klin. Wochenschr. 14:85, 1877.

16. Schiassi, B.: La cure des varices du membre inférieur par l'injection intraveineuse d'une solution d'iode, Sem. Med. Paris 28:601, 1908.
17. Smith, F. L.: Varicose veins: Complications and results of treatment of 5,000 patients, Milit. Surg. 85:514, 1939.
18. Trendelenburg, F.: Ueber die Unterbindung der Vena saphena magna bei Unterschenkelvaricen, Beitr. Klin. Chir. 7:195, 1890.
19. Waugh, J. M.: Ligation and injection of great saphenous veins, Proc. Staff Meet. Mayo Clin. 16:832, 1941.

6 / The Surgical Management of Recurrent Varicose Veins

JERE W. LORD, JR., M.D.

Professor of Clinical Surgery, New York University School of Medicine and Chief, Vascular Surgery, Cabrini Health Care Center, Columbus Hospital Division, New York, New York

THE TITLE SUGGESTS that some therapeutic maneuver had been instituted for the initial control of varicose veins and was less than successful. Recurrence to be dealt with here is that which followed surgical intervention. In some circles, sclerotherapy is considered as definitive treatment for large varicosities with incompetent valves, as well as for smaller ones only of cosmetic significance. Before discussing the surgical management of recurrent varicose veins we should consider known causes for recurrence so that therapy will evolve on a rational basis.

Of all this earth's mobile creatures, only the human animal with his penchant for standing erect is afflicted by this abnormal state. According to one authority, not one instance of varicosities has been observed in horses, dogs, cats and other four-legged animals. It may be a valid philosophical tenet that "once varicose veins, there will always be varicose veins." I believe that those individuals who develop dilated veins have either a structural weakness of the venous wall or of the valves or both. Hence if no postoperative care is given following a thorough surgical procedure, then the majority of patients will sooner or later exhibit new varicosities, which at first are small, then grow and become clinically significant. As long as postoperative patients continue to spend some 16 hr out of 24 sitting or standing, recurrences are inevitable. It may be useful to think of varicosities as one does of dental caries and to suggest the need for careful follow-up at regular intervals exactly as our dental colleagues do.

Other causes of recurrent varicose veins are far less important but should be considered in each patient with this problem.

1. Occasionally a patient with the primary defect in one system will develop incompetence of the valves of another system and will require a primary operation in the newly involved area.

2. Some patients who suffered an old deep venous phlebothrombosis have compensated well but have a tendency to develop hypertension in the communicating veins with subsequent failure of their valves and secondary dilatation of small subcutaneous veins.

3. A variant of the above is the patient who has congenitally defective valves of the deep femoropopliteal veins which persistently cause an overload on the superficial veins and early recurrences. This group of patients is helped by conscientious use of elastic stockings postoperatively as are those in group 2.

4. Several patients in our experience developed recurrent varicose veins following a thorough procedure wherein the underlying problem was an unrecognized traumatic arteriovenous fistula.

CASE 1. — M. B., a 47-year-old mother of six children, was assaulted by a knife-wielding psychotic and suffered several lacerations of the neck, chest and lower extremities. Approximately 1 year later varicosities appeared in the right lower extremity and a thorough procedure of high ligation and stripping was performed. One year later recurrence was noted and the patient was advised to have another operative procedure by one surgeon and injections only by the original surgeon. When seen in consultation the author followed a time-honored practice of placing the disk of a stethoscope over all scars from original lacerations and was rewarded by a loud, continuous bruit over the right lower extremity below the knee anterolaterally. An angiogram revealed a traumatic arteriovenous fistula between the anterior tibial artery and vein with marked enlargement of the superficial femoral artery (Fig 6 – 1). Following excision of the fistula, all varicosities cleared and the patient has remained well for the past 2 years.

CASE 2. — F. R., a 73-year-old man, had been operated upon for a right inguinal hernia 1 year earlier and when seen in consultation for the treatment of varicosities and edema of the right lower extremity was found to have a thrill and continuous bruit over the inguinal scar. An angiogram showed a traumatic arteriovenous fistula between the epigastric artery and vein which was cured by quadruple ligation of these small vessels. Edema and varicosities cleared promptly postoperatively.

5. Some patients with congenital arteriovenous fistulas develop varicosities in the lower extremity and require resection of the veins. Usually there is little difficulty in recognizing the true nature of the problem and when possible, excision of the fistulas and resection of the varicosities will lead to a cure. More often the congenital fistulas cannot be removed completely and varicosities will recur. Sclerother-

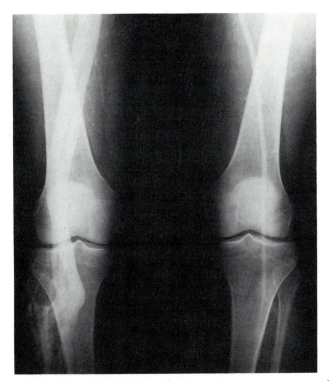

Fig 6–1.—This arteriogram shows the traumatic arteriovenous fistula between the anterior fibial artery and vein. Note enlargement of the femoral and popliteal arteries.

apy will be helpful to a greater or lesser degree and reoperation sometimes will be necessary.

6. In one patient in our series, recurrent varicosities were noted in a 21-year-old girl within 2 years of a thorough bilateral stripping procedure. When seen in consultation she exhibited an elevation of the venous pressure in the arms as well as in the legs. Thorough work-up showed that the patient's underlying problem was a chronic constrictive pericarditis and the varicosities cleared following pericardiectomy. In some eight patients undergoing pericardial resections, which the author performed between 1948 and 1961, this patient was the only one whose primary complaint was varicose veins. Several others exhibited marked ascites with some dilatation of the veins of the lower extremities, but in these patients the problem was obvious.

7. Finally, one of the common causes of recurrence following operative intervention is inadequate high ligation of the greater saphe-

nous. Although the author does not believe in exposing the femoral vein as a routine maneuver, it is important to ligate and transfix the vein within 1 cm of the femoral vein and ligate all of the tributaries which join the greater saphenous vein in this area. If a branch joins at or near the junction of the saphenous and femoral veins, then I prefer to leave that branch alone. Injury to the femoral vein will be followed by consequences far worse than the potential harm of leaving such a branch uninterrupted.

Discussion

The surgical management of varicose veins has as its bedrock a thorough search for the primary reason for the recurrence. If most of the above causes are ruled out, then I reserve a secondary operation for those few patients in whom I am unable to control the recurrences by sclerotherapeutic maneuvers. As in many other areas, failure of a primary operation to control varicosities when coupled with careful follow-up and injections when necessary, is due to a less than optimal operation in the first place. In addition to a proper high ligation of the greater saphenous, thorough stripping through multiple incisions in the thigh and lower extremity is necessary. In some patients the greater saphenous will bifurcate into two major branches in the thigh coursing in a parallel fashion to the lower leg. Both branches should be stripped independently. I am not one of those who like the "giant" strip from the internal malleolus to the groin with one or two intervening incisions. This maneuver sometimes will leave large varicosities associated with a major branch and require an early secondary operation.

Summary

The role of surgical management of recurrent varicose veins depends on a careful search for the cause of the recurrence and then application of the appropriate procedure. Ideal management of the patient with varicose veins will include an accurate diagnosis, a thoroughly performed operative procedure and careful and persistent postoperative checkups to treat new varicosities with appropriate sclerotherapeutic techniques.

7 / Compression Sclerotherapy of Varicose Veins

JOHN T. HOBBS, M.D., F.R.C.S.

Consultant Surgeon and Senior Lecturer, St. Mary's Hospital Medical School, London, England

IN A STUDY of more than 4,000 healthy Swiss workers (average age, 46 years) the prevalence of all types and grades of varicose veins was 57% for men and 68% for women; chronic venous insufficiency was found in 19% of men and in 25% of women.[1]

Varicose veins and their complications tend to overburden the surgical resources of most hospitals and, because of the cost both in time and finance, interest in injection treatment, which had been maintained in central Europe, has been renewed in the British Isles during the last two decades.

History of Sclerotherapy

Sclerotherapy first was used by Chassaignac in 1853 when he inject-ed ferric chloride into varicose veins.[2] Many substances were intro-duced, and by the early part of this century the treatment of varicose veins by sclerotherapy had become established and was in wide-spread use. However, there were many complications and the results were not uniformly good, while surgery was becoming more extensive with flush saphenofemoral ligation and thorough removal of the dilat-ed superficial veins; treatment by injection therefore was abandoned and the poor results were due to inadequate methods. Previously, less effective sclerosants were injected with the patient standing and com-pression was seldom applied; this resulted in a large thrombus which soon resolved allowing the vein lumen to reopen and, rarely, the thrombus migrated proximally as an embolus. The recanalization frequently was associated with valve destruction, so that poor injection treatment was worse than no treatment. These results brought the method into disrepute. However, with adequate techniques even the grossest varicose veins can be completely eliminated by sclerosing therapy.

Sclerotherapy has continued to be practiced in central Europe and during the last two decades Fegan[3, 4] has modified the method and established a larger clinic in Dublin and the success of his enthusiastic approach has resulted in a revival of sclerotherapy. The injection of varicose veins in a planned method and combined with the use of compression bandages was first employed in Paris by Linser[5] and Sicard.[6, 7] McAusland,[8] working in Liverpool, reported excellent results in 10,000 patients treated in this manner. Brunstein,[9] of New York, stressed the importance of the empty vein technique combined with compression bandages and immediate ambulation. For four decades Sigg[10, 11] in Basle and Tournay[12-14] in Paris have used this method effectively in many thousands of patients, and both workers use 3% sodium tetradecyl sulphate.

Many of the earlier sclerosing agents produced undesirable side effects and so these caustic and toxic agents were difficult to use. Reiner[15] demonstrated that sodium tetradecyl sulphate was more active and yet less toxic than any previously used agent; it is a stable and soluble chemical of low viscosity which can be injected easily through the finest needles. Reiner demonstrated that, although the activity was greater than other agents, the perivenous inflammatory response was less and this localized destruction of the vein intima is the reason for its success. Other workers have confirmed that 3% sodium tetradecyl sulphate is a more effective and safer agent than those previously used.[16-24]

McAusland[8] stressed the empty vein technique and after the injections applied firm pressure and bandages which allowed only small clots with less likelihood of recanalization. Orbach[19] emphasized that the vein must be occluded by intimal destruction and fibrosis and not by thrombus, and that firm compression for at least 3 weeks was necessary.

Indications for Injection of Varicose Veins

Varicose veins can be treated by one of four methods: (1) no treatment, but the patient is reassured that the veins are unlikely to give rise to symptoms and complications, or else the symptoms are due to some other cause; (2) elastic stockings to control symptoms and hide the veins but not to provide a cure; (3) injection; and (4) surgery.

If the veins are to be eliminated, then the method used must be either injection or surgery. There is a place for both methods and good results will be achieved only when there is careful assessment and planning of the treatment, together with precise execution. Varicose veins are treated badly either because the wrong method is used and no matter how well it is done it cannot succeed or because the right method is performed badly. To overcome these problems the surgeon must be competent in both methods and equally enthusiastic if he is to select and execute the most effective plan for treatment.

For injection therapy to succeed when large veins are treated, the veins must be compressed for several weeks to prevent blood and thrombus collecting in the lumen before permanent obliterating fibrosis has formed. Therefore all veins can be treated by injection provided that compression bandages can be applied and maintained in position for an adequate period of time.

It is apparent that injection-compression therapy is not indicated when there is either saphenofemoral or saphenopopliteal incompetence, because the termination of both the long and short saphenous veins cannot be adequately compressed. It is also difficult to maintain compression on the upper thigh, particularly when the leg is fat.

Proximal incompetence of either the long or short saphenous veins is treated best by limited surgery in the first instance, and this should relieve most of the symptoms. Any residual veins can be dealt with by injection. Having dealt with the termination of either the long or short saphenous veins by surgery, it is a simple matter to pass a stripper distally and remove the short saphenous vein down to just above the lateral malleolus and the long saphenous vein down to just below the knee. There is no reason to remove the long saphenous vein from the lower leg because this not only achieves little, but frequently results in damage to the saphenous nerve. The incompetence of the long saphenous system distally involves the anterior tibial tributary and more often the posterior tibial tributary which communicates directly with the more important perforating veins of the lower leg.

If general anesthesia is contraindicated, then an effective method of treatment is first to carry out a flush ligation of the saphenofemoral junction or saphenopopliteal junction under local anesthesia, and then to treat the remaining vein problems by injection, but this usually causes more inconvenience and more discomfort to the patient.

Frequently seen in female patients is a large vein meandering down the front of the thigh to the lateral aspect of the knee, and then to the side or back of the lower leg; invariably this is associated with an incompetent saphenofemoral junction which may not be apparent in a well covered thigh, but the long saphenous vein is not involved. This

TABLE 7-1.—RECOMMENDED TREATMENT FOR DIFFERENT
VEIN PROBLEMS

TYPE OF VEIN PROBLEM	PERCENTAGE OF PATIENTS		BEST PRIMARY TREATMENT
Trivial cosmetic veins	22		
Dilated superficial veins	8		
Lower leg perforating veins	5	39	Injection-compression
Post-thrombotic syndrome	4		
Long saphenous vein only	55		
Short saphenous vein only	5	61	Surgery
[Both long and short saphenous veins]	[5]		(35% required secondary injection)

situation is dealt with best by a proximal ligation under local anesthesia followed by injection-compression therapy of the dilated veins. Treatment by injection without proximal control usually results in an excessive thrombophlebitic reaction which is painful and is liable to produce skin staining, and the result may only be temporary because the thrombus allows recanalization.

The results of a random trial in which surgery and injection treatment were compared[24] showed that in 39% injection was the best primary treatment and although 61% required surgery, 35% of these required supplementary injections to achieve a perfect cosmetic result. The indications are summarized in Table 7–1 and show that injection treatment is an essential part of the management of many vein problems, being required in 74% of all patients seen during the random trial.

Treatment of Varicose Veins by Injection

The principle of injection treatment is to place a small volume of an effective sclerosant in the lumen of the vein which is compressed to prevent the formation of thrombus, and this compression must be maintained until permanent fibrosis has obliterated the lumen. Good results depend upon careful technique, and the important points of treatment are (1) where to inject, (2) how to inject and (3) how to bandage.

All those practitioners obtaining good results recommend the injection of small volumes into an empty vein which is then compressed for a sufficient period of time by properly applied bandages. Consistently good results can be obtained and complications are rare once details have been mastered.

Varicose vein problems are common and are seen in the general surgical clinics where they tend to receive insufficient attention because of their relatively less serious nature. For good results, I believe that the vein patient should be dealt with in a special clinic, staffed by trained assistants and nurses, and where the equipment is properly set out; by so doing large numbers can be seen and treated.

At the first visit a full history is taken and recorded on a specially designed, $8\frac{1}{2} \times 10$ inch card. The patient is then examined while standing on a couch so that the examiner can sit comfortably on a stool. The veins are drawn onto the chart on the back of the record card. The veins are carefully assessed by palpation and the "sliding finger" method to determine "points of control." I have not found it necessary to use the tourniquet test. The "points of control" are marked with a felt-tip pen and are intended to include all sites where incompetent perforating veins join the superficial veins. The nearer the injection is made to the perforating vein the more sure is the result, but with good compression the results will be good as long as the involved segment is injected, because the sclerotic process may extend to the point where there is flow in the deep veins.

The patient then lies down on the couch and the veins are injected at the marked points with 3% sodium tetradecyl sulphate (Sotradecol, S.T.D., Trombovar). Using disposable 2-ml syringes fitted with 25 gauge $\times$ 16 mm needles, 0.5 ml (maximum 0.75 ml for very large "blowouts") of 3% sodium tetradecyl sulphate is injected into the empty vein at the "points of control." B-D Plastipak syringes fitted with 25 gauge $\times$ 16 mm needles were found to be very effective and reliable. When more injections were made at the patient's first visit, repeated courses of treatment were required less often; the number of injections now averages about 10 per leg. When large veins are injected the leg is elevated to 45 degrees. Great care is taken to place the needle tip in the vein lumen and the segment of vein is then isolated between the index and ring fingers (Fig 7 – 1); as the injection is made the tip of the middle finger is placed over the tip of the needle to monitor the injection and ensure that there is no perivenous leak of sclerosant. Before injection the plunger is withdrawn and a small volume of blood is aspirated into the hub of the needle. Venous blood can be identified by its color and the absence of pulsation. If there is pulsa-

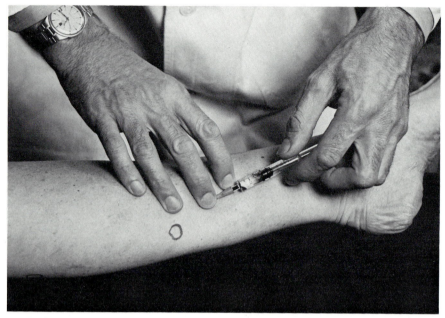

Fig 7–1.—Placement of needle in vein and injection of sclerosant. Note blood in hub of syringe and the middle finger monitoring the site of injection.

tion, which I have observed on two occasions, or if the color of the blood is very bright suggesting the possibility that it might be arterial, the needle is removed; injections are never made when there is the slightest doubt about the needle being in the vein lumen.

Because of the large number of injections it is not easy to use the large sponge rubber pads of Fegan's technique, and I was recently reassured when it was shown that those large pads had no significant advantage over bandages alone.[25] At first dental rolls were used, but sometimes the hard corners produced blistering which occasionally resulted in pressure pigmentation of the skin. Cotton wool balls were found to be very satisfactory and are conveniently and economically supplied in bags of 250 large or 500 small size; several large balls were used when there was a thick subcutaneous fatty layer at the injection site, but on thin legs a single small ball was sufficient and over bony prominences it was pulled out to prevent excessive pressure. The pads were retained in place by a small strip of 2.5-cm (1-inch) wide nonirritant hypoallergic surgical adhesive tape (Dermicel or Micropore) (Fig 7–2). This tape must never be applied with ten-

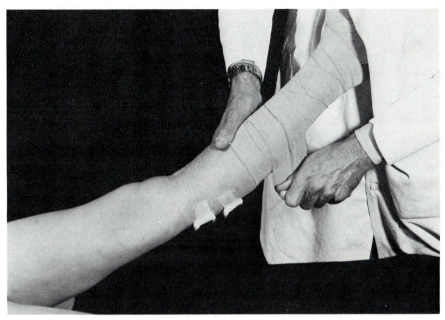

Fig 7–2.—A 7.5-cm Elastocrepe bandage being applied to leg over wool pads, which are held in place by Dermicel tape.

sion, to avoid surgical tape trauma,[26] and tension is unnecessary because pressure is applied by the bandage.

The leg then is bandaged firmly using 7.5-cm and 10-cm cotton crepe with limited stretch (Elastocrepe). The 7.5-cm bandage is applied from the head of the metatarsals up to the midcalf. Over this the 10-cm bandage is placed (see Fig 7–2) and the application of the bandages is an important and most difficult part of the treatment. The bandage must be smooth with steadily reducing pressure up the leg. The bandage is applied carefully using one hand to feel the tension and the active hand is moved to adjust the tension of the edges so that there are no loose or tight turns; the bandage must be firm and remain in place to be effective. If it is too tight it will cause the patient to wake from sleep and have to get up and walk. If the patient thinks that the bandage is uncomfortably tight on getting up from the treatment couch it is better to remove the bandage until the pain is relieved and then to reapply it.

Finally, the bandages are covered by a length of flesh-colored elasticized tubular stockinette (Tubigrip), size G4X, which is as effective as an elastic stocking, but is much cheaper and is readily available. The Tubigrip is easily applied by means of an applicator, and finished by folding the ends inside; this leaves a smooth neat appearance which holds the bandage in place (Fig 7 – 3).

The patient is instructed to walk immediately and to increase this distance over the first few days until several miles are walked each day. If the bandages feel tight when sitting the patient should alternatively plantarflex and dorsiflex the ankle joint; if tight when standing, lifting rhythmically onto the toes will relieve the discomfort. If the bandages feel tight when rising from bed or a chair the discomfort is immediately relieved by walking round the room. Some instructions are given on the appointment card to help and to reassure the patient.

After 3 weeks the patient returns for the legs to be examined and rebandaged. Although the injections and bandaging were made while the leg was elevated, an "intravascular hematoma" sometimes occurs, and is no disadvantage provided that it is evacuated at this stage when the local pressure pads are removed. The hematoma is felt as a fluctuant, often tender, swelling and is stabbed with a 19 gauge × 50 mm needle and the contents are evacuated by pressure between the two index fingers.

After 6 weeks, or 5 for smaller veins, the bandages are removed and

Fig 7–3.—Completion of bandaging of lower leg with flesh-colored elasticized tubular bandage in place.

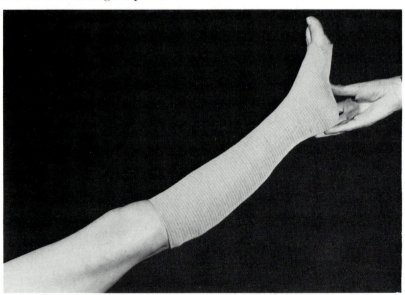

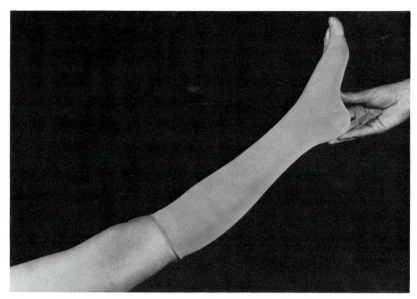

Fig 7–4. – Knee-length Scholl Duoten elastic stocking.

Fig 7–5. – A tubular elastic bandage with posterior foam strip (Tubipad) applied over the knee, when the whole leg is bandaged.

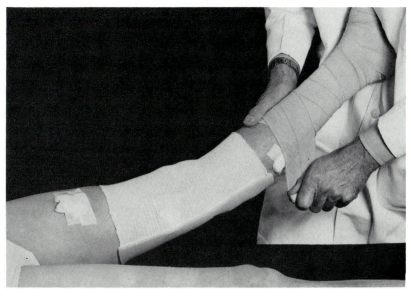

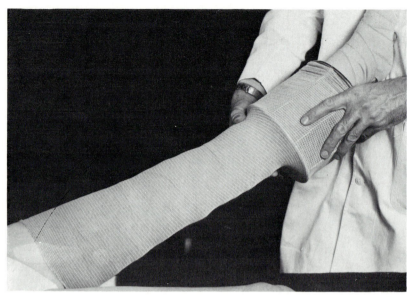

Fig 7–6.—The flesh-colored tubular elastic bandage being applied over the bandages.

a strong, two-way stretch elastic stocking (Scholl Duoten) is worn during the day for another 4 or more weeks (Fig 7–4).

If veins above the knee are also injected, or if any veins injected below the knee are seen to continue over the knee, then the thigh must also be bandaged. A length of elasticized tubular stockinette-type bandages which includes a strip of porous and inert foam padding (Tubipad) (25 cm long or one third of a pack), size P5, is reversed and placed over the knee and under the bandages to increase mobility and prevent slipping of the bandage (Fig 7–5). The bandages are then continued up to the thigh and over the knee pad. The Tubigrip is then placed over the bandages using an applicator (Fig 7–6) and remains in place more efficiently if attached to a suspender belt. During treatment the patients can continue in their normal occupations with minimal discomfort.

Complications

Complications rarely occur when the method is applied correctly; however, there are occasional problems, and particularly during the initial period when the technique is being perfected. In general, the complications are less serious and less frequent than those associated with surgical treatment. The complications include: (1) allergic response to the sclerosant; (2) toxic effects of an overdose of sclerosant; (3) incorrect placement of the sclerosant; (4) intravenous hematoma and spreading thrombophlebitis; (5) thromboembolic phenomena; (6) problems of bandaging; and (7) late complications.

Allergic reactions are rare and are usually confined to scattered urticarial blotches on the skin, particularly on the leg which has been injected. More seriously there is swelling of the lips and tongue and mild bronchospasm has been seen. These reactions promptly respond to intravenous antihistamine (Piriton, 10 mg). Toxic reactions are seen when too many injections of too large volumes are given at a single visit. The toxic reaction includes malaise with thirst, shivering, headaches and sometimes chest pain or epigastric discomfort.

If there is leakage from the injected vein, or if the injection is made into the subcutaneous tissue, an ulcer results from the necrosis of fat and skin. This punched-out necrotic area may be as large as 1 cm in diameter, and is surrounded by an inflammatory reaction. A thick scab forms and the ulcer is slow to heal, leaving a thin depressed scar often with surrounding pigmentation. Injection into peripheral nerves have been reported; these rare events have been characterized by sudden severe pain which lasts for several days, but no abnormality is seen on examination of the limbs.

An inadvertent intra-arterial injection has been reported on five occasions and in all there was gangrene of portions of the foot resulting in partial amputations. The prevention of extravenous injections depends on great care with regard to the technique of injection; the initial stab must be accurate, there must be easy aspiration of blood into the needle hub, and care must be taken that the needle and syringe are not moved during the actual injection.

An intravascular hematoma is occasionally seen when a large vein is injected and the compression has been inadequate. This intravascular clot is tender and if not evacuated may lead to discoloration of the overlying skin, and eventually recanalization can occur. The problem is overcome by evacuation of the hematoma using a large needle stab or small scalpel point incision.

Deep vein thrombosis has occurred but is rare and is not seen when the injection volumes are small and there is good compression. The few cases of pulmonary embolism have occurred in patients with large long saphenous veins and particularly when fat thighs could not be properly bandaged. Such cases are best treated by surgery.

The most difficult part of the technique is the application of bandages and during the first year that the treatment is in use patients frequently return because bandages are too tight or too loose. The bandages must be smoothly firm, but not painfully tight.

The later complications include skin staining, persistent tenderness at the injection site, the development of fresh venules or venous flares and the recurrence of varicose veins. Skin staining may fade even after 1 or 2 years, and with good technique is rarely seen. Tenderness at the site of the injection may persist for up to 3 months and often follows an intravascular hematoma, particularly in fat legs.

Recurrent varicose veins occur when the technique is applied incorrectly and in legs where the bandages cannot provide adequate compression. Proximal incompetence of the long and short saphenous veins requires surgery, and it is not possible to compress large veins in fat thighs.

Results of Treatment

The results of a random trial in which surgery was compared with injection were recently reported.[24] The overall results from the two methods of treatment showed that, at 1 year, injection therapy is more effective with a very high cure rate, but this begins to fall at 2 years and this failure rate increases markedly during the 4th, 5th and 6th years after treatment. At 1 year, surgery showed a lower success rate, but this did not fall as rapidly with time. The falloff in the success of treatment by injection—compression occurred despite repeated courses of treatment if there was proximal incompetence. It was soon obvious that a long follow-up was necessary before any conclusions could be reached with regard to the best primary treatment for varicose veins.

To determine the reasons for failure in each of the two treatment groups the results were further analyzed. There is considerable disagreement as to a reliable classification of varicose veins because of considerable overlap. Therefore, an arbitrary classification was made to differentiate three distinct groups: group 1, dilated superficial veins; group 2, incompetence of the lower leg perforators only; and group 3, involvement of the long and short saphenous systems.

When reconsidered in these three groups the results of the two methods of treatment showed marked differences. It was immediately apparent that dilated superficial veins and incompetent lower leg perforating veins are best treated by injection-compression.

When there is involvement of the saphenous systems, the early results (1 year) of treatment by injection-compression are good, but this success is not maintained for longer than 2 or 3 years, so that by 4 years the results of injection treatment show a very low success rate and a rapidly increasing failure rate. With a longer follow-up it soon became clear that surgery provided a much more permanent cure. Injection-compression treatment failed when there was gross incompetence of the saphenofemoral junction, and this reflected the experience of many phlebologists who have found that for this group of patients, injection treatment needed to be repeated after 4 or 5 years to maintain the good early results. In this large group of patients with incompetence of the proximal saphenous systems, good results were obtained from surgery, which need not be extensive since a flush saphenofemoral ligation with stripping of the long saphenous vein down to the upper part of the calf caused minimal disability after a 24-hr hospital stay, and, in most cases, resulted in complete relief of symptoms. Residual veins on the lower part of the leg often disappeared during the next few months after surgery, and if they persisted they could easily be treated by injection-compression at subsequent visits.

Proximal incompetence was present in 60% of the 746 patients seen consecutively during the period of the trial and it is this group who benefit most from surgical treatment. When there is proximal incompetence, combined treatment offered the best long-term results and it was apparent that surgery should be carried out first because, in addition to a better result, the injection therapy, if required, was simpler and confined to the lower part of the leg.

Based on the results of the random trial, a third phase, the trial of selection was begun in 1968 and to date more than 4,000 legs have been treated by the combined approach. The complementary use of surgery and sclerotherapy has proved to be very effective.

Summary

Varicose veins with their complications tend to overburden the surgical resources of most hospitals. Although sclerotherapy was first used in 1853, it was not until the early part of this century that this treatment became established and in widespread use. Later, the method fell into disrepute.

There are specific indications for injection of varicose veins and, in fact, there is a place for both injection and surgery. Injection-compression therapy is not indicated if there is saphenofemoral or saphenopopliteal incompetence.

The careful technique required of injection therapy is detailed in this presentation. The overall results of this treatment have shown that, at 1 year, injection therapy is effective and has a high cure rate. The failure rate, however, increases markedly during the 4th, 5th and 6th years after treatment.

REFERENCES

1. Da Silva, A., Widmer, L. K., Martin, H., Mall, T. H., Glais, L., and Schneider, M.: Varicose veins and chronic venous insufficiency, Vasa, 3:118, 1974.
2. Chassaignac, E.: *Nouvelle Methode pour le Traitment des Tumeurs Haemorrhoidales* (Paris: Balliere, 1885).
3. Fegan, W. G.: Continuous compression technique of injecting varicose veins, Lancet 2:109, 1963.
4. Fegan, W. G.: Treatment of Varicose Veins by Injection Sclerotherapy as Practiced in Dublin, in Hobbs, J. T. (ed.): *Treatment of Venous Disorders of the Lower Limb* (Lancaster: MTP Press, 1976).
5. Linser, P.: Ueber die konservative Behandlung der Varicen, Med. Klin. 12:897, 1916.
6. Sicard, J. A.: Quoted by McAusland.[8]
7. Sicard, J. A. and Gaugier, L.: Treatment of varices by sclerosis inducing injections (sodium salicylate and others), Presse Med. 34:689, 1926.
8. McAusland, S.: Modern treatment of varicose veins, Med. Press. 201:1, 1939.
9. Brunstein, I. A.: Prevention of discomfort and disability in treatment of varicose veins, Am. J. Surg. 54:362, 1941.
10. Sigg, K.: Treatment of varicosities and accompanying complications (ambulatory treatment of phlebitis with compression bandage), Angiology 3:355, 1952.
11. Sigg, K.: Treatment of Varicose Veins by Injection Sclerotherapy as Practiced in Basle, in Hobbs, J. T. (ed.): *Treatment of Venous Disorders of the Lower Limb* (Lancaster: MTP Press, 1976).
12. Tournay, R.: Indications et resultats de la methode sclerosante dans la traitment des varices, Bull. Med. Paris 45:73, 1931.
13. Tournay, R.: Traitment des varices: Chirurgie ou injections sclerosantes, Bull. Soc. Med. Practiciens, Lille, June, 1937.
14. Tournay, R.: 4th International Congress of Phlebology, Lucerne, Sept. 20, 1971.
15. Reiner, L.: Activity of anionic surface compounds in producing vascular obliteration, Proc. Soc. Exp. Biol. Med. 62:49, 1946.
16. Cooper, W. M.: Clinical evaluation of sotradecol, sodium alkyl sulfate solution in injection therapy of varicose veins, Surg. Gynecol. Obstet. 83:647, 1946.
17. Hirschmann, S. R.: Sclerosing therapy of varicose veins with sotradecol (sodium tetradecyl sulfate), N.Y. State J. Med. 47:1367, 1947.
18. Dingwall, J. A., Lin, D. T. W., and Lyon, J. A.: Use of sodium tetradecyl sulfate in sclerosing treatment of varicose veins; experimental and clinical study, Surgery 23: 599, 1948.
19. Orbach, E. J.: Clinical evaluation of new technic in sclerotherapy of varicose veins, J. Int. Coll. Surg. 11:396, 1948.
20. Merlen, J. F.: A new sclerosing agent for varicose veins: Tetradecyl sulphate of sodium, Bull. Soc. of Phlebog. 3:23, 1949.
21. Solomons, E.: Treatment of varicose veins in pregnancy: Critical survey of injection treatment based on 600 cases treated at Rotunda Hospital, Ir. J. Med. Sci. 353, August, 1950.
22. Blenkinsopp, W. K.: Comparison of tetradecyl sulphate sodium with other sclerosants in rats, Br. J. Exp. Pathol. 49:197, 1968.

23. Hobbs, J. T.: The treatment of varicose veins. A random trial of injection-compression therapy versus surgery, Br. J. Surg. 55:777, 1968.
24. Hobbs, J. T.: Surgery and sclerotherapy in the treatment of varicose veins, Arch. Surg. 109:793, 1974.
25. Fentem, P. H., Goddard, M., Gooden, B. A., and Yeung, C. K.: Control of distension of varicose veins achieved by leg bandages, as used after injection sclerotherapy, Br. Med. J. 2:725, 1976.
26. Dorton, H. E.: Surgical tape trauma, Surg. Gynecol. Obstet. 118:363, 1964.

Discussion: Chapters 4 through 7

PROF. NORMAN BROWSE: Doctor Lord, I really must object to the comment about not tying the saphenous vein flush with the femoral vein. If you have decided that incompetence at that point is the main cause of the patient's symptoms, you are just not doing the operation which you should do if you do not tie the vein flush with the femoral.

Another point was made that did not come over very clearly. That is, why are the patients having any treatment at all? A lot of patients with enormous veins have no symptoms. If we are operating for cosmetic purposes, then removing the dilated superficial group of veins that Mr. Hobbs talked about can be accomplished by any procedure. But, if the patients have symptoms of pain and swelling, the postphlebitic syndrome, then it is important to find the prime abnormality. How this is treated is a matter of choice. As long as the abnormality is discovered, it can be fixed in some way, whether by injection or with a piece of string.

DR. LEONEL VILLAVICENCIO: I want to call attention to some damage that we have observed during surgery on varicose veins. We have stained the lymphatics with a patent blue and have demonstrated spillage of this dye into the transverse surgical incisions used for removal of the varicosities. Also, on lymphangiograms, some spillage of the dye can be seen after surgery for varicose veins.

We have extended this study and want to call to the attention of the audience that, even though we do our vein surgery carefully and extensively, we do a lot of damage to the lymphatic system.

DR. WILEY BARKER: It is of interest to me that several years ago when I was first doing varicose vein surgery, Dr. John Homans pointed out that the saphenofemoral junction is usually higher and more medial than you expect, which is fortunate because, if one makes the incision higher and more medially, he will probably avoid much damage to the lymphatic system in the groin.

DR. ELIAS HUSNI: I would like to raise one question relative to

104

thrombosis in preexistent varicose veins. Superficial thrombophlebitis should be managed aggressively to prevent extension of the process into the deep venous system, and pulmonary embolism. We reviewed all cases of varicose veins on our service over a 10-year period. As can be noted from Table 1, there were no instances of pulmonary embolism when the thrombosed superficial veins were removed. This contrasts sharply to the experience in those treated conservatively. Anticoagulation is avoided and a probable second hospital stay is eliminated in patients treated aggressively.

Ligation and stripping and subfascial ligation of perforators was done in each surgical group. Note absence of pulmonary embolism in the patients with thrombophlebitis of superficial veins when these patients were treated surgically.

Over a 10-year period, we had 212 cases of thrombosis involving long and/or short saphenous veins or their communicators. Of these, 77 were treated medically without the use of anticoagulants. Eleven per cent of these developed pulmonary emboli, one of which was fatal. One hundred thirty-five patients were treated surgically without any pulmonary embolism. Over the same period, elective surgery was done on 602 cases of incompetence of these same veins with a 0.6% incidence of pulmonary embolism, none fatal.

DR. E. CRAIG HERINGMAN: I would like to pose two questions to the panel. We occasionally see patients with large networks of varices on the posterior aspect of the thighs, high up. I would like to ask the panel how they handle these veins. I think they occur from pelvic varices and from incompetent valves in pelvic veins.

The other question is: in view of the fact that so many patients now are requiring cardiac bypass operations, has anybody on the panel changed his method of operation in order to try to preserve some of the saphenous vein?

TABLE 1.–COMPARISON OF MEDICAL AND SURGICAL
TREATMENT OF PRIMARY VARICOSE VEINS (1965–1975)

CLINICAL DIAGNOSIS	NO. OF CASES	MANAGEMENT (NO.)	NO. WITH PULMONARY EMBOLISM
Incompetence (long ± short saphenous veins)	602	Medical (0) Surgical° (602)	0 4 (0.6%)
Thrombosis (long ± short or communicators)	212	Medical (77) Surgical° (135)	9 (11%) 0

°Ligation and stripping + subfascial ligation of perforators

DR. MICHAEL HUME: I hate to dissent from the general agreement about the importance of incompetence of the long saphenous system at the groin and the emphasis upon careful dissection at that level, but the last remark prompted me to rise and say that sparing of the main trunk of the saphenous vein in my opinion is an overriding consideration. It is fairly seldom diseased if one considers that it is usually the tributaries, rather than the main saphenous trunk, that are varicose.

I have followed a different operation and symbolically retired my stripper many years ago. We look for the incompetent perforating vein with the ultrasound probe. We deal with these, excise them by subcutaneous dissection and remove the dilated tributaries of the saphenous vein. However, we try to leave the saphenous in place in case it is needed later. I may be a minority of one in this room, but the operation hasn't proved to be badly taken. The results are good, and we are glad we have spared what is very often a normal structure, the main trunk of the saphenous vein.

DR. JOHN OLWIN: In closing my discussion, I resolved to ask just the question that has been asked. In recent years, I have cringed every time I have pulled out that stripper. Recently, I have been stripping to just below the knee. Most of the troublesome perforators and most of the varicosities are below the knee.

I agree that the greater saphenous vein is not usually diseased. Even in patients with severe varicosities, it is not diseased. The outside wall is a little thicker, that is all.

As far as the posterior aspect of the thigh is concerned, these veins are there because of incompetency in the pelvic veins. I confess that I think they are of little value functionally.

Lastly, I think that eventually we will eliminate the surgeon when we find out what varicose veins are all about as far as etiology is concerned.

DR. WILEY BARKER: Doctor Olwin, if you preserve the vein in the thigh, do you interrupt the saphenofemoral junction?

DR. JOHN OLWIN: I do interrupt the vein at the saphenofemoral junction, and I don't know what happens to it subsequently. If there is any knowledge that can be applied to this, I would be grateful.

DR. WILEY BARKER: I can tell you once in a while we get a red hot phlebitis in that isolated saphenous vein. Most of the time, it just lies quiescent.

DR. JOHN OLWIN: In my manuscript, I mention that I give heparin routinely for the first 24 hr in all of these patients. I give it continuously in a dilute solution for the first 24 hr. Fortunately, I haven't had the experience that Doctor Barker just mentioned.

DR. KARL LOFGREN: Regarding the large afflictions on the posterior aspect of the thigh, if these cause symptoms, I favor excision. Follow the veins to incompetent perforating veins, which often are associated with this type of problem.

As far as sparing the saphenous vein, my cardiovascular colleagues at the Mayo Clinic tell me that a varicose saphenous main channel is useless for bypass procedures because of tortuosity, irregularity in the wall and weakness, in general. Therefore, we do not hesitate to remove true varicose saphenous main channels. We diagnose this by palpation, by filling that is evident with the tourniquet. If the vein is normal in caliber and appears normal, we do not remove it.

There are two types of patients which we see: one with the saphenous main channel incompetency, the other with very large, tortuous, incompetent tributaries. Particularly in a situation like that, we have spared the saphenous main channel.

As far as stripping up to the knee, we have not done that. Actually, stripping the vein below the knee does not generally remove the perforating veins which, as you know, are mainly part of the posterior arch tributary over the medial lower third of the leg.

DR. JERE LORD: Doctor Hume is an extraordinarily bright surgeon, and I normally agree with him 100%, but I think Doctor Lofgren has answered the question well. I never take out a greater saphenous vein for varicose veins unless the tourniquet test shows that the valves are insufficient. We have used about 40 of these veins for peripheral bypasses as homologous grafts and have found about a third of them form false aneurysms. I don't think such veins would be very good to use around the heart.

In regard to Professor Browse, I don't want you to think that I tie the greater saphenous vein willy nilly somewhere within 2–6 inches of the groin. The tie is within 1 cm of the femoral vein in every instance. I think that is very important. I have not had a pulmonary embolus from that area that I can describe. I do not think our recurrence rate is any higher than that of other surgeons.

DR. WILEY BARKER: I would like to make one final point. I have been very fond of the use of the metal clips described by Peter Samuels. The larger clip applied across the saphenofemoral junction parallel to the femoral vein makes a very neat closure of the saphenofemoral junction. It causes minimal hemodynamic interference and minimal intimal damage.

MR. JOHN HOBBS: First, I agree with Professor Browse that up to one third of the patients in the vein clinic need only reassurance as adequate treatment. These people have other problems. They have veins on their legs, but they also may have arterial claudication, pain referred from their lumbar spine or other joints. These people obviously won't benefit from treating their veins.

Damage to the lymphatics goes along with damage to the saphenous nerve. If you strip only to the knee, you don't see this damage. Also, if you strip down, you cause less damage, and you also get a better strip of the tributaries.

Regarding veins high on the posterior thigh, these can be complex problems. In my group of patients with what I called significant vulvar veins, there were women who had veins on the posterior thigh. In 5,000 patients, 155 cases (4%), which matches figures in Switzerland, had these vulvar veins. In these patients, we perform a venogram using a small needle in one of the veins.

Several causes for vulvar veins have been demonstrated. Some are secondary to pelvic tumor and some are collaterals for iliac vein occlusion. Others arise from the saphenofemoral junction via the posterior-medial vein. Also, there is a group arising by the internal pudendal, the gluteal or the obturator vein coming from the pelvis. Doctor de Takats recognized this when he described in his book the post-thrombotic syndrome in the pelvis. For this, he recommended ligation of the internal iliac vein. There is a group of people which gynecologists recognize as having a psychosomatic disease. Treatment of this, if due to saphenofemoral incompetence, is surgery on the leg veins. Local problems can be treated effectively with injection. If they are bilateral with pelvic symptoms like dyspareunia, then hysterectomy cures all of the symptoms.

We have this fight in Europe regularly on the problem of stripping the long saphenous vein or saving it for arterial surgery, or the replacement of peripheral arteries. Of course, most patients with vein problems are women and statistically they don't need arterial replacements. Also, the number of people requiring treatment for veins is huge, whereas, the total number who need arterial reconstructions is really very small. I think this point has been overemphasized.

DIAGNOSIS OF VENOUS THROMBOSIS

Introduction

MANY OBJECTIVE METHODS are generally available which allow accurate diagnosis of deep venous thrombosis. This is fortunate because clinical diagnosis of this condition is notoriously unreliable. As new, noninvasive or minimally invasive methods have emerged, it has been necessary to compare them with an older, established, well-defined technique — venography. In the following section, this important subject is discussed by an experienced surgeon and a talented peripheral vascular radiologist. Following this, Doppler ultrasound, impedance plethysmography, and phleborheography are detailed by investigators who know the potential utility and limitations of each method. This section concludes with a discussion of radioisotope localization of thrombi and the role of the noninvasive laboratory in determining patient management.

8 / Phlebography in the Diagnosis of Venous Thrombosis

HARVEY L. NEIMAN, M.D.

Department of Radiology, Northwestern University Medical School, Chicago, Illinois

IN RECENT YEARS, the use of noninvasive clinical tests such as transcutaneous Doppler ultrasound, radionuclide venography, ^{125}I-fibrinogen uptake and impedance plethysmography has changed the spectrum of indications for lower extremity venography. Each of these tests has narrowed the indication for contrast examination. Venography remains, however, the standard for judging the newer procedures and retains a definite clinical usefulness; only contrast venography provides direct evidence for the presence of thrombus.

In our institution, the present indications for venography are: (1) cases with clinical findings and noninvasive tests in variance with each other; (2) definitive pulmonary emboli but negative clinical or noninvasive tests suggesting the presence of nonocclusive thrombi or thrombus; (3) failure to respond to heparin therapy or previous surgical treatment; (4) patients with previous venous disease with a new thrombotic event; (5) when the cause of lower extremity swelling is obscure, or the presence of external compression by tumor mass is suspected; (6) prior to vena caval interruption in an attempt to ascertain the source of emboli or the possibility of vena caval duplication; and (7) recurrent pulmonary emboli after vena caval interruption surgery.

Although venography was introduced in humans by Berberich and Hirsch,[1] it was not until the later 1930s that its frequent use was advocated.[2, 3]

Technique

Numerous techniques have been described for performing venography, each with supposed advantages.[4-11] Few of these techniques, however, concern themselves with normal lower extremity venous hemodynamics. With the patient in the upright or semiupright position, normal venous flow dynamics are such that contrast material injected into a superficial vein of the foot enters both the deep and superficial venous systems. Maximal filling, therefore, without flow artifacts, occurs in the erect or semierect position.[12, 13] The use of a tourniquet is unnecessary and may in fact result in incomplete filling of portions of the deep system such as the soleal veins and the anterior tibial veins. Complete filling of the venous system is also dependent upon the use of large volumes of contrast material and an extremity which is completely relaxed and non-weight-bearing.[10]

The examination is begun with the patient in a semierect position, approximately 45 degrees from the horizontal. Unless contraindicated, both lower extremities are studied to rule out the possibility of occult disease in the nonsymptomatic leg. Each leg, however, is examined individually. Since weight-bearing is not allowed on the leg being examined, a box is placed under the opposite foot; this then carries the patient's entire weight. In addition, a rolled towel is placed under the Achilles tendon of the examined foot in order that no pressure is exerted on the calf muscles. No tourniquets are used during the standard examination.

A 19 or 21 gauge butterfly needle is inserted into a vein on the dorsum of the foot, preferably on the medial aspect distally. For the usual examination, approximately 100 ml of 60% meglumine diatrizoate is used. If prominent varices are present, wrapping the leg with an elastic bandage may decrease the overall need for contrast material by compressing the superficial venous spaces. Even so, increased amounts are usually necessary. Injecting contrast material under fluoroscopic control has been found to be generally unnecessary, and only overhead films are obtained. Fifty milliliters of contrast material is injected and an anterioposterior, externally rotated oblique view and lateral views of the leg are obtained. The lateral view of the leg is particularly important to demonstrate the posterior tibial and soleal veins.[14-16] Seven inch by 17 inch radiographs are taken with the use of an overhead tube using exposures in the range of 70 kv.

The tilt table is then lowered to approximately 20 degrees and an additional 50 ml of contrast material is injected. Anterioposterior and externally rotated oblique views of the thigh are obtained. Attention is paid to overlapping the radiographs of the leg in order to completely visualize the popliteal vein. Keeping the knee slightly flexed sometimes results in better popliteal vein filling.[17]

The table is then brought to the horizontal position to demonstrate the upper femoral and iliac veins. Gentle application of pressure to the calf allows for a surge of contrast material into the desired areas and an anterioposterior view of the pelvis is then obtained. A Valsalva maneuver during this time may help to visualize the proximal portion of the profunda femoris and internal iliac veins (Fig 8–1). This technique demonstrates the profunda femoris vein in approximately 50% of cases.[10] In the remainder of cases, a flow defect from the profunda femoris vein is almost always seen and is a secondary sign of its patency. Frequently, a portion of the lower inferior vena cava is also seen. However, visualization is not optimal and if clinically significant disease is a consideration, a bolus of contrast material should be injected percutaneously into the femoral vein.

Fig 8–1—Renal transplant recipient with acute onset of swelling in the left leg. Note the filling of the internal iliac vein and profunda femoris vein. Proximal extent of the thrombus is demonstrated (*arrows*).

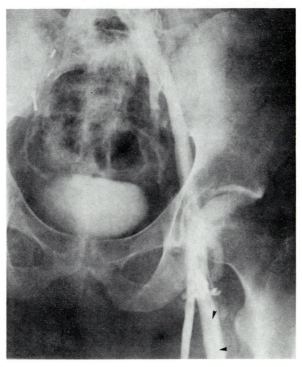

Occasionally, there may be preferential filling of the superficial venous system with poor visualization of either part or all of the deep venous system. It is in this situation that a tourniquet is applied at the ankle and a repeat injection of approximately 50 ml of contrast material is made. This technique forces contrast into the deep venous system and allows visualization of intraluminal thrombus (Fig 8–2). Although this procedure is particularly uncomfortable for the patient with deep venous thrombosis, it absolutely confirms the diagnosis and excludes the possibility of faulty needle placement.

Only rarely is a cutdown with cannulation of a saphenous vein nec-

Fig 8–2 — A, without a tourniquet, contrast material preferentially enters the superficial venous system. **B,** with a tourniquet at the ankle, the entire extent of the deep venous thrombosis is demonstrated.

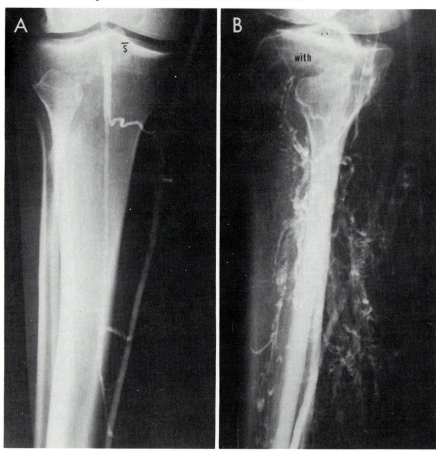

essary. Intraosseous phlebography has not proved to be necessary in any case. Transpopliteal venography has been advocated for studying the femoral and iliac veins when femoral vein catheterization is not possible.[18]

Following examination, the patient is placed in a slight Trendelenberg position and 100–200 ml of heparinized saline is infused in order to adequately remove the contrast material and minimize its irritating effect on the veins. Gentle massage and mild exercise of the foot may also be utilized. By these techniques, there has been a paucity of postvenography inflammatory complications.

Anatomy

There are four groups of veins in the lower extremity. The veins of the foot consist of a dense network of vessels with numerous communications. In the leg there are three paired deep veins which parallel the arteries. These veins join to form the popliteal vein behind the knee. This vein then continues as the femoral vein, into which the profunda femoris vein drains in the proximal thigh. The popliteal vein is usually, although not always, unpaired.

The superficial venous system, located in the subcutaneous tissue, consists of the greater saphenous vein emptying into the femoral vein and the lesser saphenous vein emptying into the popliteal vein.

The deep muscle veins in the calf vary in size and number. The soleal veins (Fig 8–3) empty into the posterior tibial and peroneal veins, while the gastrocnemius veins drain into the popliteal vein. Finally, the communicating veins are also demonstrated and connect the superficial and deep venous systems perforating through the fascia. These may be prominent in the leg but are quite infrequent in the thigh.

A normal vein on phlebographic study demonstrates a sharp, smooth margin with a rather straight or slightly curved course. A normal vessel has minimally tapered contours and a varying number of valves. The exact degree of visualization of a particular vein is somewhat dependent on the amount of contrast material injected as well as the cooperation of the patient in having a completely relaxed, non-weight-bearing extremity. The deep veins vary greatly in width and may be sacculated, beaded or uniform. In the normal individual, the deep venous system is seen in its entirety and the absence of visualization of a segment is a significant finding. Particular attention must be paid to the soleal veins, which play an important role in the genesis of thrombosis.[15,16] In patients without thrombosis, these veins have a

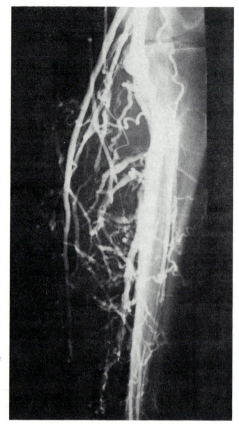

Fig 8–3—Lateral view of the leg demonstrating the soleal veins.

unique appearance, being either long and spindle-shaped, or short and bag-like.[9]

Venographic Criteria of Thrombosis

In cases of acute deep venous thrombosis, several signs may be present. The most significant of these is constant filling defects within the opacified vein (Fig 8–4).[19, 20] This is the sine qua non of acute thrombi. The intraluminal defect may be central or eccentric and may be elongated or ovoid shaped. Long segment thrombus may present as "railroad-tracking" with the thrombus occupying the center of the vessel and the contrast material being seen as a white rim at the periphery (Fig 8–5). As the thrombus ages, a portion of the contrast rim is lost, indicating adhesion (Fig 8–6).

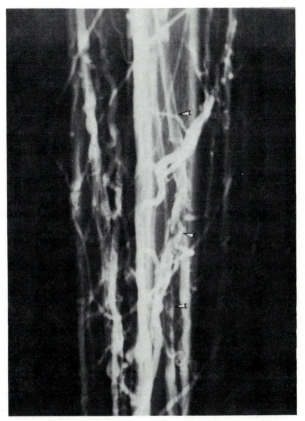

Fig 8–4.—Intraluminal filling defects (*arrows*) are present in multiple deep calf veins.

A second finding is abrupt cut-off of a normally filled venous channel. The vessel may be filled more proximally, separated by a nonopacified segment.

Diversion of flow from a segment of the entire deep venous system is further evidence of thrombosis.[10] A conscientious effort therefore must be made to identify each of the elements of the deep venous system in order to exclude diversion of flow from one of its branches. Occasionally, visualization of only the superficial venous system is seen. While this is good circumstantial evidence of acute deep vein thrombosis caused by thrombus formation in the appropriate vein as well as by compression from associated swelling, it is in this situation that a tourniquet is applied and additional contrast material is inject-

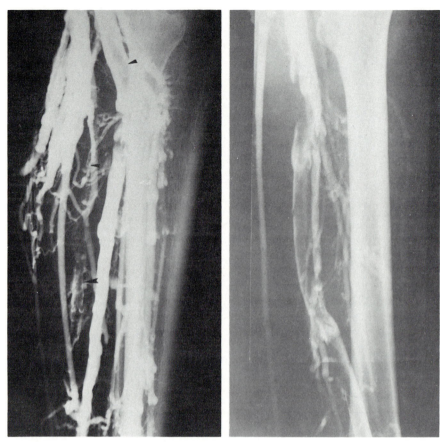

Fig 8–5 (left). — Thrombus occupies the center of several veins with contrast material appearing as a white rim (*arrows*). Note that the proximal extent of the thrombus is demonstrated in the popliteal vein.

Fig 8–6 (right). — Long segment thrombosis in the femoral vein with adherence at several sites.

ed. This latter technique forces contrast material into the deep venous system and directly demonstrates the site of disease. Tiny corkscrew collateral channels frequently are seen by this maneuver and innumerable small deep veins containing thrombus are visualized (see Fig 8–2).

Delineation of the entire extent of the thrombus is important because a nonadherent, free floating tail, particularly in the iliofemoral area, is more likely to cause pulmonary embolus (see Figs 8–1 and 8–6).[21] This ability of contrast venography to "stage" the disease pro-

cess is clearly an advantage over the noninvasive tests. Rational therapy then can be based on demonstration of both the proximal and distal
extent of the disease process.

Chronic disease is characterized by the presence of completely or
partially recanalized vessels. Partial recanalization results in narrowed, irregular, tortuous, valveless venous channels and/or variably
developed multiple corkscrew collateral vessels (Figs 8–7 and 8–8).
The intraluminal filling defect usually is absent. With complete recanalization, there is restoration of a straight, wide lumen but with loss of
valves or valve function, or the presence of duplicated vessels (Fig
8–9).[22, 23] External compression by tumor mass or soft tissue swelling
causes extraluminal compression or displacement of venous structures and occasionally complete occlusion. Intraluminal filling defects
are absent.

Several changes may be present in the venogram which simulate

Fig 8–7 (left).—Lower extremity phlebogram showing thrombus (*arrows*)
extending into the greater saphenous vein and filling of prominent collateral
veins.
Fig 8–8 (right).—Very prominent development of collateral veins (*arrows*)
in patient with history of chronic thrombosis. *R*=right side.

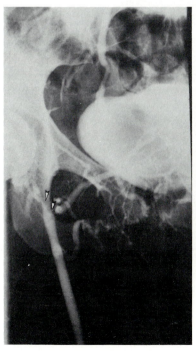
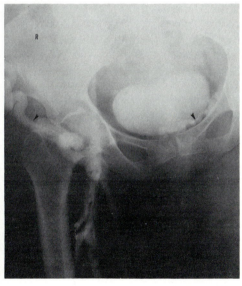

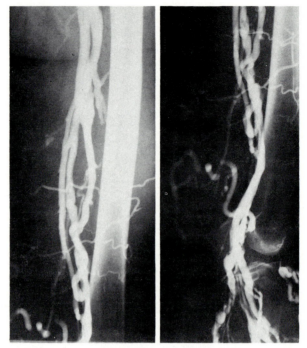

Fig 8–9.—Multiple channeled, tortuous, valveless reorganized femoral vein.

disease. Injection into a superficial vein of the proximal foot or ankle may not fill the deep plantar veins of the foot and therefore fail to fill the deep venous system. This appearance gives the spurious impression of diversion of flow into the superficial venous system. Fluoroscopy is particularly helpful in this situation, as is the use of tourniquets. False signs of deep venous thrombosis also may be seen if there is contraction of the calf muscles or external compression on the calf with subsequent diversion of flow. Disease in the popliteal veins can also be simulated by the same mechanism.[17] Flow defects from nonopacified blood into the contrast-filled column are seen most commonly at the junction of the profunda femoris vein and femoral vein and can simulate intraluminal filling defects. The defect, however, is inconstant and should appear somewhat different on the two views of this area.

Contrast venography is the most accurate method for the evaluation of the venous system of the lower extremity because it directly visualizes the veins. It is extremely unlikely that a thrombus in the iliofemoral region or in the area of the main veins of the calf would be missed. Although it is almost impossible to create an adequate model by which to judge contrast venography, subjective evaluation with clinical follow-up and/or operative findings confirm its accuracy.[8, 10, 16] The most practical advantage of phlebography is that it not only demonstrates the extent of the disease process but allows evaluation of the adherence of the thrombus as well.

Complications

Although complications are rare, the study is not entirely without risks. Inadvertent extravasation of contrast material at the injection site is associated with pain and a burning sensation. This problem, however, should be minimal. In reviewing the last 100 cases of lower extremity venography, there was one case of cardiovascular collapse. The patient was successfully resuscitated without further sequelae. There has been no evidence that phlebography in patients with deep venous thrombosis has precipitated pulmonary embolism. This reflects the experience of others.[8, 24, 25] There were several mild reactions of pruritus and urticaria following the injection of contrast material, which cleared promptly in all patients with symptomatic treatment. There have been two cases in which patients experienced tenderness and swelling in the lower extremity lasting up to 3 days. In both, the veins were not cleared of contrast material with heparinized saline. The low morbidity from contrast venography compares well with that of other authors.[10, 11, 25] The possibility, however, of contrast venography giving rise to acute thrombosis has been questioned. In a recent study by Albrechtsson and Olsson,[26] an alarming incidence of thrombosis documented by ^{125}I-fibrinogen uptake testing following venography was reported.

Summary

Venography remains the standard for judging newer procedures which intend to diagnose venous thrombosis. Indications for venography are concrete, the technique has become standardized and the anatomy has been well-described. Constant filling defects remain the most important diagnostic sign, although other abnormalities are helpful. Chronic venous insufficiency is characterized by completely or partially recanalized vessels. Complications of the procedure should be well under 3% if proper precautions are taken.

REFERENCES

1. Berberich, J., and Hirsch, S.: Die rontgenologische Darstellung der Arterien und Venem im lebenden Menschen, Klin. Wochenschr. 49:226, 1923.
2. Dos Santos, J. C.: La phlebographie directe: Conception, technique, premiers resultats, J. Int. Chir. 3:625, 1938.
3. Mahorner, H. A.: A method of obtaining venograms of the veins of the extremities, Surg. Gynecol. Obstet. 76:41, 1943.
4. Bergvall, U.: Phlebography in acute deep venous thrombosis of the lower extremity, Acta Radiol. Diagn. 11:148, 1971.
5. Brodelius, A., Lorinc, P., and Nylander, G.: Phlebographic techniques in the diagnosis of acute deep venous thrombosis in the lower limb, Am. J. Roentgenol. 111: 794, 1971.
6. Carlson, P. A.: Phlebography of the lower extremity and pelvic region, Am. J. Surg. 118:632, 1969.
7. Halliday, P.: Phlebography of the lower limb, Br. J. Surg. 55:220, 1968.
8. Thomas, M. L.: Phlebography, Arch. Surg. 104:145, 1972.
9. Nicolaides, A. N., Kakkar, V. V., Field, E. S., et al.: The origin of deep-vein thrombosis: A venographic study, Br. J. Radiol. 44:653, 1971.
10. Rabinov, K., and Paulin, S.: Roentgen diagnosis of venous thrombosis in the leg, Arch. Surg. 104:134, 1972.
11. Rogoff, S. M., and DeWeese, J. A.: Phlebography of the lower extremity, JAMA 172:1599, 1960.
12. Greitz, T.: The technique of ascending phlebography of the lower extremity, Acta Radiol. 42:421, 1954.
13. Lindblom, K.: Phlebographische Untersuchung des Untereschenkels bei Kontrastinjektion in eine subkutane Vene, Acta Radiol. 22:288, 1941.
14. Thomas, M. L., and Carty, H.: The value of the lateral projection in the diagnosis of venous thrombosis of the calf, Clin. Radiol. 25:459, 1974.
15. Kiely, P. E.: A phlebographic study of the soleal sinuses, Angiology 24:230, 1973.
16. Nicolaides, A. N., Kakkar, V. V., and Renney, J. T. G.: The soleal sinuses: Origin of deep vein thrombosis, Br. J. Surg. 87:860, 1970.
17. Arkoff, R. S., Gilfillan, R. S., and Burhenne, H. J.: A simple method for lower extremity phlebography—pseudo-obstruction of the popliteal vein, Radiology 90:66, 1968.
18. Harrell, J. E., and Grollman, J. H., Jr.: Transpopliteal venography: A new approach to the femoral and iliac veins and inferior vena cava, Radiology 90:985, 1968.
19. Thomas, M. L., McAllister, V., and Tonge, K.: The radiological appearance of deep venous thrombosis, Clin. Radiol. 45:199, 1971.
20. Zachrisson, B. E., and Jansen, H.: Phlebographic signs in fresh post-operative venous thrombosis of the lower extremity, Acta Radiol. (Diagn.) 14:82, 1973.
21. Kistner, R. L., Ball, J. J., Nordyke, R. A., et al.: Incidence of pulmonary embolism in the course of thrombophlebitis of the lower extremities, Am. J. Surg. 124:169, 1972.
22. Rosch, J., Dotter, C. T., Seaman, A. J., et al.: Healing of deep venous thrombosis: venographic findings in a randomized study comparing streptokinase and heparin, Am. J. Roentgenol. 127:553, 1976.
23. Lipchik, E. O., DeWeese, J. A., and Rogoff, S. M.: Serial long term phlebography after documented lower leg thrombosis, Radiology 120:563, 1976.
24. Sander, R. J., and Glaser, J. L.: Clinical uses of venography, Angiology 20:388, 1969.
25. Wesolowski, S. A., Greenfield, H., Sawyer, P. N., et al.: Diagnostic value of phlebography in venous disorders of the lower extremity, J. Cardiovasc. Surg. (Suppl.) 133, 1965.
26. Albrechtsson, U., and Olsson, C. G.: Thrombotic side effects of lower limb phlebography, Lancet 1:723, 1976.

9 / Diagnosis of Venous Thrombosis by Phlebography

A. N. NICOLAIDES, M.S., F.R.C.S., F.R.C.S.E.

Senior Lecturer and Honorary Consultant Surgeon to the Cardiovascular Unit and Director of the Vascular Laboratory, St. Mary's Hospital Medical School, London, England

PHLEBOGRAPHY has been the standard by which all other diagnostic methods are assessed. It may not be as sensitive as the ^{125}I-fibrinogen test, but it offers direct visualization of the venous system, of the nature and extent of the pathologic process and information about whether a thrombus is young or old and loose or adherent to the venous wall.

The Development of Phlebography

Early experimental attempts to demonstrate veins by the injection of iodinated oily substances such as Lipiodol[1, 2] or water-soluble halogen salts such as strontium bromide[3] were unsatisfactory. Oily substances produced fat emboli and halogen salts produced severe pain, thrombi and hypersensitivity. It was the developments in urography which supplied the contrast media suitable for angiography. The discovery of Uroselectan (sodium salt of 2-oxo-5-iodopyridine-N-acetic acid) and Abrodil (sodium salt of mono-iodomethane-sulphonic acid) resulted in further research in phlebography.[4] Though Uroselectan and Abrodil did not produce thrombi, they still produced severe pain around the injection area. This final drawback was eliminated with the development of another preparation called Perabrodil (3,5-diiodo-4-pyridone-N-acetic acid and diethanolamine) which proved to be completely harmless to the vessels, caused no pain and gave a good contrasting effect.[4]

123

In 1938, using Perabrodil, dos Santos was able to demonstrate that phlebography was valuable in confirming the diagnosis of suspected deep venous thrombosis.[5] He exposed a vein just posterior to the lateral malleolus and injected 20 ml of Perabrodil (50%) over 50–60 sec. He took several pictures of the leg, thigh and pelvis at the end of the injection at 50-, 70- and 90-sec intervals.

In 1940, Bauer introduced the technique in Sweden with certain modifications.[6] He described in detail the radiographic topography of the normal veins of the lower limb and the radiographic patterns in patients with fresh and old thrombosis. He found phlebography a valuable diagnostic aid in confirming the presence and determining the extent of clinically suspected thrombi.

The method of dos Santos and Bauer was "free flow phlebography" which filled the entire system of the leg, both the superficial and deep veins. Though used by others[7-10] there was considerable difficulty in interpreting the films. In 1942, Hellstein recommended that a tourniquet be applied around the ankle to prevent filling of the superficial system.[11] This was also adopted by Bauer in the same year.[12]

The inconvenience of having to cut down on a vein in every case was criticized by Welch, Faxon and McGahey, who recommended that injection be made into any superficial vein in the foot, with a tourniquet placed above the ankle to obliterate the superficial circulation.[13] 1942

In subsequent years several variations and combinations of the above techniques emerged. Some authors recommended the Trendelenburg position with a cuff at midthigh to delay flow,[9] while others maintained that a tourniquet should be placed at the level of the saphenous opening.[14] All of these methods gave variable results and seldom produced pictures of the iliac veins or inferior vena cava. In 1949, Moore argued that the medium was too dilute in the common iliac veins to give any pictures (30 ml of 35% Pyelosil). He prevented dilution by blood from the opposite limb by placing a tourniquet around the thigh of that limb, and attempted to slow the venous return from the pelvis and limb by a Valsalva maneuver just before the release of the thigh tourniquet on the side being radiographed. Thus he "always obtained good films of the iliac veins and sometimes of half or more of the inferior vena cava itself."[15]

In 1951 Dow reviewed the world literature and assessed the value of phlebography in acute thrombosis. He tried systematically several techniques, and found that the best results were obtained by injecting 20 ml of 35% Diodone into a vein on the foot and using two tourniquets, one around the ankle and another just above the knee.[16] He also demonstrated that none of the techniques investigated would fill all of the deep veins of the leg in every case. The experience of more recent years suggests that too little contrast medium was injected.

In the 1940s and 1950s many radiologists examined their patients in the erect position to prevent layering of the contrast medium.[17-19] In 1962, using a similar technique, Almen and Nylander were able to fill the muscular veins and study the effect of muscular contraction and relaxation.[20] In recent years the same method has been used in patients with acute deep venous thrombosis.[21]

Pelvic phlebography was mainly performed either by direct intravenous or indirect intraosseous injection.[22-27] In 1967 these techniques were reassessed and described in detail by Lea Thomas and Fletcher[28] who studied the venous collaterals in external and common iliac obstruction.[29]

General Principles of Ascending Phlebography

The variations described above, when combined, produce a large number of permutations so that today it is practically impossible to find two centers using exactly the same technique. We maintain that, provided a technique can demonstrate the deep venous system from the muscular veins of the calf to inferior vena cava clearly with the minimum of discomfort to the patient and without any complications, it is quite acceptable. However, over the years several general principles of technique have emerged about which there is agreement among most radiologists.

A venipuncture on the dorsum of the foot using a 21 gauge or 19 gauge wide bore needle is satisfactory. It is preferable near the base of the big toe rather than the rest of the dorsum of the foot where the skin is lax; thus extravasation of contrast medium will be detected quickly and the injection stopped. The person injecting must look at the site of injection and stop immediately when extravasation is suspected. Most radiologists agree that a cuff at the ankle will prevent filling of the superficial veins unless there are incompetent calf perforators. A cuff above the knee is preferable to a cuff below the knee because it produces better visualization of the popliteal vein, particularly if the knee is slightly flexed. In addition it allows time to obtain several views of the veins distal to it. The use of an image intensifier allows the films to be exposed at the optimum time and provides the opportunity to decide to take several views of a suspicious area. The more contrast is injected the better the results. However, contrast media are hypertonic and irritant and elevation of the limb, active muscular contractions and injection of heparin saline at the end of the examination are essential measures to avoid superficial thrombophlebitis and deep venous thrombosis. Ideally a venogram should be performed under full heparin cover (see Complications).

Technique of Ascending Phlebography Used by the Author[30, 31]

The patient lies supine on a horizontal x-ray table. A scalp vein infusion needle (21 gauge thin wall, 20 gauge bore) is introduced into a vein on the dorsum of the foot, preferably near the base of the big toe. A 2.5-cm wide pneumatic cuff is placed on the ankle to prevent any filling of the superficial veins. A similar cuff is placed midthigh to occlude the femoral vein and another cuff is placed on the opposite thigh to diminish the venous return and consequent dilution of the contrast medium in the inferior vena cava. An Elastocrepe bandage is placed on the leg slowly and firmly, but not any tighter than a bandage is normally applied as a dressing in the ward. (The purpose of this bandage is to empty the muscular veins so that they will be filled by retrograde flow when the bandage is removed.) The ankle cuff is then inflated to 120 mm Hg (140 mm Hg may be necessary in an edematous ankle) and the midthigh cuff to 200 mm Hg (Fig 9–1). The latter does

Fig 9–1.—Pneumatic cuffs and bandage on patient's leg at the beginning of the examination.

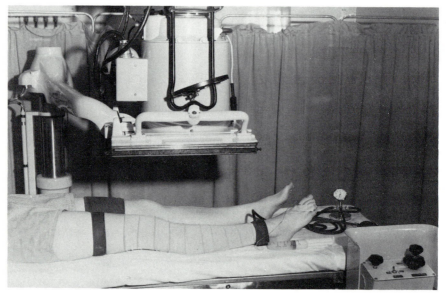

not occlude the arterial flow because of the narrowness of the cuff, but does occlude the femoral vein. The needle is attached to a syringe filled with 60 ml of 60% meglumine iothalamate (Conray 280). A second syringe is available. The contrast medium is injected as the bandage is removed and then its progress is watched on the image intensifier. Approximately 30 ml is injected over 3 min. The slower the injection the less the discomfort to the patient. This is possible because the thigh cuff allows only a minimum loss of contrast medium which is seen on the image intensifier to ascend in the tibial veins and to fill the soleal veins in a retrograde fashion. At this stage, films of the leg and lower thigh are taken in two planes (Figs 9–2 and 9–3). The midthigh cuff then is deflated, the injection of contrast is continued and films of the femoral vein are taken (Fig 9–4). The ankle cuff then is removed and the cuff on the opposite thigh is inflated to 100 mm Hg.

Fig 9–2 (left).–Normal phlebogram. A large soleal vein is obvious.
Fig 9–3 (right).–Normal phlebogram, lateral view. A large soleal vein is obvious.

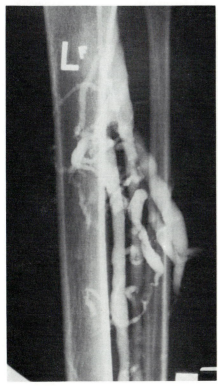 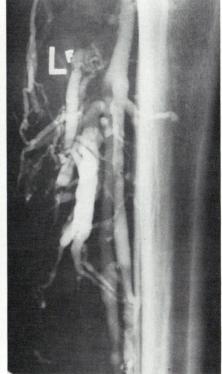

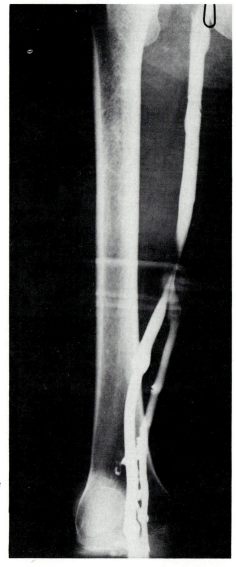

Fig 9–4.—Normal femoral vein as demonstrated by the technique described in the text. The midthigh cuff has been partially deflated.

The patient is asked to do a Valsalva maneuver and the contrast medium is followed into the external iliac vein and inferior vena cava. The examiner's hand is run along the long saphenous vein in the leg and thigh, emptying it into the femoral just before a film is taken (Fig 9–5). If a thrombus is seen, or suspected, on the image intensifier, at

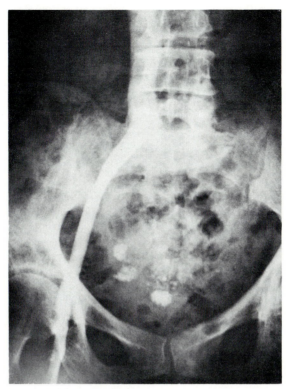

Fig 9–5.—Normal external iliac vein and inferior vena cava uniformly filled with contrast medium.

least two films are taken. A total of 80–120 ml of contrast medium is injected. Finally the veins are cleared by leg elevation, active plantar flexion and dorsiflexion of the foot and by injecting 150 ml of normal saline containing 5,000 units of heparin. Complete clearance is confirmed by fluoroscopy. The heparin is omitted if the patient is adequately anticoagulated by a continuous heparin infusion.

Percutaneous Iliac Phlebography

In a small proportion of patients (less than 3%) it is not possible to obtain good visualization of the iliac veins and inferior vena cava with ascending phlebography and yet it is essential to do so. A not infrequently encountered example is the patient with gross edema and iliofemoral vein occlusion in whom anticoagulants are contraindicated and an interruption procedure for the inferior vena cava is contemplated. A cavogram through a percutaneous injection into the contralateral common femoral vein is indicated.

Intraosseous Phlebography

This has been used to study the venous collaterals in iliac vein obstruction,[29] but it is not used for routine diagnostic purposes. It requires a general anesthetic and there is a theoretical but serious possibility of osteomyelitis and fat embolism.[32, 33]

DIAGNOSTIC CRITERIA

The value of phlebography in the diagnosis of deep venous thrombosis became fully established in 1963 when De Weese and Rogoff

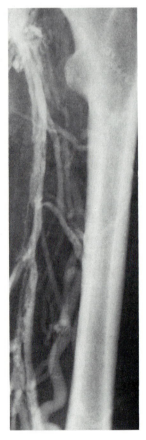

Fig 9–6. – A recanalized femoral vein with an irregular wall.

analyzed the phlebograms of 100 limbs with deep venous thrombosis and postulated the following criteria:

The unequivocal diagnosis of deep venous thrombosis was based on: (1) the presence of well defined filling defects in opacified veins; (2) the demonstration of these defects on at least two radiographs. Non-visualisation of one or more calf veins was not considered diagnostic of thrombosis since, in normal extremities, these veins are frequently not all visualised. Non-visualisation of the femoral vein with good opacification of the proximal and distal veins and the presence of collaterals was considered evidence of thrombotic obstructions.[34]

Loose thrombus appears as a cylindrical filling defect surrounded by a thin white line of contrast medium. Obliteration of the white line of contrast indicates adherence to the wall.[32] The use of the image intensifier and obtaining several views of the same vein just before and after a Valsalva maneuver help distinguish most artifacts from thrombus. Fresh thrombus fills most of the venous lumen but is not adherent to the wall. Old thrombus is partly adherent to the wall and partly lysed so that it produces the appearance of a recanalized vein with irregular wall (Fig 9–6).

Complications

Extravasation of contrast medium may produce local tissue damage and ulceration of the skin.[35] The author has seen five cases during the years 1969–1976. In all five, there was marked obstruction of the veins with edema of the foot. Ulceration occurred in four. Hyaluronidase was injected immediately when extravasation was noticed in the subcutaneous tissues in the fifth patient and ulceration did not occur. However, there was extensive blistering of the skin. It cannot be overemphasized that great care should be taken to avoid this complication and the person injecting the contrast should be aware of this. It is preferable to stop and postpone the examination rather than risk this complication.

Thrombosis due to the contrast medium is another serious complication. Minimal pain, tenderness or swelling on the day following the venogram has been observed in a small number of patients.[35] These symptoms are rarely severe and clear within 3 days of heparin therapy. Massive pulmonary embolus following phlebography has not been reported since 1942.[36] In 50% of patients who had phlebography of varicose veins associated with recurrent leg ulcers on the day before operation, Cranley found fresh thrombi not only in the superficial but also in the subfascial veins at operation.[37] This was despite the routine flushing of the veins with heparinized saline. In a recent study

Albrechtsson and Olsson have reported that in 20 of 61 patients with initially normal phlebograms, uptake of ^{125}I-fibrinogen in the legs subsequently increased. In 4 (7%) cases, independent examinations (pulmonary scintigram or a new phlebogram) demonstrated a thromboembolic or a thrombotic process.[38] These results confirm the suspicion entertained by some that thrombosis may be caused by phlebography.

Although serious thrombotic complications are uncommon, every care should be taken to prevent them (see Technique of Ascending Phlebography).

Information Obtained from Phlebography

In a series of 246 phlebograms performed by the author in 228 hospital patients with symptoms and signs suggestive of deep venous thrombosis, the soleal sinuses were demonstrated in 240 (97%). The soleal sinuses were not demonstrated in six patients with massive edema and very tense limbs. In these six patients contrast medium could not be made to enter the deep veins of the calf.

Thrombi were demonstrated in only 131 (57%) patients (137 limbs) out of the 228 with clinically suspected deep venous thrombosis. The remaining 97 patients (91 limbs) had a completely normal deep venous system. These results emphasize the fact that if one relies on

Fig 9–7.—The distribution and extent of thrombi in 137 phlebograms with thrombosis. The horizontal fields represent calf, popliteal, superficial femoral, common femoral and iliac veins.

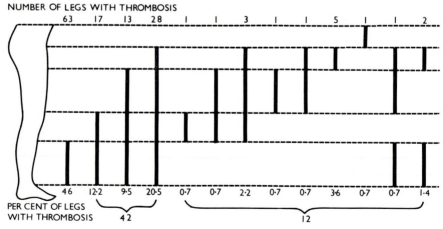

NUMBER OF LEGS WITH THROMBOSIS

63   17   13   28   1   1   3   1   1   5   1   1   2

4·6   12·2   9·5   20·5   0·7   0·7   2·2   0·7   0·7   3·6   0·7   0·7   1·4

PER CENT OF LEGS WITH THROMBOSIS   42   12

clinical signs alone, one would be treating 40% of the patients unnecessarily with anticoagulants which are expensive and have complications. Of the 97 patients who had clinical but not phlebographic evidence of thrombosis, there were 34 (35%) in whom the signs could be attributed to causes other than deep venous thrombosis. They were congestive cardiac failure, superficial thrombophlebitis, venous insufficiency, muscle strain, cellulitis, hematoma of the calf and cramp. In the remaining 63 (65%) patients a cause for the signs could not be found.

The distribution and extent of thrombi in 137 phlebograms with thrombosis are summarized in Figure 9–7 and some examples are illustrated in Figures 9–8 through 9–16. The fact that in 46% of the limbs (see Fig 9–7) the thrombi were confined to the calf means that at least in a proportion of patients thrombi can start there. It can be

Fig 9–8 (left). – Thrombus confined to a soleal vein.
Fig 9–9 (right). – Thrombi confined to soleal veins.

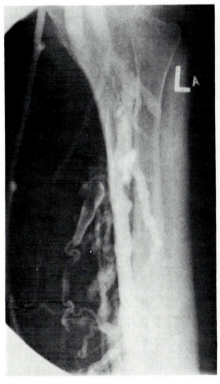
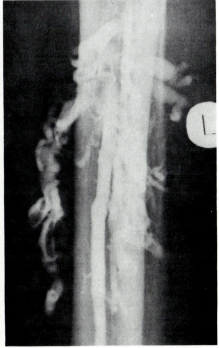

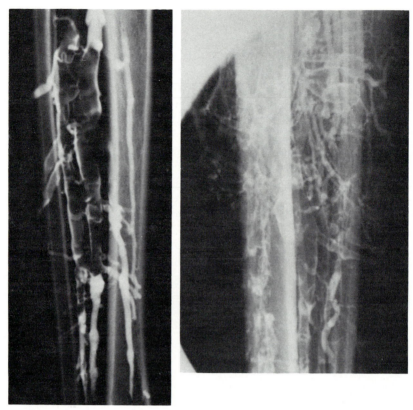

Fig 9–10 (left). – Thrombi present in the soleal and tibial veins.
Fig 9–11 (right). – Thrombi present in all the muscular and tibial veins.

argued that the presence of thrombi in the calf whenever there is proximal thrombosis may be due to peripheral extension of thrombi arising in more proximal veins. However, this does not happen, as shown by studies using the ^{125}I-fibrinogen test in surgical,[39] obstetric,[40] gynecologic[41] and medical[42] patients. These studies have in fact shown that in the early postoperative period and the first week after admission to hospital thrombi start in the calf and extend proximally.

Thrombi started at sites more proximal to the calf in 12% of limbs. These limbs constituted one fifth of all of the limbs in which the thrombotic process involved veins proximal to the calf. It has been demonstrated that it is thrombi in the veins proximal to the calf that give rise to clinical pulmonary emboli[43] and that thrombi confined to the calf may produce only small silent emboli.[44]

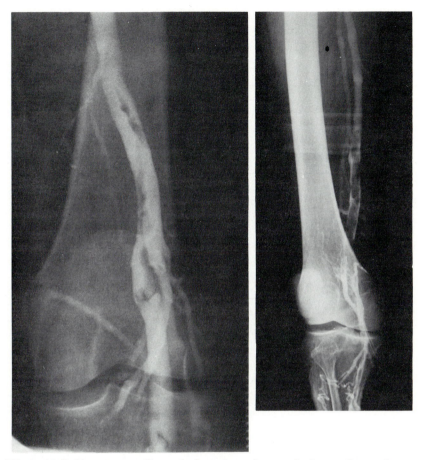

Fig 9–12 (left). — A partially occluding thrombus in the lower femoral vein.

Fig 9–13 (right). — Thrombus in the lower third of the superficial femoral vein in a limb which had thrombi in the soleal, tibial and popliteal veins. The thrombus is not firmly attached to the wall of the femoral vein so that contrast medium flows around it.

The results of this series are not incompatible with the results of the ^{125}I-fibrinogen test in hospital patients and anatomicopathologic studies based on postmortem examinations. The data support the evidence that thrombi can start practically anywhere in the venous tree of the lower limb. They also support the findings of the ^{125}I-fibrinogen test that the majority of thrombi start in the calf. The apparently different results obtained by the ^{125}I-fibrinogen test, phlebography and postmortem examination[45-51] can be accounted for by the fact that

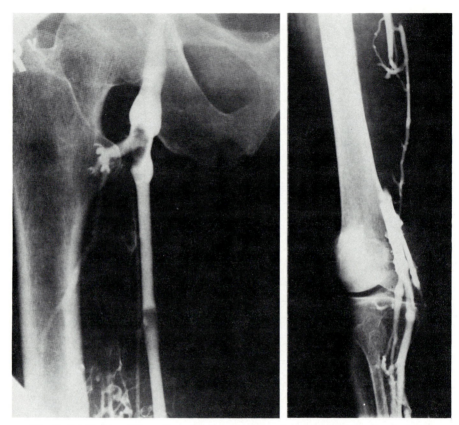

Fig 9–14 (left). – Thrombus in the common femoral and profunda femoris vein in a patient who had myocardial infarction 2 weeks earlier.

Fig 9–15 (right). – Thrombus confined to the superficial femoral vein in a patient who had a hip prosthesis 4 weeks earlier. On this occasion the patient was readmitted with clinical pulmonary embolism and a tender calf. There was not any thrombosis in the calf or pelvis on phlebography.

these investigations have been performed in completely different groups of patients at different times in relation to operation and bed rest. In addition postmortem studies are by their nature performed in a selected group of "high risk" patients. Patients who die are seriously ill, often in shock. The incidence of deep venous thrombosis in patients with hypotension is high (62%)[42] and their poor peripheral perfusion may result in stasis and consequently thrombosis not only in the calf but also in the proximal veins and their valve pockets (see Figs 9 – 14 through 9 – 16).

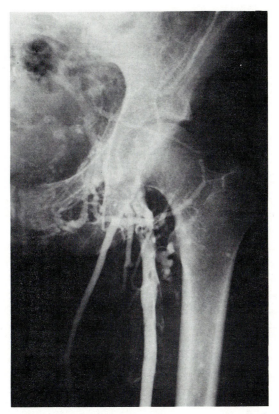

Fig 9–16. — Iliofemoral thrombosis in a patient who had spinal fusion 3 weeks earlier.

As far as prevention is concerned one important fact emerges: 78% of the thrombi which are above the knee and constitute a danger of large pulmonary embolism have their origin in the calf. If one can therefore prevent the thrombi that start in the calf one may be eliminating 78% of the thrombi that constitute a risk to life.

As far as management is concerned, the presence of thrombosis in the popliteal or more proximal veins suggests that the patient is at great risk of pulmonary embolism and prompt treatment should be instituted. Information whether the thrombus is young or old, adherent to the venous wall or not will also help decide which method of therapy should be used.

Phlebography remains the best method for confirming or excluding deep venous thrombosis because it provides a quick answer with the maximum of visual information. However, it cannot be used as a screening method because it is invasive, it requires skilled medical personnel, it is uncomfortable to the patient and it carries a small but significant morbidity.

Summary

Phlebography has been the standard by which all other diagnostic methods are assessed. Although it may not be as sensitive as ^{125}I-fibrinogen, it does offer direct visualization of the venous system, of the nature and extent of the pathologic process and information on whether a thrombus is young or old, loose or adherent. Many methods are available but those which demonstrate the deep venous system from the muscular veins of the calf to the inferior vena cava clearly are acceptable. The author favors the technique of ascending phlebography and, in less than 3%, the examination is supplemented by percutaneous iliac phlebography. Intraosseous phlebography is not utilized routinely, and unequivocal diagnosis of deep venous thrombosis is based on presence of well-defined filling defects being demonstrated on two radiographs or nonvisualization of a femoral vein with good opacification of proximal and distal veins and presence of collaterals. Complications include extravasation, usually associated with marked obstruction of the veins and thrombosis, symptoms of venous thrombosis which are rarely severe and clear within three days of heparin therapy. In a series of 246 phlebograms in 228 patients, thrombi were demonstrated in 57% and the remaining patients had completely normal deep venous systems.

Phlebography remains the best method for confirming or excluding the presence of deep venous thrombosis. It provides a quick answer with maximum visual information.

REFERENCES

1. Sicard, J. A., and Forestier, J.: Methode générale d'exploration radiologique par l'huile iodée (Lipiodol), J. Radiol. Electrol. 6:390, 1922.
2. Sicard, J. A., and Forestier, J.: Radiognostic rachidien Lipiodolé, Presse Med. 31: 1446, 1923.
3. Berberich, J., and Hirsh, S.: Die rontgenographische Darstellung der Arterien und Venen am lebenden Menschen, Klin. Wochenschr. 2:2226, 1923.
4. Bauer, G.: Phlebographic diagnosis of spontaneous thrombosis — the history of phlebography, Acta Chir. Scand. (Suppl.) 73, 1942.
5. dos Santos, J. C.: La phlebographie directe, J. Int. Chir. 3:625, 1938.
6. Bauer, G.: A venographic study of thromboembolic problems, Acta Chir. Scand. (Suppl.) 61, 1940.
7. Dougherty, J., and Homans, J.: Venography: A clinical study, Surg. Gynecol. Obstet. 71:697, 1940.

8. Fine, J., Frank, H. A., and Starr, A.: The value of venography as a diagnostic aid in deep venous thrombosis and pulmonary embolism, Ann. Surg. 116:574, 1942.

9. Mark, J.: Venography: Its use in differential diagnosis of peripheral venous circulation, Ann. Surg. 118:469, 1943.

10. Lesser, A., and Raider, L.: Venography with fluoroscopy in venous lesions of the lower limb, Radiology 41:157, 1943.

11. Hellstein, W. O.: Phlebographic studies and heparin treatment in thromboembolic disease, Acta Chir. Scand. (Suppl.) 73, 1942.

12. Bauer, G.: A roentgenologic and clinical study of the sequels of thrombosis, Acta Chir. Scand. (Suppl.) 74, 1942.

13. Welch, C. E., Faxon, H. H., and McGahey, C. E.: The application of phlebography to the therapy of thrombosis and embolism, Surgery 12:162, 1942.

14. De Bakey, M., Schroeder, G. F., and Ochsner, A.: Significance of phlebography in phlebothrombosis, JAMA 123:788, 1943.

15. Moore, H. D.: A new method of venography with particular reference to its use in varicose veins, Br. J. Surg. 37:78, 1949.

16. Dow, J. D.: Venography of the leg with particular reference to acute deep thrombophlebitis and to gravitational ulceration, J. Fac. Radiol. 2:180, 1951.

17. Lindblom, K.: Phlebograpische Untersuchung des Unterschenkels bei Kontrastinjektion in eine subcutane Vene, Acta Radiol. (Stockh.) 22:288, 1941.

18. Lofstedt, S.: Om tekniken vid flebografi i benet, Nord. Med. 31:1535, 1946.

19. Scott, H. W., and Roach, I. F.: Phlebography of the leg in the erect position, Ann. Surg. 134:104, 1951.

20. Almen, T., and Nylander, G.: Serial phlebography of the normal lower leg during muscular contraction and relaxation, Acta Radiol. 57:264, 1962.

21. Haeger, K., and Nylander, G.: Acute phlebography, Triangle 8:18, 1967.

22. Farinas, D. L.: Abdominal venography, Am. J. Roentgenol. 58:599, 1947.

23. Greitz, T.: Phlebography of the normal leg, Acta Radiol. 44:1, 1955.

24. Helander, C. G., and Lindbom, A.: Venography of the inferior vena cava, Acta Radiol. 52:257, 1959.

25. Fukuta, K.: A study of pelvic venography, Nagoya J. Med. Sci. 23:17, 1960.

26. Goldstein, M., van Hoorn, M., and van der Stricht, J.: La phlebographie pelvienne. Technique et indications, Acta Chir. Belg. 63:885, 1964.

27. Schobinger, R. A.: *Intraosseous Venography* (New York: Grune and Stratton, 1960).

28. Thomas, M. L., and Fletcher, W. L.: The technique of pelvic phlebography, Clin. Radiol. 18:399, 1967.

29. Thomas, M. L., Fletcher, G. W. L., Cockett, F. B., and Negus, D.: Venous collaterals in external and common iliac vein obstruction, Clin. Radiol. 18:403, 1967.

30. Nicolaides, A. N., Kakkar, V. V., Field, E. S., and Renney, J. T. G.: The origin of deep vein thrombosis: A venographic study, Br. J. Radiol. 44:653, 1971.

31. Nicolaides, A. N.: The prevention of post-operative deep venous thrombosis, Jacksonian Prize Essay, 1972.

32. Thomas, M. L.: Phlebography, Arch. Surg. 104:145, 1972.

33. Thomas, M. L., and Tighe, J. R.: Death from fat embolism as a complication of intraosseous phlebography, Lancet 2:1415, 1973.

34. De Weese, J. A., and Rogoff, S. M.: Phlebographic patterns of acute deep venous thrombosis of the leg, Surgery 53:99, 1963.

35. Rabinor, K., and Paulin, S.: Roentgen diagnosis of venous thrombosis in the leg, Arch. Surg. 104:134, 1972.

36. Homans, J.: Thrombosis as a complication of venography, JAMA 119:136, 1942.

37. Cranley, J. J.: Diagnostic Tests for Venous Thrombosis, in Cranley, J. J. (ed.): *Vascular Surgery, Vol. II, Peripheral Venous Diseases* (New York: Harper & Row, 1975).

38. Albrechtsson, U., and Olsson, C. G.: Thrombotic side-effects of lower limb phlebography, Lancet 1:723, 1976.

39. Flanc, C., Kakkar, V. V., and Clarke, M. B.: The detection of venous thrombosis in the legs using ^{125}I-labeled fibrinogen, Br. J. Surg. 55:742, 1968.
40. Friend, J., and Kakkar, V. V.: The diagnosis of deep vein thrombosis in the puerperium, J. Obstet. Gynaecol. Br. Commonw. 77:820, 1970.
41. Ballard, R. M., Bradley-Watson, P. J., Johnstone, F. D., Kenney, A., McCarthy, T. G., Campbell, S., and Weston, J.: Low doses of subcutaneous heparin in the prevention of deep vein thrombosis after gynaecological surgery, J. Obstet. Gynecol. 80:469, 1973.
42. Nicolaides, A. N., Kakkar, V. V., Renney, J. T. G., Kidner, P. H., Hutchison, D. C. S., and Clarke, M. B.: Myocardial infarction and deep vein thrombosis, Br. Med. J. 1:432, 1971.
43. Kakkar, V. V., Howe, C. T., Flanc, C., and Clarke, M. B.: Natural history of deep vein thrombosis, Lancet 2:230, 1969.
44. Browse, N. L., and Thomas, M. L.: Source of non-lethal pulmonary emboli, Lancet 1:258, 1974.
45. Virchow, R.: *Cellular Pathology* (London: Churchill, 1860).
46. Aschoff, L.: *Lectures in Pathology* (New York: Hoeber, 1924).
47. Homans, J.: Thombosis of deep veins of lower leg causing pulmonary embolism, N. Engl. J. Med. 211:993, 1934.
48. Rossle, R.: Uber die Bedentung and Entstehung der Wandenvenenthrombosen, Virchows Arch. f. pathol. Anat. 300:180, 1937.
49. Neumann, R.: Ursprungszentren und Entwicklungsformen der Bein-Thrombose, Virchows Arch. f. pathol. Anat. 301:708, 1938.
50. Hunter, W. C., Krygier, J. J., Kennedy, J. C., and Sneeden, V. D.: Etiology and prevention of thrombosis of the deep leg veins, Surgery 17:178, 1945.
51. Gibbs, N. M.: Venous thrombosis of the lower limb with particular reference to bedrest, Br. J. Surg. 45:209, 1957.

Discussion: Chapters 8 and 9

MR. A. N. NICOLAIDES: Most people who are working in this field agree that phlebography remains the best method for confirming or excluding suspected deep venous thrombosis. It provides a quick answer with a maximum of visual information. There are as many methods of ascending phlebography as there are radiologists. Details of the technique do not really matter as long as visualization is very good and as long as maximum information comes from the venograms with the least discomfort to the patient and with the least number of complications.

Like Doctor Neiman, we are worried about complications. The morbidity is very low. In the last 6 years, in a series of more than 1,000 venograms, we have seen four ulcers from extravasation on the dorsum of the foot. In a fifth case, we injected hyaluronidase straight away, and there was no loss of skin. I recommend this to you if such an event should occur.

In all five cases, the injection was done on the lateral aspect of the foot. So, this is not recommended. We prefer setting a needle in a vein near the big toe. Also, I would like to add that an extravasation of this degree occurred when a junior member of the team was doing the venogram.

We are rather worried about occurrence of deep venous thrombosis after venography. We became very much aware of this problem from Doctor Cranley's publication where his team performed phlebography in patients with varicose veins prior to operation, and when they operated, they found a large number of thrombi in many of the veins.

We are also aware of the important study of isotopically discovered thrombi after venography. In this study, if the venogram was normal, they used radioactive fibrinogen testing afterward. They detected a high incidence of postvenography thrombosis. So, now we are beginning to do venography under full cover of heparin. I would like to finish by presenting to you a short, but cautionary tale.

A little girl of six was admitted to our hospital with massive femoral thrombosis of the left leg following chickenpox. She was treated with streptokinase for 5 days with a very dramatic improvement. She was subsequently treated with heparin, and then went to oral anticoagulant therapy. During this period, we did another venogram in order to find out how effective our clearance of the veins was. I think this was our mistake. Twelve hours later, she developed massive deep thrombosis of the whole leg with venous gangrene of the toes. We went back to large doses of heparin. The final outcome was better than we expected. With the exception of the tip of the big toe, there was a complete recovery. But it was a vivid experience nevertheless.

DR. EDWIN SALZMAN: I think I should speak in defense of venography and make two points. First, the finding of development of positive fibrinogen scans following a negative venogram has been raised as evidence of the frequency of venous thrombosis as a complication of venography. But you should be aware that our experience and the experience of the McMaster University at Hamilton, Ontario, suggests that a positive fibrinogen scan in a person who has had a venogram does not mean that the patient has postvenography thrombosis. It would appear the contrast media can induce the laydown of radioactive fibrinogen. Thus, there will be a positive scan in a substantial number of patients. When we had the opportunity to repeat phlebography in a number of these patients, we found that many did not have a complicating thrombus. Some did; most did not. Therefore, I would emphasize that a positive scan after venography is not evidence of complicating thrombus.

Second, regarding Mr. Nicolaides' tragic case: I think that the case is perhaps as much a condemnation of the failure to follow the therapy with heparin as it is a complication of phlebography.

DR. EUGENE STRANDNESS: In regard to the Swedish study that was just reported, in patients with normal venograms with positive fibrinogen scans, there were seven individuals with repeat studies. The investigators demonstrated thrombi in four. Furthermore, the report, I think from Ed Salzman's institution, would suggest that, if you perform a number of phlebograms, the chance of developing clinical thrombophlebitis is in the range of 10%. If a repeat examination is carried out, thrombi will be demonstrated in about 60% of these patients.

The risk of deep venous thrombosis after phlebography is actually higher than is the risk after having a major surgical operation. At McMaster University Medical Center, only 2.9% had venous thrombosis. I think a word of caution is in order here about the relative risks of venography. Although I think there is virtually no report about the presence of deep venous thrombosis after phlebography, I am sure in some cases existing thrombophlebitis is actually made worse.

I believe that venography is the best test, but if you look at it carefully, it is not without its risks.

DR. HARVEY NEIMAN: I think that the comments emphasize what I said. Venography is the definitive test but we have to use it with caution and be aware of the risks that are involved in the study.

10 / The Place of Occlusive Impedance Plethysmography in the Diagnosis of Venous Thrombosis

H. Brownell Wheeler, M.D., Nilima A. Patwardhan, M.D., and Frederick A. Anderson, Jr., M.S.

Department of Surgery, University of Massachusetts Medical School, Worcester, Massachusetts

In 1959, Dr. Geza de Takats[1] clearly defined the dilemma which confronts the clinician dealing with thromboembolic disease. In order to prevent major pulmonary embolism, the physician must prescribe "early intensive management of peripheral venous thrombosis." On the other hand, early peripheral venous thrombosis may be "either symptomless or accompanied by such vague and nonspecific symptoms that a positive diagnosis (on clinical grounds alone) is impossible." This basic clinical dilemma has led to the current widespread interest in noninvasive diagnostic procedures for deep vein thrombosis.

In the years since de Takats defined this clinical problem, several noninvasive methods have been developed for the diagnosis of deep thrombophlebitis. The multiplicity of techniques now available for this purpose has created confusion as to the proper place of each in clinical practice. Which is the best procedure for a particular patient? Are the various methods complementary or competitive? The following presentation attempts to define the place of impedance plethysmography in the diagnosis of venous thrombosis.

Background

Plethysmography is a time-honored technique for physiologic study of the circulation, first having been described by Glisson in 1622. Venous occlusion plethysmography was first introduced in 1905 by Brodie and Russell[2] for study of arterial blood flow. These authors inflated a pressure cuff around the leg sufficiently high to occlude venous return, but not high enough to affect arterial inflow. This technique subsequently was modified by Hewlett and van Zwaluwenburg[3] and became a standard method for assessment of arterial blood flow. The accuracy of the method was improved by use of an arterial occlusion cuff just distal to the plethysmograph, as first suggested in 1938 by Grant and Pearson.[4]

The application of plethysmography to the study of venous disease, and particularly venous thrombosis, is much more recent. Widespread interest in the use of plethysmography for the diagnosis of venous thrombosis was stimulated in the United States by early results reported with impedance plethysmography[5, 6] and by results reported from Europe using water displacement, air cuff or strain gauge plethysmography.[7-9] A wide variety of plethysmographic techniques have now been described. All rely, at least in part, on some method of temporary venous outflow occlusion. The maximum rate of outflow following release of venous occlusion is the most valuable single measurement.

Our own laboratory now has over 8 years of experience using impedance plethysmography for the diagnosis of venous thrombosis. The objective has consistently been to develop a simple test, one which can be done reliably at a patient's bedside by a technician. Our earliest studies concentrated on the use of respiratory maneuvers to increase intra-abdominal pressure and thereby produce temporary venous outflow obstruction. Several investigators published favorable corroborative studies,[10-13] but others found the method unreliable.[14, 15] The inability of some patients to take adequately deep breaths to obstruct venous return was stated to be the fundamental weakness in the method.[16]

From these reports it became clear that a more standardized form of temporary venous outflow occlusion was necessary in order to produce consistent results which could be reproduced in any hospital by the average laboratory technician. A thigh cuff inflated to slightly above venous pressure therefore was employed to produce venous outflow occlusion. The details of the testing procedure, the instrumentation and the method of interpretation were simplified. During the past 4 years, this technique has produced uniformly reliable results and has remained standardized.

Technique

Occlusive impedance plethysmography is carried out with the patient resting flat in bed. The leg to be tested is placed on a pillow, and the foot of the bed is elevated just enough to facilitate venous drainage from the lower leg. The calf should be slightly above heart level. The patient should be comfortable and the leg muscles should be relaxed. Patients usually assume a comfortable, relaxed position when the foot is slightly rotated externally and the knee is slightly flexed. This position usually is facilitated by having the patient shift his weight chiefly to the hip on the side being tested.

Circumferential electrodes are placed around the calf, with their inner margins approximately 10 cm apart. A 7-inch wide pneumatic cuff with a rigid backing is then placed around the lower thigh with its lower edge at least 2 inches above the knee joint. The cuff should not be applied tightly and should easily admit a finger between the cuff and the skin when the cuff is deflated.

The electrodes are connected to an electrical impedance plethysmograph with a current frequency of 22 kHz and a current strength of 1 ma. The pneumatic cuff is connected to an air pressure system which

Fig 10–1.—Impedance plethysmographic tracings on a 27-year-old man with suspected pulmonary embolism. In the right leg there is a slow rise in venous volume following temporary venous occlusion, consistent with reduced peripheral blood flow. The venous outflow is prompt. On the left side, venous outflow is delayed, consistent with venous thrombosis.

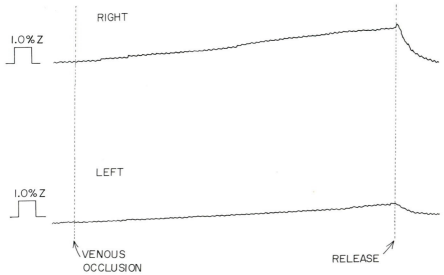

RIGHT

1.0% Z

LEFT

1.0% Z

VENOUS
OCCLUSION

RELEASE

allows rapid inflation and deflation. The pneumatic cuff is then inflated to a pressure of 45 cm H_2O for 45 sec. This allows full distention of the venous system in most patients. Occasionally, the pressure needs to be maintained longer in order to obtain the maximum venous volume increase. This is particularly true in patients with peripheral vasoconstriction. Longer periods of venous occlusion should be employed in patients who have only a small increment in venous volume which is still slowly increasing at 45 sec. In such patients, the period of occlusion should be prolonged to as much as 2 min.

The cuff pressure then is released. The cuff must deflate promptly because the rapidity of outflow during the first 3 sec is the single most important measurement in the detection of venous thrombosis. Any mechanical delay in the deflation of the cuff might cause a delay in the outflow rate simulating venous thrombosis.

The increase in venous volume following inflation of the cuff is measured from the strip chart recording. The decrease in venous volume during the first 3 sec following release of the cuff also is measured. These two variables, termed venous capacitance (VC) and venous outflow (VO), then are plotted as a function of each other on a

Fig 10–2.—Graph of venous capacitance plotted against venous outflow in 3 sec in the patient whose tracings are shown in Fig 10–1. The right leg falls in the normal range, but the left leg is consistent with venous thrombosis. Pulmonary angiogram confirmed pulmonary emboli. Phlebography was considered unnecessary.

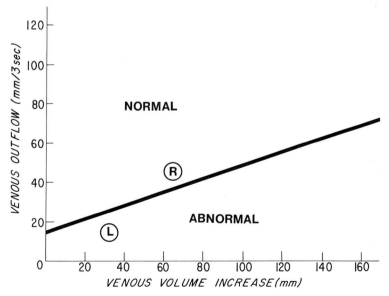

scoring graph. Ranges of normal and abnormal have been determined from earlier studies.[17-19] Interpretation is based upon where the specific test result falls on the scoring chart (Figs 10 – 1 and 10 – 2).

Initial test results are sometimes poorer than those observed in succeeding tests. This "warm-up" effect is observed most dramatically in patients with increased venous tone. Accordingly, unless good normal responses are obtained initially, the test should be repeated three to five times. Final interpretation of results should be based upon the best test obtained. Both mechanical and physiologic factors may decrease the magnitude of venous volume changes, but they cannot artificially improve the test results.

Whenever an abnormal test is obtained, the operator also should be sure that no mechanical venous obstruction exists. This sometimes is produced inadvertently when the electrodes or the pneumatic cuff are applied too tightly to the leg. It has also been seen occasionally in patients with unusually tight clothing or bandages.

Clinical Results

Using the instrumentation, testing procedure and method of interpretation described above, our overall accuracy for detection of iliac, femoral or popliteal thrombosis is 96% (254/264 correlations with phlebography).[20] The sensitivity was 97% (77/79 limbs with thrombosis of the iliac, femoral or popliteal veins demonstrated by phlebography). The specificity was 96% (177/185 limbs with normal phlebograms). However, these results have been criticized because many patients were admitted to the study on the basis of clinical signs or symptoms, possibly representing advanced stages of thrombosis, and because phlebograms were not obtained consecutively on all patients, introducing the possibility of bias in the selection of patients for phlebography. Another criticism has been the lack of a blind experimental design.

An excellent prospective, consecutive, blind study of this method of occlusive impedance plethysmography has been reported recently by investigators at McMaster University.[19] These investigators also arrived at an overall accuracy of 96% (510/530 correlations with phlebography). The sensitivity in their series was 93% (124/133 limbs with proximal vein thrombosis). The specificity was 97% (386/397 limbs which were normal on phlebography). The slightly lower sensitivity in this study is probably due to the larger number of early asymptomatic thrombi detected by ^{125}I-fibrinogen.

When variations of the methodology, instrumentation or interpretation of impedance plethysmography have been employed by other investigators, the results have been less uniform, although still favorable.[21, 22] Additional corroboration of the physiologic principles underlying occlusive impedance plethysmography has also come from the use of water displacement, air cuff and strain gauge plethysmography.[7-9, 23, 24] The large and well-studied series of Cranley et al.,[25, 26] which employed both respiratory maneuvers and multiple recording air cuff plethysmographs, demonstrates the pathophysiologic effects of venous thrombosis particularly well.

When thrombi are hemodynamically insignificant, they cannot be detected by impedance plethysmography. The small, isolated calf vein thrombus is overlooked. Unless thrombosis involves several calf veins, there is little effect on venous dynamics. In our series, only 21% of the patients with calf vein thrombosis were detected (7/33 venograms). Failure to detect hemodynamically insignificant clots has not posed a risk with respect to subsequent pulmonary embolism in our experience.[20]

The test is also ineffective in the diagnosis of old phlebitis. As time goes by, many patients with old phlebitis develop adequate collateral outflow channels, or sometimes recanalize the thrombosed major veins. In either event, venous outflow improves with time in the majority of patients and the test may revert to normal, even if a major vein remains thrombosed. Only 29% of patients with radiographic evidence of old phlebitis were detected as abnormal (15/52 phlebograms).

Patients with old thrombophlebitis who have abnormal impedance phlebograms usually have persistent major venous outflow obstruction without adequate collateral formation. These patients sometimes can be distinguished from those with fresh thrombosis by observing the presence or absence of respiratory excursions with the leg slightly below heart level. These respiratory waves are obliterated in the presence of fresh major venous thrombosis, but may return later due to collateral development. The presence of good respiratory excursions in the face of impaired venous outflow suggests chronic rather than acute venous occlusion.

Since occlusive impedance plethysmography is merely a modified form of classical venous outflow plethysmography, which has been used for many years to assess arterial blood flow, the results of venous occlusion plethysmography are understandably influenced by a variety of factors which markedly alter arterial blood flow. Shock, marked peripheral vasoconstriction, low cardiac output, arterial occlusive disease and other factors which affect peripheral blood flow determine the rate of increase in blood volume following temporary venous out-flow occlusion.

With a markedly reduced blood volume increase following cuff compression, the rate and magnitude of outflow following cuff release naturally is diminished. Although it is uncommon for false positive results to be obtained due to vasoconstriction and/or decreased peripheral blood flow, decreased capacitance and outflow values are observed frequently when these conditions are present. Interpretation of tests in patients with peripheral vasoconstriction or other factors known to reduce peripheral blood flow must be made with this fact in mind. In such a patient, a normal test result can be relied upon. However, an equivocal or abnormal test preferably should be repeated when the patient's peripheral blood flow has been restored to normal. If this is not possible, a phlebogram should be done to corroborate the impedance findings.

Impedance tests also reflect interference with venous outflow due to extrinsic mechanical compression. This occasionally is seen with cancer of the pelvis. Venous compression also can be produced by a large hematoma, a Baker's cyst, tight clothing or bandages or any other cause of extrinsic compression of major veins.

Perhaps the commonest but most subtle form of extrinsic compression is increased muscle tension in the calf. Contraction of the calf muscles squeezes the calf veins and reduces the volume of blood they can hold. For this reason, it is important to be sure that the patient is comfortable and that his leg muscles are thoroughly relaxed.

Discussion of Clinical Applications

Clinically Suspected Deep Vein Thrombosis

The best established use of occlusive impedance plethysmography is the evaluation of patients with clinically suspected deep vein thrombosis. Many patients have nonspecific signs or symptoms which suggest the possibility of deep vein thrombosis, but a large number of these patients ultimately prove to have some other cause for their signs or symptoms. The clinician knows that a major thrombus may exist in a patient with minimal symptoms, but he still may hesitate to subject a patient with minimal symptoms to the expense and unpleasantness of a phlebogram. What should a physician do when a young woman on oral contraceptives come to his office with mild calf tenderness? Or when he sees a postoperative patient who has significant ankle swelling after a femoropopliteal arterial reconstruction or a medial meniscectomy? Or after a myocardial infarction? The clinician needs some quick and simple but accurate procedure to establish the diagnosis of venous thrombosis or else to rule it out.

When a patient has even minimal physical findings which are due to major vein thrombosis, impedance plethysmography shows a markedly abnormal response. Similar physical findings due to other causes do not affect the plethysmographic response. The accuracy of occlusive impedance plethysmography in patients with clinically suspected deep vein thrombosis is extremely high. The method provides immediate and accurate diagnosis and rapid assessment of the risk of major pulmonary embolism, even in patients with minimal clinical findings.

SCREENING PATIENTS AT RISK

Previous work with ^{125}I-fibrinogen has identified patient populations at high risk with respect to the development of thrombophlebitis. Use of prophylactic anticoagulants has markedly diminished the incidence of thrombosis in these patients. Since patients in known high-risk categories now receive routine prophylaxis, the yield on plethysmographic screening has been relatively low. At the present time we employ this procedure only to screen those high-risk patients in whom prophylactic anticoagulation is deemed contraindicated or those patients who appear to have a significant risk of thromboembolic disease despite the use of prophylactic anticoagulants.

EVALUATION OF SUSPECTED PULMONARY EMBOLISM

Since the overwhelming majority of pulmonary emboli arise from thrombi in the leg veins, it is not surprising that the incidence of abnormal impedance tests has been stated to be over 90% in patients with proved pulmonary emboli.[27] Our own experience corroborates this high rate of correlation. Routine impedance plethysmography on patients clinically suspected of having pulmonary embolism often reveals abnormal tracings, even in asymptomatic extremities. On the other hand, a normal impedance tracing in a patient suspected of having pulmonary embolism casts doubt on this diagnosis. The test provides a simple way to help assess the likelihood of suspected pulmonary embolism.

EVALUATION OF ANTICOAGULANT THERAPY

In the long-term treatment of patients with deep vein thrombosis, the question frequently arises as to how long oral anticoagulants should be continued. This is particularly true if there are bleeding complications or if there is difficulty in controlling the prothrombin time. In the past, we have been reluctant to discontinue oral anticoagulants for several months following proven deep vein thrombosis. More recently, our policy has been somewhat more flexible and guided in part by the results of impedance plethysmography, as well as by any difficulties encountered in anticoagulant management. If the test shows perfectly normal venous dynamics, we are more inclined to omit oral anticoagulants when there is any difficulty in their management. On the other hand, if the plethysmographic tracing shows marked venous outflow obstruction, we are reluctant to discontinue anticoagulants for fear that the persistent venous stasis might predispose to recurrent thrombosis.

VENOUS THROMBOSIS OF THE UPPER EXTREMITIES

Although venous thrombosis is much less common in the upper extremities than in the lower extremities, the technique of occlusive impedance plethysmography can be carried out on the arm as well as the leg. The discrepancy between normal and abnormal tracings is even more striking than in the leg. Although the diagnosis of subclavian, axillary or brachial vein thrombosis is often apparent clinically, in dubious cases impedance plethysmography provides a quick and accurate assessment of the regional venous dynamics. With increasing use of subclavian venous catheters, more patients are being encountered with venous outflow obstruction of the upper extremity. Early and accurate diagnosis and prompt treatment of venous thrombosis is obviously desirable in the upper extremity, as well as in the lower extremity.

TOTAL HIP REPLACEMENT

The high incidence of fatal pulmonary embolism in early reported series of total hip replacements has resulted in great interest in the early diagnosis of venous thrombosis in these patients. Occlusive impedance plethysmography has been employed for this purpose by several investigators. Hume et al.[28] reported 32 patients who underwent phlebography and impedance plethysmography after hip surgery. No clinically significant clots were overlooked by impedance plethysmography. In 44 patients with hip surgery reported by Hull et al.[19] the sensitivity for proximal vein thrombosis was 88%, and the specificity was 84%. Larger series are necessary before the exact accuracy of this technique can be assessed in patients with hip surgery. At present the method appears quite promising, but perhaps somewhat less sensitive and less specific than in patients with clinically suspected venous thrombosis.

Relationship to Other Diagnostic Methods

As experience is gained with a variety of methods to diagnose venous thrombosis, it appears that their relationship may be more complementary than competitive. Each has certain advantages and certain limitations. Although impedance plethysmography has become the standard noninvasive diagnostic procedure for venous thrombosis in our hands, phlebograms are still essential in the management of some patients. Doppler examination is still employed as an adjunct to physical examination, and ^{125}I-fibrinogen scans will continue to be employed for special study groups.

DOPPLER EXAMINATION

Doppler examination of the venous system can be done at the patient's bedside and is the most rapid noninvasive diagnostic test for venous thrombosis. Vascular surgeons who carry pocket Doppler flowmeters for the evaluation of the peripheral arterial system usually employ the same instrument to examine the venous system in patients in whom they are concerned about the possibility of deep vein thrombosis. The impressions are subjective, and the reliability doubtless varies from one observer to another. Each examiner must assess the validity of his conclusions in view of his own past experience.

We view this procedure as a valuable extension of the physical examination. Although we do not base a diagnosis of venous thrombosis on Doppler examination alone, this technique provides useful information which is easy to obtain and helpful to correlate with the patient's clinical findings or with impedance plethysmography. However, unlike others,[21] we do not feel it is necessary to corroborate the impedance test with Doppler examination.

^{125}I-FIBRINOGEN SCANNING

^{125}I-fibrinogen scanning is unquestionably the most reliable prospective method to detect formation of calf clots. It has been of great value in studying the natural history of venous thrombosis, identifying high risk patient groups and evaluating various methods of prophylaxis. It will doubtless continue to be useful for these same purposes. We do not use this method for patients with clinically suspected deep vein thrombosis because of the delay in obtaining results and because of the inability to detect thrombi which originate in the groin and pelvis. Although these thrombi are much less frequent than calf vein thrombi, they are also a much greater threat to the patient.

Although impedance plethysmography overlooks early calf vein thrombosis, the incidence of clinically detected pulmonary embolism in patients with normal impedance tests has been extremely low (0.3%).[20] We conclude that the treatment of isolated calf thrombi with full heparinization is more hazardous than the thrombi themselves. For this reason we do not use ^{125}I-fibrinogen for routine clinical screening. We continue to feel that it is the best available method for investigative studies in which the detection of early calf vein thrombosis is essential.

PHLEBOGRAPHY

Phlebography continues to be desirable in the management of some patients with possible thromboembolism, despite the availability of impedance plethysmography. Although we no longer feel that phlebograms are routinely necessary to corroborate the diagnosis of venous thrombosis in patients with abnormal impedance tracings, we still like to obtain phlebograms in some patients, particularly when there may be some pathophysiologic factors which could influence the tracings. For example, bilateral abnormal impedance tracings in a patient with hypotension should not be assumed to represent venous thrombosis without a corroborative phlebogram. Reduction in peripheral blood flow and severe peripheral vasoconstriction might affect the tracing in such a patient.

When clinical findings point toward venous thrombosis and when the impedance tracing confirms this impression, we are quite comfortable in beginning treatment without phlebography. Conversely, when there is an abnormal impedance tracing with no clinical evidence to suggest thrombosis, we like to have a corroborative phlebogram before committing the patient to full-dose heparinization.

As to other types of plethysmography, we have had no clinical experience. In the research laboratory, we have studied mercury strain gauge and air cuff plethysmography and compared the measurements so obtained with those of impedance plethysmography. We have found no reason to change our methodology and prefer to use techniques and equipment which are now quite well studied and documented as to their reliability.

Conclusion

Fresh thrombosis in major veins alters their physiologic function in characteristic ways. The resting venous volume is increased, the venous capacitance is decreased and the maximum venous outflow rate is markedly diminished. These changes in venous function are measured easily at the bedside using impedance plethysmography with temporary venous outflow occlusion.

This simple, noninvasive procedure now has become a well-established method for the diagnosis of fresh thrombosis in the popliteal, femoral or iliac veins. The same technique also can be used to diagnose thrombosis of the brachial, axillary or subclavian veins. The method is simple and safe for the patient and can be done by a technician at the bedside. There is an overall accuracy of roughly 96%, when the testing procedure, instrumentation and method of interpretation are similar to those described herein.

Occlusive impedance plethysmography does not detect isolated calf clots. However, clinically significant pulmonary embolism in patients with normal impedance plethysmography is extremely rare. This observation corroborates the impression of most investigators that clinically significant pulmonary emboli usually arise from the iliac, femoral or popliteal veins. To date, the chief use of impedance plethysmography has been to confirm or deny the presence of clinically suspected deep vein thrombosis.

Acknowledgments

The phlebograms in this study were performed by Dr. Karl Benedict, Jr., and the Department of Radiology, St. Vincent Hospital, Worcester, Massachusetts. Doctor Joseph A. O'Donnell was a major collaborator during the early phases of this work. The instrumentation was provided by the Cintor Division of Codman and Shurtleff, Inc., Randolph, Massachusetts, 02368.

REFERENCES

1. de Takats, G.: *Vascular Surgery* (Philadelphia: W. B. Saunders Company, 1959).
2. Brodie, T. G., and Russell, A. E.: On the determination of the rate of blood flow through an organ, J. Physiol. 32:47P, 1905.
3. Hewlett, A. W., and van Zwaluwenburg, J. G.: The rate of blood flow in the arm, Heart 1:87, 1909.
4. Grant, R. T., and Pearson, R. S. B.: The blood circulation in the human limb: Observations on the differences between the proximal and distal parts and remarks on the regulation of body temperature, Clin. Sci. 3:119, 1938.

5. Mullick, S. C., Wheeler, H. B., and Songster, G. P.: Diagnosis of deep venous thrombosis by measurement of electrical impedance, Am. J. Surg. 119:417, 1970.
6. Wheeler, H. B., Mullick, S. C., Anderson, J. N., and Pearson, D.: Diagnosis of occult deep vein thrombosis by a non-invasive bedside technique, Surgery 70:20, 1971.
7. Eiriksson, E.: Plethysmographic studies of venous diseases of the legs, Acta Chir. Scand. (Suppl.) 398:7, 1968.
8. Aschberg, S.: Crural venous obstruction or incompetence, Acta Chir. Scand. (Suppl.) 436:1, 1973.
9. Hallbook, T., and Gothlin, J.: Strain gauge plethysmography and phlebography in diagnosis of deep venous thrombosis, Acta Chir. Scand. 137:37, 1971.
10. Gazzaniga, A. B., Pacella, A. F., Bartlett, R. H., and Geraghty, T. R.: Bilateral impedance rheography in the diagnosis of deep vein thrombosis of the legs, Arch. Surg. 104:515, 1972.
11. Connolly, J. E., and Gazzaniga, A. B.: Newer techniques to detect venous thrombosis with special reference to electrical impedance plethysmography, Surg. Clin. North Am. 54:69, 1974.
12. Seeber, J. J.: Impedance plethysmography: A useful method in the diagnosis of deep vein thrombophlebitis in the lower extremity, Arch. Phys. Med. Rehabil. 55: 1730, 1974.
13. Nadeau, J. E., Demers, R., Skinner, B., and McLean, L. D.: Impedance phlebography: Accuracy of diagnosis in deep vein thrombosis, Can. J. Surg. 18:219, 1975.
14. Steer, M. L., Spotnitz, A. J., Cohen, S. I., Paulin, S., and Salzman, E. W.: Limitations of impedance phlebography for diagnosis of venous thrombosis, Arch. Surg. 106:44, 1973.
15. Dmochowski, J. R., Adams, D. F., and Couch, N. P.: Impedance measurement in the diagnosis of deep venous thrombosis, Arch. Surg. 104:170, 1972.
16. Schulman, R. H., Friedman, S. A., and Degenshein, G.: Impedance phlebography: Critical evaluation in its relations to inspiratory capacity, Circulation 48:1295, 1973.
17. Wheeler, H. B., O'Donnell, J. A., Anderson, F. A., and Benedict, K., Jr.: Occlusive impedance phlebography: A diagnostic procedure for venous thrombosis and pulmonary embolism, Prog. Cardiovasc. Dis. 17:199, 1974.
18. Wheeler, H. B., O'Donnell, J. A., Anderson, F. A., Penney, B. C., Peura, R. A., and Benedict, K., Jr.: Bedside screening for venous thrombosis using occlusive impedance plethysmography, Angiology 26:199, 1974.
19. Hull, R., van Aken, W. G., Hirsh, J., Gallus, A. S., Hoicka, G., Turpie, A. G., Walker, I., and Gent, M.: Impedance plethysmography using the occlusive cuff technique in the diagnosis of venous thrombosis, Circulation 53:696, 1976.
20. Wheeler, H. B., and Patwardhan, N. A.: Evaluation of Venous Thrombosis by Impedance Plethysmography, in Madden, J., and Hume, M. (eds.): Venous Thromboembolism: Prevention and Treatment (New York: Appleton-Century-Crofts, Inc., 1976), pp. 33–50.
21. Yao, J. S. T., Henkin, R. E., and Bergan, J. J.: Venous thromboembolic disease, Arch. Surg. 109:664, 1974.
22. Johnston, K. W., Kakkar, V. V., Spindler, J. J., Corrigan, T. P., and Fossard, D. P.: A simple method for detecting deep vein thrombosis: An improved electrical impedance technique, Am. J. Surg. 127:349, 1974.
23. Hallbook, T., and Ling, L.: Plethysmography in the diagnosis of acute deep vein thrombosis, Vasa 3:263, 1974.
24. Barnes, R. W., Collicot, P. E., Mozersky, D. J., Sumner, D. S., and Strandness, D. E., Jr.: Noninvasive quantitation of maximum venous outflow in acute thrombophlebitis, Surgery 72:971, 1972.
25. Cranley, J. J., Canos, A. J., Sull, W. J., and Grass, A. M.: Phleborheographic technique for diagnosing deep venous thrombosis of the lower extremities, Surg. Gynecol. Obstet. 141:331, 1975.

26. Cranley, J. J., Gay, A. Y., Grass, A. M., and Simeone, F. A.: A plethysmographic technique for the diagnosis of deep venous thrombosis of the lower extremities, Surg. Gynecol. Obstet. 136:385, 1973.
27. Sasahara, A. A.: Current problems in pulmonary embolism: Introduction, Prog. Cardiovasc. Dis. 17:1, 1974.
28. Hume, M., Kuriakose, T. X., Jamieson, J., and Turner, R. H.: Extent of leg vein thrombosis determined by impedance and I[125] fibrinogen, Am. J. Surg. 129:455, 1975.

11 / Diagnosis of Venous Thrombosis by Doppler Ultrasound

DAVID S. SUMNER, M.D.

Professor and Chief, Section of Peripheral Vascular Surgery, Southern Illinois University School of Medicine, Springfield, Illinois

IN 1959, Satomura described a method for detecting blood flow transcutaneously with ultrasound using the Doppler effect.[23, 24] Clinicians, who quickly recognized the potential value of this remarkable instrument for studying peripheral vascular disease,[22, 28, 30] found the method to be particularly well suited for the diagnosis of acute venous thrombosis.[26, 31, 34] The rationale is simple: mechanical obstruction produced by the intraluminal thrombi alters the venous flow pattern, and these alterations are readily detected by the Doppler.

Although other noninvasive methods have been developed for diagnosing thrombophlebitis, Doppler ultrasound has several distinct advantages over most of them. The equipment is simple to operate, inexpensive and portable. Venous surveys can be made rapidly and easily at the bedside with minimal discomfort to the patient. Furthermore, in experienced hands, the Doppler has been shown to be remarkably accurate especially in regard to disease of the major deep veins of the leg.[1, 8, 11, 15, 25, 32, 35]

Instrumentation

Currently, there are several commercially available ultrasonic flowmeters that can be adapted to the study of venous disease. In these devices, a piezoelectric crystal mounted at the end of a hand-held probe is driven to emit a continuous beam of ultrasonic energy with a frequency of 5–10 MHz. The sound is coupled to the skin by means of a water soluble gel and is then transmitted through the underlying skin and subcutaneous tissues. When the sound waves strike an acoustic interface, a portion of the ultrasonic energy is reflected back toward the probe. If the reflecting object is stationary, the backscattered signal will have the same frequency as the incident sound beam; if, on the other hand, the object is in motion, the frequency of the reflected sound will be shifted in accordance with the Doppler principle. The frequency of sound reflected from erythrocytes moving away from the probe will be lower than the transmitted frequency, while that reflected from erythrocytes moving toward the probe will be increased. A second piezoelectric crystal mounted adjacent to the transmitting crystal receives the backscattered sound. The transmitted and reflected signals then are mixed to produce a beat frequency that is equal to the Doppler frequency shift and proportional to the velocity of the moving blood cells. Since this beat signal is in the audible range it can be amplified to drive a set of earphones or a loudspeaker. Alternatively, it can be passed through a zero-crossing frequency to voltage converter to produce an analogue signal suitable for recording on a strip chart.

These instruments can be made to sense direction of blood flow by introducing a 90-degree phase shift prior to flow detection.[13, 16, 29] Forward and reverse flow can be displayed on separate meters located on the instrument panel, demonstrated qualitatively on separate channels on a strip chart or differentially recorded on a single channel. This circuitry does not separate the audio channels. However, recently introduced "outphasing" flowmeters do permit complete separation of the audio signals so that forward flow is delivered to one speaker and reverse flow to another.[20]

CHOICE OF EQUIPMENT

For all clinical venous examinations, the audible output is sufficient. Recordings are required only for future documentation. Likewise, it is seldom necessary to use a directional Doppler since the character and timing of the signals can usually be relied on to distinguish between forward and reverse flow. Thus, a simple unidirectional Doppler with an audio output will provide all of the necessary diagnostic information in most cases of suspected acute venous thrombosis.

Because of their simplicity and portability, pocket-sized Doppler flowmeters with stethoscopic earphones are especially useful for ward work. However, in the laboratory, the clinician may appreciate the added information provided by the more complex instruments. A valuable feature of the "outphasing" type of directional instrument is the ability to completely cancel flow toward or away from the probe. This allows the examiner to completely eliminate confusing arterial signals so that he can focus his attention exclusively on the venous signal.

Superficial veins, such as the saphenous and the posterior tibial, are best examined with a high frequency instrument (10 MHz), but the deeper veins, such as the superficial femoral or popliteal, are most easily studied with a lower frequency device (5 MHz). The lower the frequency of the sound, the deeper it penetrates without losing energy. This feature is especially valuable when the limb being examined is fat, since adipose tissue is a relatively poor conductor of sound. Flow in a deep vein that may not even be detected with a 10-MHz instrument often provides a surprisingly strong signal with a 5-MHz device. While the lower frequency instruments have greater powers of penetration, their spatial discrimination is not as precise as that of the higher frequency devices, a fact that may cause some confusion when there are nearby collateral veins. For these reasons, the author employs both a 5 MHz and a 10 MHz Doppler in all cases studied in the laboratory.

Method of Examination

The examination is best performed in a warm room (25 C) after the subject has rested for 10 or 15 min. In cases of severe peripheral vasoconstriction, it may be necessary to use an electric blanket to stimulate blood flow. All constrictive clothing and elastic stockings must be removed.

The subject is examined in a horizontal supine position with his or her head resting on a pillow. Both legs are abducted moderately at the hip, externally rotated to a mild degree and slightly flexed at the knee. Rotation and abduction facilitate probe placement and knee flexion reduces the pressure of the popliteal tissues on the underlying vein. It is most important that the subject's legs be relaxed in order to prevent compression of the deep veins by tense muscles.

Although examination of the popliteal vein can be accomplished in the supine position, it is best performed with the patient lying prone, hands folded beneath the head, the legs flexed sharply at the knee and the feet supported by one or two pillows. This relaxes the popliteal space, allowing better access to the underlying vein.

The same principles apply to the upper extremities and neck veins. Both arms are slightly abducted from the side and externally rotated.

When the neck veins are studied, it may be necessary to remove the pillow in order to provide access for the Doppler probe. Also, rotating the subjects head slightly may facilitate the examination of the internal and external jugular veins.

The probe is pointed cephalad and held at a 45–60-degree angle to the skin. After the vein has been located, the probe angle can be modified somewhat to obtain the most powerful signal. When the angle between the sound beam and the underlying vessel approaches 90 degrees, the signal becomes low pitched and harsh. As the angle becomes more acute, the signal becomes less noisy and its frequency increases. However, decreasing the angle increases the distance between the probe and the vessel. Thus, when the angle is too acute, little signal will be received. Unlike most of the other veins of the lower limb, the popliteal vein does not parallel the skin but tends to dive anteriorly as it approaches the adductor hiatus. For this reason, reception in popliteal fossa may be improved by positioning the probe at right angles to the skin.

In order to facilitate sound transmission, the Doppler probe is coupled to the skin with a water-soluble gel. No pressure should be applied to the skin when superficial veins are being examined, and only moderate pressure need be used in examining deep veins. Because venous pressure is so low, too much external pressure will collapse the underlying veins.

Examination of the leg veins is carried out systematically. The common femoral, superficial femoral, popliteal, posterior tibial and saphenous veins are studied, usually in that order. At each level, it is important to compare the signal in one limb with that in the same vein of the other limb. This should always be done before moving distally to another area. Repeated comparisons frequently will reveal slight differences in the flow pattern that otherwise would not have been apparent.

The first step at each level is to determine the presence or absence of a spontaneous venous flow signal. Because collateral veins frequently are present, it is mandatory that the examiner be certain that he is studying the proper vein; otherwise, erroneous interpretations are inevitable. Identification is best accomplished by first locating the adjacent artery and then moving the probe in the appropriate direction until venous flow is encountered. It must be emphasized that the probe need be moved only slightly, less than a centimeter in most cases. This usually can be accomplished by shifting the skin or by merely tilting the probe. When the venous signal first becomes audible, arterial flow should still be present in the background. A combination of signals is the best assurance that the correct vein is being detected. At this point, the probe can be readjusted as necessary to reduce the arterial interference and improve the volume of the venous signal. (As mentioned before, some instruments can be adjusted to cancel the arterial signals.)

If the examiner is still in doubt regarding the identity of the vein, he may trace the signal up or down the leg. Ordinarily, major veins are relatively straight, adhering to well-defined anatomical pathways. Collateral veins, on the other hand, often follow a circuitous course and are difficult to trace. Furthermore, collateral veins are frequently more superficial than the major veins and are more easily compressed with the Doppler probe.

After the vein has been located, the examiner should listen carefully for a few moments to the signal, noting its relationship to respiration and any pulsations of cardiac origin. This is often the most revealing part of the study. Next, the quality, magnitude and timing of the signal are assessed while the subject takes a deep breath and performs a Valsalva maneuver. The last step is to augment the venous flow by gently but firmly compressing the leg at multiple levels proximal and distal to the site of the probe. With the probe over the common femoral vein, the distal thigh and proximal calf are compressed. At the popliteal level, compression sites include the calf and thigh; and at the posterior tibial region, they include the foot, calf, thigh and groin. Sometimes it may be helpful to augment the flow by having the subject flex or extend his ankle in order to empty the calf veins.

The procedure for the upper extremity is analogous to that for the lower. An orderly examination of the subclavian, axillary, brachial and forearm veins is undertaken. Venous signals at each level are compared with those at the same level in the opposite arm in regard to their spontaneous flow pattern, relationship to respiration and response to peripheral augmentation maneuvers (compression of the forearm or clenching the fist). In the neck, the examination is limited to assessing the spontaneous signals arising from the internal and external jugular veins or their tributaries.

Normal Venous Flow Patterns

Venous flow signals can be classified as "spontaneous" and "augmented." Spontaneous signals are those that are audible without supplementary measures being required to increase the velocity of venous flow. Augmented signals are those that are generated in response to compression of the limbs or are produced by muscle contraction.

SPONTANEOUS SIGNALS

In normal limbs, spontaneous signals should always be heard at the common femoral, superficial femoral and popliteal levels. With a little patience, they can be detected in most posterior tibial veins and in roughly half of the saphenous veins at the ankle. Warming the feet or calf muscle exercise will augment blood flow sufficiently to produce an audible signal in many cases in which flow was not heard on the initial attempt. Tense patients may have restricted blood flow in veins as far proximal as the superficial femoral. Efforts to reassure the patient and to reposition his limbs may be helpful. Usually, however, there is no difficulty in obtaining a spontaneous signal.

Characteristically, the audible signal is low pitched, contains a wide spectrum of frequencies and sounds much like a windstorm (Fig 11–1). In the legs of a supine individual, the signal varies with respiration, decreasing with inspiration and increasing with expiration (Fig 11–2). With each inspiration, the descent of the diaphragm causes the intra-abdominal pressure to rise, compressing the inferior vena cava and impeding venous outflow from the legs. With expiration, the diaphragm rises, abdominal pressure decreases and the blood backed up in the legs surges cephalad to fill the abdominal veins. As a rule, these phasic flow patterns can be detected in all veins, both superficial and deep, as far distally as the ankle, but they are somewhat more distinct in the popliteal and more proximal veins.

In some subjects, particularly women, this characteristic phasic flow pattern may not be pronounced, the flow in these cases assuming a

Fig 11–1.—Sonogram of femoral vein signal (probe 55 degrees to the skin). The amplitude of the signal at any given frequency is indicated by the depth of shading, the darkest being the loudest. Increments of 6 dB separate the contours. Note the low peak frequency (4,000 Hz) and the multitude of frequency levels.

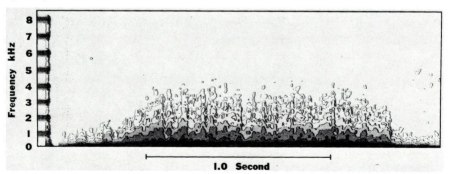

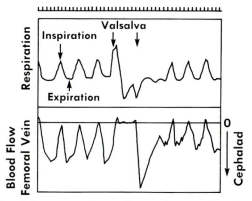

Fig 11–2. — Blood flow in common femoral vein of a 41-year-old (supine) male showing effect of respiration and Valsalva maneuver. Since the tracing was made in the differential mode with the probe pointed up the leg, venous blood flow in the normal cephalic direction produces a negative deflection. Respiration was recorded with a mercury-in-Silastic strain gauge.

more constant character. Occasionally, in a "thoracic breather," the venous flow may even increase with inspiration and decrease with expiration, responding directly to changes in intrathoracic pressure. This pattern is also observed when the subject is standing or tilted into an upright position.[14] Because of gravitational effects, the dependent veins of the abdomen and legs tend to remain distended in upright subjects so that flow is more responsive to changes in intrathoracic pressure than it is to changes in abdominal pressure.

Venous outflow will decrease markedly with a deep breath or cease altogether with a Valsalva maneuver in all normal legs even when there is little phasic response to quiet respiration (see Fig 11–2). Thus, the deep breath and the Valsalva maneuver are good tests for normal venous function. The rapid increase in intra-abdominal pressure that accompanies a Valsalva maneuver tends to displace blood out of the abdomen down the legs. When the iliofemoral valves are competent, little or no retrograde blood flow will be detected at the common femoral level prior to valve closure. However, in some otherwise normal individuals, the iliofemoral valves will be absent or functionally incompetent. In these subjects, a Valsalva maneuver will result in rather prolonged retrograde flow in the common femoral vein.

In addition to the large variations in venous flow that occur in response to respiratory movements, there are smaller pulsations that coincide with the cardiac cycle.[19, 21, 33] These pulsations may be evident as far distally as the superficial veins of the feet. They are particu-

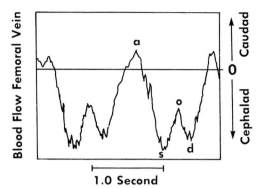

Fig 11–3. — Pulsatile blood flow in common femoral vein of a patient with mild congestive heart failure. Tracing was made during suspended respiration in the differential mode with Doppler probe pointed cephalad. Letters correspond to events in the cardiac cycle: *a*, atrial contraction; *s*, ventricular systole; *o*, opening of tricuspid valve; and *d*, ventricular diastole.

larly prominent when the central venous pressure is elevated due to congestive heart failure, tricuspid insufficiency or pulmonary hypertension (Fig 11–3).

Signals in the upper extremity also vary with respiration but may either increase or decrease with inspiration.[14] Cardiac pulsations are often quite evident and are easily detected even in the dilated veins

Fig 11–4. — Normal response to augmentation maneuvers. Differential tracings were made with subject supine. *C*, compression; *R*, release; **A**, compression distal to probe; **B**, compression proximal to probe.

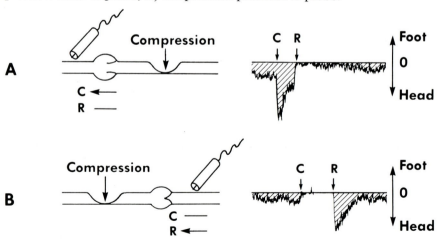

on the dorsum of the hand. In the jugular veins, pulsations of cardiac origin are particularly prominent.

AUGMENTED SIGNALS

Manual compression of the leg distal to the probe will empty the underlying veins and propel blood cephalad past the probe, thus augmenting the venous signal (Fig 11–4, A). The magnitude of the augmented signal depends on the quantity of blood displaced, on the force and velocity of the compression maneuver and the distance be-

Fig 11–5.—Venous flow signals from a 61-year-old female who presented with left iliofemoral thrombosis 1 week after repair of a right Spigelian hernia. Zero flow level is indicated on the ordinate. Normal cephalad direction of venous flow is shown by *arrows*. Time in seconds is on the abscissa. Calf compression is designated by *CC*, foot compression by *FC*. Common femoral tracings were taken by shifting probe from over the artery to over the vein. Note low volume continuous flow in left superficial femoral vein and high volume continuous flow in left saphenous vein.

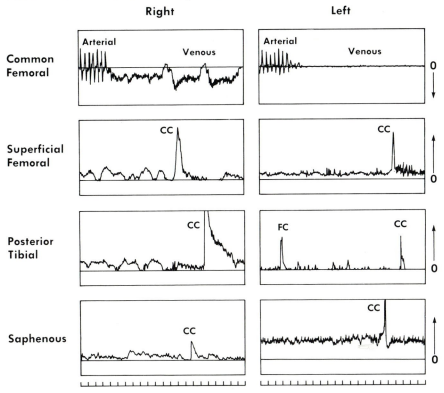

tween the probe and the compression site. If the veins are relatively empty, no augmentation will be perceptible even though the venous channels are widely patent.

With the probe over the common femoral area, distal thigh compression will always produce an augmented signal, but calf compression may not in a large number of normal limbs. At the superficial femoral and popliteal levels, calf compression will always augment the signal;

Fig 11–6.—Venous flow signals from a 69-year-old male who developed right popliteal and calf vein thrombosis after a long airplane flight. Zero flow level is indicated on the ordinate. Calf compression is designated by *CC*, foot compression by *FC*. Time in seconds is shown on abscissa. Flow signals from adjacent artery appear sporadically in tracings from right and left popliteal and posterior tibial veins. Note high volume continuous flow in right saphenous vein at the ankle.

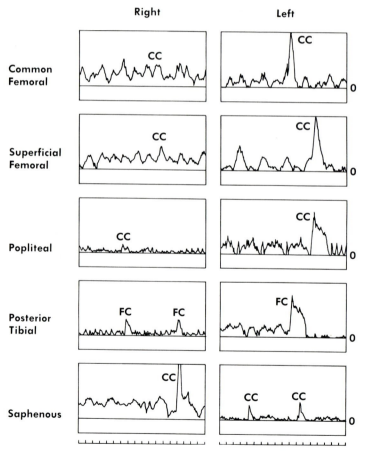

similarly, even a very light squeeze of the foot will invariably augment the posterior tibial signal (Figs 11–5 and 11–6).

In normal subjects, compression of the leg proximal to the site of the
probe results in an immediate cessation of flow; release of the compression allows the backed-up blood to escape, thereby augmenting
the signal (see Fig 11–4, B). During proximal compression, venous
valves close prohibiting retrograde flow toward the probe. When the
compression is released, these valves open allowing blood to flow
cephalad in the normal direction.

If there are no valves between the site of compression and the
probe, some blood will reflux down the vein toward the probe producing a signal coincident with the compression. Even in normal limbs,
this is commonly observed when the lower thigh is squeezed and the
probe is over the popliteal vein. Also reflux is often noted in the normal saphenous vein to midcalf when the probe is positioned at the
ankle.

Flow Patterns Associated with Venous Obstruction

Obstruction of the major venous channels can be detected in a
number of ways (Fig 11–7). Obviously, if the probe is pointed toward
a completely occluded venous segment no spontaneous or augmented
signal will be heard (see Fig 11–7, A). The main challenge to the examiner is to be certain that the probe is actually over the vein in question. As emphasized previously, the proximity of the adjacent artery is
the most reliable guide. If the examiner leaves the neighborhood of
the artery, he usually will encounter collateral venous signals and may
be misled into thinking that the major vein is patent when it is actually
occluded (Fig 11–8).

The signal heard over a patent vein peripheral to an obstruction will
vary in magnitude depending upon the availability of residual outflow
channels between the site of the probe and the obstruction. If outflow
channels are few or nonexistent, flow will markedly decrease or be
absent altogether (see Fig 11–7, B). This situation is most likely to
occur when the probe is just below the occlusion.

When, however, the probe is over a patent vein some distance below an occlusion, the signal will be "continuous," lacking the usual
phasic response to respiration (see Fig 11–7, C). It will not be interrupted by a deep breath. Even a Valsalva maneuver may fail to obliterate the signal. The continuous nature of the flow is the result of the
high venous pressure that builds up distal to the obstruction. Blood is
forced to bypass the obstruction via high resistance collateral path-

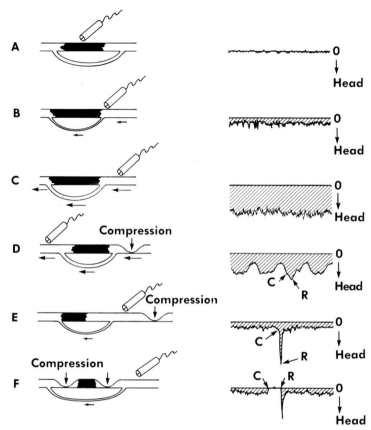

Fig 11–7. — Spontaneous (**A, B,** and **C**) and augmented (**D, E,** and **F**) venous flow patterns associated with venous obstruction. Differential tracings were made with subject supine. *C*, compression; *R*, release. Compare with normal responses in Figures 11–2 and 11–4.

ways, making the flow less responsive to the low level changes in abdominal pressure that accompany respiration.

Another way of recognizing the presence of obstruction is through the use of augmentation maneuvers. When the probe is positioned proximal or cephalad to a venous obstruction, the venous signal may be normal or reduced in volume depending upon the adequacy of the collateral inflow (see Fig 11–6). However, compression of the extremity peripheral to the obstruction site will cause little or no augmentation of the flow (see Fig 11–7, D). Total reliance on this test is apt to produce a significant number of false positive and false negative ex-

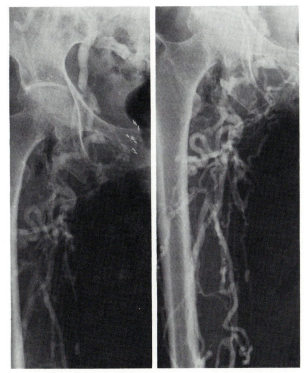

Fig 11–8.—Phlebogram showing extensive development of collateral veins in femoral and superficial femoral region in a 77-year-old female who had acute iliofemoral thrombosis 3 years previously. In such cases, the jumble of veins makes Doppler examination difficult. This particular study was interpreted accurately.

aminations. False negative studies result when there are good collateral channels around the obstruction and limb compression has been vigorous. False positive results occur when the limb veins are relatively empty so that little blood is displaced by the compression maneuver.

If the probe is over a patent vein but distal to an occlusion, compression of the limb or foot distal to the probe may produce a signal, but the volume of this augmented signal will be reduced and it will have an "abrupt" quality (see Fig 11–7, E). Similarly, when the compression site is proximal to the probe, the resulting augmentation will be abrupt and of low volume (see Fig 11–7, F). This holds true regardless of whether the occlusion is at, above or below the site of compression. Since the quality of the signal is very important in these cases, comparisons between the limbs are necessary in order to pick up subtle differences.

Although not a direct sign of venous obstruction, increased flow in superficial veins is one of the most important findings in limbs with deep venous thrombosis. Often the flow on the side of the occlusion will be several times that in the same vein of the opposite (normal) extremity (see Figs 11–5 and 11–6). This will be true even when the veins are not perceptibly dilated. Examining the saphenous vein at the ankle in cases of suspected calf vein thrombosis or the subcutaneous veins of the inguinal region in cases of iliofemoral thrombosis may be especially valuable. The increased flow in these superficial veins is merely a manifestation of their role as collateral channels bypassing areas of deep venous occlusion.

Flow Patterns Associated with Venous Valvular Incompetence

Incompetence of the deep venous valves may be congenital but is usually the result of preexisting phlebitis.[7] On the other hand, the etiology of primary varicose veins, the most common manifestation of superficial venous incompetence, remains uncertain but is thought to be on a congenital basis[10, 21] or to result from incompetent perforating veins.[9] Secondary varicose veins are merely dilated and incompetent collaterals that bypass occluded deep veins. Thus, venous valvular incompetence is not a characteristic finding in acute venous thrombosis.

Since this chapter is concerned only with the recognition of acute venous thrombosis, venous valvular incompetence is of importance only in that it may be a manifestation of preexisting phlebitis. Therefore, the Doppler findings associated with valvular incompetence will not be dealt with in any detail.

Basically there are two methods of recognizing valvular incompetence. The first of these employs the Valsalva maneuver. In the event that all veins located cardiad to the site of the probe are incompetent, a Valsalva maneuver will cause blood to flow retrograde out of the abdomen down the leg toward the probe (Fig 11–9, A). This response is most easily elicited at the common femoral area, but can be heard in both superficial and deep veins as far distally as the ankle.

The second method employs compression of the leg above the site of the probe. If the intervening valves are incompetent a retrograde surge of blood will be heard. Upon release of the compression, blood rushes back up the leg, producing a to-and-fro sound (see Fig 11–9, B).

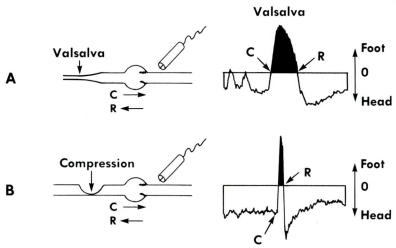

Fig 11–9.—Spontaneous (**A**) and augmented (**B**) venous flow patterns associated with venous incompetence. Differential tracings were made with subject supine. *C*, compression, either manual or by Valsalva maneuver; *R*, release of compression. Compare with normal response in Figures 11–2 and 11–4.

Although a directional Doppler is helpful in distinguishing antegrade from retrograde flow during these maneuvers, it is necessary in only a few cases. Usually the timing of the signal will suffice.

Diagnosis of Acute Deep Venous Thrombosis

Patients suspected of having deep venous thrombosis usually present with one of the following: (1) classical signs of thrombophlebitis, including swelling, tenderness and pain; (2) proved or suspected pulmonary embolus; (3) unexplained edema of the legs; (4) unexplained and often peculiar pains of the legs; (5) inflammation of the leg; (6) postoperative leg swelling or pain; (7) unexplained postoperative fever; or (8) recurrence of pain or increased swelling in a postphlebitic extremity.

In addition, it is reasonable to suspect the presence of venous thrombosis in a fairly large percentage of patients who have been confined to bed for a prolonged period or who recently have undergone a major abdominal or orthopedic operation. This is especially true if the patients are over 40 years of age, are obese, have experienced recent trauma, have a malignancy or are suffering from congestive heart failure.

Some of the conditions frequently confused with deep venous thrombosis are listed in Table 11–1. Even an astute clinician may occasionally fail to recognize these problems. More often, he will entertain the proper diagnosis but cannot, with certainty, rule out thrombosis of the deep veins. Therefore, in all cases where the diagnosis is questionable, objective studies should be obtained.

The Doppler examination is conducted in the same manner in all patient categories regardless of the depth of the clinical suspicion. As outlined earlier in this chapter, the emphasis should be on the recognition of venous obstruction rather than venous valvular incompetence. Thus, the examiner must be concerned with: (1) *absence* of flow in a particular vein, (2) presence of a *continuous* flow signal, (3) *lack or decreased augmentation* of flow with compression maneuvers and (4) *increased* flow in superficial veins.

Although some investigators rely heavily on augmentation maneuvers, in my experience augmented signals are not very dependable and should be interpreted cautiously. Furthermore, forcible compression of the leg is potentially dangerous in patients in whom there is a possibility of pulmonary embolus. For these reasons, I feel that the examination should be based primarily on spontaneous signals. Augmentation maneuvers are performed carefully (or avoided altogether in some patients) and are used only as confirmatory evidence.

Since any sudden change in venous outflow from the legs could dislodge a tenuously adherent thrombus, Valsalva maneuvers also pose some risk for the patient. Therefore, this study is restricted to those patients in whom there is little danger of pulmonary embolus.

Certain other points bear reiteration. In all cases, a complete venous survey should be performed carefully and systematically. At all sites, the examiner must think anatomically in order to be sure that he is actually studying the appropriate vein and not some collateral. He should always compare carefully the venous signals of both legs in

TABLE 11–1.—CONDITIONS
MIMICKING ACUTE DEEP
VENOUS THROMBOSIS

Edema: cardiac, metabolic, postoperative, etc.
Lymphedema
Ruptured muscle with subfascial hematoma
Ruptured synovial cyst
Cellulitis, lymphangitis, inflammatory lymphedema
Myositis
Superficial thrombophlebitis
Trauma

order to detect slight differences in the flow pattern that may provide a necessary clue to the diagnosis.

A final word of caution: at all times the examiner should avoid overstating his findings. If there is any doubt whatsoever regarding the diagnosis, one must not hesitate to obtain a phlebogram. A definitive diagnosis, whether positive or negative, is much too important to both the physician and the patient to neglect any approach that will achieve this end.

Iliofemoral Thrombosis

When the thrombus is confined to the iliac veins, the common femoral signal is continuous and not interrupted by a deep breath or Valsalva maneuver, and usually has a reduced volume. Findings over the more peripheral veins will be similar.

More commonly, both the iliac and common femoral vein will be involved. In these cases, no signal will be detected over the common femoral vein as the probe is shifted medially away from the arterial signal (see Fig 11–5). Further exploration in the groin region usually will reveal a number of collateral veins with more-or-less continuous, rather high-pitched signals. Although these collateral signals may be quite loud, they are usually easily obliterated with slight skin pressure and they always defy any attempts to be traced for more than a few centimeters.

Depending upon the distal extent of the thrombus, the superficial femoral signal will be absent, will be audible only with compression maneuvers or will be continuous (see Fig 11–5). Signals over the popliteal and posterior tibial veins will be similar. Augmentation of the posterior tibial flow by foot or calf compression will produce a low-pitched, low-volume, abrupt signal—if this vein is patent (see Fig 11–5).

Another typical finding is increased flow in small subcutaneous veins in the groin or upper thigh. Increased flow often is present in the saphenous vein at thigh or ankle level (see Fig 11–5).

Superficial Femoral Thrombosis

Thrombosis of the superficial femoral vein is seldom an isolated finding.[5, 18] Usually, there are accompanying clots in the common femoral and/or popliteal below-knee veins. In cases of isolated superficial femoral thrombosis, no venous signals will be detected immediately adjacent to the superficial femoral artery even with augmentation maneuvers, but collateral signals are frequently found a centimeter or so away. It is therefore absolutely necessary to be certain of the identity of the venous signal by the techniques described above. Signals in the popliteal and posterior tibial vein will be similar to those described under "Iliofemoral Thrombosis."

POPLITEAL-TIBIAL THROMBOSIS

Depending upon the extent of proximal involvement, signals in the popliteal vein may be relatively normal, reduced in volme, present only with augmentation or entirely absent.

If the posterior tibial vein at the ankle is thrombosed, no signal will be detected even with augmentation. Occasionally, there are prominent superficial collateral veins that can be confusing. However, these veins will not be immediately adjacent to the artery and are quite easily compressed by the probe. Often, one or more of the posterior tibial venae comitantes will be patent at ankle level despite occlusions more proximally in the calf. In this event, there is seldom a spontaneous signal and the augmented signal will be of low pitch, low volume and abrupt (see Fig 11–6).

ACUTE THROMBI ASSOCIATED WITH POSTPHLEBITIC SYNDROME

Patients who have had previous episodes of phlebitis are more prone to develop repeat thrombi than the general population. These cases constitute the greatest challenge to the Doppler technique. Fresh thrombi may even escape detection on the phlebogram.

Recognition of chronic venous insufficiency may or may not be difficult. In the well developed case, the clinical signs of venous stasis are diagnostic, and the Doppler examination is only confirmatory. In other cases in which clinical signs are minimal or absent altogether, the Doppler may be helpful in making the diagnosis. The examination is based on the recognition of both venous obstruction and venous valvular incompetence.

Recanalized veins and collateral veins present a confusing picture and may be mistaken for the normal deep veins if they are in proximity to the appropriate artery (see Fig 11–8). As mentioned previously, collateral veins may be recognized by their irregular course and occasionally by their superficial location (allowing easy compressibility). The rate of flow may be low or increased. Most of the dilated collateral veins and recanalized veins will display valvular incompetence. The same is true of the major deep veins that have remained patent despite injury to their valves by the phlebitic process. Valvular incompetence is easily detected by the techniques outlined earlier in this chapter.

Obviously, when the examiner is faced with such a confusing picture, he cannot make the diagnosis of superimposed acute thrombophlebitis unless he has detailed knowledge of the preexisting flow patterns. However, when such information is available, the diagnosis may be possible. For example, if it were known that the superficial femoral vein had been patent at the last examination and is no longer so, the conclusion would be that this vein had clotted off in the interim. On the other hand, if the examination has not changed, it is usually safe to assume that the patient's current symptoms are related to chronic venous insufficiency. When confusion remains, phlebograms must be obtained and examined for evidence of fresh clot among the postphlebitic changes.

LIMITATIONS

Since the Doppler examination depends upon the recognition of distorted flow patterns in those major veins that exist in continuity from the periphery to the heart, clots lodged in venous tributaries will escape detection. Among those veins that are inaccessible to the Doppler are several that frequently harbor thrombi: (1) the internal iliac and pelvic veins, (2) the profunda femoris vein and (3) the venous sinusoids within the calf muscles. Fortunately for the examiner, thrombosis of these veins is frequently associated with thrombosis of veins easily studied with the Doppler.[5] Thus, there are fewer false negative examinations than would otherwise occur.

In order to avoid this source of error, some investigators recommend using the ^{125}I-fibrinogen uptake test in conjunction with the Doppler examination. They rely on the Doppler in the iliac and femoral regions and on the isotope in the calf region. Another approach is to obtain a phlebogram of those limbs where the Doppler findings are negative but clinical suspicion remains high. Parenthetically, it might be pointed out that failure to detect small clots localized to the soleal or gastrocnemial sinusoids is seldom of immediate consequence since virtually all significant emboli arise from the popliteal or larger veins.

Thrombi in the anterior tibial vein also will escape detection with the usual Doppler study. Occasionally, the anterior tibial vein will be involved in the absence of posterior-tibial thrombi. Examination of the anterior tibial vein is difficult owing to its rather deep location in the calf. Spontaneous signals seldom are heard. However, the vein

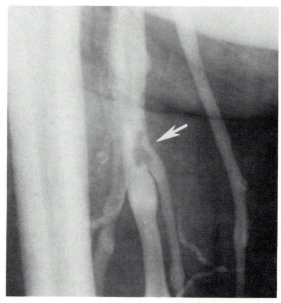

Fig 11–10. — Phlebogram of right leg of a 57-year-old female with a postoperative pulmonary embolus. A nonocclusive thrombus located at the junction of the superficial femoral vein and a tributary (*arrow*) was missed on Doppler examination. Otherwise phlebograms of both legs were negative.

usually can be detected by augmentation maneuvers after the examiner has located the anterior tibial artery. Absence of augmentation is presumptive evidence of obstruction.

Because the Doppler detects only the presence or absence of venous flow and only roughly its quantity, it is conceivable that a long, narrow clot originating in a valvular sinus of a major vein could escape discovery. Since such clots are prone to break away to form pulmonary emboli, failure to recognize their existence is perhaps the most serious of the potential limitations of the Doppler technique (Fig 11–10). Several reports indicate that it is possible, at least occasionally, to detect nonadherent thrombi on the basis of alterations in the venous flow pattern.[1, 6, 11] Unfortunately, there is no information in the literature documenting how frequently such thrombi are recognized.

SOURCES OF ERROR

Aside from the limitations discussed above, there are several other diagnostic pitfalls that the examiner should be aware of.

Previous Thrombophlebitis

The diagnostic difficulties encountered with the postphlebitic limb already have been alluded to. Errors can be avoided only by having knowledge of the preexisting venous flow patterns.

Poor Sound Transmission

Sound transmission through excessively fat legs, through hematoma and through scar tissue is poor. Allowances must be made when these conditions prevail. Use of a low frequency instrument (5 MHz) may improve the signal reception.

Excessive Pressure on the Probe

Although deep veins are relatively resistant to compression, occasionally they will be collapsed by local pressure exerted on the probe, thus giving the false impression of venous occlusion. Superficial veins collapse with the slightest external pressure. Consequently, when they are examined, the probe should not actually touch the skin but be coupled only through the acoustic gel. Ordinarily, unless a deep vein is being studied, the probe should just barely indent the skin. Occasionally, however, for a very deep vein, it may be necessary to apply considerable pressure.

Continuous Venous Signals

Although a nonfluctuating, continuous venous signal may indicate proximal obstruction, the examiner should be cognizant of other causes. In patients with congestive heart failure, the veins within the abdominal cavity may remain distended throughout the respiratory cycle despite periodic fluctuations of abdominal pressure. As a result, the venous signal in the legs will not fluctuate normally with respiration but will be relatively continuous. The presence of prominent cardiac pulsations is a clue to this situation.

Inflammatory processes within the leg may produce such high rates of venous flow that the signal becomes nearly continuous. The excessively high volume of flow and the typical physical findings of inflammation help differentiate this situation from the low volume continuous flow pattern associated with proximal obstruction.

Sluggish Venous Flow

Absence of a spontaneous venous signal can be due to reduced velocity of blood flow, especially in cases of peripheral vasoconstriction. Augmented signals also may be somewhat reduced. Comparison with the signal at the same level in the opposite limb should prevent the examiner from making an erroneous diagnosis of venous obstruction. Warming the legs or having the patient flex and extend his feet may increase blood flow sufficiently to produce a spontaneous signal.

Extrinsic Compression

Tense muscles in the calf or thigh can compress the underlying veins, reducing or abolishing the spontaneous signal. Flexing the legs at the hip and knee and reassuring the patient may avoid this problem.

External compression at the popliteal level is particularly troublesome. Even when all deep veins are completely patent, the signal at the popliteal and posterior tibial level may be absent or continuous and display poor augmentation. Knee surgery, ruptured popliteal cysts (Baker's cysts) and local hematomas from ruptured muscle bellies are the primary offenders. The presence of a perfectly normal superficial femoral signal suggests extrinsic compression rather than thrombosis. If uncertainty persists, a phlebogram should be obtained.

Iliac vein occlusion may be suspected when the inferior vena cava or pelvic veins are subjected to extrinsic compression by tumors, scar tissue or ascites. In these cases, the femoral vein will be patent and a good spontaneous, albeit continuous, signal will usually be obtained. When the iliac vein is thrombosed, the common femoral vein is usually also occluded.[5, 18]

Difficulties in the Popliteal Area

Even under the best of circumstances, the popliteal vein may be difficult to examine. Results must be interpreted with this in mind. Not only is the vein superficial to the artery, making it easy to compress, but it moves from lateral to medial across the popliteal space from above downward. Also, numerous other veins are crowded into the popliteal space. Tributaries include the sural veins, the lesser saphenous vein, and occasionally the anterior tibial vein. A glance at a venogram will reveal the complexity of the venous anatomy in this area.

Inexperience

Perhaps this is the most frequent cause of error. Careless, hastily performed examinations by persons unskilled in the techniques inevitably will lead to a high incidence of false positive and false negative studies.[1, 15]

Superficial Venous Thrombosis

Ordinarily, superficial thrombophlebitis is easily diagnosed clinically. The elongated patch of swollen, tender, skin with an underlying firm cord is typical. Consequently, the major role of the Doppler in these cases is to rule out concomitant deep venous involvement. However, occasionally localized erythema due to trauma, fat necrosis, cellulitis, vasculitis or lymphangitis may pose a problem in differential diagnosis.

Superficial thrombophlebitis is the presumptive diagnosis when no spontaneous or augmented venous signal can be heard over the area of inflammation, provided it is known that a vein passes through the region. On the other hand, if the inflammation is due to lymphangitis, cellulitis, etc., a venous signal should be readily demonstrated and may even display increased flow.[3] Prominent arterial flow signals in the area of inflammation may cause some confusion, but they should be easily differentiated from venous signals by their pulsatility and by the direction of blood flow.

Results

A number of investigators have evaluated the accuracy of Doppler ultrasound for diagnosing deep venous thrombosis by comparing the findings with those shown on phlebography. As shown in Table 11–2, the overall accuracy in more than 1,000 studies was 88%, ranging from 49 to 96%. The incidence of false positive diagnoses varied from 0 to 50% and of false negative diagnoses, from 0 to 52%. Inaccuracies appear to be increased when the examination is limited to the more proximal veins and when augmented signals are overemphasized.[2, 27]

Most of the errors have occurred in the below-knee examination. Of 78 false negative studies reported in the literature, 57 (73%) were the result of erroneous interpretations of popliteal and/or below-knee studies.[4, 8, 11, 12, 15, 17, 25, 32, 35] Because of these experiences, it is often stated that the Doppler technique is satisfactory for diagnosing

TABLE 11-2.—ACCURACY OF DOPPLER DIAGNOSIS OF
VENOUS THROMBOSIS

AUTHOR (DATE)	NO. OF STUDIES	% FALSE POSITIVE	% FALSE NEGATIVE	% OVERALL ACCURACY
Evans (1970)[8]	200	0	13	91
Milne et al. (1971)[17]	35	50	52	49
Sigel et al. (1972)[25]	248	19	12	86
Strandness and Sumner (1972)[32]	57	5	21	91
Yao et al. (1972)[35]	50	6	13	92
Holmes (1973)[11]	71	15	0	96
Johnson (1974)[12]	32	17	42	63
Barnes et al. (1975)[1]	122	8	4	94
Bolton and Hoffman (1975)[4]	76	21	24	78
McCaffrey et al. (1975)[15]	118	10	3	96
Total	1009	12	13	88

venous thrombosis above the knee, but that it is ineffectual below the knee.

In my opinion, these conclusions are unwarranted. True, isolated thrombi in the soleal and gastrocnemial sinusoids will be missed, but those within the posterior tibial veins should, in most cases, be detected. In a recent study, Barnes and his associates[2] found that the Doppler technique was accurate in 84% of limbs with below-knee disease. While the incidence of false positive studies was appreciable (32%), most of the false positive diagnoses were associated with other conditions which altered the venous flow velocity in the calf: for example, subfascial hematoma, cellulitis and muscle paralysis.

During the past year, the author has personally performed Doppler evaluations on 225 patients referred for consultation because of known or suspected venous disease. Of these, six were seen because of varicose veins, 53 for chronic venous insufficiency, and the remainder, 166, for acute deep venous thrombosis. Fifty-eight (35%) of the patients referred for suspected acute deep venous thrombosis had positive Doppler findings. Thirty had iliofemoral thrombosis and 28 had popliteal-tibial disease. Those patients (65%) with negative Doppler findings had suspected or proved pulmonary embolus, unexplained edema or pain in the legs, postoperative swelling in a limb following hip or knee surgery, pain in a postphlebitic extremity, or one of the diagnoses listed in Table 11-1.

Phlebograms were performed on 49 limbs at the discretion of the referring physician (Table 11-3). The overall accuracy was 94%

TABLE 11–3.—COMPARISON OF DOPPLER
FINDINGS WITH PHLEBOGRAPHY IN
49 LIMBS

| | PHLEBOGRAPHY | | |
	POSITIVE	NEGATIVE	TOTAL
Doppler Positive	20	2	22
Doppler Negative	1	26	27
Total	21	28	49

(46/49). There were 2/22 false positive studies (9%) and 1/27 false negatives (4%).

One of the false positive examinations was in a 52-year-old female who had persistent calf pain in her right leg for 2 months following a knee operation. Venous flow signals were entirely normal at all sites except over the right posterior tibial vein. Here the signal was not present spontaneously and the augmented flow, though present, was reduced in volume. The phlebogram was entirely negative. The other false positive examination occurred in a 74-year-old female who noted continual pain and swelling in her left ankle for 2 weeks after discharge from the hospital. All flow signals were normal except those in the left posterior tibial region where they were not spontaneously audible and were poor even with augmentation. Except for some incompetent perforators, the phlebogram was entirely negative.

The single false negative study was in a 47-year-old female who had undergone a left knee operation 1 month previously. After discharge she developed pleuritic chest pain and evidence of a pulmonary embolus on lung scan. Two days prior to my examination, she began having pain and tenderness in the left calf. Doppler flow signals were essentially normal at all levels, but the posterior tibial flow was more sluggish on the left side than on the right. Also, the left saphenous flow was somewhat more vigorous than that on the right. However, it was felt that these findings were not sufficiently marked to be diagnostic. The phlebogram showed very minimal deep venous thrombosis with a few clots located distally in the posterior tibial vein.

Conclusion

The use of Doppler ultrasound to diagnose deep venous thrombosis may be compared to the use of the stethoscope to diagnose cardiac disorders. With both instruments, experience, interpretive skill and clinical acumen are necessary to provide consistently good results.

These skills can be cultivated with a little patience and practice. Hasty, impatient and careless use of the instrument will result in many erroneous diagnoses and quickly cause the examiner to lose interest in the method.

Although several non-invasive methods have been developed for diagnosing thrombophlebitis, Doppler ultrasound has several distinct advantages over the others. When properly employed, it provides a convenient, rapid, accurate and inexpensive method for diagnosis of deep venous thrombosis. Simple nondirectional Doppler instruments with audio output are adequate for use in diagnosis of venous disease. The venous flow signals which are heard can be classified as spontaneous and augmented. Comparison of the signals between limbs is essential to the evaluation. Absence of flow, presence of continuous flow, lack of or decreased augmentation and increased flow in superficial veins are characteristic findings when the Doppler examination is performed in diagnosis of venous thrombosis. The examination has limitations when thrombosis is present in major tributary veins such as the internal iliac, profunda femoris, or calf muscle venous sinuses. Accuracy of the method ranges from 49 to 96% with an overall accuracy in more than 1,000 studies of 88%. Below-knee examinations account for 73% of all errors.

REFERENCES

1. Barnes, R. W., Russell, H. E., and Wilson, M. R.: *Doppler Ultrasonic Evaluation of Venous Disease, a Programmed Audiovisual Instruction* (2d ed.; Iowa City: University of Iowa, 1975) pp. 1–251.
2. Barnes, R. W., Russell, H. E., Wu, K. K., and Hoak, J. C.: Accuracy of Doppler ultrasound in clinically suspected venous thrombosis of the calf, Surg. Gynecol. Obstet. 143:425, 1976.
3. Barnes, R. W., Wu, K. K., and Hoak, J. C.: Differentiation of superficial thrombophlebitis from lymphangitis by Doppler ultrasound, Surg. Gynecol. Obstet. 143:23, 1976.
4. Bolton, J. P., and Hoffman, V. J.: Incidence of early post-operative iliofemoral thrombosis, Br. Med. J. 1: 247, 1975.
5. Diener, L.: Origin and Distribution of Venous Thrombi Studied by Postmortem Intraosseous Phlebography, in Nicolaides, A. N. (ed.): *Thromboembolism: Etiology, Advances in Prevention and Management* (Baltimore: University Park Press, 1975) pp. 149–166.
6. Doig, R. L., and Browse, N. L.: Rapid propagation of thrombus in deep vein thrombosis, Br. Med. J. 4:210, 1971.
7. Edwards, E. A., and Edwards, J. E.: The effect of thrombophlebitis on the venous valve, Surg. Gynecol. Obstet. 65: 310, 1937.
8. Evans, D. S.: The early diagnosis of deep-vein thrombosis by ultrasound, Br. J. Surg. 57: 726, 1970.
9. Fegan, W. G.: *Varicose Veins: Compression Sclerotherapy* (London: Heinemann, 1967).
10. Gunderson, J., and Hauge, M.: Hereditary factors in venous insufficiency, Angiology 20: 346, 1969.

11. Holmes M. C. G.: Deep venous thrombosis of the lower limbs diagnosed by ultrasound, Med. J. Aust. 1: 427, 1973.

12. Johnson, W. C.: Evaluation of newer techniques for the diagnosis of venous thrombosis, J. Surg. Res. 16: 473, 1974.

13. Kato, K., and Izumi, T. A.: A new ultrasonic Doppler flowmeter that can detect flow directions, Med. Ultrason. 5:28, 1970.

14. Lewis, J., Hobbs, J., and Yao, J.: Normal and Abnormal Femoral Vein Velocities, in Roberts, C. (ed.): *Blood Flow Measurement* (London: Sector Publishing Ltd., 1972) pp. 48–52.

15. McCaffrey, J., Williams, O., and Stathis, M.: Diagnosis of deep venous thrombosis using a Doppler ultrasonic technique, Surg. Gynecol. Obstet. 140: 740, 1975.

16. McLeod, F. D., Jr.: Directional Doppler demodulation, 20th Ann. Conf. on Engineering in Med. and Biol. 27: 1, 1967.

17. Milne, R. M., Gunn, A. A., Griffiths, J. M. T., and Ruckley, C. V.: Postoperative deep venous thrombosis. A comparison of diagnostic techniques, Lancet 2:445, 1971.

18. Nicolaides, A. N., and O'Connell, J. D.: Origin and Distribution of Thrombi in Patients Presenting with Clinical Deep Venous Thrombosis, in Nicolaides, A. N. (ed.): *Thromboembolism: Etiology, Advances in Prevention and Management* (Baltimore: University Park Press, 1975) pp. 167–180.

19. Nippa, J. H., Alexander, R. H., and Folse, R.: Pulse wave velocity in human veins, J. Appl. Physiol. 30: 558, 1971.

20. Nippa, J. H., Hokanson, D. E., Lee, D. R., Sumner, D. S., and Strandness, D. E., Jr.: Phase rotation for separating forward and reverse blood velocity signals, IEEE Trans Sonics and Ultrasonics, SU-22:340, 1975.

21. Reagan, B., and Folse, R.: Lower limb venous dynamics in normal persons and children of patients with varicose veins, Surg. Gynecol. Obstet. 132:15, 1971.

22. Rushmer, R. F., Baker, D. W., Johnson, W. L., and Strandness, D. E.: Clinical applications of a transcutaneous ultrasonic flow detector, JAMA 199: 326, 1967.

23. Satomura, S.: Study of the flow patterns in peripheral arteries by ultrasonics, J. Acoust. Soc. Japan 15:151, 1959.

24. Satomura, S., and Kaneko, Z.: Ultrasonic blood rheograph, 3rd Intern. Conf. Med. Electron., London, 1960, pp. 254–258.

25. Sigel, B., Felix, W. R., Jr., Popky, G. L., and Ipsen, J.: Diagnosis of lower limb venous thrombosis by Doppler ultrasound technique, Arch. Surg. 104:174, 1972.

26. Sigel, B., Popky, G. L., Boland, J. P., Wagner, D. K., and Mapp, E. McD.: Diagnosis of venous disease by ultrasonic flow detection, Surg. Forum 18:185, 1967.

27. Sigel, B., Popky, G. L., Mapp, E. M., Feigl, P., Felix, W. B., Jr., and Ipsen, J.: Evaluation of Doppler ultrasound examination. Its use in diagnosis of lower extremity venous disease, Arch. Surg. 100: 535, 1970.

28. Stegall, H. F., Rushmer, R. F., and Baker, D. W.: A transcutaneous ultrasonic blood-velocity meter, J. Appl. Physiol. 21: 707, 1966.

29. Strandness, D. E., Jr., Kennedy, J. W., Judge, T. P., and McLeod, F. D., Jr.: Transcutaneous directional flow detection: A preliminary report, Am. Heart J. 78: 65, 1969.

30. Strandness, D. E., Jr., McCutcheon, E. P., and Rushmer, R. F.: Application of a transcutaneous Doppler flowmeter in evaluation of occlusive arterial disease, Surg. Gynecol. Obstet. 122:1039, 1966.

31. Strandness, D. E., Jr., Schultz, R. D., Sumner, D. S., and Rushmer, R. F.: Ultrasonic flow detection. A useful technic in the evaluation of peripheral vascular disease, Am. J. Surg. 113: 311, 1967.

32. Strandness, D. E., Jr., and Sumner, D. S.: Ultrasonic velocity detector in the diagnosis of thrombophlebitis, Arch. Surg. 104:180, 1972.

33. Strandness, D. E., Jr., and Sumner, D. S.: *Hemodynamics for Surgeons* (New York: Grune & Stratton, 1975).

34. Sumner, D. S., Baker, D. W., and Strandness, D. E., Jr.: The ultrasonic velocity detector in a clinical study of venous disease, Arch. Surg. 97:75, 1968.

35. Yao, S. T., Gourmos, C., and Hobbs, J. T.: Detection of proximal-vein thrombosis by Doppler ultrasound flow-detection method, Lancet 1: 1, 1972.

12 / Diagnosis of Deep Venous Thrombosis by Phleborheography

JOHN J. CRANLEY, M.D., ARTHUR J. CANOS, M.D., AND
KRISHNAMURTHI MAHALINGAM, M.D.
*Kachelmacher Memorial Laboratory for Peripheral Venous Diseases and
the Department of Surgery, Good Samaritan Hospital, Cincinnati, Ohio*

PHLEBORHEOGRAPHY is a practical, highly reliable, noninvasive method of diagnosing deep venous thrombosis of the lower extremities.[1-6] Mainstream occlusive thrombi from the popliteal to the vena cava are regularly diagnosed and clots that involve several centimeters of the venous trunks below the knee usually are detected. Clots lying outside the main venous stream and some small clots in veins in the infrapopliteal area elude detection.

Since 1971 nearly 10,000 extremities have been tested for venous thrombosis at Good Samaritan Hospital or in our private office. We have come to rely on the phleborheograph in selecting patients for admission and in deciding whether or not to administer anticoagulant therapy. However, only a subgroup of 570 extremities with phleborheographic confirmation of the diagnosis comprises the statistical basis of this report. The phleborheographic technique currently is being employed in 16 other hospitals. Participating physicians report results substantially similar to ours.

Principles Involved

REDUCTION OF RESPIRATORY WAVES IN DEEP VENOUS THROMBOSIS

Normal breathing produces a rhythmic increase and decrease in the volume of the lower extremity, which is transmitted to the phleborheograph and recorded as an oscillation on the tracing synchronous with the wave produced by a recording cuff placed around the chest. Called respiratory waves, these oscillations are present in all normal extremities. Acute deep venous thrombosis obliterates or significantly reduces the size of the respiratory waves. With the development of collateral circulation, waves that have been absent usually reappear and those that have been smaller become larger. The change is noticeable in approximately 2 weeks. However, although these new waves appear or become larger, they may differ from normal waves in that they are relatively small and may be more rounded in configuration. In a patient with femoroiliac thrombophlebitis, it is a significant finding that respiratory waves may be visible in tracings from the leg if the veins of the leg are patent, despite the absence of waves in the thigh. On the basis of these findings, it is deduced that the respiratory influence travels down the limb through the collateral veins. Of special interest is the fact that respiratory waves in the lower extremity are usually larger in amplitude when the patient lies on his left side than those obtained when he is supine. Occasionally, also, the respiratory waves are larger when the patient lies on his right rather than on his left side. There is no full explanation for this phenomenon (see below).

Interference with Blood Outflow from Extremity

Deep venous thrombosis interferes with the normal outflow of blood from the extremity in response to rhythmic compression. Similar to active muscle contraction on walking, intermittent compression of the extremity propels blood proximally. A recording cuff proximal to the site of compression detects the momentary damming up of

Fig 12–1.—The lower extremities must be below heart level. This distends the veins and permits better transmission of hydraulic impulses.

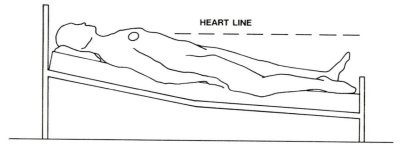

blood when venous thrombosis or extraluminal compression blocks its exit. Indicative of the blockage, a rise in base line of the volume recorder takes place. However, whenever compression is applied to the normal extremity when no impediment to venous outflow is present, the base line remains level. This phenomenon localizes the site of thrombosis. If the thigh tracing shows a stepwise rise while the calf is being compressed, the level of the obstruction to the deep veins is located above the thigh cuff. Rarely, external compression may be to blame. Otherwise, intraluminal thrombosis is present.

Similarly, if there is obstruction at or above the recording cuffs, compression of the foot causes a rise in base line of phleborheographic tracings from the leg. A rise in base line is unequivocal evidence of venous obstruction, with no known exceptions.

COMPRESSION OF THE CALF

Compression of the calf has two results: blood is propelled up the unobstructed extremity, and blood is siphoned out of the normal foot. When the calf is compressed, a recording cuff on the foot shows a fall in base line. Absent or less than normal foot emptying in the presence of a rise in base line and absent respiratory waves is indicative of acute deep venous thrombosis. More subject to artifacts than the others, this maneuver nevertheless permits detection of a normal tracing at a glance.

Technique

The patient lies quietly in bed with the lower extremities approximately 10 degrees below heart level (Fig. 12–1). The first four cuffs of the phleborheograph are for recording only (Fig. 12–2). Cuff 1 is placed around the thorax. Cuff 2 is applied to the midthigh, cuff 3 to the upper part of the calf and cuff 4 to the midcalf. Cuff 5 on the lower calf and cuff 6 on the foot are used to record transmitted impulses and also to apply compression. There are two operational modes: runs A and B. In run A, all cuffs on the thigh and leg record the responses to compression of the foot by applying pressure to the foot cuff. In run B pressure is applied to the lower calf (cuff 5). All other cuffs record the response, including the cuff on the foot (cuff 6), which records changes in pedal volume. In applying the cuffs care must be taken to place the bladder of the cuff dorsally. Otherwise, artifacts will result from the extremity resting on the bladder.

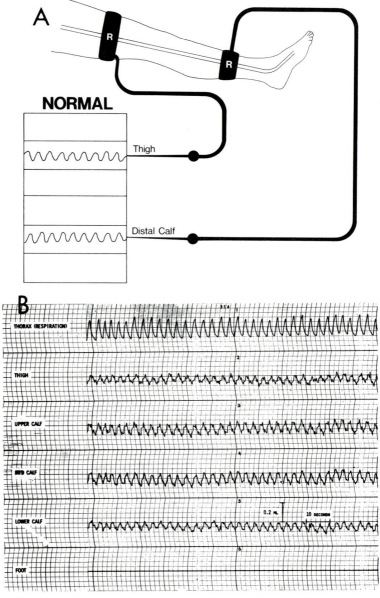

Fig 12–2.—**A,** diagram showing recording cuff on thigh and lower calf. **B,** normal tracing. *First line* is from pneumatic cuff placed around epigastrium to record actual respiration. Tracings of thigh, upper calf, midcalf and lower calf show large respiratory waves always seen in a normal subject. The *sixth channel* is for application of pressure, nonfunctioning at this setting.

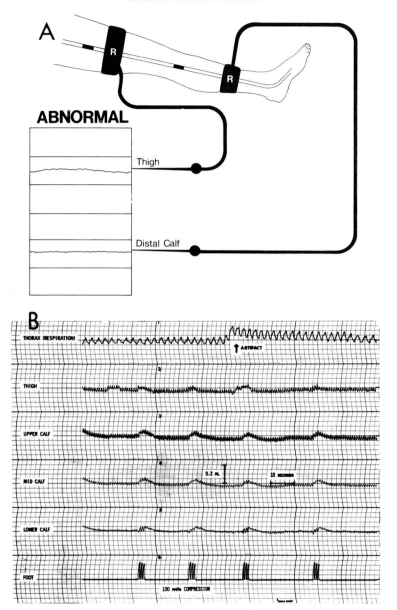

Fig 12–3.—A, diagrammatic representation of clots in deep veins obliterating the normal respiratory waves. **B,** tracing of actual subject to demonstrate absence of respiratory waves in thigh, upper calf, midcalf and lower calf in a patient with acute deep thrombophlebitis. A rise in baseline also is seen each time the foot is compressed.

RUN A: FOOT COMPRESSION

The recording cuffs are automatically inflated to 10 mm Hg pressure. The chart speed is 2.5 mm/sec. Calibration is performed by adjusting the amplification so that the 0.2-ml volume calibrator causes a 2-cm pen deflection. Respiratory waves are observed first. Following this, the compress control is operated, and three short bursts of pressure – 100 mm Hg – are delivered to the foot (cuff 6), 0.5 sec in duration and at 0.5-sec intervals. About 40% of the pressure is expended in inflating the cuff, so that actually only about 60 mm Hg of pressure is exerted on the foot.

While the recording pen may move erratically with application of pressure, in a normal extremity the base line remains level. If there is interference with the outflow of blood from the extremity, the base line rises with each successive compression as the extremity swells; this is caused by the blood damming up (Fig 12–3). If this occurs, time is allowed for the pen to return to the base line before the next series of compressions is applied. This maneuver is repeated at least three times, but if there is any interference with the tracing for any reason whatever, pressure may be applied as often as necessary.

If the respiratory waves appear to be smaller than usual, the patient is turned on his left side with both knees slightly flexed, the right leg lying behind the left. This maneuver increases the size of the respiratory waves; however, in a patient with acute deep venous thrombosis, changing his position does not restore the obliterated waves.

RUN B: CALF COMPRESSION

The recording cuff on the lower part of the calf (cuff 5) now becomes a compression cuff, while the cuff on the foot (cuff 6) is converted to a recording cuff. In this run, operating the compress control automatically causes 50 mm Hg of pressure to compress the cuff on the calf three times, similar to compression of the foot in run A. Again, about 40% of this pressure is expended in inflating the cuff, so that actually only about 30 mm Hg of pressure is exerted on the calf.

Emptying of the foot is observed. This decrease in volume of the foot is demonstrated in the tracing (cuff 6) by a fall in base line. This test is repeated at least three times. Time must be allowed for the pen to return to its base line before the next application of pressure. In a fully normal extremity, the pen base line falls at least 3 cm, corresponding to a 0.3-ml volume change under a cuff whose dimensions are 9 ×17 cm.

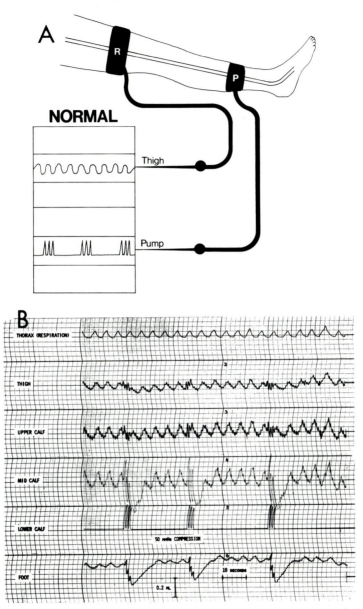

Fig 12–4. – **A,** diagrammatic tracing of normal limb. Application of pressure to calf does not influence the baseline of the recording taken from the thigh. This is because there is no obstruction to the flow of blood from the limb. **B,** actual tracing. Compression of the lower calf does not produce a rise in baseline of the thigh or upper calf tracing. Reduction of volume in midcalf and foot is explained in Figure 12–8.

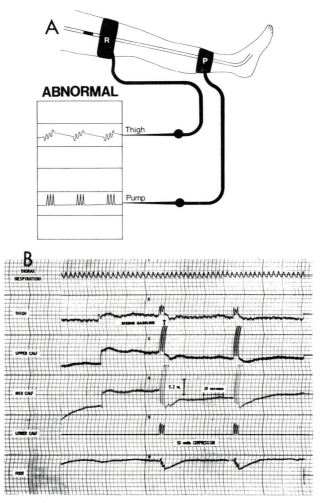

Fig 12–5.– **A,** diagrammatic tracing of clot in deep femoral vein. Pressure applied to calf forces blood proximally causing a rise in baseline, as shown in thigh recording, reflecting a minute swelling of thigh due to obstruction to outflow of blood from the limb. **B,** actual tracing demonstrating rise in baseline of tracing in upper calf and thigh as calf is compressed. Rise in baseline of thigh and upper calf (*tracings 2* and *3*) as the thigh is compressed (*tracing 5*). Also shown is lack of normal emptying of foot, absence of respiratory waves in foot, midcalf and upper calf and small visible respiratory waves in thigh. This suggests that the clot extends above the thigh recording cuff but is not typical of occlusion of common femoral vein.

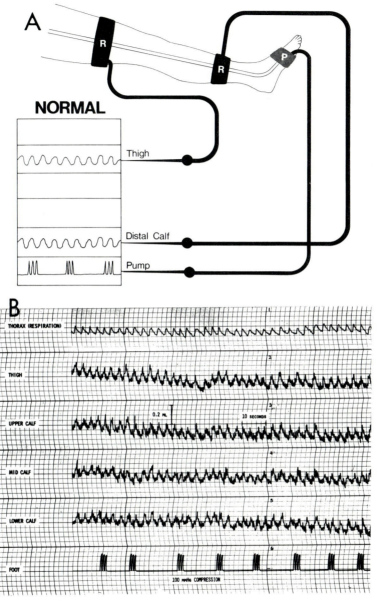

Fig 12–6.—**A,** diagrammatic representation of application of pressure to foot while recording from calf and thigh in a normal subject. **B,** actual tracing demonstrating large respiratory waves in thigh, upper calf, midcalf and lower calf; also note absence of rise in baseline each time compression is applied to the foot.

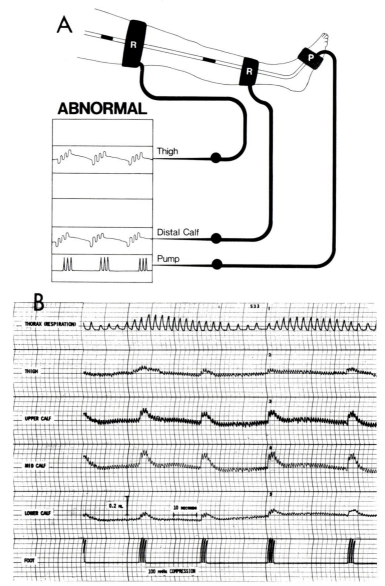

Fig 12–7.—**A,** diagrammatic representation of application of 100 mm Hg of pressure to foot, causing a rise in baseline in the volume recorder when there are clots in the deep venous system. **B,** actual tracing demonstrating rise in baseline in entire extremity each time pressure is applied to foot, indicating obstruction. Also note absence of respiratory waves, indicating that the process is acute. Also shown is the fact that this patient has Cheyne-Stokes respiration (*tracing 1*).

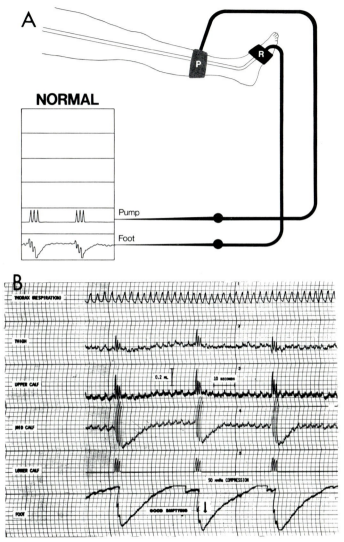

Fig 12–8.— A, diagrammatic representation of fact that application of pressure to calf reduces volume in foot as blood is siphoned out of foot and up the extremity. **B,** actual representation of normal subject. Note that there is excellent and prompt emptying of foot each time the calf is compressed. This emptying is mimicked in the midcalf. There is no distinct rise in baseline in thigh or upper calf. Respiratory waves are clearly visible in thigh and leg. All of these factors indicate a normal extremity. It is also of interest that the filling time of the foot, approximately 18 sec (nine 2-sec lines), is significantly longer than that seen in the postphlebitic limb.

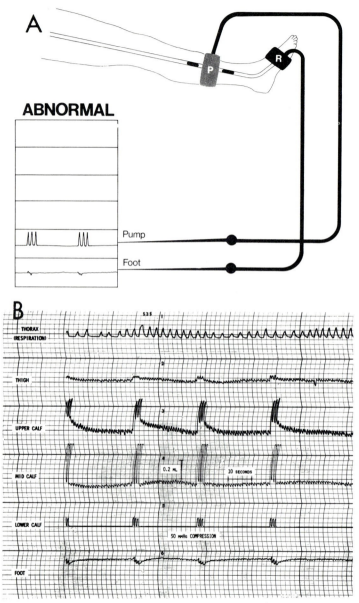

Fig 12–9.–A, diagrammatic representation of abnormal tracing demonstrating that the normal emptying of foot is reduced or absent in the patient with deep venous thrombosis. **B,** actual tracing demonstrating poor emptying of foot. This also shows a rise in baseline in thigh, upper calf and midcalf, and absence of respiratory waves. This is typical of a patient with acute deep venous thrombosis.

As the lower part of the calf is compressed, the recording from the midcalf normally falls somewhat, mimicking the fall in base line of the foot. On the other hand, the base line of the tracing from the upper part of the calf and lower part of the thigh remains level (Fig. 12–4). However, if any obstruction to the deep venous system exists above the recording cuff, a rise in the base line occurs that is progressive with each compression (Figs. 12–5, 12–6 and 12–7). In extensive thrombophlebitis this may be a sharp, abrupt rise; on the other hand, a stepwise rise of whatever magnitude is significant (Figs. 12–8 and 12–9).

The phleborheograph has three frequency function settings: respiration, phleborheography and pulse. If the arterial pulses are large, it may be difficult to identify the respiratory waves. Setting the function switch to respiration filters out the arterial pulse and permits clear visualization of the respiratory waves. At this function setting, a false rise in pen base line may be observed during foot and calf compression. This is accounted for by the additional time at this function setting for the pen to return to its base line.

For study of the arterial circulation, the function switch can be changed to pulse. Thus the phleborheograph becomes a five-channel pulse volume recorder. At this function setting the instrument can also be used as a five-channel digital plethysmograph.

Results

In the developmental stages of our work, which terminated in January 1974, 412 tests were done using a standard polygraph. Since then, an instrument especially designed for diagnosing deep venous thrombosis, the phleborheograph, has been in regular clinical use at Good Samaritan Hospital. It is a reassuring commentary on the basic soundness of the fundamental thesis that the results in both the experimental and clinical series have turned out to be identical after exclusion of technical and interpretational errors. Mechanization of the equipment has eliminated much of the work formerly done manually by the technician, an improvement that insures more uniformity in positioning and inflating the pressure cuffs on the extremity under study.

Presently, 570 extremities of patients in whom the diagnosis of acute deep venous thrombosis was suspected have been evaluated by phlebography as well as phleborheography. The change in correlation rates has been minimal: 96% using the polygraph and 97% using the phleborheograph. Similarly, the change in percentage of inherent errors has been barely perceptible, for both series approximately 5% false negatives and 1.5% false positives. All false negatives were in

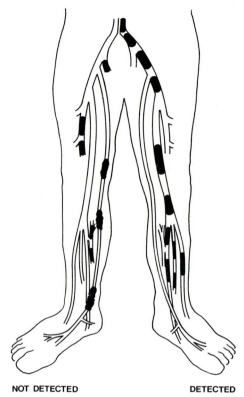

NOT DETECTED   DETECTED

Fig 12–10.–Diagrammatic demonstration of clots not detected by this method on the right side and those detected on the left side. Clots in the saphenous system, the soleal veins and an isolated clot in the deep femoral vein or the hypogastric vein are not detected. On the left side are shown clots that are detected, i.e., clots in the anterior and posterior tibial, peroneal, popliteal, femoral, external and common iliac veins and the vena cava. (From Cranley, J. J.: *Vascular Surgery. Vol. II: Peripheral Venous Diseases* [Hagerstown, Md.: Harper & Row, 1975]. Used by permission.)

veins of the leg below the popliteal. In a group of 43 phlebograms visualizing clots limited to the infrapopliteal area, 12 (28%) went undetected by phleborheography (Fig. 12–10).

Discussion

Advantages of Phleborheography

The advantages of this modality may be divided into two categories, those pertaining to the method and those pertaining to the equipment.

The Method

This method is noninvasive and painless and involves physiologic principles. It is performed by a technician in 20–45 min, and the recordings are interpreted by a physician. Approximately 80% of the tracings can be sight-read by an experienced physician; the remaining 20% require close scrutiny. The test permits one to distinguish clearly between acute and chronic processes. Actually, the test measures only two variables. The first is the presence or absence of obstruction in the deep venous system. The second is the measurement of the collateral venous circulation as indicated by the presence or absence and the size and configuration of the respiratory waves. If there is evidence of obstruction without respiratory waves, the process is acute. If there is obstruction in the presence of small respiratory waves, the process is subacute. If there is obstruction in the presence of large respiratory waves, the process is chronic. Serial tracings show the gradual transition from the acute occlusion to the development of the chronic state or to the dissolution of the thrombi. It is helpful to keep the tracings for future reference.

The Equipment

Advantages of the phleborheograph are that the method is mechanical, capable of precise volumetric calibration. The equipment is an adaptation of the basic Grass polygraph, which has proved reliability over a 30-year period. The versatility of the polygraph is carried over into the phleborheograph. For example, the equipment may be used with a photocell on the fingertip or on the earlobe. The photocell is highly sensitive and produces large wave forms whose characteristics may be studied. It is not, however, capable of being calibrated volumetrically. A digital oncometer may be applied to the finger to study volumetric changes in the digit as a digital plethysmograph. This may be calibrated volumetrically. An encircling cuff, such as that used in the standard technique on the limbs, may be made for the fingers or toes and thus one can observe the amplitude of the pulsation which may be calibrated volumetrically as related to the size of the cuff used.

A uni- or bidirectional Doppler ultrasonic flowmeter may be connected to the phleborheograph and a permanent tracing made. Analysis of simultaneous tracings made by the Doppler technique, which is related to flow, and the cuff technique, which is related primarily to pressure changes, may offer hope of eliciting more information. If desired, an electrocardiograph panel may be inserted and the time relationship between the cardiac pulse and other tracings in the limb may be studied.

DISADVANTAGES

The greatest problems in the development of phleborheography have been due to the fact that the technique is new and must be learned, and that interpretation of the tracings is not always easy. Although it is possible to describe in writing technical guidelines and the involved principles, it is not possible to become adept at this method by studying the literature alone. Actual experience is necessary. Some physicians find this unacceptable for various reasons. However, all physicians and technicians who have learned the method to date have supported the manufacturer's decision to make the learning experience a condition of sale.

The technician must learn to recognize an abnormal pattern and then to maneuver the patient to various positions to see if the tracing reverts to normal. If it does, the tracing is considered normal. On the other hand, if the tracing is positive, it is impossible to make it appear to be normal by any maneuvering of the patient's position. The fact that the tracing may be normal, for example, when the patient lies on his left side and abnormal when he is supine indicates that the main venous channels are compressed in certain positions. The most common example is compression of the popliteal vein by the extended knee. This phenomenon has been documented radiologically by Arkoff et al.[7] Similarly, flexion of the thigh may compress the femoral vein in the inguinal area. Many times it is not possible to determine why the veins are compressed in a particular position. However, we have come to believe that the tracing is an accurate reflection of the physiologic status of the venous tree at the moment of recording. It is revealing some actualities of the physiologic state previously unrecognized.

The technician must be aware of these hemodynamic vagaries. He must also recognize that misapplication of the cuff may produce mechanical artifacts. For example, if the bladder of the cuff lies under the limb, gross artifacts can be produced. If the compressing cuff does not fit snugly on the limb, compression of the bladder will not propel blood up the limb and thus cause a rise in base line in the presence of deep venous thrombosis. With 4 or 5 days of training and study of several hundred illustrative tracings, the physician will experience little difficulty in reading most phleborheograms. However, there can be no question that those who interpret tracings daily soon develop expertise that cannot be gained otherwise. The experienced person is able to detect an artifact not apparent to others and to recognize minor changes in the tracing as being indicative of an abnormality that is entirely missed by a casual observer.

Some of the more common subtle changes may be listed here: (1) A patient with a very small occluding thrombus may have a rise in base line with normal appearing respiratory waves just as is seen in the patient with the postphlebitic syndrome. This combination is also apparent immediately following surgical ligation of a vein. In other words, there is an occlusion with good collateral circulation. In such instances, the clinical history is valuable. (2) A second point of importance is that any rise in base line that is consistently present is significant, even though the rise may be of small size. Thus, a clot in a limb with large venous collaterals will show a less obstructed pattern than one with small collateral venous channels. (3) The patient with the typical clinical postphlebitic syndrome almost invariably shows some evidence of deep venous obstruction and a well-developed collateral circulation. On the other hand, in some limbs with acute deep venous thrombosis, the phleborheographic pattern gradually becomes normal. This is interpreted to mean that there has been complete recanalization of the clot. It is not possible to obtain confirmatory phlebograms on most such patients who have left the hospital and are asymptomatic.

A thrombus that is attached to a vein wall but does not occlude the vein is not detected by phleborheography. This may explain the significantly higher incidence of deep vein thrombosis as detected by the radioactive fibrinogen uptake test than by this method. On the other hand, it is questionable whether such a thrombus is clinically significant until the vein is occluded and the soft jelly-like clot forms on the head of the thrombus.

A patient with the typical postphlebitic syndrome may develop an area of acute deep venous thrombosis that is difficult to detect early. The reason is that the respiratory waves, being very large due to the postphlebitic syndrome, may be reduced significantly in size but still appear to be within normal limits. In order to detect it, the physician must have a high index of suspicion if a patient with chronic deep venous insufficiency develops new symptoms. His course should be followed carefully.

A final problem that has surfaced during our 5 years of work on this project is the patient who develops some symptoms of deep venous thrombosis, for example, due to muscular vein thrombosis, and who may have a normal phleborheogram. One or 2 weeks later, he has a major venous thrombosis that may be missed entirely if a second phleborheogram is not obtained. In the presence of symptoms that persist, or if the physician suspects deep venous thrombosis, it is well to repeat the test in 3–5 days.

Phleborheography has proved to be a practical and highly useful method of detecting deep venous thrombosis by us and by all those who are currently using it. It is not a perfect method in that small clots below the knee are not always detected. It requires a carefully trained, alert technician. It is a fact that some patients with proved pulmonary embolism may be found to have a normal phleborheogram and indeed, a clearly patent venous tree from ankles to the vena cava by phlebography. Whether or not these thrombi have come from a hidden source, such as the hypogastric vein, or from the main trunks and have broken off completely, leaving an empty vein, cannot be demonstrated at this time. All in all, however, phleborheography has proved highly useful to us not only in diagnosing deep venous thrombosis but also in helping us improve our understanding of the physiology of the venous circulation of the lower extremities.

Summary

Phleborheography has reached the state of development where it can be said to be a practical, highly reliable noninvasive method of diagnosing deep venous thrombosis of the lower extremities. A 5-year experience examining nearly 10,000 extremities at the Good Samaritan Hospital has caused us to rely on the phleborheograph in selecting patients for admission for treatment of deep venous thrombosis. A subgroup of 570 extremities with phlebographic confirmation of the diagnosis comprises the statistical basis of this report. There has been a 97% correlation of diagnoses using the phleborheograph and phlebography. There have been approximately 5% false negatives and 1.5% false positive examinations. All false negative examinations were in veins of the leg distal to the popliteal.

Some problems with the method include the diagnosis of a thrombus which is not totally occlusive and the patient with typical postphlebitic syndrome who develops an acute deep venous thrombosis may also be difficult to detect early. Nevertheless, phleborheography has proved to be a practical and highly useful method of detecting acute deep venous thrombosis.

REFERENCES

1. Cranley, J. J.: *Vascular Surgery. Vol. II: Peripheral Venous Diseases* (Hagerstown, Md.: Harper & Row, 1975), Chapter 4.

2. Cranley, J. J., Gay, A. Y., Grass, A.M., and Simeone, F. A.: A plethysmographic technique for the diagnosis of deep venous thrombosis of the lower extremities, Surg. Gynecol. Obstet. 136: 385, 1973.
3. Cranley, J. J.: Phleborheography, R. I. Med. J. 58: 111, 1975.
4. Cranley, J. J., Canos, A. J., Sull, W. J., and Grass, A. M.: Phleborheographic technique for diagnosing deep venous thrombosis of the lower extremities, Surg. Gynecol. Obstet. 141:331, 1975.
5. Cranley, J. J., Canos, A. J., and Sull, W. J.: Diagnosis of deep venous thrombosis: Fallibility of clinical symptoms and signs, Arch. Surg. 111:34, 1976.
6. Cranley, J. J., Canos, A. J., and Mahalingam, K.: in Madden, J. L., and Hume, M. (eds.): *Venous Thrombosis: Prophylaxis and Treatment* (New York: Appleton-Century-Crofts, 1976), Chapter 8.
7. Arkoff, R. S., Gilfillan, R. S., and Burhenne, H. J.: A simple method for lower extremity phlebography: Pseudo-obstruction of the popliteal vein, Radiology 90: 66, 1968.

Discussion: Chapters 10 through 12

DR. EUGENE STRANDNESS: I think one lesson is to be learned. Every diagnostic technique has its problems. That includes fibrinogen as well as all of the noninvasive tests. I don't think these tests should be considered to be in conflict with each other, but should be considered to be complementary.

Noninvasive tests, as far as we know, have no adverse effects, but the problem of the false positive and false negative errors is important. If you look at the literature very carefully, and if you look at the places that are doing these tests in the best possible manner, the false positive rate will be in the range of 10%, and the false negative rate will also be in the range of 10%. Translated to patients, this means one in 10 patients will have a thrombus that might be missed and, similarly, one in 10 was labeled with having the disease when it was absent.

The basis for the false negative result is thrombi located in segments which are not accessible to the techniques. A profunda femoris vein cannot be visualized by any of the noninvasive techniques. As a matter of fact, venography is noneffective here also. Similarly, we cannot detect any of the clots that arise in the pelvis unless they involve the major iliac veins themselves.

False positive tests probably occur when the examination is improperly performed or there are coexisting conditions that interfere with venous outflow from the limbs. These have been summarized in recent papers by Dr. Robert Barnes.

The question is, can we fully rely on the tests and proceed with or without treatment on the basis of the tests alone. This is where clinical judgement is required. I think it is important, as has been emphasized by Doctor Wheeler and Doctor de Takats, not to put clinical judgement aside in favor of instrumentation.

Under any circumstance when you strongly suspect that either a patient has venous thrombosis and the tests fail to show this, or the reverse is true, and your therapeutic decision is going to be very criti-

206

cal, we would strongly recommend that a phlebogram be carried out. However, we are firmly convinced that, if the noninvasive techniques are carried out with the same dedication as a good phlebogram, these tests will be very useful in the bedside clinical evaluation of patients with suspected deep venous thrombosis.

DR. JOHN PFEIFER: We have utilized in an office noninvasive laboratory for the past two years both the impedance technique and the phleborheography (PRG) technique of Doctor Cranley. In the past two years, we have done a great many studies with PRG. In that group of patients, we have had two false positives, both of which could be interpreted retrospectively as having been old venous disease with inadequate collateralization where the tracings were misread, giving us an accuracy with the PRG of approximately 96%.

A very important side benefit of this unit in the office is that it has reduced our admissions to the hospital for deep vein thrombi by approximately 50% in the past 2 years. In those patients where we were clinically convinced we were dealing with deep vein thrombosis and did not believe the negative PRG tracing, when we admitted the patient to the hospital, we found that the venograms were negative and the patient did not have deep vein thrombosis.

Our experience with the impedance technique has not been as good. We have had a higher rate of inaccuracy. Approximately 15% false negative and 15% false positive results were obtained, but our study with impedance techniques has not been as tightly controlled as Doctor Wheeler's.

Our experience with the Doppler examination has been that it is very difficult to get an accurate reading. Again, we have not applied the enthusiasm or the precision to this technique that Doctor Sumner has.

DR. STEVEN DOSICK: We have found at the Medical College of Ohio a difference in the accuracy rates between the different Doppler instruments. We reported originally an accuracy of 95% at the American Heart Association meeting with a 5 MHz unit. The 9 MHz unit, when used in our hands on 50 patients, has shown a 15% lower accuracy rate. The penetration at the popliteal and femoral is not very deep, as compared to the 5 MHz unit. I think when you are comparing studies, you may be comparing apples and oranges unless you take into consideration the type of unit used.

DR. WILLARD JOHNSON: I would like to ask Doctors Wheeler and Cranley about the role of arterial insufficiency in regard to their false positives. Is there an ankle Doppler pressure that may preclude an accurate examination?

DR. FRANK MURPHY: We have been using Doctor Cranley's phleborheograph in the past year and one-half, and found it very useful as a screening test, especially on outpatients. You have a concept that a patient has phlebitis or no phlebitis, you run this test, the respiratory waves are good, and you can safely say the patient does not have phlebitis.

We have done 200 studies and we have done 30 venograms. We cross-check both ways. Clinically, if we have evidence of phlebitis, and our phleborheogram says no, we do a venogram. If the phleborheogram says positive and clinically we say no, we do a venogram. In the 30 venograms, we have missed two thrombi, both in the calf veins. We have not missed any from the popliteal vein. So, we are very pleased with this instrument, and would recommend it for use in the office and also in postoperative patients.

DR. LAZAR GREENFIELD: I would like to ask the authors on noninvasive techniques two questions. First, if they are willing to anticoagulate a patient for a long period of time on the basis of a single study and, second, whether or not there is any correlation between the extent of disease as documented by their studies and pulmonary embolic episodes.

DR. WILLIAM BAKER: As moderator, I would like to ask a few questions. First, Doctor Sumner, your statistics are very impressive. Were the results obtained by you or did a technician obtain those results? Do you think a technician can get as accurate results as an interested physician? Second, I would like to ask everybody what they do with a patient with known chronic venous disease who comes in with the question of new, acute thrombophlebitis.

DR. BROWNELL WHEELER: The patient who has had old phlebitis who comes in with a question of fresh phlebitis is a difficult patient. We find that often these patients have normal tests on plethysmography. In that case, we are reassured, but we often end up getting a phlebogram to be absolutely sure.

My first general comment would be that I think there is no point in Doctor Sumner buying Doctor Cranley's phleborheograph. It is obvious that he does very well indeed with the Doppler. All of the techniques work very well in the hands of people who are used to them and most familiar with them. Now, Doctor Sumner did talk about experienced hands. The examination that he does is more complex than the original one described by Sigal. He commented on some variability in results, which certainly has been our experience, too. I think his is a very good technique for screening as an extension of physical examination.

I carry a pocket Doppler and use it for venous disease. I have the phleborheograph which works well and gives a lot of associated information. It is also a multichannel recorder which has a lot of potential for other uses.

Our own emphasis has been to try to develop a rather central test that is idiot-proof and has general practicability.

I was interested in the discussants' comments on differences in Doppler equipment. You might be comparing apples and oranges. I was also interested in Doctor Pfeifer's comments about 15% false negative and false positive results with impedance. He does use different instrumentation. As far as I know, the figures for everybody using the equipment, the technique and the method of interpretation that I described are the same.

With respect to Doctor Johnson's question about arterial insufficiency and its effect on plethysmographic techniques: the only difference it makes is that it may take longer to accumulate venous volume after inflation of the cuff. Sometimes in patients like that, we like to leave the cuff inflated for up to 2 min., rather than the normal 45 sec. Other than that, it makes no difference whatsoever.

We haven't done a correlation of Doppler ankle pressures, but I don't think there is a Doppler ankle pressure below which you cannot do this test, provided you wait long enough.

With respect to Doctor Greenfield's questions, he asked, are you willing to anticoagulate on the basis of your test. Absolutely, but only in the context of clinical judgment as emphasized by Doctor Strandness. I use the results of the test like I would use the result of any laboratory test. A white count of 10,000 means something different than one of 5,000, or one of 20,000 in a clinical context. An impedance result that is on a diagonal line which separates all normal from abnormal results has a totally different meaning from one way up or way down, depending on the clinical context. On the basis of clinical judgement, I will anticoagulate or will not anticoagulate on the basis of that test in a given clinical situation.

As to the extent of disease versus the incidence of pulmonary embolism: the feeling I have is that most of the clinically significant pulmonary emboli come from femoral, popliteal or iliac veins. I am more worried about the ones up around the groin than those lower down. However, our test will give an abnormal result all of the way from the popliteal vein right up to the femoral vein.

DR. LOWELL BROWN: Doctor Sumner, how long does it take you to do your Doppler examination?

DR. DAVID SUMNER: I was very interested in the remarks about the type of Dopplers that are used. Actually, I think you can get very good results with any type of Doppler that you want to use, but the 5 MHz does have the advantage of having a greater penetration. Therefore, it is easier in some heavier patients to hear the venous flow in the superficial femoral vein or the popliteal vein with the 5 MHz unit. It is not as good for examination of the posterior tibial vein.

If you want to detect clots below the knee, the 10 MHz Doppler applied very lightly to the skin; actually, just coupled to the skin with the gel, is by far the best method of examining that vein. In about 95% of the normal people, you can hear a good phasic flow signal in that way. If I am doing tests in the laboratory, I use the 5 MHz unit and the 10 MHz or the 9 MHz Doppler units simultaneously.

How long it takes me to do the examination depends on the type of patient. Some are very easy, and it will only take about 10 min. Some may take as long as 25 min because, if the examination is not clear cut, you must examine all sites carefully and repeat the examination.

Doctor Baker asked, did I do those tests or did a technician. The ones I selected for this presentation were ones that I had done personally and not the ones that the technician had done. There are skilled technicians around this country who can perform the Doppler examination with the same degree of accuracy.

Doctor Baker also asked about old thrombophlebitis. That is, indeed, one of the confusing areas. However, there are usually enough clues that distinguish between an old and an acute thrombophlebitis. The presence of the collaterals will give a clue, for example. If there is any question, we would do a phlebogram on such patients.

Doctor Greenfield asked, do we anticoagulate on the basis of these studies. The answer is that we anticoagulate or don't anticoagulate on the basis of the studies. Only about one fourth of the patients will undergo a venogram. It ends up that the ones that I order are about one tenth of the studies which would have been done before the Doppler. So, that is the final diagnostic technique in most of the patients that I see. As to the extent of the disease and pulmonary embolism: a number of the patients with pulmonary embolism will have a negative Doppler study.

DR. JOHN CRANLEY: In answer to the first question, arterial disease and lymphatic disease have no effect on the phleborheographic test for thrombosis. In answer to the second question, the patient is treated or not treated with anticoagulant therapy on the basis of the test. This is one of our problems. We would like to continue to obtain phlebograms frequently enough in order to document results. However, the confidence of our staff in this test is such that it is getting more and more difficult to obtain confirmatory phlebograms in our hospital.

In answer to the third question, we have seen pulmonary emboli in a patient with a negative phleborheogram and with a negative phlebogram. We have seen a positive phleborheographic test become negative immediately after lodgment of a pulmonary embolus. Formerly, we thought some clot always remained in the vein. Today, we believe this is not always true. In some instances the whole clot may break loose.

Finally, we do make an attempt to locate the clot by the phleborheographic technique. If the acute clot occludes the femoral or iliac vein, the location is rarely in doubt. If the test shows an acute obstruction in the leg, we like to determine whether or not it extends into the popliteal, and if so, how high. If a patient is examined with phlegmasia cerulea dolens with clotting of all the major veins, there may be no respiratory waves visible and indeed, not even a rise in base line on distal compression. In this case, squeezing the calf does not cause blood to flow up the leg because all the large veins are clotted.

13 / Diagnosis of Venous Thrombosis by the ¹²⁵I-Fibrinogen Test

A. N. NICOLAIDES, M.S., F.R.C.S., F.R.C.S.E.

Senior Lecturer and Honorary Consultant Surgeon to the Cardiovascular Unit and Director of the Vascular Laboratory, St. Mary's Hospital Medical School, London, England

AND

JOHN T. HOBBS, M.D., F.R.C.S.

Consultant Surgeon and Senior Lecturer, St. Mary's Hospital Medical School, London, England

THE RADIOACTIVE FIBRINOGEN test is now regarded as the most sensitive method for detecting the presence of a developing thrombus and whether it is extending or lysing. The test is based on the experimental demonstration that ¹³¹I-fibrinogen injected into the circulation is incorporated into a forming thrombus as ¹³¹I-fibrin (Fig 13–1) which can be detected by an external scintillation counter.[1, 2] The feasibility of this method first was demonstrated in a patient who received 90 μCi of ¹³¹I-fibrinogen 1 hr before treatment of varicose veins by injection sclerotherapy in July 1961, in Boston.[3] Subsequently the test was used to confirm the presence of deep venous thrombosis which had been clinically diagnosed.[4] In 1965 ¹²⁵I was used instead of ¹³¹I as the radioactive label.[5] ¹²⁵I has a longer half-life (60 days) than ¹³¹I (8 days) and it emits much lower energy gamma radiation so that lighter and more mobile apparatus can be used. The accuracy of the test has been confirmed by venography[6, 7] and by using a ratemeter[8] it has become a simple test suitable for routine screening of a large number of patients.

The authors have so far used this test in over 1,000 patients and the information presented here is based not only on a review of the literature, but also on their own experience.

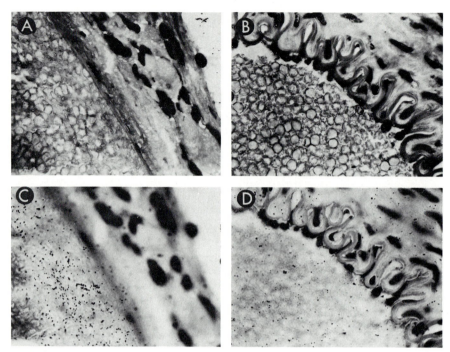

Fig 13–1.—Autoradiographs of long saphenous vein containing thrombus, and of saphenous artery of rabbit; × 670. **A** (vein) and **B** (artery) 2 days after 50 μCi ^{131}I-fibrinogen. **C** (vein) and **D** (artery) 3 days after 46 μCi ^{131}I-fibrinogen. (From Hobbs.[2])

Quality of ^{125}I-Fibrinogen

Human fibrinogen is obtained from a selected pool of donors whose blood has been used on at least five occasions without any occurrence of serum hepatitis in the recipients and in whom Australian antigen cannot be demonstrated at the time of collection.

Initially most workers had to label the fibrinogen themselves. It was soon realized that the "jet iodination" technique[9] was the best method of labeling because it produced the minimum of denaturation of the fibrinogen, although only 30–50% of the isotope was tagged to the protein. Labelling with a higher efficiency using the "chloramine-T" method was associated with considerable denaturation of the fibrinogen molecule. This was obvious because the fibrinogen would be removed from the circulation quickly and the radioactivity over the heart and legs would become too low within 24–48 hr.

These problems soon were overcome and in England there is now an excellent commercially available preparation of high clotability and Australian antigen-free ^{125}I-fibrinogen (Radiochemical Centre, Amersham). A single dose (1.1 mg fibrinogen labelled with 100 μCi of ^{125}I) provides enough radioactivity for scanning the patient's legs for 1 week.

Details of the Method

The thyroid gland is saturated by sodium iodide (100 mg) given orally 24 hr or intravenously one-half hour before intravenous injection of 100 μCi of ^{125}I-fibrinogen. The same dose of sodium iodide is administered daily for 3 weeks.

The first measurement of radioactivity is made at least 2 hours after the injection of the ^{125}I-fibrinogen. This is for two reasons. During that time any denatured fibrinogen will be removed from the circulation and considerable equilibration will occur between the intravascular and extravascular fibrinogen. Counts taken immediately after the injection tend to produce high readings over the heart and relatively low readings over the legs so that a false increase in the radioactivity in the legs may be detected 24 hr later. Subsequently, the radioactivity can be measured daily, but in practice it has been found sufficient to obtain counts every other day. If there are indications of thrombosis then counting should be performed daily to see whether the thrombus is extending, remaining stationary or lysing.

The radioactivity is measured over the heart at a site marked in the 4th left intercostal space, 2.5 cm from the sternal edge, at 5-cm intervals along the surface markings of the femoral vein in the thigh and the back of the calf from the popliteal fossa to the ankle. During counting the legs are elevated 30 degrees to prevent venous pooling and to give access to the back of the calf. If the legs were not elevated, misleadingly high readings would be obtained in patients with varicose veins.

Although early workers expressed the results as absolute counts[1, 5, 6] it has been found that the diagnosis of deep venous thrombosis was easily established if the results were expressed as a percentage of the heart count.[7, 8] This is because the radioactivity in the legs disappears approximately at the same rate as the radioactivity in the heart. Therefore, in the absence of thrombosis the percentage radioactivity at any position in the leg will be the same from day to day. In practice there is a tendency for the percentage radioactivity to increase slightly from day to day. This does not exceed 2% per day (16% in 8 days) (Fig. 13–2).[10] This is because the clearance of the extra-

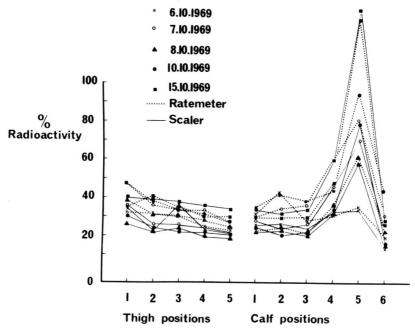

Fig 13–2.—Readings of limb counts obtained simultaneously by both a ratemeter and a scaler. They are expressed as percentages of the heart count.

vascular fibrinogen is slower than the clearance of the intravascular and the ratio of the extravascular to intravascular fibrinogen is higher in the leg than at the heart.[10]

Criteria for the Diagnosis of Thrombosis

The diagnosis of thrombosis is made whenever the percentage radioactivity is increased by 20 or more at the same position on two different days or between adjacent positions on the same day provided this increase persists for more than 24 hr. These criteria have been established using venography as the objective arbiter of the presence of deep venous thrombosis.[7, 8, 10, 11]

In order to test these criteria 20 patients with postoperative thrombosis and 20 patients without were randomly selected from the general surgical patients scanned routinely with a scintillation counter (scaler).[10] Venography was performed in all. The radioactivity was expressed as a percentage of the heart count and the increase in the percentage radioactivity at the site and on the day thrombosis was

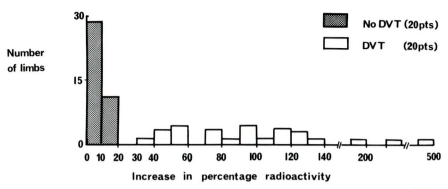

Fig 13–3.—The increase in the percentage counts on the day thrombosis was detected. The presence of thrombosis was confirmed by venography. *DVT*, deep venous thrombosis.

diagnosed was noted. In the patients without thrombosis the greatest reading at any point during the period of scanning was also noted. The increase of these percentage readings was plotted against the numbers of limbs (Fig 13–3). It can be seen that in all normal limbs the maximum increase in any of the percentage readings was never greater than 20. However, whenever there was thrombosis, the increase was greater than 30 on the day the thrombosis was diagnosed. On subsequent days the increase in the percentage radioactivity at the sites of thrombosis was even greater. In 18 of the 20 limbs with thrombosis it became over 100%.

In 10% of limbs there is a transient increase in the radioactivity which is greater than 20%, but returns to normal within 24 hr. Venography has always failed to demonstrate the presence of deep venous thrombosis in these limbs. This is the reason that any increase in the percentage radioactivity greater than 20 will be considered as evidence of thrombosis only if it persists for more than 24 hr.

Scaler versus Ratemeter

There is no doubt that a scaler is more accurate than a ratemeter as far as individual readings are concerned.[12] However, in the presence of thrombosis the increase in the percentage radioactivity is so high (see Figs 13–2 and 13–3) that a ratemeter will not fail to detect it. This is because on subsequent days as the absolute count over the heart decreases, the absolute count over the thrombus increases, resulting in such a high percentage radioactivity that the diagnosis will not be missed. A ratemeter is usually lighter and less expensive than a

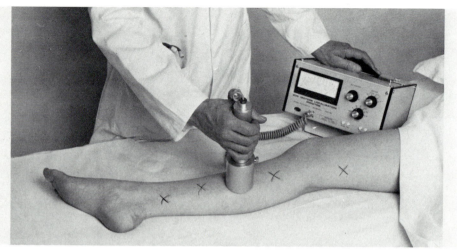

Fig 13–4.—Ratemeter with scintillation detector probe (Pitman model 235N isotope localization monitor).

scaler.[8, 11] If provided with a percentage scale the results could be obtained directly as a percentage of the heart count. The Pitman 235 isotope localization monitor is the one most extensively used in England (Fig 13–4).

Sensitivity and Specificity

Venography performed in 233 patients with a positive ^{125}I-fibrinogen test from several centers[6, 7, 13-19] has demonstrated the presence of thrombosis in 217 (93%). However, the test is by no means specific for deep venous thrombosis. Any inflammatory condition such as superficial thrombophlebitis, hematoma, wounds, fractures, ulceration, cellulitis and arthritis will result in an increase in the radioactivity. Unless such causes are excluded by careful examination of the patient's legs the test would lead to false positive findings.

The presence of edema can also produce an increase in the percentage of radioacitivty, but this occurs uniformly in all of the positions counted over the extent of the edema. This is often the case after total hip replacement. The diagnosis of deep venous thrombosis in the presence of edema can be made with certainty only if an increase of 20% or more in the radioactivity occurs in relation to adjacent points on the same leg (Table 13–1).

The ^{125}I-fibrinogen test will not detect any thrombosis in the region

TABLE 13-1.—INDIVIDUAL READINGS OF RADIOACTIVITY IN THE LEG AFTER ADMINISTRATION OF ^{125}I-FIBRINOGEN IN A CASE OF VENOUS THROMBOSIS*

LEG POSITIONS	% OF HEART-COUNT		DAYS AFTER OPERATION				
	PREOPERATIVE	POSTOPERATIVE	1	2	3	4	5
Right leg							
Thigh: 1	32	48	38	48	37	36	28
2	31	37	32	38	40	24	22
3	30	34	33	34	26	23	27
4	24	35	29	33	30	22	23
5	23	28	25	28	30	21	17
Calf: 1	32	30	23	36	30	25	24
2	24	35	25	43	30	28	18
3	28	37	26	38	36	24	20
4	31	41	39	45	48	31	27
5	35	81	64	95	130	124	116
6	20	22	25	45	28	25	24
Left leg							
Thigh: 1	30	44	33	43	48	31	26
2	27	37	28	39	50	32	37
3	28	37	29	36	50	22	28
4	28	40	34	38	29	25	24
5	21	34	27	28	38	36	22
Calf: 1	24	39	37	30	30	24	38
2	31	37	35	31	56	68	74
3	28	24	31	56	80	103	119
4	27	83	71	80	96	116	130
5	25	67	49	70	82	105	100
6	14	33	19	21	25	32	30

*From Hobbs and Nicolaides, 1971.[11]
An increase of more than 20 in the readings was found, within a few hours after operation, in the right calf at position 5 and this persisted for several days. At the same time, a similar rise in readings was found in the left calf at positions 4 and 5. On subsequent days, there were increases in readings at positions 3 and 2, indicating that the thrombotic process was spreading. In neither leg did the thrombus propagate into the thigh.

of the groin and pelvis because of the high background radioactivity in the bladder.

Precautions and Contraindications

Fibrinogen is a blood product and its administration carries a small but finite risk of serum hepatitis. The benefit from the test must always be balanced against this risk. The authors are not aware of any case of hepatitis following the injection of ^{125}I-fibrinogen obtained from screened donors who are under medical surveillance. This is also the experience of others.[20, 21, 24]

Although the radiation dose received by the patient is very small (total body dose: 1.7×10^{-4} rad/μCi) the use of the test should be avoided in the persons under 30 and women of child-bearing age.

Saturating the thyroid gland with sodium iodide is essential in order to minimize the radiation received by the thyroid.

Information Obtained by the 125I-Fibrinogen Test

The 125I-fibrinogen test has demonstrated that the incidence of deep venous thrombosis is much higher than previously thought and that it varies with different groups of patients (Table 13–2). Half of the patients with thrombosis do not have any symptoms or signs.[6, 7, 10] In addition the 125I-fibrinogen test has provided answers to several questions.

WHEN DO THROMBI OCCUR?

By screening a large number of patients with the 125I-fibrinogen test it was demonstrated that 45% of the thrombi started on the day of op-

TABLE 13–2.—INCIDENCE OF DEEP VENOUS THROMBOSIS IN PATIENTS STUDIED WITH THE 125I-FIBRINOGEN TEST

TYPE OF PATIENTS	INCIDENCE (%)	REFERENCE
General surgical	35	Flanc et al., 1968[6]
	35	Negus et al., 1968[7]
	30	Kakkar et al., 1970[26]
	41	Williams, 1971[27]
	42	Gordon-Smith et al., 1972[28]
	23	Nicolaides et al., 1972[29]
	14	Gallus et al., 1973[30]
Patients undergoing thoracotomy	26	Nicolaides et al., 1972[29]
Gynecologic	17	Friend, 1971[31]
	15	Bonnar and Walsh, 1972[32]
	29	Ballard et al., 1973[33]
Obstetric	4	Friend, 1971[31]
Patients with fractured neck of femur	47	Field et al., 1972[34]
	54	Kakkar et al., 1972[35]
	56	Gallus et al., 1973[30]
Patients undergoing elective hip operations	42	Gallus et al., 1973[30]
	37	Nicolaides et al., 1974[36]
Patients undergoing prostatectomy	30	Nicolaides et al., 1972[37]
	38	Mayo et al., 1972[38]
Patients with myocardial infarction	34	Murray et al., 1970[39]
	38	Nicolaides et al., 1971[40]
	29	Handley et al., 1972[41]
	17	Warlow et al., 1973[42]
	22	Gallus et al., 1973[30]
Medical patients in shock	68	Nicolaides et al., 1971[40]
Patients having aortoiliac reconstruction	30	Angelides et al., 1976[43]

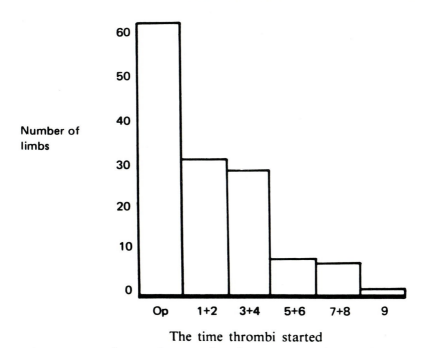

The time thrombi started

Fig 13–5. — Time of onset of venous thrombosis in general surgical patients.

eration, 43% during the first 4 postoperative days and the remaining 12% during the subsequent 5 days.[10, 22] The time thrombosis was first detected is shown in Figure 13–5. Bilateral thrombosis tended to occur in the early postoperative period. With the exception of two patients, whenever thrombi occurred in both limbs, they occurred within 24 hr of each other.[10]

WHERE DO THROMBI START?

The site in the legs where the increased radioactivity first occurs in patients studied with the ^{125}I-fibrinogen test is the site where a thrombus starts. Of 330 general surgical patients studied before and after operation, deep venous thrombosis developed in 98 (29.7%) patients.[10, 23] In 89% of the patients with thrombosis the radioactivity was detected first in the calf. In 6.5% it was detected first in the popliteal fossa and in 4% in the thigh (Fig 13–6).

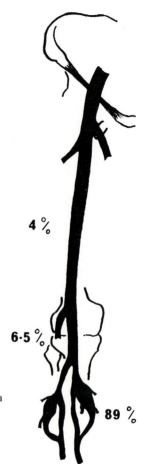

4 %

6·5 %

89 %

Fig 13–6.–Site of origin
of thrombi as detected by
[125]I-fibrinogen test.

What Is the Fate of Thrombi?

The early natural history of postoperative thrombosis has been
studied using the ^{125}I-fibrinogen test.[13] The majority of thrombi (78%)
either lyse spontaneously or remain localized to the calf, while only
22% extend into and proximal to the popliteal vein. Large clinical
pulmonary emboli occur in patients in the latter group[13] and only
small silent emboli in patients with thrombi confined to the calf.[24]
Thus for the first time it has become possible to select the patients
whose life is at risk.

WHAT IS THE EFFICACY OF PREVENTIVE MEASURES?

The 125I-fibrinogen test has been a powerful tool used in numerous clinical trials designed to determine the efficacy of different methods of prevention. Because of the inaccuracy of clinical signs the 125I-fibrinogen test has enabled us to evaluate prophylaxis with a greater accuracy.

WHICH PATIENTS NEED PROPHYLAXIS?

Clinical factors thought to be associated with a high incidence of deep venous thrombosis have been recorded in 674 surgical patients studied with the 125I-fibrinogen test. Age, varicose veins, previous deep venous thrombosis, severity of operation, infection and the surgical specialty were good predictors of the risk of thrombosis. Using these clinical factors it was possible to calculate the risk for any patient and obtain guidelines about the patients that need prophylaxis. It has been suggested that patients over the age of 40 who have major operations and patients over the age of 60 having any operation have a risk of deep venous thrombosis greater than 6% and therefore should receive prophylaxis.[25]

Practical Uses and Current Status

It is obvious from the above that the 125I-fibrinogen test is a useful research tool. It is used extensively in studies of the incidence of deep venous thrombosis and in clinical trials of the prevention of thrombosis.

With the increased awareness of the dangers of venography, the 125I-fibrinogen test is used more frequently in the diagnosis of established thrombosis in patients presenting with symptoms and signs. In a study of 102 patients with signs of deep venous thrombosis the test gave a correct diagnosis in 78% of the 85 legs shown to contain thrombus by phlebography and only 10% of false negative results in the 195 legs examined. The false negative results occurred in patients with phlebographically very old thrombi.[21] The main disadvantage is that it may take 24–48 hr to make the diagnosis.

Finally, the 125I-fibrinogen test is useful in the management of limited deep venous thrombosis detected in the calf of patients who are ambulant. Provided the patient's legs are scanned for 1 week treatment is not necessary because the majority of these thrombi will lyse spontaneously.[13] It does not matter if the established thrombus in the calf, demonstrated by phlebography, does not become radioactive. Any proximal extension will incorporate ^{125}I-fibrinogen and will be detected. If the increased radioactivity extends up to the popliteal fossa, then full anticoagulation therapy with heparin should be commenced and the patient should be confined to bed. Such proximal extension will occur in 15–20% of patients.[13]

The information obtained from studies in which the ^{125}I-fibrinogen test was used has revolutionized our approach to deep venous thrombosis, is responsible for our better understanding of the pathogenesis and natural history of the condition and has resulted in the progress in the prevention and management which has been observed during the last 5 years.

REFERENCES

1. Hobbs, J. T., and Davies, J. W. L.: Detection of venous thrombosis with ^{131}I-labelled fibrinogen in the rabbit, Lancet 2:134, 1960.
2. Hobbs, J. T.: External measurement of fibrinogen uptake in experimental venous thrombosis and other local pathological states, Br. J. Exp. Pathol. 43:48, 1962.
3. Hobbs, J. T.: Unpublished data, 1961.
4. Palko, P. D., Nansen, E. M., and Fedoruk, S. O.: The early detection of deep vein thrombosis using ^{131}I-tagged human fibrinogen, Can. J. Surg. 7:215, 1964.
5. Atkins, P., and Hawkins, L. A.: Detection of venous thrombosis in the legs, Lancet 2:1217, 1965.
6. Flanc, C., Kakkar, V. V., and Clarke, M. B.: The detection of venous thrombosis of the legs using ^{125}I-labelled fibrinogen, Br. J. Surg. 55:742, 1968.
7. Negus, D., Pinto, D. J., Le Quesne, L. P., Brown, N., and Chapman, M.: ^{125}I-labelled fibrinogen in the diagnosis of deep vein thrombosis and its correlation with phlebography, Br. J. Surg. 55:835, 1968.
8. Kakkar, V. V., Nicolaides, A. N., Renney, J. T. G., Friend, J., and Clarke, M. B.: ^{125}I-labelled fibrinogen test adapted for routine screening for deep-vein thrombosis, Lancet 1:540, 1970.
9. McFarlane, A. S.: In vivo behaviour of ^{131}I-fibrinogen, J. Clin. Invest. 42:346, 1963.
10. Nicolaides, A. N.: The Prevention of Postoperative Deep Venous Thrombosis, Jacksonian Prize Essay, Royal College of Surgeons of England, 1972.
11. Hobbs, J. T., and Nicolaides, A. N.: The Diagnosis of Acute Deep Vein Thrombosis With 125-Iodinated Fibrinogen, in Zeitler, E. (ed.): *Diagnostik mit Isotopen bei arteriellen und venosen Durchblutungsstorungen der Extremitaten* (Bern: Hans Huber, 1971).
12. Charkes, N. D.: ^{125}I-Fibrinogen scanning, Lancet 1:1191, 1973.
13. Kakkar, V. V., Howe, C. T., Flanc, C., and Clarke, M. B.: Natural history of deep vein thrombosis, Lancet 2:230, 1969.
14. Lambie, J. M., Barber, D. C., Dhall, D. P., and Matheson, M. A.: Dextran 70 in prophylaxis of postoperative venous thrombosis. A controlled trial, Br. Med. J. 2:144, 1970.
15. Pinto, D. J.: Controlled trial of an anticoagulant in the prevention of venous thrombosis following hip surgery, Br. J. Surg. 57:348, 1970.
16. Kakkar, V. V.: The diagnosis of deep vein thrombosis using the ^{125}I-fibrinogen test, Arch. Surg. 104:152, 1972.
17. Milne, R. M., Gunn, A. A., and Griffiths, J. M. T.: Postoperative deep venous thrombosis, Lancet 2:445, 1971.

18. Bonnar, J., and Walsh, J.: Prevention of thrombosis after surgery by British dextran 70, Lancet 1:614, 1972.

19. Hume, M., and Gurewich, V.: Peripheral venous scanning with 125I-tagged fibrinogen, Lancet 1:845, 1972.

20. Kakkar, V. V., and Corrigan, T. P.: Detection of deep vein thrombosis: Survey and current status, Progr. Cardiovasc. Dis. 17:207, 1974.

21. Browse, N. L., Clapham, W. F., Croft, D. N., Jones, D. J., Thomas, M. L., and Williams, J. O.: Diagnosis of established deep vein thrombosis with the 125I-fibrinogen uptake test, Br. Med. J. 4:325, 1971.

22. Nicolaides, A. N.: Prevention of deep vein thrombosis, Geriatrics 28:69, 1973.

23. Nicolaides, A. N., and Gordon-Smith, I.: A Rational Approach to Prevention, in Nicolaides, A. N. (ed.): *Thromboembolism* (Lancaster: Medical and Technical Publishing, 1975).

24. Browse, N. L., Glemenson, G., and Croft, D. N.: Fibrinogen detectable thrombosis in the legs and pulmonary embolism, Br. Med. J. 1:603, 1974.

25. Nicolaides, A. N., and Irving, D.: Clinical Factors and the Risk of Deep Venous Thrombosis, in Nicolaides, A. N. (ed.): *Thromboembolism* (Lancaster: Medical and Technical Publishing, 1975).

26. Kakkar, V. V., Howe, C. T., Nicolaides, A. N., Renney, J. T. G., and Clarke, M. B.: Deep vein thrombosis of the leg — is there a "high risk" group?, Am. J. Surg. 120: 527, 1970.

27. Williams, H. T.: Prevention of postoperative deep vein thrombosis with perioperative subcutaneous heparin, Lancet 2:950, 1971.

28. Gordon-Smith, I. C., Grundy, D. J., Le Quesne, L. P., Newcombe, J. F., and Bramble, F. T.: Controlled trial of two regimes of subcutaneous heparin in prevention of postoperative deep vein thrombosis, Lancet 1:1133, 1972.

29. Nicolaides, A. N., Dupont, P. A., Desai, S., Lewis, J. D., Douglas, J. N., Dodsworth, H., Fourides, G., Luck, R. J., and Jamieson, C. W.: Small doses of subcutaneous sodium heparin in preventing deep vein thrombosis in major surgery, Lancet 2:890, 1972.

30. Gallus, A. S., Hirsh, J., Tuttle, R. J., Trebilcock, R., O'Brien, S. E., Carroll, J. J., Minden, J. H., and Hudecki, S. M.: Small subcutaneous doses of heparin in prevention of venous thrombosis, N. Engl. J. Med. 288:545, 1973.

31. Friend, J.: Personal communication, 1971.

32. Bonnar, J., and Walsh, J.: Prevention of thrombosis after pelvic surgery by British Dextran 70, Lancet 1:614, 1972.

33. Ballard, R. M., Bradley-Watson, P. J., Johnstone, F. D., Kenney, A., McCarthy, T. G., Campbell, S., and Weston, J.: Low doses of subcutaneous heparin in the prevention of deep vein thrombosis after gynaecological surgery, J. Obstet. Gynaecol. 80: 469, 1973.

34. Field, E. S., Nicolaides, A. N., Kakkar, V. V., and Crellin, R. Q.: Deep vein thrombosis in patients with fractures of the femoral neck, Br. J. Surg. 59:377, 1972.

35. Kakkar, V. V., Corrigan, T., Spindler, J., Fossard, D. P., Flute, P. T., Crellin, R. Q., Wessler, S., and Yin, E. T.: Efficacy of low doses of heparin in prevention of deep vein thrombosis after major surgery, Lancet 2:101, 1972.

36. Nicolaides, A. N., Dupont, P. A., Parsons, D., Appleburg, M., Horan, F. T., Esau, K. M., and Walker, C. J.: Small dose subcutaneous sodium heparin in preventing deep venous thrombosis after elective hip surgery, Br. J. Surg. 61:320, 1974.

37. Nicolaides, A. N., Field, E. S., Kakkar, V. V., Yates-Bell, A. J., Taylor, S., and Clarke, M. B.: Prostatectomy and deep-vein thrombosis, Br. J. Surg. 59:487, 1972.

38. Mayo, M. E., Halil, T., and Browse, N. L.: The incidence of deep vein thrombosis after prostatectomy, Br. J. Urol. 43:738, 1971.

39. Murray, T. S., Lorimer, A. R., Cox, F. C., and Lawrie, T. D. V.: Leg vein thrombosis following myocardial infarction, Lancet 2:792, 1970.

40. Nicolaides, A. N., Kakkar, V. V., Renney, J. T. G., Kidner, P. H., Hutchison, D. C. S.,

and Clarke, M. B.: Myocardial infarction and deep vein thrombosis, Br. Med. J. 1: 432, 1971.

41. Handley, A. J., Emerson, P. A., and Fleming, P. R.: Heparin in the prevention of deep vein thrombosis after myocardial infarction, Br. Med. J. 2:436, 1972.
42. Warlow, C., Beattie, A. G., Terry, G., Ogston, D., Kenmure, A. C. F., and Douglas, A. S.: A double-blind trial of low doses of subcutaneous heparin in the prevention of deep-vein thrombosis after myocardial infarction, Lancet 2:934, 1973.
43. Angelides, N., Nicolaides, A. N., Fernandes e Fernandes, J., Bowers, R., Lewis, J.: Incidence of deep venous thrombosis in patients having aortoiliac reconstruction, Br. J. Surg. 64:517, 1977.

14 / Isotope Venography

RICHARD H. DEAN, M.D.

*Department of Surgery, Vanderbilt University Medical Center,
Nashville, Tennessee*

ALTHOUGH THE IMPORTANCE of pulmonary thromboembolism has been recognized for years, it continues as a common, potentially lethal disorder, occurring in almost any age and clinical setting. This was emphasized recently in Coon's autopsy series, which showed no significant change in the prevalence of pulmonary emboli between his study (12.3%) and a similar series obtained 20 years previously (13.6%).[4] Contributing to this unaltered prevalence are the frequent absence of preliminary clinical signs of venous thrombosis. This is emphasized by recent studies showing the absence of clinical signs in over two thirds of patients with venous thrombosis.[3, 16] Further, when present, physical findings accurately predict the presence of venous thrombosis in only one third of patients.[2, 13] Clearly, then, improved methods of screening high risk patients for venous thrombosis are necessary. Although contrast venography continues to be the definitive diagnostic tool, there is justified reluctance to its routine use in screening large numbers of patients for venous thrombosis. Whereas the ^{125}I-tagged fibrinogen uptake test has provided valuable information on the development of deep vein thrombosis in high risk patients, its clinical utility is also limited. Since the test must be initiated prior to thrombus formation it has no value as a screening test for established venous thrombosis. Further, the ^{125}I-labeled fibrinogen uptake test is less accurate when evaluating larger veins such as the common femorals, iliacs and vena cava. To overcome the requirement of initiating the study prior to clot formation Kempi et al.[12] have evaluated the use of ^{99}Tc-streptokinase for the isolation of deep vein thrombi. Since streptokinase induces thrombolysis it should show increased concentration in areas of venous thrombosis. Although their study showed an

89% correlation with the results of contrast venography, its clinical application requires more investigation.

The Doppler ultrasound velocity detector combined with impedance plethysmography[21] and phleborheography[6] have correlated well with contrast venography and are gaining widespread acceptance as screening test for venous thrombosis. Applicable to almost any clinical setting, these noninvasive tests have added new versatility to the accurate detection of venous thrombosis. None of these studies, however, give data regarding pulmonary embolism.

The frequency of silent pulmonary emboli, without preceding evidence of venous thrombosis, has been stressed by Coon and Collier.[5] In a study of 595 autopsies they found that only 10% of patients had clinical signs of venous thrombosis prior to death from pulmonary embolism. This stresses the need for evaluating both the peripheral venous system and the pulmonary vasculature in all such patients. In this regard, an accurate method for the simultaneous definition of pulmonary emboli and their site of origin would be a significant addition to the diagnostic armamentarium of the clinician.

The potential use of radiopharmaceuticals for this purpose was first reported by Webber and his associates in 1969.[18] In this report they observed areas of increased radioactivity in the axillary regions of some patients undergoing lung scanning with ^{99m}Tc macroaggregates of albumin (MAA). Finding these "hot spots" in areas of previous endothelial damage by intravenous catheters, they proposed that an attraction existed between these areas of clot and the isotope, and suggested its potential use for venographic evaluation of the lower extremities. Webber and Victery[20] subsequently measured the electrophoretic mobility and surface charges of MAA and clots and theorized that the hot spots were, at least in part, the result of opposing surface charges on the two particles causing an accumulation of the isotope on the clot surface. Following these observations, series reported by Webber et al.,[19] Duffy et al.[8] and others[7, 15] documented the clinical applicability of limb scanning for venous thrombosis with ^{99m}Tc-MAA when performing pulmonary scans. Unfortunately, the irregular shape of MAA has led to its frequent entrapment in venous valves of the legs resulting in a high incidence of false positive hot spots on delayed imaging. This problem can be averted by using ^{99m}Tc-pertechnetate which has a high correlation with the results of contrast venography.[1, 10] The constant recirculation of ^{99m}Tc, however, precludes its use for pulmonary perfusion scanning and therefore defeats the original advantage of this technique.

These disadvantages of both ^{99m}Tc-MAA and ^{99m}Tc led Henkin and his associates[9] to investigate the use of human albumin microspheres (HAM) as a further refinement in this technique. In this method, 15 μ to 30 μ HAM of uniform spherical shape are tagged with ^{99m}Tc. This particle size does not recirculate and is also ideal for lung scanning.[14] Using this modification in technique the authors found no false positive hot spots in their study of 25 limbs. They suggested that the disappearance of false positive hot spots was secondary to a reduction of total surface area and, thereby, a reduction in surface charge on the microspheres when compared to the macroaggregates. Although the attraction of the MAA and HAM for the clot surface remains incompletely understood, the loss of false positive hot spots when using HAM supports its preferential use. Further, the availability of ^{99m}Tc-HAM for routine pulmonary perfusion scanning and the ease of leg imaging suggests that this technique may have widespread application in the simultaneous evaluation of venous thrombosis and pulmonary embolism.

Technique

Isotope venography is performed using a gamma scintillation camera equipped with either a 4,000- or 16,000-hole collimator. Human albumin microspheres are labeled with ^{99m}Tc to give a final concentration of 4.0 mCi/ml. Patients are placed supine on a portable cart. With two tourniquets placed just above each ankle, a 23-gauge butterfly needle, attached to a 3-way stopcock and a syringe of heparinized saline, is inserted into a dorsal vein of each foot.

With the camera positioned to image the iliac veins and lower vena cava 0.5 mCi of ^{99m}Tc-HAM is injected into each pedal vein followed by a 5-ml flush of heparinized saline. Following visualization of this level the patient is moved and the technique is repeated with the camera first centered over the thigh and then the calf to assess venous flow at these levels. A cobalt 57 marker is placed lateral to the patellar region for identification of this level. Images are recorded on both Polaroid film and digital videotape. Following a 5-min delay after the last injection of isotope, leg scans are repeated at each level to detect any retained increased radioactivity (hot spots). Additional data which can be obtained during isotope venography includes measurement of transient times from injection until the first appearance of isotope in the field of view. Following the completion of limb scanning the needles are removed and the patient is repositioned for a standard four-view camera pulmonary perfusion scan.

Interpretation

The normal pathway of isotope flow through the lower extremity venous system is depicted in Figure 14–1. Since pressure injections are not employed the isotope follows the normal deep venous drainage of the foot. After entering the calf one or two channels of venous flow are identified. These then coalesce into the common channel of the popliteal vein. On thigh imaging, the single column of radioactivity in the superficial femoral vein is found. Finally, scanning of the pelvic region shows the flow in both iliac veins and vena cava. Frequently there is a greater isotopic opacification of the external than the

Fig 14–1.—Drawing of the normal pathway of isotope drainage from the foot following ^{99m}Tc-HAM injection with the associated leg scan depicting a normal isotope venogram.

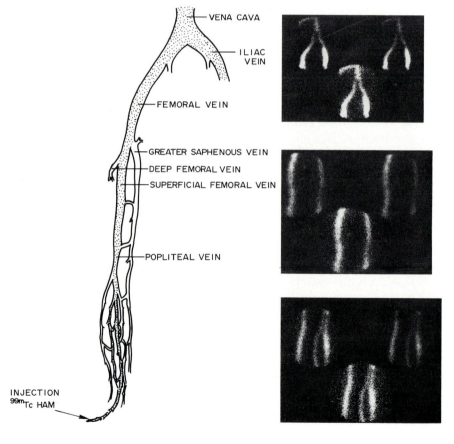

VENA CAVA

ILIAC VEIN

FEMORAL VEIN

GREATER SAPHENOUS VEIN
DEEP FEMORAL VEIN
SUPERFICIAL FEMORAL VEIN

POPLITEAL VEIN

INJECTION
^{99m}Tc HAM

common iliac veins, suggesting a hang-up of the ^{99m}Tc-HAM in the external iliac vein from a partially occluding clot in the external iliac vein. In the absence of other abnormal findings such as collateral venous drainage or delayed hot spots, however, it is secondary to the addition of nonvisualized internal iliac flow at that level diluting the isotope concentration in the common iliac vein. Barnes et al.[1] have suggested that the absence of this normal dilutional effect of the internal iliac vein effluent may suggest the presence of thrombi occluding pelvic venous drainage.

Based on the criteria listed in Table 14–1, interpretation of the study can be categorized as: (1) normal, (2) suspicious for venous thrombosis or (3) definitively positive. The finding of delayed transit of the isotope in one limb and the opacification of multiple venous channels on calf imaging are suspicious but not pathognomonic of venous thrombosis. Since incompetency of venous valves can lead to opacification of multiple venous channels in the calf and the demonstration of both the superficial femoral and the saphenous vein in the thigh, these findings, by themselves, do not necessarily mean that thrombi are present.

Findings considered definitely positive for venous thrombosis, however, include the loss of visualization of a segment of the venous system with or without the demonstration of collateral channels, and the appearance of hot spots on delayed imaging of the respective levels. These findings are particularly conclusive when demonstrated in the thigh or pelvic image. Since the superficial femoral vein should be uniformly opacified, a segmental loss of visualization of this vein, especially when collateral channels are identified, unequivocally establishes the diagnosis of venous thrombosis in this segment (Fig 14–2). Likewise, the appearance of pelvic collaterals is pathognomonic for ileofemoral venous thrombosis. Contrast cavography from a femoral injection site normally may show the internal iliac system secondary to reflux from the pressure injection. Since the isotopic visualization of this segment only follows the physiologic pathway of

TABLE 14–1.—CRITERIA FOR INTERPRETATION
OF ISOTOPE VENOGRAM

CATEGORY	CRITERIA
Suspicious	Prolonged transit time in one limb
	Opacification of multiple calf venous channels
Abnormal	Nonvisualization of a venous segment
	Demonstration of venous collaterals in thigh or pelvis
	Retained "hot spots" on delayed imaging

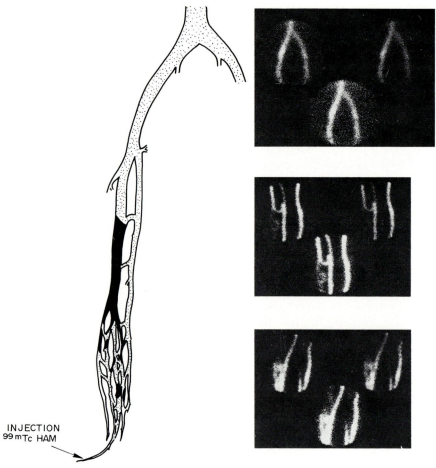

Fig 14–2. — Drawing depicting flow of the ⁹⁹ᵐTc-HAM represented in the accompanying isotope venogram. Note the absence of visualization of the popliteal and distal superficial femoral vein. The proximal femoral vein is opacified by a large collateral from the saphenous vein.

venous drainage, any demonstration of collateral veins in the segment is indicative of venous thrombosis (Fig 14–3).

Although no investigation has defined a relationship between complete reendothelialization of the clot surface and the loss of hot spots on delayed imaging, the finding of hot spots suggests the presence of a nonendothelialized surface with an attraction to the ⁹⁹ᵐTc-HAM. Therefore, hot spots, if present, suggest recent venous thrombosis. In patients with a history of venous thrombosis, this is particularly im-

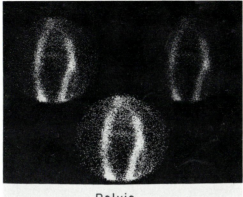

Pelvis

Fig 14–3. — Isotope venogram of patient with left femoral vein thrombosis showing opacification of the common iliac vein by a pelvic collateral. Note the abnormally medial pathway of ^{99m}Tc-HAM from the left lower extremity.

Fig 14–4. — Demonstration of "hot spots" on delayed scanning of the right calf of the patient depicted in Figure 14–2. This finding confirms the presence of fresh clot.

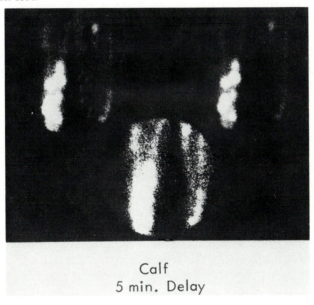

Calf
5 min. Delay

portant, for other abnormal findings may be on the basis of old thrombosis. Only hot spots will confirm the presence of recently deposited venous thrombi (Fig 14-4).

Comments

The compelling need for better understanding of pulmonary thromboembolism requires a more aggressive diagnostic evaluation of high risk patients. Clearly, clinical impressions alone are sufficiently misleading to dictate a policy requiring diagnostic confirmation of both venous thrombosis and pulmonary embolism. While contrast venography remains the definitive study for venous thrombosis, it gives no information regarding embolization of such clots. Similarly, the cost, necessity for experienced radiologic personnel, frequent patient discomfort and potential risk of chemical phlebitis limit its liberal use in screening for venous thrombosis. Additionally, visualization of pelvic veins and vena cava is frequently poor when a pedal injection site is used, thereby creating the need for both pedal and femoral injections to completely evaluate the venous system of the lower extremity. The advent of isotope venography circumvents these disadvantages of contrast studies while simultaneously allowing pulmonary perfusion scanning for pulmonary emboli. Further, recent comparative studies show excellent correlation between isotope venography using ^{99m}Tc-HAM and contrast venography. In a study of 34 limbs Yao and his associates[22] showed an 89% correlation between the results of isotope and contrast venography. In studying 46 limbs by both methods in our center we have found a 96% correlation. Thirty-three limbs were normal by both isotope and contrast venography. Likewise, the contrast venogram gave confirmation in 11 of 13 abnormal isotope venograms. The two false positive isotope studies had multiple calf veins opacified with delay hot spots identified. Contrast venography in these individuals revealed venous valvular incompetency with varicosities but no thrombi.

Although no false negative leg scans were found in our comparative study, the calf veins defy accurate assessment. Blood flow from the foot will be preferentially directed away from totally occlusive thrombi in the calf. Similarly, only those veins receiving blood from the injected pedal vein will be identified. Since no information is available regarding the unopacified calf veins, the presence of occluding clots in these veins cannot be excluded.

Although the correlation with contrast venography is salutory and supports the clinical use of isotope venography, the chief advantage of this method is the ability to perform simultaneous peripheral venography and pulmonary scanning. Thus, with the single study, pulmonary emboli can be identified while investigating likely sites of their origin. Nine patients in our group had pulmonary emboli shown by lung scan. Deep vein thrombosis extending, at least, into the thigh was proved by isotope venography in five (55%) of these. Three of the remaining four patients had multicentric calf vein thrombi present. Likewise, Yao and his associates[22] found pulmonary emboli primarily associated with proximal deep venous thrombosis and multicentric thrombi in their series of isotope venograms. Similarly, Walker,[17] in an exhaustive study, found that 49% of pulmonary emboli originated from iliofemoral venous thrombosis. Although Kakkar et al.[11] have stressed the importance of calf vein thrombi, they suggested that the greatest danger is in their proximal propagation and subsequent embolization. Clearly, the routine use of radionuclide venography when obtaining lung scans may give important additional epidemiologic information regarding the relative embolic potentials of thrombi at the respective levels.

At present, radionuclide venography with simultaneous lung scanning using ^{99m}Tc-HAM appears to be an important addition to the diagnostic evaluation of pulmonary thromboembolism. The ease of obtaining leg scans while assessing the pulmonary vasculature supports its use in patients studied for pulmonary emboli. Likewise, the observed correlation with the results of contrast venography suggests its clinical applicability as a means of localizing the site of venous thrombosis while also screening for unsuspected pulmonary embolism.

Summary

The chief advantage of isotope venography is the ability to perform simultaneous peripheral venous examination and pulmonary scanning. Thus, pulmonary emboli can be identified while investigations are directed at the sites of origin of venous thrombosis. The technique is performed using a gamma scintillation camera equipped with either a 4,000- or 16,000-hole collimator. Human albumin microspheres are labelled with ^{99m}Tc to give a final concentration of 4.0 mCi/ml. Using a two tourniquet technique, a 23-gauge needle is inserted into the dorsal vein of each foot and injection is accomplished. Images are recorded on both Polaroid film and digital video tape. Findings considered definitely positive for venous thrombosis include loss of visualization of a segment of the venous system with or without demonstration of collateral channels and the appearance of hot spots on delayed imaging. The hot spots suggest presence of a nonendothelialized surface with attraction to the ^{99m}Tc human albumin microspheres. Such findings suggest recent venous thrombosis and this finding is particularly helpful in patients with a history of venous thrombosis. Radionuclide venography with simultaneous lung scanning appears to be an important addition to the diagnostic evaluation of patients with pulmonary thromboembolism.

REFERENCES

 1. Barnes, R. W., McDonald, G. B., Hamilton, G. W., Rudd, T. G., Help, W. B., and Strandness, D. E., Jr.: Radionuclide venography for rapid dynamic evaluation of venous disease, Surgery 73:706, 1973.
 2. Bergan, J. J., et al.: Prevention of pulmonary embolism, Arch. Surg. 92:605, 1966.
 3. Browse, N.: Deep vein thrombosis: Diagnosis, Br. Med. J. 4:676, 1969.
 4. Coon, W. W.: The spectrum of pulmonary embolism, Arch. Surg. 111:398, 1976.
 5. Coon, W. W., and Collier, F. A.: Clinicopathologic correlation in thromboembolism, Surg. Gynecol. Obstet. 109:259, 1959.
 6. Cranley, J. J., Gay, A. Y., Grass, A. M., and Simeone, F. A.: A plethysmographic technique for the diagnosis of deep venous thrombosis of the lower extremities, Surg. Gynecol. Obstet. 136:385, 1973.
 7. Driedger, A. A., Reid, B. D., and Heagy, F. C.: Lung and leg scanning with ^{99m}Tc-labelled albumin macroaggregates, Can. Med. Assoc. J. 111:403, 1974.
 8. Duffy, G. J., D'Auria, D., Brien, T. G., Ormond, D., and Mehigan, J. A.: New radioisotope test for detection of deep venous thrombosis in the legs, Br. Med. J. 1: 712, 1973.
 9. Henkin, R. E., Yao, J. S. T., Quinn, J. L., III, and Bergan, J. J.: Radionuclide venography (RNV) in lower extremity venous disease, J. Nucl. Med. 15:171, 1974.
10. Hobbs, J. T., Highman, J. M., and Yao, S. T.: The investigation of the iliac veins by an ultrasound technique and by radioscanning with a gamma camera, J. Vasc. Dis. 1:170, 1972.
11. Kakkar, V. V., et al.: Low dose of heparin in prevention of deep vein thrombosis, Lancet 2:699, 1971.
12. Kempi, V., Van Der Linden, W., and Von Scheele, C.: Diagnosis of deep vein thrombosis with ^{99m}Tc-streptokinase: a clinical comparison with phlebography, Br. Med. J. 4:748, 1974.
13. McLachlin, J., Richards, T., and Paterson, J. C.: An evaluation of clinical signs in the diagnosis of venous thrombosis, Arch. Surg. 85:738, 1962.
14. Poulose, K. P., et al.: Diagnosis of pulmonary embolism: Correlative study of clinical scan and angiographic findings, Br. Med. J. 3:67, 1970.
15. Rosenthall, L.: Combined inferior vena cavography, iliac venography, and lung imaging with ^{99m}Tc albumin macroaggregates, Radiology 98:623, 1971.
16. Sevitt, S., and Gallagher, N. A.: Prevention of venous thrombosis and pulmonary embolism in injured patients, Lancet 2:981, 1959.
17. Walker, M. A.: The natural history of venous thromboembolism, Br. J. Surg. 59:753, 1972.
18. Webber, M. M., Bennett, L. R., Cragin, M., and Webb, R., Jr.: Thrombophlebitis — demonstration by scintiscanning, Radiology 92:620, 1969.
19. Webber, M. M., Pollak, E. W., Victery, W., Cragin, M., Resnick, L. H., and Grollman, J. H., Jr.: Thrombosis detection by radionuclide particle (MAA) entrapment: Correlation with fibrinogen uptake and venography, Radiology 111:645, 1974.

20. Webber, M. M., and Victery, W.: MAA-studies of electrophoretic mobility and charge: Relationship to thrombosis affinity, J. Nucl. Med. 14:463, 1973.
21. Yao, J. S. T., Henkin, R. E., and Bergan, J. J.: Venous thromboembolic disease, Arch. Surg. 109:664, 1974.
22. Yao, J. S. T., Henkin, R. E., Conn, J., Jr., Quinn, J. L., III, and Bergan, J. J.: Combined isotope venography and lung scanning, Arch. Surg. 107:146, 1973.

Discussion: Chapters 13 and 14

DR. KENNETH HETZEL: Doctor Dean mentioned the diagnostic criteria of collateralization, appearance of hot spots and nonvisualized segments of vessels. In the venogram shown here, it is apparent that the patient demonstrates collateralization which is also seen on the contrast venogram. However, the same patient in other views has retained hot spots of radioactivity.

Some in this field have questioned the interpretation of hot spots being called a forming thrombus. They feel that these may be a valvular structure in the vein. Others say that experimental evidence of hot spot thrombi in the laboratory is lacking. Indeed, when we sectioned experimental thrombus, we identified no nuclear source macroaggregates. However, we went to the animal laboratory and set up a model to produce a type of thrombus which has platelets, granulocytes and ages with time. As it does this, the platelets degranulate and fibrin matrices form. Then, we took human albumin microspheres as provided by the 3M Company and instead of labeling them with a translucent radioisotope, we used fluorescent dye so visual microscopy could identify the location of the albumin within the thrombus. It was found that the fluorescent dye and microspheres were well incorporated within the thrombus.

The interesting part about this is that we see some microspheres on the surface in the area of sticky platelet mass while others are in a deep red cell mass.

We currently are conducting a study based on this finding, in which it appears that white cells recognize the microspheres as a foreign body. This may be an immunologic response, but it may be simply a charge phenomenon. The microspheres in this case are carrying a slight positive charge whereas leukocytes have a slight negative charge. We are investigating charge-altered microspheres and their effect on localization of venous thrombosis in animals.

238

15 / Role of the Vascular Laboratory in the Diagnosis of Venous Thrombosis

WILLIAM S. GROSS, M.D., BONNO VAN BELLEN, M.D., JAMES K. CREASY, M.D., MARIAN F. MCNAMARA, M.D., JOHN J. BERGAN, M.D. AND JAMES S. T. YAO, M.D., PH.D.

Blood Flow Laboratory, Division of Vascular Surgery of the Department of Surgery, Northwestern University Medical School, Chicago, Illinois

SEVERAL NONINVASIVE vascular laboratory testing methods are now in standard use for the diagnosis of deep venous thrombosis. Numerous investigators have reported high degrees of accuracy using phleborheography,[1] Doppler ultrasound[2-4] and impedance plethysmography.[5-7] Since the establishment of the vascular laboratory at the Northwestern University Medical Center, our approach to patients presenting with venous thromboembolic events has been the use of combination testing techniques by means of Doppler ultrasound and impedance outflow examination. Based on our previous experience, the diagnostic accuracy of the combined test, when compared with venography, is 95%.[8] This high degree of accuracy in detecting the presence of deep venous thrombosis should allow the physician to base therapeutic judgment on the results of the noninvasive test. However, it appears that the therapeutic implications of this test and the indications for its usage have not been adequately clarified to the primary care physicians who refer patients to the vascular diagnostic laboratory.

This study was undertaken to determine the effects that noninva-

Supported by Grant No. HL-16253-61, National Heart and Lung Institute and the Northwestern University Vascular Research Fund.

239

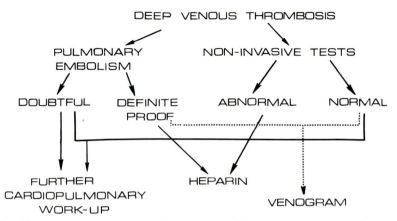

Fig 15–1.—Diagnostic and therapeutic scheme in patients with venous thromboembolism.

sive testing methods have had on the diagnostic work-ups as well as therapy delivered by primary care physicians.

Materials and Methods

Hospital records of 197 patients referred by primary care physicians with the clinical diagnosis of deep venous thrombosis were reviewed. All of these patients were examined in the Blood Flow Laboratory following the diagnostic scheme illustrated in Figure 15–1. One hundred and forty-four patients had normal venous examinations and 53 patients had abnormal results (Table 15–1). The presenting symptoms of 144 patients with normal venous examinations are outlined in Table 15–2. All patients whose records were selected for review had periods of follow-up of at least 1 year.

Details of Doppler ultrasound and impedance plethysmography techniques have been reported previously.[4] In essence, flow velocity waveforms were recorded over the common femoral and popliteal veins by means of a directional Doppler (Parks Electronics Laboratory

TABLE 15–1.—RESULT OF NONINVASIVE
VENOUS EXAMINATION IN 197 PATIENTS WITH
SUSPECTED DEEP VENOUS THROMBOSIS

Normal test result	144
Abnormal test result	53
Total	197

TABLE 15-2.—PRESENTING SYMPTOMS OF 144 PATIENTS
WITH NORMAL VENOUS EXAMINATIONS

SYMPTOM	NO. OF PATIENTS
Leg pain only	75
Leg pain with swelling	33
Leg swelling only	8
Chest pain	17
Shortness of breath	7
Other	4
Total	144

Model 806, 10 MHz). Posterior tibial vein patency was determined by the calf and foot squeeze maneuver.[4] Careful attention was also given to both the response to the Valsalva maneuver in the common femoral vein and bidirectional flow at the common femoral, popliteal and posterior tibial veins in an effort to demonstrate venous valvular incompetency. The impedance outflow examination was carried out using an impedance plethysmograph (Codman IPG-200 Impedance Plethysmograph, Cintor Co.). Usually, a total of five or six measurements was done in each limb before and after a brief period of active or passive exercise. Both the right and left limbs were studied in all patients. Hospitalized patients with a history of prolonged bed rest were routinely subjected to a brief period of active or passive exercise after the initial impedance examination. Impedance outflow testing then was repeated since it often returned to normal after the induced exercise (Fig 15-2).

Fig 15-2.—Return of venous outflow after exercise in a patient with prolonged bed rest. **A,** before exercise; **B,** after exercise.

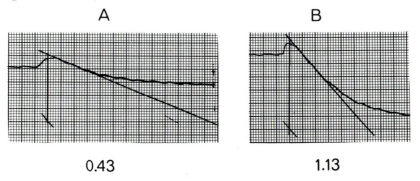

A   B

0.43   1.13

Diagnostic Criteria

Figure 15–3 illustrates the typical Doppler ultrasound and impedance outflow test results in normal and abnormal subjects. The absence of respiratory modulation in the common femoral and popliteal
veins combined with an abnormal impedance outflow test signified

Fig 15–3.–A, normal and abnormal impedance outflow examinations.
B, normal and abnormal Doppler examinations. *(Continued.)*

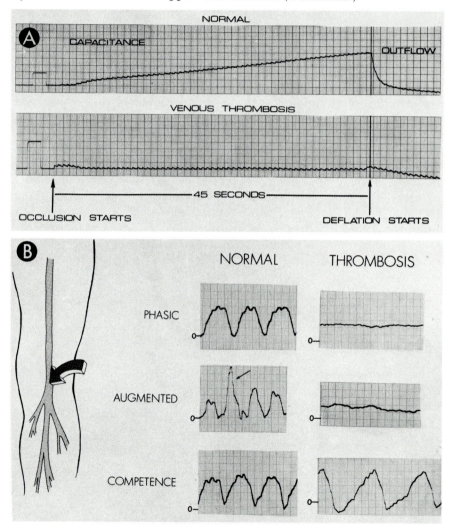

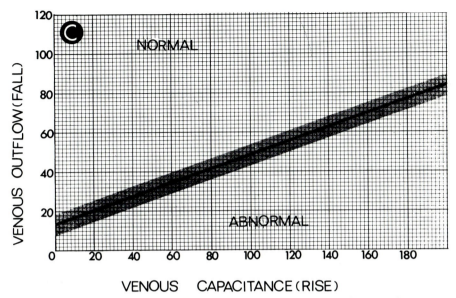

Fig 15–3 (cont.).— C, graph for charting abnormal and normal venous outflow.

the presence of acute deep vein thrombosis. Prominent cardiac pulsation, when seen in the common femoral or popliteal venous flow tracing, indicated the presence of right-sided heart failure or tricuspid insufficiency. In all of these patients, the impedance plethysmographic outflow test was abnormal bilaterally. When prominent cardiac influence was seen in the venous flow tracings at the common femoral vein, recording from the jugular or brachial vein was then performed. The demonstration of similarity in all of these tracings further docu-

Fig 15–4.— Prominent cardiac pulsation seen in Doppler venous flow tracings (common femoral vein) in a patient with documented tricuspid insufficiency. The impedance outflow was also abnormal bilaterally. Identical ultrasound tracing also was seen in the brachial vein recording.

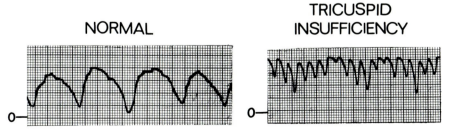

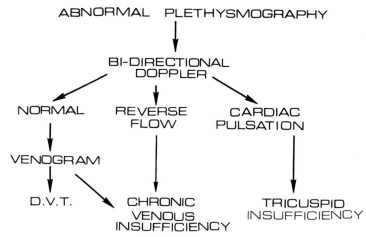

Fig 15–5. — Diagnostic maneuvers in patients found to have normal Doppler and abnormal impedance outflow testing *D.V.T.*, deep venous thrombosis.

mented the influence of cardiac disease on venous flow dynamics and physiologically clarified the impedance plethysmography result (Fig 15–4).

In patients with normal femoral and popliteal venous flow waveforms by Doppler examination, but an abnormal impedance plethysmograph outflow test, diagnostic maneuvers as depicted in Figure 15–5 were used. A unilateral abnormal impedance plethysmographic recording in the symptomatic leg, in patients without cardiac disease or prolonged bed rest, indicated the presence of thrombosis, usually at the popliteal or calf vein level. Venography in these cases was obtained only if the clinician wished to confirm the diagnosis. In bilaterally abnormal impedance plethysmography studies, attention was paid to the presence of valvular incompetency. If there was no evidence of venous valvular incompetency, it was recommended that venography be obtained for further identification of deep venous thrombosis below the popliteal vein level.

Data Analysis

Data analysis was done according to the results of the venous examination. Hospital records on these patients were reviewed and analyzed according to the method of treatment following the performance of noninvasive tests along with the early and late outcome of the pa-

TABLE 15–3. — RESULT OF TREATMENT AND ANATOMICAL SITES
OF VENOUS THROMBOSIS BY NONINVASIVE TESTING
IN 53 PATIENTS WITH ABNORMAL VENOUS EXAMINATION

Anatomical site	
Iliofemoral	21
Femoropopliteal	20
Calf	12
Total	53
Treated with heparin	53
Death (Iliofemoral)	1

tient. Particular attention was directed to an analysis of the therapy
started in response to the test results.

ABNORMAL VENOUS EXAMINATION

In all 53 patients with abnormal test results, heparin therapy was
begun by the primary care physician. One patient with the diagnosis
of iliofemoral venous thrombosis suffered a fatal pulmonary embolus.
Interestingly, none of these patients suffered any major hemorrhagic
complications of their anticoagulant therapy. In this group of patients,
it appears that the combination of clinical evaluation and the results of
noninvasive testing led to the institution of appropriate therapy
(Table 15–3).

NORMAL VENOUS EXAMINATION

One hundred and forty-four patients were analyzed (Table 15–4).
In 108 patients who were referred to the vascular laboratory because
of clinical suspicion of deep venous thrombosis, no therapy was given
by the primary care physician after the initial report of a normal venous examination. None of these 108 patients suffered lower extremi-

TABLE 15–4. — MODE OF THERAPY AND RESULT
IN 144 PATIENTS WITH NORMAL VENOUS EXAMINATION

MODE OF THERAPY	NO. OF PATIENTS
Heparin begun before test	36
Heparin discontinued after test	(21)
Heparin continued after test°	(15)
Not treated	108
Total	144
°6 patients with bleeding complications.	

ty sequelae, and there was no evidence of thromboembolic events during early or late follow-up.

Thirty-six patients had heparin therapy instituted prior to the performance of noninvasive testing for deep venous thrombosis. In 21 of these 36 patients, heparin therapy was discontinued after the report of a normal venous examination to the primary care physician. Fifteen patients continued to receive heparin; in 6 of these 15 patients, major hemorrhagic complications developed. Three of these six patients had normal venograms. One patient in this group receiving heparin therapy experienced hematuria which led the referring physician to seek urologic consultation and an exhaustive work-up was undertaken. This work-up was negative and subsequently led to hematologic evaluation including bone marrow aspiration. The therapeutic approach to this patient is most puzzling.

Table 15–5 shows the final diagnoses on 144 patients with a normal venous examination. Although 15 patients had a diagnosis of deep vein thrombosis, none of these patients had objective evidence to confirm or deny the diagnosis.

Comment

This study confirms the potential usefulness of noninvasive testing as a guide in the diagnosis and therapy of venous thromboembolism.

TABLE 15–5.—FINAL DIAGNOSES IN PATIENTS WITH NORMAL NONINVASIVE VENOUS EXAMINATION

FINAL DIAGNOSIS	NO. OF PATIENTS
Superficial thrombophlebitis	16
Deep vein thrombosis	15
Chronic venous insufficiency	15
Leg pain, unknown etiology	15
Congestive heart failure (tricuspid insufficiency)	8
Chronic obstructive pulmonary disease	4
Angina pectoris	7
Myocardial infarction	2
Neuropathy	16
Soft tissue trauma	8
Cellulitis	5
Arthritis conditions	12
Vasculitis	4
Sickle cell ulcer	1
Arterial occlusive disease	4
Psychogenic pain	7
Other	4
Total	144

The fact that none of the patients with normal results who were untreated suffered further thromboembolic events makes it apparent that appropriate decisions regarding therapy can be made on the basis of the data obtained by Doppler ultrasound and impedance plethysmography. Heparin therapy in these normal individuals is not only inappropriate but may lead to significant complications and the added expense of prolonged hospitalization. As with all laboratory tests, noninvasive testing for venous thrombosis must be utilized with sound clinical judgment, and must be related to the clinical evaluation of each patient. It must be emphasized that all current noninvasive tests are designed to detect hemodynamic changes as a result of thrombus occluding venous flow. When the thrombus is small and nonocclusive, these noninvasive tests will be of limited value. Therefore, in patients presenting with pulmonary symptoms but without leg symptoms, the finding of a normal venous examination does not rule out the presence of a nonocclusive thrombus serving as the source of the pulmonary embolus, and venography may be indicated.

Most venous thrombi are occlusive and therefore are detectable by noninvasive testing techniques. Unlike other investigators, we favor the combined use of both Doppler ultrasound and impedance plethysmography because of the ability of Doppler ultrasound to detect pulsatile flow characteristics in the presence of severe right-sided heart failure. It appears that a high percentage of false positive results as reported by Hull et al.[7] who used the impedance technique alone, were in patients who had cardiac disease. Prominence of cardiac pulsations observed in the venous flow tracings by Doppler ultrasound examination have been reported as an indication of tricuspid insufficiency[9] and, therefore, because of high venous pressure, impedance outflow testing will be abnormal in this group of patients.

The finding of abnormal venous outflow in patients confined to bed for a prolonged period of time deserves further clarification. It is possible that prolonged bed rest may result in loss of muscle tone which, in turn, alters the venous compliance and hence, the venous outflow. Loss of muscle tone as seen in patients with spinal cord injury appears to be a good example that confirms this observation. Our preliminary study[10] found the majority of spinal cord injured patients to have normal Doppler but abnormal impedance outflow examinations. None of these patients had evidence of calf vein thrombosis on venography. In patients subjected to prolonged bed rest, a brief period of exercise to increase the muscle (or venous) tone will often result in a return to normal in outflow testing.

The analysis of 144 patients with normal venous examinations is of particular interest. One hundred and eight patients received no anti-coagulant treatment and were either discharged or denied admission to the hospital for further workup. None of these patients returned with further symptoms or pulmonary embolus over a follow-up period of 1 year. This finding suggests that noninvasive testing is a valid tool and, when used along with sound clinical judgment, will spare unnecessary hospital admission and expense. The continued use of heparin despite invasive and noninvasive tests which refuted the diagnosis of venous thrombosis is difficult to understand. Of interest is the high incidence (40%) of bleeding complications in this group of patients. It would appear that further education about the diagnosis of venous thrombosis and the therapeutic implications of noninvasive testing is necessary.

Review of the final diagnoses of 144 patients with normal venous examinations further illustrates the fallibility of using clinical signs in establishing the diagnosis of acute deep venous thrombosis, since all of these patients were initially referred by the primary care physician in order to document the results of their physical findings. Other investigators have recorded a similar observation.[11]

In dealing with patients with suspected deep venous thrombosis, we have recommended a general scheme of diagnosis and therapy for the primary care physician (see Fig 15–1). We feel that this approach will lead to appropriate therapeutic judgment and better patient care. In patients presenting with pulmonary symptoms felt to be secondary to a pulmonary embolus, a thorough objective evaluation including perfusion ventilation lung scan and, if necessary, pulmonary angiography, should be carried out (see Fig 15–1). In all patients with objective documentation of pulmonary embolus, noninvasive testing is performed in order to locate the source of the embolus and aid in further diagnostic and therapeutic judgments. If the diagnosis of pulmonary embolism is in doubt, a normal venous examination would help to eliminate the possibility and steer the patient to further cardiopulmonary work-up for his chest symptoms. In patients presenting with lower extremity symptoms only, noninvasive testing is done and the results dictate the patient's further therapy. Pulmonary work-up has been reserved only for those patients with respiratory symptoms compatible with pulmonary embolus. Heparin therapy is instituted in all patients with abnormal test results and in those patients with documented pulmonary embolism. This therapeutic outline has been most satisfactory.

Obviously, venography still has an important role in the diagnosis and management of patients with suspected venous thromboembolism. In cases where unequivocal documentation of pulmonary embolus is present but noninvasive testing for deep thrombosis is normal, venography is carried out to locate the source of the embolus. Most importantly, when strong clinical suspicion is in disagreement with the noninvasive test results, or when the results are equivocal, venography is undertaken.

It is our conclusion that the noninvasive testing methods for deep venous thrombosis are useful in bridging the diagnostic gap between clinical examination and venography. We feel that the high degree of accuracy and reliability of the noninvasive testing methods is most acceptable. These tests should be ordered to confirm the suspicion of deep venous thrombosis determined by physical examination. Follow-up of patients with normal noninvasive test results seems to indicate that therapeutic decisions can be made on the basis of these results. In addition, the inappropriate use of heparin appears to lead to significant complications and added hospital expense.

Summary

Several noninvasive vascular laboratory tests are now in standard use in the diagnosis of acute deep vein thrombosis. This study was designed to assess the utility of these tests by the primary care physician who referred the case for study. Special emphasis has been placed on (1) the influence of the testing upon the treatment phase of the patient by his physician and (2) the short-term outcome and 1 year follow-up of these patients.

In our laboratory, a combination of Doppler ultrasound and impedance outflow testing has been used. Analysis has been completed on 197 patients. Normal venous examinations were defined as normal Doppler ultrasound and normal impedance outflow testing. In 144 patients in this category, 36 had heparin therapy instituted prior to examination and in 21 of these, heparin was discontinued after laboratory evaluation. Fifteen patients continued through the full course of anticoagulant treatment and six of these developed significant complications of therapy. None of the 129 patients without anticoagulant treatment had further venous problems during 1 year of follow-up.

REFERENCES

1. Cranley, J. J., Canos, A. J., Sull, W. J., and Grass, A. M.: Phleborheographic technique for the diagnosis of deep venous thrombosis of the lower extremities, Surg. Gynecol. Obstet. 141:331, 1975.
2. Sigel, B., Popky, B., Wagner, D., et al.: Comparison of clinical and Doppler ultra-

sound evaluation of confirmed lower extremity venous disease, Surgery 64:332, 1968.

3. Dean, R. H., and Yao, J. S. T.: Hemodynamic Measurements in Peripheral Vascular Disease, in Ravitch, M. M. (ed.): *Current Problems in Surgery* (Chicago: Year Book Medical Publishers, Inc., August, 1976).

4. Barnes, R. W., Russell, H. E., Wu, K. K., and Hoak, J. C.: Accuracy of Doppler ultrasound in clinically suspected venous thrombosis of the calf, Surg. Gynecol. Obstet. 143:425, 1976.

5. Johnston, K. W., and Kakkar, V. V.: Plethysmographic diagnosis of deep vein thrombosis, Surg. Gynecol. Obstet. 139:41, 1974.

6. Wheeler, H. B., O'Donnell, J. A., Anderson, F. A., Jr., and Benedict, K., Jr.: Occlusive impedance phlebography: A diagnostic procedure for venous thrombosis and pulmonary embolism, Cardiovasc. Dis. 17:199, 1974.

7. Hull, R., Van Aken, W. G., Hirsh, J., Gallus, A. S., and Hoicka, G.: Impedance plethysmography using the occlusive cuff technique in the diagnosis of venous thrombosis, Circulation 53:696, 1976.

8. Yao, J. S. T., Henkin, R. E., and Bergan, J. J.: Venous thromboembolic disease: Evaluation by new methodology, Arch. Surg. 109:664, 1974.

9. Brickner, P. W., Scudder, T., and Weinrib, M.: Pulsating varicose veins in functional tricuspid insufficiency, Circulation 25:126, 1962.

10. Yao, J. S. T.: Unpublished data.

11. Barnes, R. W., Wu, K. K., and Hoak, J. C.: Fallibility of the clinical diagnosis of venous thrombosis, JAMA 234:605, 1975.

Discussion: Chapter 15

DR. VICTOR BERNHARD: I would like to congratulate Doctor Gross and his associates on presenting a very important facet of all of the discussions we have heard today. I agree with their results. We do exactly the same things in terms of noninvasive evaluation of our patients, come up with practically identical results, and have a 95% accuracy when compared with venography.

The scheme of management which says that something very objective is required before continuing anticoagulation therapy is also correct.

This paper emphasizes that a knowledgeable physician or surgeon who understands the physiology and pathology of the problems identified by noninvasive techniques must intercede between the nameless faceless report and the patient to make sure that an appropriate conclusion is derived from the studies. It also is important to recognize that these tests cost money. They must be properly ordered or a lot of data which is unnecessary will accrue.

DR. BROWNELL WHEELER: This is a particularly important paper because it addresses the issue of influence of the quality of care. We know that all of the tests work in the hands of people who are familiar with them and highly motivated to perform them. But, the question is, does this really get through to the practice of medicine which is dependent upon the prescriptions of doctors who are not familiar with the tests. The answer is, it does, if you educate your primary physician. This paper makes that point beautifully.

Doctor Bernhard emphasized the issue of cost. That is very appropriate because there is so much concern now about the high cost of medical care. This is new technology. Instruments cost money; patients are billed for each test that is done. Nevertheless, I think that the screening test for venous thrombosis could save an enormous amount of money. There are an awful lot of patients who are treated for venous thrombosis who don't have it. The bills get to be very high, indeed.

Also, if these tests are used as Doctor Gross and his co-workers do, in lieu of venography, much money is saved. Thus, vascular laboratory tests can actually be cost-saving and not just add more and more to the cost of medical care.

DR. JOHN PFEIFER: Just one comment on cost. There has been a great deal of stress on noninvasive labs in the hospital setting. As I mentioned previously, we have now used our lab for 2 years in an outpatient or office setting, and we found that the cost saving is really quite sizeable. The charge to a patient for a phleborheogram is $35.00.

We have been impressed with our clinical inaccuracy in diagnosing a deep vein thrombosis. Prior to the advent of noninvasive testing, we had to admit even the equivocal or the marginal cases to hospital and presumptively treat them with heparin or at the very least do a venogram to confirm our diagnosis.

We find that approximately 50% of the patients we see in the office with a suspect deep vein thrombosis are proving by phleborheography to be negative and, therefore, are not admitted to hospital.

The last time we assessed the cost of hospitalization for routine management of a simple deep vein thrombosis, it was approximately $1,000. Now, I think the trade-off of a $35.00 noninvasive phleborheogram for $1,000 worth of heparin therapy and bed rest in hospital is really quite significant, and I think we must consider these factors in this new age of federalism that we now approach.

DR. VICTOR deWOLFE: I would just like to reemphasize the last two comments, and tell about the patient who comes in with so-called chronic thrombophlebitis. All of us know there is no such thing as chronic thrombophlebitis. Thrombophlebitis may be recurring, but it is not chronic.

We also know if a patient did have five or six episodes of recurrent thrombophlebitis, he would definitely present with chronic venous insufficiency. He would have a swollen leg, dilated superficial veins, perhaps secondary varicose veins. However, we find that many of these people appear with normal looking extremities. They may have tight calf muscles and hamstrings, we learn that they have been hospitalized five or six times for chronic thrombophlebitis, and we find it very difficult to convince the patients and their physicians that they do not have thrombophlebitis. In the past, we have used venography to prove to the patient and to the physician that there was no thrombophlebitis. In this era of noninvasive tests, the examinations are going to be very helpful in this type of patient. I agree that it will definitely save a great deal of money.

DR. STEVEN DOSICK: I can give you some figures from outpatients we have been seeing in our laboratory. We found that 66% of the patients that we saw in the lab were normal. These patients have been sent back to the physician, whom we called right away. I think we have significantly reduced hospitalizations, and have given these patients a great deal of help.

As we all know, patients who have had venograms are loathe to have them again. However, if they have a noninvasive test, they are much happier about the whole situation.

DR. HENRY BERKOWITZ: In light of the two comments that just preceded me, I would like to ask the general question that is often asked of me. That is, since these patients do not have phlebitis, what do they have?

DR. JOHN CRANLEY: I would like to try to answer that question. The first answer you must give is that just because you don't know the diagnosis doesn't prove that they have deep venous thrombosis. I estimate that 70% of the patients sent to me in my office with the diagnosis of deep venous thrombosis don't have it, and 50% of the patients sent to the hospital with thrombophlebitis don't have it. And I get a little bit irked when people say to me, "Well, what *do* they have?" We don't always know. But taking differential diagnoses in the order of the frequency of their occurrence, the first is hemorrhage of the muscle, or spontaneous muscle hemorrhage. This is very common. We have 400 or 500 patients with this syndrome in our files. It can be diagnosed by the history of an instantaneous onset of pain that is much more severe than that which occurs with deep venous thrombosis. A few days after onset, ecchymosis may appear.

The second most common differential diagnosis in our practice has been recurrent cellulitis of the limb. When a patient reports that he has had phlebitis 10 or 15 times, the probability is that he has not had it at all. What he has had is recurrent cellulitis of the limb. Some of these patients are hospitalized each time and treated with anticoagulant therapy in the mistaken belief that they have deep venous thrombosis.

The third differential diagnosis in our experience is gravitational swelling. Anyone who sits or stands for a long time may develop swelling of the limb. In debilitated patients or those with painful limbs, such swelling is aggravated. One of the most interesting phases of this study has been the opportunity to study patients with massive swelling of the limb who do not have deep venous thrombosis. A typical case is the patient who returns to the Emergency Room 2 weeks after a hip operation with what appears to be phlegmasia alba dolens. A phleborheogram is obtained that is negative. The referring physician cannot believe this, and so we are able to persuade him to let us obtain a phlebogram. In all such instances to date, the phlebogram has been negative. The explanation is simply an accumulation of gravitational fluid in the patient who sits and watches television all day and evening.

VENOUS THROMBOEMBOLIC DISEASE

Introduction

WHILE VENOUS PHYSIOLOGY is important and varicose veins are a nuisance, and the diagnosis of venous thrombosis is vexing, none of these subjects carry the grave connotation that hangs over the general topic of venous thromboembolism. Pulmonary embolism strikes down the young and old alike. It does not respect the wealthy or the mighty. As indicated by Simon Sevitt below, venous thromboembolism may be an epidemic sweeping Western civilization.

In the section which follows, thrombolytic therapy is discussed by an authoritative source, and heparin therapy by its most lucid apologist. Doctor Sasahara has summarized the current approach to the patient problem using all technical advances heretofore advocated, and the Northwestern group has summarized a large experience with caval interruption. Finally, Mobin-Uddin has presented the current status of the caval umbrella and Greenfield, the fantastic idea of performing percutaneous pulmonary embolectomy.

16 / Pathology and Pathogenesis of Deep Vein Thrombi

SIMON SEVITT, M.D., F.R.C.P.I., F.R.C. PATH.

Consultant Pathologist, Birmingham Accident Hospital,
Birmingham, England

DEEP VEIN THROMBOSIS in the lower limbs is a relatively common condition and is particularly important because of the risk of pulmonary embolism. Most cases arise during the course of another illness, and a connection with confinement to bed and advancing age has been known for a long time. Injured, orthopedic, gynecologic, obstetric and surgical subjects are at risk, but also many medical patients such as those with heart attacks, congestive cardiac failure, acute strokes, paraplegia and tetanus. Occasionally deep vein thrombosis occurs as a primary state in healthy ambulant men and women without apparent cause, and it is now a recognized hazard in patients taking therapeutic estrogens and in women taking contraceptive estrogens. Other recognized predisposing factors are obesity and previous thrombosis. There is also a statistical association between venous thrombosis and blood group A.[11] Evidence has accumulated that venous thrombosis and pulmonary embolism have been increasing progressively in Western society at least since the end of the Second World War, and wave-like changes in its incidence have been recorded in Central Europe with periods of high frequency attributed to prosperity and of low frequency to times of scarcity. Other reports indicate that the incidence is considerably greater in most European countries and North America than in countries in Africa, Asia and South America. These differences are not likely to be genetic in origin because those of Negro and European origin in the United States of America have similar high rates whereas, for example, African Negroes and Japanese have similar low rates. Environmental differences in activity and diet may be responsible, and recent reports indicating a rising incidence of venous thromboembolism after childbirth and surgery in parts of Asia and Africa support this contention. Consequently the pathogenesis of deep vein thrombosis is likely to be complex. Thrombogenic factors are not likely to be restricted to specific effects of trauma or surgery, such as the release of a tissue thromboplastin.

The thrombotic process is abacterial and noninflammatory, and the distinction drawn by some workers between so-called thrombophlebitis and phlebothrombosis (deep vein thrombosis) is not justified. Any inflammatory changes in the vein wall are secondary to the thrombi. Deep vein thrombi are usually bilateral even in patients with injury restricted to one lower limb, but in only a minority do they produce symptoms or signs referable to the limbs, such as pain or swelling. This has been demonstrated by anatomical dissections of the lower limb veins at necropsy and by phlebography and radioactive scanning after injecting ^{125}I-fibrinogen. Thrombosis is silent in the majority of limbs and subjects with thrombi, and this explains the frequency of

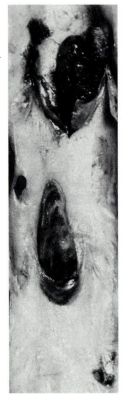

Fig 16–1.—Two small primary thrombi in valve pockets of a common femoral vein.

unheralded embolism, that is, embolism not preceded by limb signs of thrombosis.

Pathology

Deep vein thrombi vary from a few millimeters in length to long tubular masses filling main veins. They are formed in veins greater than 1 or 2 mm in diameter and generally in large or medium-sized vessels. They begin as microscopic nidi, grow by an additive process and become visible. The small thrombi are found commonly in valve pockets (Fig 16–1) throughout various deep veins of the leg and thigh and in saccules of soleal veins. It is from these that the long tubular structures grow.

Figure 16–2 illustrates the process of thrombus growth. At first, growth is by propagation in the direction of the venous stream by the deposition of successive layers of thrombus coagulum from the blood, and by this means the primary microscopic nidus becomes visible (see Fig 16–2, A and B). Addition of further layers, both longitudinally (see Fig 16–2, C) and circumferentially, increases the length and

Fig 16–2. — Diagram illustrating the propagation of a deep vein thrombus from a nidus in a valve pocket (**A**) and the deposition of successive layers of fibrin, platelets, etc. (**B** and **C**). Retrograde extension occurs when there is venous blockage from propagation (**D**).

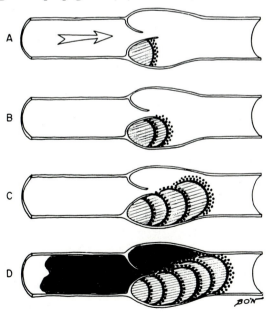

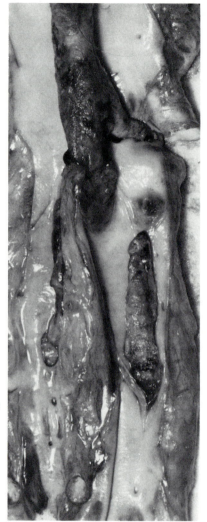

Fig 16–3.—Propagating deep vein thrombus in the common femoral vein (*top*) taking origin from valve pockets at the junction of the deep femoral and superficial femoral veins. Note also the smaller independent propagating thrombus in the deep femoral vein (*right*).

diameter of the thrombus (Figs 16–3 to 16–6). Such thrombi at first are attached to the vein only at their points of origin and float almost freely in the blood stream, which explains their ease of detachment. Contraction helps to prevent venous blockage; serum is squeezed out and a relatively dry, firm structure is formed. The initial attachment is fibrinous, but endothelial-fibrocyte invasion from the intima soon occurs when anchoring begins. Propagation may cease at any time and

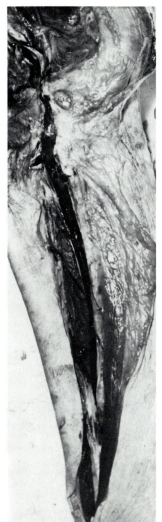

Fig 16–4.—Long confluent thrombus in the common and superficial femoral veins propagating into the external iliac vein (*top*).

later recommence, when fresh thrombus-coagulum is deposited on organizing or even organized material.

With further propagation, venous obstruction may occur and this often leads to retrograde thrombosis back to the next tributary (see Fig 16–2, D). In this way long confluent thrombi in deep thigh veins or leg veins develop (see Fig 16–4). In short, thrombi consist of a centrally directed propagating head, an elongating body, one (or two)

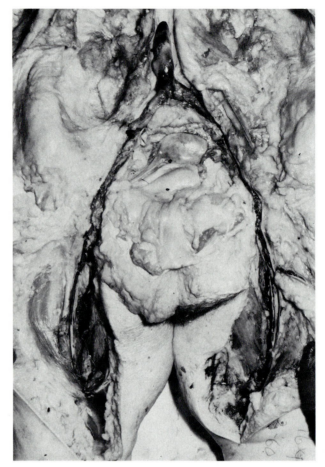

Fig 16–5.—Bilateral iliofemoral thrombi propagating into the lower part of the inferior vena cava.

points of original attachment and sometimes a peripheral retrograde tail. The head is not a fixed part, but it grows and changes as new material is deposited on its surface from the flowing blood, while the body is made up of successive deposits which once formed the head.

STRUCTURE OF THROMBI

All thrombi, whether venous, arterial or cardiac, are formed in flowing blood by an additive process, and this explains their layered structures. All contain a fibrin network, clumps of platelets, red cells and

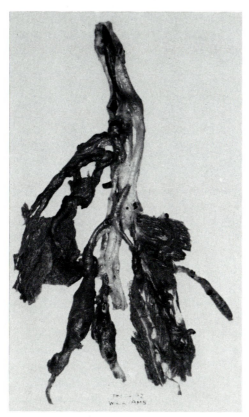

Fig 16–6. — Dissection of the calf showing extensive thrombosis of soleal veins with several dilated thrombosed sinuses. Also note thrombi in the posterior tibial veins.

granular leukocytes, though the relative amounts differ widely. Platelets commonly predominate in recent arterial thrombi and heart-valve vegetations, while most venous thrombi are red structures dominated by large amounts of erythrocytes trapped in a fibrin network, but with many clumps of platelets present especially at the propagating ends. Structural differences are influenced by underlying vascular lesions and speed of blood flow, by venous, arterial or cardiac location, and by the size and age of the thrombi. Nevertheless, present evidence points to closely packed clumps of platelets with narrow fibrin borders (Fig 16–7) as the *building blocks* of all enlarging thrombi, whatever their origin and location. Their formation is likely to involve both the coagulation mechanism and platelet aggregation. These structures will be referred to as platelet-fibrin units.

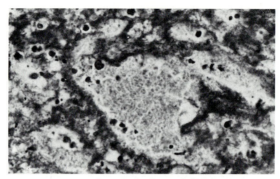

Fig 16–7.—Platelet-fibrin "building blocks" of growing thrombi. Each pale zone is composed of closely packed platelets (with a few leukocytes) and is surrounded by a narrow rim of fibrin. This extends into a peripheral network

STRUCTURE OF VENOUS THROMBI

The surface of a nonadherent venous thrombus is often slightly granular and it has fine circumferential striations known as the lines of Zahn, which are external evidence of lamination. Most are dark red from many red cells, but some are pink or whitish depending on the relative content of red cells, leukocytes and platelets. The propagating end is sometimes expanded—the so-called serpent's head—and is often pink or pale. Isolated pale zones or bands often interrupt the red surface. Lamination is usually evident when a thrombus is cut through.

Histologically, numerous red cells trapped in a fibrin mesh are often dominant, but the phenomenon of layering is also characteristic (Fig 16–8). Layering is prominent in recently propagated thrombi. Red cell masses are laminated circumferentially and longitudinally and seams of fibrin lie within or between them or connect leukocyte or platelet areas with red cell zones. Such thrombi also contain foci of closely packed platelets often surrounded by granular leukocytes and fringed by a narrow rim of fibrin (Figs 16–7 and 16–9). These features are best made out by differential staining with the phospho-tungstic-acid-hematoxylin technique or one of the Mallory trichrome stains such as the acid-picromallory method.

Platelet masses are usually large and prominent in the propagating head (Fig 16–10) or newly formed layers (see Fig 16–9). Though some may appear isolated, close scrutiny and serial sectioning reveals many interconnections. In propagating areas, the platelet masses have a complex coral-like arrangement as noted origi-

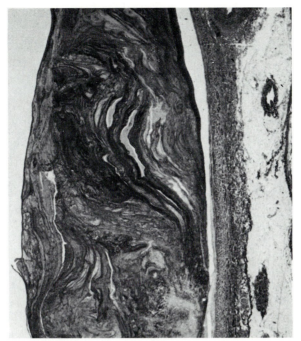

Fig 16–8.—Laminated structure of a femoral vein thrombus cut longitudinally. Vein wall on the right. Picromallory; ×6.6.

nally by Aschoff in 1924.[1] The individual platelets though closely packed are not fused; commonly their outlines and membranes are preserved even at the histologic level. Electron microscopy of deep vein thrombi has not been reported. The close fringing by fibrin is an important feature (platelet-fibrin units) and the platelet-aggregate together with its fibrin border may be considered the structural unit or building block of *growing* thrombi. The fibrin border connects peripherally with a fibrin reticulum entangling red cells and leukocytes, though a few fibrin strands may also pass into or across the platelet clump. Many clumps contain a few large mononuclear cells often packed with phagocytosed platelets.

The intimacy between the platelet-aggregates and the bordering fibrin is the key to thrombus growth, while the lamination indicates the manner of growth. The structure of the fibrin-bordered platelet clumps points to the release of a fibrin-forming substance from the platelets to account for the peripheral fibrin, and a platelet-clumping substance during fibrin formation to account for further platelet masses. Thrombin release could account for both (see below).

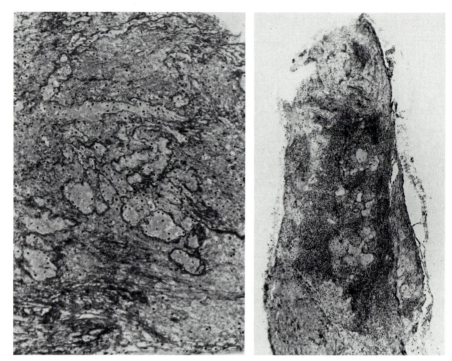

Fig 16–9 (left). — Multiple platelet-fibrin units (building blocks) in a growing venous thrombus. Many units communicate with each other in an irregular corraline fashion. Picromallory; ×120. (Reduced to ⁴/₅.)

Fig 16–10 (right). — Proximal end of the thrombus in Fig 16–12 showing multiple platelet-fibrin units characteristic of recent growth. Picromallory; ×48. (Reduced to ⁴/₅.)

VALVE POCKET THROMBI AND NIDUS STRUCTURE

The structure of valve pocket thrombi was studied to ascertain the nature of the nidi from which they grow and their manner of growth to visible thrombi.[20, 21] Most recent ones have two main architectural zones, namely (1) a red area restricted distally in the pocket and located by the vein wall (Figs 16–11 and 16–12) and (2) a larger white region which comprises most of the length of the thrombus and often covers the red area (Figs 16–10 and 16–12). The white coagulum is propagated growth; its structure includes many well-defined platelet-fibrin units along much of its length (see Fig 16–10) which often cover the red area (see Fig 16–12, left). The overlying valve cusp nearly always remains free and unattached to the thrombus, indicative

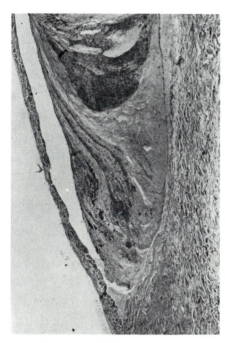

Fig 16–11. — Valve pocket thrombus. Note the pale-stained "red area" by the vein wall (*right*). It is covered by propagated thrombus proximally (*above*) and on the surface facing the valve leaf (*left*). Phosphotungstic-acid hematoxylin; ×30. (Reduced to ⅘.)

Fig 16–12. — Distal end of a valve pocket thrombus. The large "red area" (pale-stained) on the *right* is partly adhering to the vein wall and is covered (on the *left*) by propagated thrombus facing the valve cusp. Picromallory; ×30. (Reduced to ⅘.)

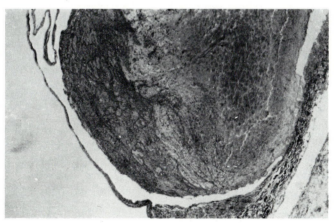

of fibrinolytic activity. The white coagulum is clearly secondary growth similar in structure to that seen in propagating thrombi.

On the other hand, red areas are relatively circumscribed zones located distally in the thrombus by the vein wall (see Fig 16–12, right) and their structure is dominated by red cells with fibrin laminas. They may or may not contain a few platelet-fibrin units, which are tiny when present. These red areas which vary in size are likely to be or to contain the initial structures (nidi) of valve pocket thrombi. Their location distally in the pocket by the vein wall is the first to become anchored to and organized by fibrocytic cells from the vein. Hence this is the oldest and original part of the thrombus.

The platelet-poor or platelet-free structure of the red areas does not suggest an important role for platelets in the formation of thrombus-nidi. This is unlike recent hemostatic plugs and experimental thrombi on damaged endothelium in which platelet masses laid down on the damaged vein wall predominate initially.[5, 18] It is also unlike *recent* thrombi in arteries with atheromatous disease where platelets also predominate initially. However, these platelet structures soon become

Fig 16–13 (left).—Apparently empty valve pocket containing a fusiform mass of crowded red cells with some leukocytes lying against the vein wall (*right*). Hematoxylin and eosin; ×120. (Reduced to ¾.)

Fig 16–14 (right).—Valve pocket containing small masses of polymorphs. Picromallory; ×48. (Reduced to ¾.)

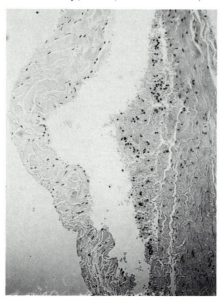
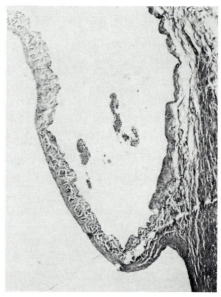

replaced by a predominantly fibrin structure often with many red cells. Consequently a dynamic changing structure may also be involved in the nidi of deep vein thrombi. This counsels caution in underestimating the possible role of platelets.

In an attempt to overcome the static limitations imposed by the histology of valve-pocket thrombi, the microscopic contents of apparently empty femoral valve pockets were investigated to help decide the nature of the initial nidus.[20, 21]

Examination by serial histology of apparently empty valve pockets excised from main femoral veins revealed various small condensed antemortem structures. Of these, condensed foci of red cells often containing some leukocytes (Fig 16–13) were frequent. Tiny fibrin fragments surfaced by endothelial cells were also frequent but were considered to be the remnants of aborted thrombi. The red cell foci must have been deposited into the pocket by eddy currents at the pocket mouth. A few pockets contained tiny circumscribed platelet clumps or small masses of leukocytes similarly deposited (Fig 16–14). Possibly any of these could represent the unstable nidi from which thrombi grow. Stability is achieved through fibrin formation and growth occurs following local interaction between the coagulation sequence and platelet clumping.

VEIN WALL

The studies did not reveal preceding intimal damage or inflammation in the vein wall or valve cusps at the site of small thrombi. Any changes found could be attributed to organization of former thrombi or to technical artifacts. Intimal thickenings are not uncommon in this region but they are probably the endproducts of previous thrombi. Further, there was little difference between the histology of vein walls with and without recent thrombi, and the lining of valve pockets without thrombi was no different from those with tiny thrombus fragments.

Location of Deep Vein Thrombi and Primary Sites of Origin

Venous dissection studies at necropsy have demonstrated thrombi in a variety of locations in the thigh and leg (see Figs 16–3 to 16–6).[6, 13, 22, 23] Independent thrombi may be found in various deep veins of the leg, thigh and pelvis in some limbs and continuous thrombi in other limbs. Thrombi in calf veins are often distinct and separate from thrombi in thigh veins. Thrombosis in calf muscles generally involves the soleal veins, especially the sinuses (see Fig 16–6) and less often veins of the gastrocnemius muscle. Often the former are associated with thrombi in posterior tibial veins, but one can occur without the other. Thrombi in iliac and femoral veins may be independent or continuous. Iliac or femoral vein thrombi may occur without calf vein thrombi and vice versa, or both may be present in the same limb. Thrombosis of the external iliac vein often is associated with thrombosis of the common femoral vein but it may be isolated, while a thrombus in the profunda femoral vein may be isolated or may extend into the common femoral vein. A popliteal vein thrombus is usually continuous with thrombi in the posterior tibial veins, but occasionally it is isolated. It is important to note that thrombosis of the superficial femoral vein rarely occurs as an isolated phenomenon. Usually it is continuous with a long thrombus in the common femoral vein which indicates that it formed by retrograde extension after proximal venous blockage and not by propagation from calf veins. Occasionally, however, it is continuous with a thrombus in the popliteal vein or popliteal and posterior tibial veins as if it had formed by central propagation. Rarely the inferior vena cava is involved through propagation of thrombi from one or both common iliac veins (see Fig 16–5).

These dissection studies resolved the previous conflict concerning the sites of origin of deep vein thrombi. In one view, still unfortunately prevalent, thrombi originate only in calf veins and propagate to the thigh. Another concept regarded thrombi as arising first in the iliofemoral channel and then spreading to the leg through retrograde extension. The dissection studies have shown that the one concept does not exclude the other. Further, the varied patterns of thrombosis can be explained only on the basis that thrombi may begin at one or more of several sites.

Six main primary sites of origin are now recognized.[23] These are shown in Figure 16–15 and consist of (1) the iliac vein, generally the external iliac just above the inguinal ligament, (2) the common femoral vein including the mouths of the medial and lateral circumflex tributaries, (3) the deep femoral vein usually at a valve cusp near its termination, (4) the popliteal vein near the adductor ring where there is a relatively large valve, (5) the posterior tibial veins and (6) the intramuscular veins of the calf, particularly the soleal veins. The concept of multiple independent sites of origin is supported by the occurrence of small isolated thrombi usually in valve-cusps (see Fig 16–1) at the various points. Thrombosis at one site is often independent of thrombosis elsewhere and thrombi may arise in one, two or more of them. Their subsequent extension in the leg or thigh or both is responsible for the variety of thrombus patterns seen at necropsy dissection.

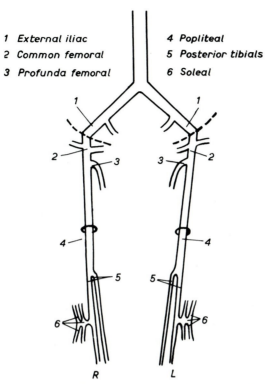

1 External iliac   4 Popliteal
2 Common femoral   5 Posterior tibials
3 Profunda femoral   6 Soleal

Fig 16–15.—Diagram of the primary sites of origin of deep vein thrombi in the lower venous tree. The six main sites in the thigh and calf are independent of each other, although thrombosis is frequent at two or more of them. The thrombi extend from these loci of origin.

Thrombi in calf veins are usually the earliest and most frequent manifestation of deep vein thrombosis, and there is evidence that the independent thigh vein thrombi form later in many subjects.[6, 23] This may have relevance to their pathogenesis in some cases, since thrombogenic substances released from calf vein thrombi might initiate independent thigh vein thrombi under certain conditions like venous stasis. Though calf vein thrombi usually form earlier than thigh vein thrombi, the latter are more dangerous because of major embolic detachment.

SIGNIFICANCE OF MULTIPLE PRIMARY SITES OF ORIGIN

The multiple independent sites of thrombus origin and especially the independent loci of origin in deep leg and thigh veins indicate that anatomical peculiarities of the lower venous tree together with the dynamics of a slowed venous stream decide where the thrombi begin to form, especially in the horizontal position of bedrest. The sites of election can be explained by a disturbance of normal laminar blood flow at valves and saccules induced by venous stasis. Turbulence is produced, a phenomenon similar to the eddies of a river at a bend, and there is experimental evidence that the direction of flow at the periphery of a slowed stream may be even locally reversed from that in the center. Flow studies in excised venous segments[4] showed that when perfusion was from below, the stream eddied at the free borders of the valve cusps, and when india ink was injected into the valve pockets, it lay in a stagnant pool with little movement or diffusion into the moving perfusate. In extracorporeal shunts, turbulent flow produces silting of formed elements, especially platelets, and their deposition on the wall at eddy zones.[15] Likely favorite sites for eddies are all valve pockets, especially large ones, dilated sinuses like those in the soleal veins, the termination of the posterior tibial veins when compressed by the tendinous origin of the soleus muscle, the common femoral veins because of the multiple streams of inflow and the external iliac veins because of the acute change in flow direction above the inguinal ligament. Thus, only venous anatomy and disturbances of flow promoted by stasis can explain the primary sites of deep vein thrombogenesis.

Pathogenesis

Since the time of Virchow, venous stasis has been recognized as the major predisposing factor in most cases of deep vein thrombosis. Whether or not "hypercoagulable" blood changes are necessary is still debated, though many of the findings reported are likely to be the results of thrombosis rather than its cause. The need for primary damage to the venous intima is questionable. Since Eberth and Schimmelbusch, concepts of venous thrombogenesis have been dominated by the controversy concerning the presence or absence of intimal lesions, and recent studies have been complicated by the belief that every thrombus begins at the site of endothelial injury. However, present evidence indicates that venous thrombi form on normal endothelium.

Venous Stasis

The connection between venous stasis and thrombi, though strong, rests on circumstantial evidence. The frequency of deep vein thrombosis at necropsy is closely related to advancing age and duration of bed rest, and the preconditions of venous stasis—immobilization of a lower limb in a plaster cast, sitting still with the limbs dependent, congestive cardiac failure and so on—are those which occur in the variety of medical, surgical, traumatic and other subjects prone to thrombosis.

Both the linear speed of venous flow along the lower limbs assessed with radioactive isotopes[30] and the rate of clearance of injected radio-opaque material[13] are greatly reduced when the limbs are supine, horizontal and still. Further, the blood volume of the limbs increases during recumbency due mainly to venous dilatation, probably because the deep veins behave like passive tubes, their emptying depending on calf muscle contraction. Moreover there is phlebographic evidence that the points of maximum stasis along relatively stagnant channels are the valve pockets and venous saccules.[13] Clearance of the injected radiopaque medium was particularly delayed in circumscribed foci corresponding to valve pockets in thigh veins and venous saccules in deep calf veins.

The term stasis implies either a reduced linear velocity (centimeters per minute) or a reduced rate of venous return (volume per minute) and the latter of course is dependent on the arterial perfusion of the limbs. Dilation of veins is particularly important for a fall in linear velocity, but in operation cases at least, reduction of arterial perfusion of the limbs also seems important.[2] Thus the reduced linear velocity is due to venous dilatation, combined in many cases with a fall in arterial perfusion of the lower limbs.

THROMBOGENIC EFFECTS OF VENOUS STASIS

Complete cessation of flow does not produce thrombosis in vessels, at least in carefully ligated segments, though it has been reported that a combination of isolation and partial obstruction of a vein segment for more than 24 hr often led to thrombosis.[17]

The disturbance of laminar flow induced by slowing of the venous return, including the production of turbulence and eddies and the pooling of blood at particular sites, already has been referred to. A number of other effects with thrombogenic potential may also occur at the particularly stagnant foci:

1. The silting into valve pockets and venous saccules of platelets, leukocytes and red cells.

2. The accumulation within the pockets and saccules of activated blood clotting factors either released locally or already arrived from a

distance, by retarding their dilution. The experimental production of stasis thrombosis by injection of serum has particular relevance to this possibility.

3. The local accumulation of adenosine diphosphate (ADP) derived from the silted red cells and leukocytes.

4. Preventing the arrival from a distance of substances like anti-thrombin and plasma ADPase which inhibit fibrin formation and ADP-induced platelet aggregation.

5. Possibly the production of hypoxia in endothelium lining valve pockets.

SERUM-INDUCED STASIS THROMBI

The various experimental methods for producing venous thrombi which utilize intimal damage seem to have little bearing on what happens in deep vein thrombosis, and the concept has been advanced in recent years primarily by Wessler[28] that venous thrombi may develop by a combination of vascular stasis and altered coagulability of the blood without intimal damage. This was based on an experimental model in which ligatures are placed proximally and distally on a freed segment of a large vein, then serum free of thrombin is injected into another vein and the ligatures are tied a few moments later.[27] A red worm-like thrombus forms within the isolated segment. The serum activity is transient, as if it is destroyed or removed, and thrombi do not form if there is undue delay in tying off the vascular segment. Such stasis thrombi consist of red cells enmeshed in a fine fibrin network and contain only scattered platelets and leukocytes. Their structure is that of a blood clot formed in a tube. Unlike natural thrombi, they are not laminated and there are no clumps of platelets or polymorphs. However, when the thrombi are exposed to flowing blood, varying amounts of platelets, leukocytes and fibrin adhere to the surface. The thrombogenic properties of the serum were ultimately traced to the presence of certain activated coagulation factors now believed to be important for the early stages of intrinsic clotting, that is, activated clotting factors XII (Hageman), XI and IX. These are present as inactive precursors in normal plasma but are activated during clotting. Subsequent studies[29] showed that activated factor X has very powerful thrombogenic power and indicated that activation of this highly unstable factor in vivo is likely to be particularly important as a thrombogenic intermediary. Other studies showed that techniques other than serum infusion can also trigger thrombosis in areas of venous stasis, such as the injection of surface-active agents like celite,[26] long-chain saturated fatty acids[3] and the endotoxin of certain gram-negative bacilli.[25] These presumably work through their power to activate parts of the clotting mechanism.

When the possible role of ADP in producing stasis-thrombi was studied, even relatively large doses given intravenously failed to produce thrombi in isolated venous segments, though a marked reduction in the circulating platelet count occurred.[24] Thus ADP-induced platelet aggregation is unlikely to be an initiating factor in the pathogenesis of stasis thrombosis.

Hypothesis of Pathogenesis (Fig 16–16)

The full explanation is likely to be more complex than the following account, details of which are elaborated elsewhere.[9]

As already noted, red cells and fibrin predominate in the structure of the nidus from which a venous thrombus grows and platelets are

Fig 16–16. — Outline of an hypothesis of deep vein thrombogenesis (nidus formation) on normal intimal endothelium under conditions of venous stasis.

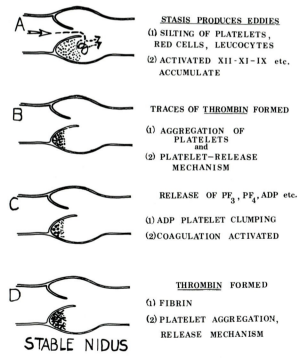

A

STASIS PRODUCES EDDIES
(1) SILTING OF PLATELETS,
RED CELLS, LEUCOCYTES
(2) ACTIVATED XII - XI - IX etc.
ACCUMULATE

B

TRACES OF THROMBIN FORMED
(1) AGGREGATION OF
PLATELETS
and
(2) PLATELET—RELEASE
MECHANISM

C

RELEASE OF PF_3, PF_4, ADP etc.
(1) ADP PLATELET CLUMPING
(2) COAGULATION ACTIVATED

D

THROMBIN FORMED
(1) FIBRIN
(2) PLATELET AGGREGATION,
RELEASE MECHANISM

STABLE NIDUS

relatively few or absent histologically. Formed elements, especially red cells, are silted into the valve pocket or saccule by eddy currents promoted by slowing of the venous stream (stage A). The silted elements are unstable at first and are liable to be washed away with an increase in venous flow. Stability is ensured by the formation of fibrin (stage D) which is dependent on the generation of thrombin. The thrombin is formed locally but cannot be washed away because of the flow disturbance. Generation of sufficient thrombin to transform fibrinogen to fibrin probably depends on intermediary reactions (stages B and C), the power of thrombin to clump platelets at weak concentrations and the consequent platelet-release mechanism which makes platelet thromboplastin (PF3) available for the coagulation mechanism. By this means more thrombin is generated. At present, only local generation of thrombin can explain stabilization of the nidus on intact endothelium and its subsequent growth to a thrombus.

Two methods are possible for the initial appearance of thrombin, namely (1) through the carriage of activated coagulation factors from a distance (stage A) or (2) by their local formation. The former is in accord with the experimental production of venous thrombi under conditions of stasis following the injection of serum into the general circulation (see above). Consequently the carriage from afar of activated factors involved in the early stage of intrinsic coagulation, that is, activated factors XII, XI or IX, might trigger the coagulation sequence in the stagnant pools of valve pockets, activate factor X and lead to the generation of a little thrombin. Factor XII may not be essential since the original patient with congenital deficiency of this factor (Mr. Hageman) died of pulmonary embolism.[19] The work indicating that subcutaneous injections of heparin, in dosage which fails to affect whole blood clotting time, have the power to prevent postoperative calf vein thrombi[12] is consistent with and supports the present concept of deep vein thrombogenesis. Small amounts of heparin in the blood probably have the ability to inhibit traces of thrombin and thereby prevent the thrombogenic process. Further, heparin has been shown to enhance the normal inhibitory power of plasma against purified activated factor X[31] and may thereby help neutralize the appearance of traces of activated factor X.

This concept presupposes a continual or at least intermittent activation of the early stage procoagulant factors in the vascular system and a normal mechanism for their removal. The latter has been demonstrated, the liver and reticuloendothelial system being largely responsible, but the former is still hypothetical. The possibility is worth considering that atheromatous lesions in the lower aorta and major arteries of the lower limbs contribute to the initiation process by activating procoagulant factors in the blood flowing over them. This would help to explain the susceptibility of middle-aged and elderly patients to deep vein thrombi. However it cannot be the whole explanation since young subjects without significant atheroma may also develop deep vein thrombi. Further, it would not explain the occurrence of venous thrombosis in young women taking contraceptive estrogens. In them, estrogen-induced changes in the coagulation mechanism or platelet-behavior may be operative, thrombosis probably occurring during the stasis of normal nocturnal bedrest. However the precise mechanism is unknown as yet.

An alternative initiating mechanism is the onset of platelet aggregation through the local release of ADP from the red cells and leukocytes silted into the valve pockets. The process might continue to thrombin generation following platelet degranulation and the release of platelet thromboplastin (PF3) with consequent activation of the intrinsic clotting mechanism. Against the role of extrinsic clotting as an initial pathway are the reports of venous thromboembolism in patients with congenital deficiency of factor VII,[7, 8] the experiments which failed to produce stasis thrombi after injecting large doses of ADP (see above) and also the uncertainty concerning the increased availability of PF3 by ADP action on platelets. On the other hand ADP may be involved as a supplementary mechanism following the initial action of thrombin (stage C). Release of platelet factor 4 might also be a factor (stage C), since this can precipitate fibrinogen, and its injection produces evidence of intravascular coagulation in in vivo experiments.

The final outcome is also determined by the balance between thrombogenic and fibrinolytic mechanisms, not shown in Figure 16–16. Favoring thrombosis is the demonstration that little fibrinolytic activity develops in the veins of the leg after the production of stasis,[16] and that there is a relatively prolonged period of inhibited fibrinolysis following an early transient activation in injured patients[10] and others exposed to stress. In circumstances favorable to thrombogenesis, the nidus once formed is strengthened by fibrin through further release of thrombin. Growth occurs through the successive deposition of layers of aggregated platelets and fibrin with entangled red cells and leukocytes. Soon this becomes the propagating head and the original nidus area remains or is transformed into a structure containing much fibrin, many red cells and few platelet clumps.

Fibrin contraction is probably important for nidus stabilization and growth, since serum containing thrombin would be locally released. Its action is likely to be potentiated by the release from degranulated platelets of platelet-aggregating substances like ADP and adrenaline, and coagulation activators (PF3 and PF4). Thrombogenesis is likely to be arrested at any stage by an increase in venous return with abolition of eddy currents, and with consequent dilution and neutralization of locally released thrombogenic and platelet aggregating substances.

Summary

Deep vein thrombi begin as microscopic nidi generally in valve pockets throughout various veins of the leg, thigh and pelvis. Growth is by an additive process through the repeated deposition of thrombus-coagulum from the flowing blood. Thereby they become layered structures. Venous stasis and eddying of flow are the main predisposing mechanisms for formation and growth. Thrombi can form independently in various deep thigh and leg veins and bilateral thrombosis is common. Growth can occur from each primary site by forward propagation, and later by retrograde extension after venous blockage. Thereby long tubular structures are formed. Thrombi form earlier and more commonly in calf veins than in thigh veins. Growth is characterized histologically by lamination and by multiple platelet masses closely rimmed by fibrin—the "building blocks" of all thrombi. The structure of these platelet-fibrin units indicates that biochemical interaction between platelets and the coagulation mechanism is the key to growth. Repeated activation of the coagulation sequence and of platelet aggregation following the liberation of small amounts of thrombin is the probable explanation.

The structure of valve pocket thrombi indicates that the nidus of origin is located distally in the pocket near the vein wall, that it is laid down on normal venous endothelium and is formed mainly of red cells and fibrin. Platelet collections are either absent or are few and small in contrast with their prominence in the growing parts of thrombi.

REFERENCES

1. Aschoff, L.: *Lectures on Pathology* (New York: Hoeber, 1924), Chapter 11.
2. Browse, N. L.: Effect of bedrest on resting calf blood flow of healthy adult males, Br. Med. J. 1:1721, 1962.
3. Connor, W. E., Hoak, J. C., and Warner, E. D.: Fatty Acids and Thrombus Formation, in Sasahara, A. A., and Stein, M., (eds.): *Pulmonary Embolic Disease* (New York: Grune & Stratton, 1965).
4. Cotton, L. T., and Clarke, C.: Anatomical localization of venous thrombosis, Ann. R. Coll. Surg. Engl. 36:214, 1965..
5. French, J. E.: The structure of natural and experimental thrombi, Ann. R. Coll. Surg. Engl. 36:191, 1965.

6. Gibbs, N. M.: Venous thrombosis in the lower limbs with particular reference to bedrest, Br. J. Surg. 45:209, 1957.
7. Godal, H. C., Madsen, K., and Nissen-Meyer, R.: Thromboembolism in patients with local proconvertin (Factor VII) deficiency, Acta Med. Scand. 171:325, 1962.
8. Hall, C. A., Rapaport, S. L., Ames, S. B., and De Groot, J. A.: A clinical and family study of hereditary proconvertin (Factor VII) deficiency, Am. J. Med. 37:172, 1964.
9. Hume, M., Sevitt, S., and Thomas, D. P.: *Venous Thrombosis and Pulmonary Embolism* (London: Oxford Press, and Cambridge, Mass.: Harvard Press, 1970).
10. Innes, D., and Sevitt, S.: Coagulation and fibrinolysis in injured patients, J. Clin. Pathol. 17:1, 1964.
11. Jick, H., Slone, D., Westerholm, B., Inman, W. H., Vessey, M. P., Shapiro, S., Lewis, G. P., and Worcester, J.: Venous thromboembolic disease and ABO blood type, Lancet 1:539, 1969.
12. Kakkar, V. V., Field, E. S., Nicolaides, A. M., Flute, P. T., Wessler, S., and Yin, E. T.: Low doses of heparin in prevention of deep vein thrombosis, Lancet 2:669, 1971.
13. McLachlin, A. D., McLachlin, J. A., Jory, T., and Rawling, E. G.: Venous stasis in the lower extremities, Ann. Surg. 152:678, 1960.
14. McLachlin, J., and Paterson, J. C.: Some basic observations on venous thrombosis and pulmonary embolism, Surg. Gynecol. Obstet. 93:1, 1951.
15. Mustard, J. F., Murphy, E. A., Rowsell, H. C., and Downie, H. G.: Factors influencing thrombus formation *in vivo*, Am. J. Med. 33:621, 1962.
16. Nilsson, I. M.: Changes in the coagulation and fibrinolytic system predisposing to thrombosis, Acta Chirurg. Scand. (Suppl.) 387:15, 1968.
17. O'Neill, J. F.: Effects on venous endothelium of alterations in blood flow through vessels in vein walls, and possible relation to thrombosis, Ann. Surg. 126:270, 1947.
18. Poole, J. C. F.: Structural aspects of thrombosis, Sci. Basis Med. 55:1964.
19. Ratnoff, O. D., Busse, R. J., and Sheon, R. P.: The demise of John Hageman, N. Engl. J. Med. 279:760, 1968.
20. Sevitt, S.: The structure and growth of valve-pocket thrombi in femoral veins, J. Clin. Pathol. 27:517, 1974.
21. Sevitt, S.: Pathology and pathogenesis of deep vein thrombi, Proc. Roy. Soc. Med. 68:261, 1975.
22. Sevitt, S., and Gallagher, N. G.: Prevention of venous thrombosis and pulmonary embolism in injured patients. A trial of anticoagulant prophylaxis with phenindione in elderly patients with fractured necks of femur, Lancet 2:981, 1959.
23. Sevitt, S., and Gallagher, N. G.: Venous thrombosis and pulmonary embolism. A clinicopathological study in injured and burned patients, Br. J. Surg. 48:475, 1961.
24. Stuart, R. K., and Thomas, D. P. Comparative effects of ADP and thrombin in producing stasis thrombosis, Thromb. Diath. Haemorrh. 18:537, 1967.
25. Thomas, D. P., and Wessler, S.: Stasis-thrombi induced by bacterial endotoxin, Circ. Res. 14:486, 1964.
26. Thomas, D. P., Wessler, S., and Reimer, S. M.: The relationship of Factors XII, XI and IX to hypercoagulable states, Thromb. Diath. Haemorrh. 9:90, 1963.
27. Wessler, S.: Studies in intravascular coagulation. III. The pathogenesis of serum-induced venous thrombosis, J. Clin. Invest. 34:647, 1955.
28. Wessler, S.: Thrombosis in the presence of vascular stasis, Am. J. Med. 33:648, 1962.
29. Wessler, S., and Yin, E. T.: Experimental hypercoagulable state induced by Factor X: Comparison of non-activated and activated forms, J. Lab. Clin. Med. 72:256, 1968.
30. Wright, H. P., Osborn, S. B., and Edmunds, D. G.: Effects of post-operative bedrest and early ambulation on the rate of venous blood flow, Lancet 1:222, 1951.
31. Yin, E. T., Wessler, S., and Stoll, P. J.: Rabbit plasma inhibitor of the activated species of blood coagulation factor X. Purification and some properties, J. Biol. Chem. 246:3694, 1971.

17 / The Status of Thrombolytic Therapy

Hau C. Kwaan, M.D., F.R.C.P. (Edin.), F.A.C.P.

Professor of Medicine, Northwestern University Medical School, and the Hematology Section, Veterans Administration Lakeside Hospital, Chicago, Illinois

THE APPROACH to the management of thromboembolism has undergone a significant change with the advent of fibrinolytic agents. Hitherto, the therapy has been limited to the use of anticoagulants that can only prevent the propagation of the thrombus while relying on the endogenous fibrinolytic activity to effect its resolution. With exogenous fibrinolytic agents, on the other hand, one hopes to achieve a more effective direct lysis of the thrombus.[1-3] A variety of fibrinolytic agents are now available for thrombolytic therapy. Reports of clinical trials[4-14] indicate that in many thromboembolic conditions, better results were obtained with fibrinolytic agents when used in combination with anticoagulants when compared with those observed with anticoagulants alone. These results, however, are far from fulfilling the initial hopes of a rapid and complete lysis of the thrombus. A number of problems related to the modality of thrombolytic therapy, such as the optimal dosage, choice of fibrinolytic agents, supplementary administration of plasminogen, frequency and duration of doses and the optimal means of delivery of fibrinolytic agents to the site of thromboembolism, are yet to be solved before thrombolytic therapy can be accepted as a definitive measure in the management of thromboembolic diseases. In order to apply thromboembolic therapy judiciously, a thorough understanding of the mechanism of thrombus formation, propagation and resolution is essential. Some of the major factors important in the thrombogenesis are also the very same factors that impair the lysis of a thrombus. Virchow first pointed out the triad of etiologic factors,[15] namely, changes in the contents of the blood, alteration in the blood flow and abnormalities in the blood vessel wall. By the same token, lysis of a thrombus can be impaired by changes in the blood such as increase in inhibitors of fibrinolysis, decrease in plasminogen or a high fibrinogen level. Aberrant blood flow can result in a thrombus rich in platelets and thus resistant to fibrinolysis, and a damaged vascular intima loses its content of plasminogen activator and cannot contribute to local lysis of the thrombus. As a tribute to Doctor de Takats, it should be pointed out that a number of years ago he had stressed the importance of the variability of endogenous fibrinolytic response to stimuli among patients with thromboembolic disorders, and had given the term "fibrinolytic potential" to this response.[16, 17]

Greater attention has also been given recently to the relationship between the structure of a thrombus and its susceptibility to lysis. Most venous thrombi are composed mainly of fibrin and red cells with only small amounts of leukocytes and platelets. They are thus regarded as suitable for thrombolytic therapy. In contrast, most arterial thrombi are rich in platelets and leukocytes and contain less fibrin and are resistant to lysis. This general rule is, however, not always applicable. Venous thrombi very often show a high content of platelets. This is particularly true in thrombi in venous segments that previously have been the site of recurrent thrombosis. Here the pattern of blood flow has been altered by incomplete recanalization of the organized thrombus. Platelet-rich thrombi can be produced experimentally by alteration of blood flow by means of reducing the lumen size of a venous segment.[18] Such thrombi contain few fibrin strands found between layers and clumps of degranulated platelets and are resistant to fibrinolysis. Similarly, the early nidus of a venous thrombus arising from a vein valve is also composed mainly of platelets. Though the secondary thrombus that results from the propagation of the original nidus is rich in fibrin and is thus susceptible to lysis, complete resolution of the thrombus may not always be achieved.

Pharmacology

The nature of the fibrinolytic system and the pharmacology of the various fibrinolytic agents has been extensively reviewed[1, 3, 19-28] and will be discussed only briefly. Fibrinolysis in vivo is brought about by the conversion of plasminogen to plasmin by specific plasminogen activators. An internal arginylvaline bond in native plasminogen (Glu-Pg) first is cleaved to form a species of plasmin (Glu-Pm),[25] which may then autocatalytically cleave an amino terminal peptide from the heavy chain of Glu-Pm to form the final species of plasmin (Lys-Pm) (Fig 17–1). Plasminogen (Glu-Pg) may also be converted by the initial molecules of Glu-Pm or Lys-Pm to form a smaller form of plasminogen, Lys-Pg, before the final formation of Lys-Pm. This new understanding of the biochemical basis of plasminogen activation takes on a new significance since it has been found that the intermediary form of plasminogen (Lys-Pg) is more readily adsorbed onto fibrin than the native form (Glu-Pg)[26] and that the intravenous infusion of a small amount of partially activated plasminogen (containing Lys-Pg) greatly enhances the clinically demonstrable thrombolytic effects of streptokinase in patients with extensive deep vein thrombosis.[27]

In the discussion of the pharmacology of thrombolysis, naturally occurring inhibitors of fibrinolysis in the blood must be considered. It is known that these inhibitors may be elevated in the blood in patients suffering from a variety of pathologic conditions associated with a thromboembolic diathesis.[28] These inhibitors include an antiplasmin, an inhibitor against plasminogen activation and specific inhibitors against urokinase.[29, 30] Among these, the alpha-2 plasmin inhibitor[31] containing antiplasmin activity is perhaps the one with greatest clinical significance. Others include antithrombin III,[32] alpha-1 antitrypsin,[33] C1-inhibitor,[34, 35] and inter-alpha-trypsin inhibitor.[36]

The in vivo interaction between therapeutically administered plasminogen activators and these inhibitors is still not clearly understood. Obviously, the inhibitory action must be overcome before the activator can exert its action on the thrombus. The variability of inhibitor levels in different patients can thus greatly influence the effectiveness of the therapy.

The interrelationship between the fibrinolytic components in the circulating plasma and those within the thrombus is also a matter of

Fig 17–1. — Activation of human plasminogen to plasmin.

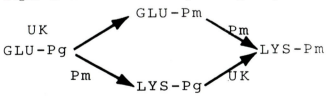

Pg = PLASMINOGEN
Pm = PLASMIN
UK = UROKINASE

intense study. According to Alkjaersig et al.[37] plasminogen is adsorbed to fibrin during the thrombus formation. Activators from whatever source (e.g., therapeutic urokinase) would convert this "in-thrombus" plasminogen to plasmin which in turn would digest the fibrin in situ. This hypothesis recently has been challenged.[38] It has been shown that the in-thrombus plasminogen may not be sufficient for the lysis of the thrombus as first thought and that adequate amounts of plasminogen from the circulating blood reaching the thrombus may be the deciding factor on the success or failure of the lysis.

THROMBOLYTIC AGENTS AVAILABLE

The fibrinolytic enzyme, plasmin, has been used in earlier phases of development of thrombolytic therapy. Preparations containing plasmin derived from streptokinase activation of plasminogen (Thrombolysin)[39] or from trypsin activation of plasminogen were shown to be able to increase significantly the plasma fibrinolytic activity. Due to many reasons, including excessive fibrinogenolysis and hypotension from activation of plasma kininogens,[22] plasmin gave way to plasminogen activators as the more popular agents were used in clinical trials. Attempts to stimulate endogenous plasminogen activator release from blood vessel wall have been made using vasoactive drugs such as nicotinic acid and its analogues,[40] sulfonylureas, phenformin, testosterone and other anabolic steroids.[41] A moderate increase in the plasma fibrinolytic activity can be achieved, but such action is usually transient. Significant thrombolysis of a major thrombus or embolus has not been convincingly demonstrated, though several reports of improvement in cutaneous vasculitis have appeared in the literature.[42] Of the available exogenous plasminogen activators, urokinase and streptokinase have undergone extensive experimental and clinical studies.

Urokinase in its natural state in the urine has a polypeptide structure with a molecular weight of 54,000.[43] This has been purified for therapeutic use with the pharmacologic preparation containing a smaller active fragment having a molecular weight of 36,000.[44] Recently, another source of urokinase was discovered in the cultures of human kidney cells.[45-47] The pharmacologic product derived from the tissue culture has a similar molecular size of 35,000. Urokinase is stable in the lyophilized from, but tends to adsorb to glass when in solution. It is thus prepared with either human albumin or mannitol for stabilization.

Streptokinase is derived from the filtrate of cultures of beta-hemolytic streptococcus and is thus antigenic in contrast to urokinase. Both are potent activators of plasminogen but have no lytic action on fibrin by themselves. As emphasized earlier, the effectiveness of these agents depends on the availability of plasminogen either trapped within the thrombus or from the circulating plasma. During fibrinolytic therapy, particularly when streptokinase is used, the continuous activation of the circulating plasminogen may lead to its depletion. New clots formed at this time would be lacking in plasminogen and thus relatively refractory to further actions by plasminogen activator.

It has been shown that streptokinase may form an equimolar complex with plasmin.[25] Such a complex acts as a plasminogen activator but does not have any fibrinolytic action of its own. Thus it is possible that during streptokinase therapy, most of the circulating plasminogen is converted to plasmin while an excess of streptokinase would then combine with the plasmin to form the streptokinase-plasmin complex. In time, both the plasminogen and any "free" plasmin would be depleted. The resulting enzymes in circulation would then consist only of potent activators, streptokinase and streptokinase-plasmin complex, none of which has any direct lytic effect on the fibrin clot. Thus, during streptokinase therapy it is important to monitor not just the activator activity but more appropriately the plasmin activity. This usually is accomplished by using the thrombin time test.[48]

MODE OF ADMINISTRATION

Either urokinase or streptokinase is usually given systemically, although attempts have been made to infuse either agent locally into a vessel proximal to the site of the thrombotic obstruction. In the case of urokinase, a loading dose of 2,000 CTA units/lb of body weight is given intravenously, followed by the continuous intravenous infusion of amounts of 2,000 CTA units/lb body weight/hr. This dosage may be adjusted in order to maintain a euglobulin lysis time[22] of 15–20 min. The individual variations to the pharmacologic effect of urokinase, namely drug resistance, are not commonly encountered. If this level of induced plasma fibrinolytic activity is maintained for 8–12 hr, most thrombi in the body that are amenable to lysis should be optimally affected. In the case of streptokinase, a different problem in dosage may arise from previous immunization to beta-hemolytic streptococcus. A high antistreptokinase antibody level may be encountered in patients having recent streptococcal infections and in those who have recently received streptokinase treatment. In these patients the initial dose is titrated in vitro by the determination of the amount of streptokinase required to lyse, in 10 min, 1.0 ml of a patient's citrated plasma, after clotting by calcium chloride. This titrated dose multiplied by the total plasma volume would be the amount of loading dose and should overcome the circulating antistreptokinase activity. In the absence of such antibody, the initial loading dose of 250,000 units should be adequate for a 70-kg adult. Since streptokinase is antigenic, the possibility of an anaphylactoid reaction must be kept in mind. As a precaution, most investigators advocate that the loading dose should be given over 30 min by slow intravenous infusion and that 100 mg of hydrocortisone should be given intravenously prior to streptokinase therapy. The loading dose is followed by a continuous intravenous infusion at the rate of 100,000 units/hr.

For simplified clinical monitoring the euglobulin lysis time method[22] provides adequate information on the pharmacologic effect of urokinase. In the case of streptokinase, however, because of the formation of streptokinase-plasmin complex as discussed above, what one would like to measure is the activity of plasmin and not that of plasminogen. Thus, the euglobulin lysis time is not suitable. Since plasmin causes proteolysis of fibrinogen, fibrinogen degradation product levels in the plasma would reflect the ultimate pharmacologic action.[49] A simplified laboratory test commonly used is the thrombin time. This should be prolonged to 2–3 times the control value.

COMPLICATIONS OF THROMBOLYTIC THERAPY

For effective therapy, the doses of thrombolytic agents may have to be sufficiently high to produce a significantly increased systemic fibrinolytic activity. An impaired hemostatic function always exists during the period of therapy. The frequency and severity of bleeding complications varies from minor oozing at sites of venipuncture to massive blood loss. This seems to depend on the care given to the invasive procedures performed immediately before and during the thrombolytic therapy. One of the most carefully documented observations of hemorrhagic complications was made during the Phase 1 Urokinase Pulmonary Embolism Trial (UPET)[4, 5] and the Phase 2 Urokinase-Streptokinase Pulmonary Embolism Trial (USPET).[50] When urokinase was given in the doses mentioned here for 12 hr, 60% of the patients were observed to have significant bleeding accompanied by a fall in their hematocrit value of 10% or more or which required the transfusion of two or more units of blood. The bleeding usually took place at cutdown sites and other locations of invasive procedures. It is noteworthy that no correlation was observed between the severity of bleeding and the degree of changes in the coagulation parameters, such as the plasma fibrinogen or plasminogen levels, or the shortening of the whole blood euglobulin lysis time. It was found in the Phase 2 USPET that among those patients receiving 24 hr of urokinase therapy, the incidence of severe bleeding was higher than among those treated for only 12 hr. Reduction of invasive procedures to a minimum and meticulous care given to any intravenous puncture would greatly reduce the bleeding complications. Recent surgical procedures, particularly those of orthopedic nature, are definite contraindications to thrombolytic therapy.

When streptokinase is used, one may encounter several additional complications that are not seen with urokinase therapy. A pyrexial reaction was observed with certain older preparations, though this is now rare with the more purified extracts. An anaphylactoid vasomotor collapse has also been reported. As a precautionary measure, a pretreatment dose of hydrocortisone (100 mg intravenously) is recommended.

COMPARABILITY OF DIFFERENT AGENTS

The relative merits of urokinase and streptokinase do not seem to be of sufficient importance to preclude the use of one agent over the other in most instances. The exception is in the case of immunologic resistance to streptokinase. Since streptokinase is derived from streptococcus, any recent infection with the hemolytic streptococcus would raise the antistreptokinase antibody level. In practice, this is not a frequent encounter. Also, for the same reason of antigenicity, streptokinase therapy cannot be repeated within a short period of time should a recurrence of thromboembolism require a second course of thrombolytic therapy.

Among the urokinase preparations, two forms derived from human urine, Winkinase with a molecular size 54,000[43] and Urokinase with a molecular size of 36,000,[44] though biophysically different were shown clinically to have the same therapeutic and pharmacologic properties. Likewise, recent comparability studies carried out clinically on the urokinase derived from tissue culture and those from urine showed no differences in their clinical behavior.[47]

RESULTS OF THROMBOLYTIC THERAPY

Pulmonary Embolism

Because spontaneous resolution of a thrombus or embolus can occur with anticoagulant therapy alone, the effectiveness of thrombolytic agents cannot be assessed with certainty. The best documented clinical trial thus far is a prospective randomized study of urokinase and streptokinase in pulmonary embolism (UPET Phase 1 and USPET Phase 2). The results were published in detail elsewhere.[4, 5, 50] Although no difference in mortality rate was found between the anticoagulant (heparin) group and the thrombolytic group, a greater degree of improvement in the hemodynamic abnormalities and in the pulmonary perfusion (as shown by the lung scan) was observed in the thrombolytic group when compared with the heparin group. The clinical changes were not as striking as the objective parameters in most cases. However, among those patients with massive embolism, the dyspnea and the accentuated pulmonary closure sound disappeared more quickly in the thrombolytic group. The difference in results between the two groups, though statistically significant 24 hr after the therapy, did not persist when the lung scan resolutions were compared again on the 7th day. This finding was not surprising since, with adequate heparin therapy, one would expect a significant degree of spontaneous fibrinolysis. The investigators in this study conclude that it is the patient with massive pulmonary embolism who is most likely to benefit from thrombolytic therapy particularly when systemic hypotension is present. Thus, in the patient in whom surgical embolectomy might be indicated, a "medical embolectomy" with thrombolytic agents may be tried instead, hoping to achieve a lower mortality.

Deep Vein Thrombosis

Though there is general agreement that thrombolytic therapy is indicated in the first attack of deep vein thrombosis, the results are even more difficult to assess than those in pulmonary embolism. The aim of therapy in this thrombotic condition is to achieve a complete resolution with little or no damage to the venous structures, thus avoiding the sequelae of chronic venous insufficiency and of recurrent thrombosis. Unfortunately, it is not always possible to establish clinically in a given case whether or not it is the first episode of thrombosis and it is unlikely that the age of the thrombus can be determined with any accuracy. It has been observed that the results of thrombolytic therapy can be correlated to the age of a thrombus with excellent results in thrombi that are "clinically" less than 24 hr old and poor in those when treatment began 96 hr after onset.[51]

Most reports cite results of improvement, documented venographically, with partial or complete lysis of the thrombi in 50–70% of the cases (Table 17–1), comparing favorably to the results of heparin

TABLE 17–1.—REPORTED RESULTS OF TREATMENT OF VENOGRAPHICALLY PROVED DEEP VENOUS THROMBOSIS OF THE LOWER LIMB*

AUTHOR	NO. OF PATIENTS	AGE OF DEEP VENOUS THROMBOSIS (DAYS)	EXTENT OF LYSIS			RANDOMIZED COMPARISON
			COMPLETE	PARTIAL	NIL	
Gallus et al.[51]	7 (H-S)	< 1	1	3	3	
	9 (H-S)	1–4	1	3	5	
	14 (H-S)	> 4	3	4	7	
Gormsen[52]	18 (S)	> 6	6	6	2	No
Gormsen and Laursen[53]	20 (H)		3	2	9	No
Browse et al.[54]	5 (S)	< 21	0	4	1	
	5 (H)		0	0	5	
Kakkar et al.[55]	10 (S)	< 4	6	1	2	Yes
	10 (H)		2	2	5	
Robertson et al.[56]	9 (S)	< 4	5	1	3	Yes
			1	0	6	

*H, heparin; S, high-dose streptokinase; S-H, combination of low-dose streptokinase and heparin.

therapy.[51-56] A more striking finding was reported recently when a different regimen of thrombolytic therapy was used. Prior to each daily administration of streptokinase, the patient first was given an intravenous infusion of plasminogen.[27] Of the 12 patients thus treated, complete lysis occurred in eight and partial lysis in the remaining four. These results are encouraging. Further randomized prospective studies using this regimen are being undertaken at this time.

Central Retinal Vein Thrombosis

Though uncommon, this form of thrombosis is of clinical interest because of a poor outcome in visual acuity of the affected eye in the untreated patient.[57] Recent trials were carried out comparing the results of four regimens of treatment: urokinase followed by heparin therapy; streptokinase followed by heparin therapy; heparin therapy alone; and no thrombolytic or anticoagulant therapy.[57] Evaluation of the merits of these various regimens was hampered by the difficulty in obtaining a sufficiently large number of patients in each group since this is not a common disease. However, the results suggest that the use of urokinase or streptokinase may provide a better chance of improvement in vision than when heparin was used alone. Again, these data need to be confirmed by further studies.

Arterial Thromboembolism

The discussion of the use of thrombolytic therapy in arterial thromboembolism is out of the scope of this article. It should be pointed out that results are generally not as encouraging as those with venous thrombi. Platelets form a major component of arterial thrombi and are not amenable to fibrinolysis. Furthermore, platelets are a rich source of inhibitors of fibrinolysis and thus can hinder the lysis of fibrin strands present around the platelet clumps within the thrombus. It is difficult to attribute any real significance to reports of the use of thrombolytic agents when the improvement was in the neighborhood of 30%.[12]

Perspective

Clearly many problems associated with the use of thrombolytic agents remain to be solved. The present recommended dose of thrombolytic agents exceeds many times the quantity of plasminogen activator required to lyse a thrombus in vitro. There is a real need for understanding the reason for such a wide discrepancy between the in vivo and in vitro doses. Reducing the amount of drug can of course greatly lower the hazards of bleeding while at the same time increasing the drug efficacy. Obviously during the transport of the drug from intravenous injection to the thrombus, much of the plasminogen activator is lost through binding and other interaction with the inhibitors. On reaching the thrombus, the degree of lysis depends on how much free plasmin can be generated. This is limited by the quantity of plasminogen available and the amounts of antiplasmins present. One promising approach is that of introduction of exogenous plasminogen to supplement the endogenous source immediately prior to the infusion of the plasminogen activator.[27] Through a better understanding of the mechanism of plasminogen activation, it is possible to first convert the plasminogen to its intermediary product, Lys-plasminogen, which has a higher affinity for the fibrin than its native form, Glu-plasminogen, and which is more readily converted to the active lytic enzyme plasmin. Search for means of converting the circulating plasminogen to the lys-form will help to achieve this aim. Another alternative theoretical consideration that must be explored is the possibility of increasing the susceptibility of the fibrin substrate to lysis. Since most thrombi are in a constant dynamic state of deposition and resolution, it may be feasible to change the nature of the secondary fibrin deposits. One attempt in this direction has been to prevent secondary fibrin deposition through the use of heparin concurrently with a low dose of streptokinase.[51] The results of this study were not conclusive, but did indicate a greater efficacy than when heparin alone was used. Another approach was the simultaneous use of a defibrinating agent such as Ancrod and a thrombolytic agent.[58] Though Ancrod can induce a fibrin clot that is highly susceptible to fibrinolysis,[59] it causes a severe depletion of the plasma plasminogen level and thus would seriously impair the efficacy of any plasminogen activator.

In conclusion, it is apparent from the many clinical reports that there is a definite place for thrombolytic therapy in dissolving venous thrombi and emboli. However, the full potential of this therapeutic approach is far from being exploited. Many problems relating to efficacy, dosage, route of administration and combination of other therapeutic modalities have yet to be solved.

Summary

Increasing use of thrombolytic agents in recent years has been reported. Most studies indicate beneficial effects in venous thrombosis and embolism. Of these, the results of clinical trials in three conditions — pulmonary embolism, deep vein thrombosis and central retinal vein thrombosis — are presented. Two agents most commonly used are urokinase and streptokinase. Problems that limit the usefulness of thrombolytic agents include drug efficacy, dosage, route of administration, combination with other therapeutic agents and frequency of bleeding complications. Some theoretical considerations on how some of these problems might be solved are discussed in this chapter.

REFERENCES

1. Fletcher, A. P., and Sherry, S.: Thrombolytic agents, Am. Rev. Pharmacol. 6:89, 1966.
2. Fearnly, G. R.: Fibrinolysis: Physiology and pharmacology, Br. Med. Bull. 20:185, 1964.
3. Kwaan, H. C., and Grumet, G. N.: The Place of Thrombolytic and Defibrinating Agents in the Treatment of Thromboembolism, in Nicolaides, A. N. (ed.): *Thromboembolism and Aetiology, Advances in Prevention and Management* (Lancaster: Medical and Technical Publishing Co., Ltd., 1975), p. 251.
4. The urokinase pulmonary embolism trial. A national cooperative study, Circulation 47:Suppl. 2:1, 1973.
5. Hyers, T. M.: Urokinase in the treatment of pulmonary embolism, Thromb. Diath. Haemorrh. Suppl. 47:165, 1971.
6. Hume, R.: Fibrinolysis in myocardial infarction, Br. Heart J. 20:15, 1958.
7. Schmutzler, R., Fritze, E., Gebauer, D., Gillmann, H., Heckner, F., Kortge, P., Van DeLoo, J., Pezold, F. A., Poliwode, H., Praetorius, F., and Zekorn, D.: Fibrinolytic therapy in acute myocardial infarction, Thromb. Diath. Haemorrh. Suppl. 47:211, 1971.
8. Verstraete, M.: Streptokinase and myocardial infarction, Br. Med. J. 4:679, 1971.
9. Amery, A., Roeber, G., Vermeullen, H., et al.: Single-blinded randomized multicentre trial comparing heparin and streptokinase treatment in recent myocardial infarction, Acta Med. Scand. (Suppl.) 505:14, 1969.
10. Heikinheimo, R., Ahrenberg, P., Honkopohja, H., et al.: Fibrinolytic treatment in acute myocardial infarction, Acta Med. Scand. 189:7, 1971.
11. Golden, L. H., Schultz, R. W., Ambrus, C. M., Dean, D. C., Lippschutz, E. J., Sanne, M., and Ambrus, L.: Streptokinase and urokinase activated plasmin therapy in myocardial infarction, Thromb. Diath. Haemorrh. Suppl. 47:217, 1971.
12. Martin, M., Schoop, W., and Zeitler, E.: Streptokinase in chronic arterial occlusive disease, JAMA 211:1169, 1970.
12. Martin, M., Schoop, W., and Zeitler, E.: Streptokinase in chronic arterial occlusive disease, JAMA 211:1169, 1970.
13. Kwaan, H. C., Dobbie, J. G., and Fetkenhour, C. L.: The Use of Anticoagulants and Thrombolytic Agents in Occlusive Retinal Vascular Disease, in Paoletti, R., and Sherry, S. (eds.): *Thrombosis and Urokinase* (New York: Academic Press, 1977), pp. 191–198.
14. Hohmann, R., Martin, M., Weigelin, E.: Fibrinolysis in retinal vein occlusions, Albrecht von Graefes Arch. Klin. Ophthalmol. 187:327, 1973.
15. Virchow, R.: *Die Cellularpathologie* (4th ed.; Berlin, 1871), p. 194.
16. de Takats, G., and Vaithianathan, T.: The fibrinolytic potential, Rev. Surg. 25:453, 1968.
17. de Takats, G.: Spontaneous fibrinolysis, Surgery 65:399, 1969.
18. Hatem, A., and Kwaan, H. C.: An in vivo model of early thrombi. II. Kinetics of thrombus growth in veins, in preparation.

19. Sherry, S., Fletcher, A. P., and Alkjaersig, N.: Fibrinolysis and fibrinolytic activity in man, Physiol. Rev. 39:343, 1959.
20. The fibrinolytic system, Pharmacology Society Symposium, Fed. Proc. 25:28, 1966.
21. Sherry, S.: Fibrinolysis, Ann. Rev. Med. 18:247, 1968.
22. Kwaan, H. C.: Disorders of fibrinolysis, Med. Clin. North Am. 56:163, 1972.
23. Kwaan, H. C.: Disorders of fibrinolysis, in Ogston, D., and Bennett, B. (eds.): *The Biochemistry, Physiology and Pathology of Hemostasis* (Aberdeen, Scotland: John Wiley & Sons, Ltd., in press).
24. Fratantoni, J. C.: Thrombolytic therapy, N. Engl. J. Med. 293:1073, 1975.
25. Robbins, K. C., and Summaria, L.: Biochemistry and fibrinolysis, Thromb. Diath. Haemorrh. Suppl. 47:9, 1971.
26. Thorsen, S.: Differences in the binding to fibrin of native plasminogen and plasminogen modified by omega-aminocarboxylic acids, Biochem. Biophys. Acta 393:55, 1975.
27. Kakkar, V. V., Sagar, S., and Lewis, M.: Treatment of deep vein thrombosis with intermittent streptokinase and plasminogen infusion, Lancet 2:674, 1975.
28. Kwaan, H. C.: Inhibitors of fibrinolysis, Thromb. Res. 2:31, 1973.
29. Rimon, A., Shamash, Y., and Shapiro, B.: The plasmin inhibitor of human plasma. IV. Its action on plasmin, trypsin, chymotrypsin, and thrombin, J. Biol. Chem. 241:5102, 1966.
30. Schreiber, A. D., Kaplan, A. P., and Austen, K. F.: Plasma inhibitors of the components of the fibrinolytic pathway in man, J. Clin. Invest. 52:1394, 1973.
31. Moroi, M., and Aoki, N.: Isolation and characterization of α_2-plasmin inhibitor from human plasma, J. Biol. Chem. 251:5956, 1976.
32. Highsmith, R. F., and Rosenberg, R. D.: The inhibition of human plasmin by human antithrombin-heparin cofactor, J. Biol. Chem. 249:4335, 1974.
33. Crawford, G. P. M., and Ogston, D.: The influence of α-1-antitrypsin on plasmin, urokinase, and Hageman factor cofactor, Biochem. Biophys. Acta 354:107, 1974.
34. Harpel, P. C., and Cooper, N. R.: Studies on human plasma C1 inactivator-enzyme interactions. I. Mechanisms of interaction with C1s, plasmin and trypsin, J. Clin. Invest. 55:593, 1975.
35. Schreiber, A. D., Kaplan, A. P., and Austen, K. F.: Inhibition by C1 INH of Hageman factor activation of coagulation, fibrinolysis, and kinin generation, J. Clin. Invest. 52:1402, 1973.
36. Gallimore, M. J.: Serum inhibitors of fibrinolysis, Br. J. Haematol. 31:217, 1975.
37. Alkjaersig, N., Fletcher, A. P., and Sherry, S.: The mechanism of clot dissolution by plasmin, J. Clin. Invest. 38:1086, 1959.
38. Sharp, A. A.: Mechanism of Fibrinolysis, in Davidson, J. F., Samama, M. M., and Desnoyers, P. C. (eds.): *Progress in Chemical Fibrinolysis and Thrombolysis*, vol. 1 (New York: Raven Press, 1975), p. 19.
39. Moser, K. M.: Thrombolysis with fibrinolysin (plasmin): New therapeutic approach to thrombo-embolism, JAMA 167:1695, 1958.
40. Wiener, M., Edisch, W., and Steele, J. M.: Occurrence of fibrinolytic activity following administration of nicotinic acid, Proc. Soc. Exp. Biol. Med. 98:755, 1958.
41. Fearnley, G. R., Chakrabarti, R., and Evans, J. F.: Fibrinolytic and defibrinating effect of phenformin plus ethyloestrenol, Lancet 1:910, 1969.
42. Dodman, B., Cunliffe, W. J., Roberts, B. E., and Sibbald, R.: Clinical and laboratory double-blind investigation on effect of fibrinolytic therapy in patients with cutaneous vasculitis, Br. Med. J. 2:82, 1973.
43. Lesuk, A., Terminellor, L., and Traver, J. H.: Crystalline human urokinase: Some properties, Science 149:880, 1965.
44. White, W. F., Barlow, G. H., and Mozen, M. M.: The isolation and characterization of plasminogen activators (urokinase) from human urine, Biochemistry 5:2160, 1966.
45. Bernik, M. B., and Kwaan, H. C.: Origin of fibrinolytic activity in cultures of the

human kidney, J. Lab. Clin. Med. 70:650, 1967.

46. Bernik, M. B., and Kwaan, H. C.: Plasminogen activator activity in cultures from human tissues. An immunological and histochemical study, J. Clin. Invest. 48:1740, 1969.

47. Barlow, G. H., and LaVera, L.: Characterization of the plasminogen activator isolated from human embryo kidney cells: comparison with urokinase, Thromb. Res. 1: 201, 1972.

48. Fletcher, P. P., Alkjaersig, N., and Sherry, S.: The maintenance of a sustained thrombolytic state in man. I. Induction and effects, J. Clin. Invest. 38:1096, 1959.

49. Kwaan, H. C., and Barlow, G. H.: Nature and biological activities of degradation products of fibrinogen and fibrin, Ann. Rev. Med. 24:335, 1973.

50. Urokinase-Streptokinase Embolism Trial. Phase 2 results. A cooperative study, JAMA 229:1606, 1974.

51. Gallus, A. S., Hirsch, J., Cade, J. F., Turpie, A. G. G., Walker, I. R., and Gent, M.: Thrombolysis with a combination of small doses of streptokinase and full doses of heparin, Sem. Thromb. Hemostasis 2:14, 1975.

52. Gormsen, J.: Streptase Treatment of Acute Phlebothrombosis, in *Symposium on Thrombolytic Therapy with Streptokinase*, Munich, 1967, pp. 41–49.

53. Gormsen, J., and Laursen, B.: Treatment of acute phlebothrombosis with streptase, Acta Med. Scand. 181:373, 1967.

54. Browse, N. L., Thomas, M. L., and Pim, H. P.: Streptokinase and deep vein thrombosis, Br. Med. J. 3:717, 1968.

55. Kakkar, V. V., Flanc, C., Howe, C. T., O'Shea, M., and Flute, P. T.: Treatment of deep vein thrombosis. A trial of heparin, streptokinase and arvin, Br. Med. J. 1:806, 1969.

56. Robertson, B. R., Nilsson, I. M., and Nylander, G.: Thrombolytic effect of streptokinase as evaluated by phlebography of deep venous thrombi of the leg, Acta Chir. Scand. 136:173, 1970.

57. Kwaan, H. C., Dobbie, J. G., and Fetkenhour, C. L.: Clinical trial of heparin, urokinase, and streptokinase in occlusive retinal vascular disease, Am. J. Ophthalmol, 1977 (in press).

58. Kwaan, H. C., and Grumet, G. N.: Potentiation of plasminogen activation by ancrod and reptilase, Fed. Proc. 32:427, 1973.

59. Kwaan, H. C.: Use of defibrinating agents ancrod and reptilase in the treatment of thromboembolism, Thromb. Diath. Haemorrh. Suppl. 54:377, 1973.

Discussion: Chapters 16 and 17

MR. LEONARD COTTON: Doctor Sevitt is much too modest to explain to us that it was he and Gibbs and McLaughlin who really started the drive toward solving problems of venous thrombosis 20 years ago. Those three people really established the basic pathology and anatomy of venous thromboembolism.

Gibbs showed that soleal sinuses were the commonest thrombotic sites. Doctor Sevitt demonstrated the valve pocket thrombi. Fascinating that these are always in one valve pocket; I wonder why. Of course, one does know that in the valve pocket there is complete stasis. If you set up a vein, put india ink in the valve and run fluid through, the india ink will stay and not be diluted.

Then, last, the question of thrombolytic therapy. I must say I find myself in a complete muddle over this. In my own institution, streptokinase was used on arterial thrombosis. We put a catheter in a femoral artery and infused it there, thinking that it is better to get the activator into the clot itself. We got the most marvelous resolution, but within a few days, the whole thing clotted up again despite the use of anticoagulants.

I am very relieved to hear that urokinase can now be made synthetically. Formerly, it was rumored that one clinical course needed the entire urine output of the Danish Army.

DR. JOHN OLWIN: I would like to speak to three points. First, the importance of early treatment for thrombosis, whenever it occurs. Ideally, we would treat prophylactically for all impending intravascular clotting. Concerning active treatment, there are many reports to indicate that whatever the mode of therapy, its institution within 48–72 hr following the onset of symptoms and signs is a most important factor in the final outcome. As Doctor Kwaan has shown, thrombolytic agents used early can restore pretherapy vision to eyes with central retinal vein thrombosis. In a classic study and report in 1956, Dr. Bertha Klein demonstrated that early treatment is most effective and late (beyond 10 days of clinical onset) is largely futile except for prevention of thrombosis in the opposite eye. To demonstrate to one-self the importance of early therapy, I would suggest that each of you be on the lookout for a hospitalized patient who under your eyes develops a full blown superficial thrombophlebitis in a varicosity and within 12 hr of its clinical appearance, you give him or her, unless contraindicated, 10,000 units of heparin intravenously and another such dose 12 hr later. You will be pleased and gratified to return the following day to find little or no evidence of thrombosis.

Regarding the effectiveness of prothrombin depressive agents, there have been many clinical studies to support their use and those investigators with qualified coagulation backgrounds have had little difficulty in administering effective therapy. It is a matter of proper control. In my own experience, there have been a number of patients with a history of recurring episodes of thrombosis and/or embolism (and in some cases, serious bleeding from hypoprothrombinemia) who, when their prothrombin levels were properly controlled, have gone years with no further difficulty. I have one such patient who has been on dicumarol for 30 years with no recurring thromboembolism.

18 / Heparin Therapy in Venous Thromboembolism

EDWIN W. SALZMAN, M.D.

Department of Surgery, Harvard Medical School and Beth Israel Hospital, Boston, Massachusetts

IN THE NEARLY 40 years since its introduction as a clinical anticoagulant in man, heparin, supplemented by long-term anticoagulation with oral vitamin K antagonists, has become the standard for treatment of patients with established venous thrombosis and pulmonary embolism. Common usage has come to dictate practice so that the administration of heparin and oral anticoagulants to patients with venous thromboembolism is virtually routine, and surgical interruption of the great veins is reserved for patients who cannot safely be given anticoagulant drugs because of a special hazard of bleeding or who suffer recurrent thromboembolic complications during anticoagulant therapy.

If one examines critically the evidence upon which this practice is based,[1] one finds an extensive literature composed primarily of uncontrolled accounts of large series of patients treated with anticoagulant drugs and a surprisingly limited body of data derived from well-controlled prospective randomized trials.

In 1960 Barritt and Jordan[2] reported a series of patients with pulmonary embolism, half of whom were initially assigned to receive intravenous heparin and an oral vitamin K antagonist and the other half to comprise a control group. After 35 patients had been studied, 10 of the 19 control patients had sustained recurrent pulmonary embolism and 5 had died, whereas no recurrent embolus had occurred in the patients who were anticoagulated. The additional 38 patients entered into the trial were all treated with anticoagulant drugs, and 1 recurrent pulmonary embolus was encountered in these patients, none of whom succumbed.

297

This study has never been repeated. Confirmation seems superfluous in view of the dramatic superiority of anticoagulation compared with no treatment at all, but it is by no means clear that the therapeutic regimen employed was optimal. Even today there is controversy regarding many aspects of the use of heparin: the ideal method for control of dosage, the optimal route and schedule of administration, the appropriate duration of treatment and other important questions. Consideration of some of these matters constitutes the substance of this report.

The mechanism of action of heparin has been clarified by work in many laboratories, culminating perhaps in the elegant series of observations by Yin et al.[3] and Rosenberg and Damus[4] and Damus et al.[5] It is now clear that heparin has little direct action as an anticoagulant but operates primarily to accelerate the action of a natural constituent of plasma, so-called antithrombin III or heparin cofactor, which forms an inactive complex with and thus inhibits the action of thrombin, activated factor X, and in fact all of the serine proteases involved in the intrinsic and extrinsic clotting systems. Like the inhibiting action of antithrombin on activated procoagulant clotting factors, activation of antithrombin by heparin is stoichiometric, not enzymatic. Since the coagulation system is an amplifying cascade, in which structural changes in the molecule of a substance present in only trace concentration in plasma (factor XII) ultimately lead to conversion into fibrin of the second most plentiful protein in plasma (fibrinogen), it is logical that prophylaxis against coagulation may be accomplished by small doses of heparin sufficient to inactivate trace quantities of procoagulants high in the coagulation cascade, whereas much larger quantities of heparin are required to interrupt the coagulation scheme once activated factor X and thrombin are present in high concentrations in the neighborhood of an established clot. This point also has important implications in the selection of methods for monitoring heparin therapy, discussed below.

Although heparin can be given in small subcutaneous doses effectively for prevention of thromboembolism in high-risk patients, its administration in therapeutic dosage is best accomplished by the intravenous route, since its absorption and duration of action when administered subcutaneously are largely unpredictable, and the incidence of local hematomas is unacceptably high when it is given by the intramuscular route. There is controversy regarding the safest and most effective schedule for administration of the drug. Administration by continuous infusion or by intermittent injection each has its champions. The issue had never been subjected to a prospective controlled trial at the time the results of heparin therapy were first critically examined in our own institution.[6] Following a survey of 100 consecutive patients who received heparin in therapeutic doses, all by intermittent intravenous injection, we discovered that one third developed a bleeding complication and one fifth developed a major hemorrhage sufficient to require transfusion or prolong hospitalization or result in interruption of therapy. There was no benefit in these patients from the use of the whole blood clotting time to control dosage. We next undertook a prospective controlled randomized trial in which intermittent injections of heparin, administered in arbitrary fixed doses or with dosage regulated by laboratory tests, were compared with the results of continuous heparin infusion. The results of this study are shown in Table 18–1. The three programs of administration appeared equally effective for control of thromboembolism; one pulmonary embolus occurred during treatment in each of the three patient groups. However major bleeding complications were encountered seven times more frequently in patients who received heparin by intermittent injection than in those who had the drug administered by continuous infusion, and if one includes among the hemorrhagic complications an unexplained fall in hematocrit of more than 6%, which was encountered four times in the patients given intermittent injections, the difference is even more striking.

The use of laboratory tests for control of dosage appeared to offer no advantage in patients who received the drug by intermittent injection. The frequency of major bleeding and of recurrent thromboembolism was the same in the two groups with intermittent injection, regardless of whether the activated partial thromboplastin time (PTT) was employed or not. It is perhaps not surprising that when the blood was totally incoagulable after an intravenous bolus, the rate of bleeding was not influenced by the extent to which the clotting test was prolonged 3 hr later. We did not examine the value of laboratory control in patients who received heparin by continuous infusion, since all patients in this treatment group had prescription of dosage according to the activated partial thromboplastin time. Basu and co-workers[7] considered this question in a series of 234 patients treated by continuous infusion and concluded that patients with recurrent venous thromboembolism had a significantly lower activated PTT than patients without recurrence, although there was no difference in the amount of heparin received by the two groups. No recurrent thromboembolic episode occurred in a patient whose PTT was within the prescribed therapeutic range. On the other hand they found no difference in either mean heparin dose or activated PTT in patients with or without a bleeding complication.

TABLE 18–1. — RESULTS OF CONTROLLED TRIAL

	HEPARIN EVERY 4 HR	HEPARIN EVERY 4 HR, PTT	INFUSION, PTT
No. of patients	68	72	69
Patients with major bleeding*	7(10%)	6(8%)	1(1%)
Most recent PTT (sec)	55, 53, 38	110, 123, 68, 52, 200, 136	56
Patients with minor bleeding	11(16%)	16(22%)	18(26%)
Total heparin dose (units) ±SD	196,600±28,290	186,930±57,700	142,240±23,640

*Including wound hematoma, intracranial hemorrhage, hemothorax, other soft tissue hematomas, and hemarthrosis, but not including 3 patients in column 1 and 1 patient in column 2 with unexplained fall in hematocrit greater than 6%.

Similar observations were made by Pitney et al.[8] in a study comparing the whole blood clotting time, the activated PTT and a plasma heparin assay based on the principle of protamine titration. In our trial, the only major bleeding complication in a patient who received heparin by continuous infusion occurred when the partial thromboplastin time was not excessively prolonged. At present we regard the use of laboratory tests for control of heparin management as desirable during continuous infusion therapy, but it should be recognized that this recommendation is tentative and that its scientific basis is somewhat flimsy.

A recent report by Bynum and Wilson[9] has challenged the contention that continuous infusion of heparin is less frequently complicated by major bleeding than is intermittent injection. They observed no difference in bleeding complications regardless of the schedule of administration in a series of 36 patients treated for pulmonary embolism. However, since they encountered 5 recurrent pulmonary emboli among their 36 patients (14%) as compared with 3 recurrences encountered in our own study (1.4% of 209 patients, of whom 86 were treated for pulmonary embolism and 91 for deep vein thrombosis), one must question the adequacy of anticoagulation in their trial.

If one elects to control heparin dosage by laboratory tests, there is no agreement in the literature concerning the most satisfactory laboratory method. Support can be found for a variety of in vitro coagulation tests, including the whole blood clotting time, the activated whole blood clotting time, the activated partial thromboplastin time, the thrombin time, the protamine titration test, the recalcification time and its activated version and other more sensitive and perhaps more specific tests for heparin action. Certainly there is reason to believe that patients vary in their response to heparin. Hirsh and associates[10] have shown that considerable variation exists in the response of clotting tests to heparin in different patients, and that, on the average, patients suffering from acute thromboembolic problems require larger quantities of heparin for an equivalent effect on in vitro clotting tests. However, selection from among the coagulation assays mentioned above, and others, appears in most instances to be made on the basis of technical considerations, such as reproducibility, convenience and economy, whereas the problem in control of heparin therapy is more likely a conceptual one. The issue is not a matter of selecting the clotting test that meets the most rigorous requirements for an in vitro bench technique. As Rosenberg has pointed out,[11] optimal dosage of heparin should in theory depend upon the local levels (at the site of thrombosis) of the activated serine proteases whose action is inhibited by this agent. In other words, the dose of heparin appropriate to a given patient's needs should be a reflection of the procoagulant tendency in the patient. The assays now employed to regulate heparin dosage are designed to test heparin's ability to activate antithrombin in a particular blood sample, and for the most part they fail to reflect the magnitude of the procoagulant stimulus that exists in the living patient. The in vivo heparin tolerance test[12] of our host, Doctor de Takats, is probably a step in the right direction. Perhaps an indication of where optimal management will lie is illustrated by the fibrinopeptide assay of Nossel and associates[13] or the assay of intermediates in prothrombin conversion recently developed by Rosenberg.[14] These tests actually detect circulating evidence of the presence of thrombin, and they can therefore give evidence of the adequacy of heparin treatment in blocking the progression of events toward fibrin formation in an individual patient. For example, Nossel has shown that the generation of fibrinopeptide A, a product of the action of thrombin on fibrinogen, is a feature of pulmonary embolism that is promptly reversed by heparin in most patients. In an occasional case, fibrinopeptide is detectable in blood samples obtained from the patient even after large doses of heparin, which may explain the periodic instances when heparin is unsuccessful in aborting the thrombotic tendency. Through such individualized studies as these, we may approach a more nearly ideal program, in which anticoagulation will provide adequate protection against thrombosis but avoid the hazard of bleeding that now attends our best efforts at prescribing heparin.

Summary

In the nearly 40 years since its introduction as a clinical anticoagulant in man, heparin supplemented by long-term anticoagulation with oral vitamin K antagonists has become the standard for treatment of patients with established venous thrombosis and pulmonary embolism. However, even today, there is controversy regarding many aspects of the use of heparin. The ideal method for control of dosage, the optimal route and schedule of administration, the appropriate duration of treatment and other important questions are dealt with in this presentation, suggesting that the administration of heparin in therapeutic dosage is best accomplished by the intravenous route, and that major bleeding complications are encountered less frequently if the drug is administered by continuous infusion. Monitoring heparin dosage by laboratory tests receives no uniform support in the literature concerning the most satisfactory laboratory method. The in vivo heparin tolerance test proposed by Doctor de Takats is probably a step in the right direction, since it reflects the magnitude of the procoagulant stimulus that exists in the living patient.

REFERENCES

1. Aggeler, P. M., and Kosmin, M.: Anticoagulant Prophylaxis and Treatment of Venous Thromboembolic Disease, in Sherry, S., Brinkhous, K. M., Genton, E., Stengle, J. M. (eds.): *Thrombosis* (Washington, D.C.: National Academy of Sciences, 1969).
2. Barritt, D. W., and Jordan, S. C.: Anticoagulant drugs in the treatment of pulmonary embolism. A controlled trial, Lancet 1:1309, 1960.

3. Yin, E. T., Wessler, S., and Stoll, P. J.: Identity of plasma activated factor X inhibitor with antithrombin III and heparin co-factor, J. Biol. Chem. 246:3712, 1971.
4. Rosenberg, R. D., and Damus, P. S.: The purification and mechanism of action of human antithrombin-heparin cofactor, J. Biol. Chem. 248:6490, 1973.
5. Damus, P. S., Hicks, M., and Rosenberg, R. D.: Anticoagulant action of heparin, Nature 246:355, 1973.
6. Salzman, E. W., Deykin, D., Shapiro, R. M., and Rosenberg, R.: Management of heparin therapy. Controlled prospective trial, N. Engl. J. Med. 292:1046, 1975.
7. Basu, D., Gallus, A., Hirsh, J., et al.: A prospective study of the value of monitoring heparin treatment with the activated partial thromboplastin time, N. Engl. J. Med. 287:324, 1972.
8. Pitney, W. R., Pettit, J. E., and Armstrong, L.: Control of heparin therapy, Br. Med. J. 4:139, 1970.
9. Bynum, L. J., and Wilson, J. E., III: Continuous vs. intermittent heparin in pulmonary embolism (abstract), Am. Rev. Resp. Dis. 113:148, 1976.
10. Hirsh, J., van Aken, W. G., Gallus, A. S., Dollery, C. T., Cade, J. F., and Yung, W. L.: Heparin kinetics in venous thrombosis and pulmonary embolism, Circulation 53:691, 1976.
11. Rosenberg, R. D.: Actions and interactions of antithrombin and heparin, N. Engl. J. Med. 292:146, 1975.
12. de Takats, G.: Heparin: The need for a flexible protocol, Am. J. Surg. 132:1, 1976.
13. Nossel, H. L., Yudelman, I., Canfield, R. D., et al.: Measurement of fibrinopeptide A in human blood, J. Clin. Invest. 54:43, 1974.
14. Rosenberg, R.: Personal communication.

Discussion: Chapter 18

DR. MICHAEL HUME: The subject of heparin is so large that a whole conference could be given to it, and Doctor Salzman has done a beautiful job in summarizing the present status of this most important drug.

We have a balance of indications and objectives between preventing recurrence of thromboembolism and avoiding hemorrhage. There isn't much free space in some patients between those two objectives.

Page 1, No. 1 of the December, 1976 volume of the *American Journal of Surgery* contains an editorial entitled, "The Need for a Flexible Regimen for Heparin Therapy." Appropriately, that editorial was written by Doctor de Takats. The flexible dosage idea has been more accepted recently since the continuous infusion has been introduced through the very fine work at the Beth Israel Hospital by Doctor Salzman.

We must consider whether we are dealing with the acute pulmonary embolism which needs a far larger dose, early in the treatment, or if we are dealing with the smaller process further along.

Regarding laboratory control, this isn't a matter so much of which one of the tests is used, whether a heparin retarded clotting time described by Doctor de Takats or an activated partial thromboplastin time. It is, instead, the implication that we will be sampling the patient's own blood during treatment.

More difficult to me than preventing recurrence is the problem of avoiding hemorrhage. We are up against a very stubborn problem and are going to have trouble if there is drug interaction. In this regard, we know we are going to have trouble in elderly, postmenopausal women and in major orthopedic operations. Hemostasis in these is different than after soft tissue operations. We have felt that the method of continuous infusion by the pump has let us get through these two difficult aspects very well.

DR. DOMINIC VERDA: All of us have heard considerable discussion the last few days on the therapy of chest and lung and leg conditions. This is good and proper for our day. On the other hand, I would like to open up a Pandora's box. This is, that the prevention of these surgical conditions might in the future prove more rewarding for our civilization.

Strange as it may seem, I was able to uncover in the German literature some work that has been very much overlooked. In 1924, a German scientist was able to report that following major surgery, the platelet population increases at the same time the clotting factor specifically decreases. This was confirmed independently by a London group when cesarean sections were carried out and the platelet count went as high as 800,000 and 1 million.

My discussion is primarily concerned with the homeostasis of platelet population. Why do we have an increased platelet count following major surgery on high risk patients? The platelet count will rise 4–5 hours after surgery. Why does this happen?

The St. Louis group was first to bring out that minidoses of heparin, even as low as 3,000 mg every 6 hours, will decrease the platelet population from, say, 600,000 down to normal. Likewise, the coagulation time goes down.

DR. CHARLES SACHATELLO: There are many physicians and surgeons who are still reluctant to use continuous intravenous heparin, and I just rise to give testimony to the fact that it is a very safe way to use heparin. We have used the continuous intravenous heparin now for almost 10 years. We have used a variable dose from 200 to 1,000 units an hour. In our experience, 1,000 units an hour, arrived at empirically, has been very effective in adults.

We have seen three groups of patients who tend not to need these doses. The woman under 100 lb does not seem to tolerate this dose, the woman over 65, and, more recently, a group of patients who have had bilateral amputation, especially high thigh amputations. I suspect it is because these people are smaller and weigh less. We have had experience with the continuous intravenous heparin in patients with gastrointestinal bleeding and have treated them successfully simply by using a lower dose continuously. I recommend this to you.

DR. VICTOR deWOLFE: I would like to describe very briefly a divergent concept that we are looking into in Cleveland. That is what we term the cause-and-effect type of thrombophlebitis. That is, the cause is an operation; the effect is the phlebitis. The cause is removed by having the operation completed. The effect is treated adequately and, therefore, we don't get it any longer. Our plan is to treat the patients for 10 days with adequate dosage of heparin and not treat them any longer with long-term anticoagulants.

We have had six recurrences of either recurrent phlebitis or recurrent pulmonary embolism. Three of these six have had surgery for malignancy. The other three were treated for only 7 and 8 days of heparin, rather than 10.

We feel that we need more cases to test further this hypothesis, but it is presented because we are working on it and I think it may have some merit.

DR. ANDREW DALE: Doctor Salzman, I would like to continue the question that has been raised about long-term treatment with warfarin. I suspect that at the moment this is something that is so poorly understood that most of us would like to sweep it under the carpet and simply not discuss it. I hope you will make some remarks in your closing about your feelings about warfarin.

Personally, I tend to agree with Doctor deWolfe and have serious doubt that warfarin is actually effective. It is, however, a standard medication in our regimen, and some physicians have even been sued for not using it.

I think we should all recognize that failure to use it does have medicolegal implications. If we actually think that there are two sides to the story, I think we should bring out the other side.

I would vote at the moment on the basis of flimsy scientific evidence that warfarin is not preventive in the management of deep vein thrombosis.

DR. EDWIN SALZMAN: We are going to discuss prophylaxis against thromboembolism later and, perhaps, the discussion of prevention with warfarin can be held to that time. Maybe Doctor Wessler will have more to say about its use in therapy later, when he has an opportunity to close.

DR. NORMAN BROWSE: I would just like to object to the word "treatment" when we talk about giving heparin to these patients. When you give heparin to patients who have established pulmonary embolism, who have established deep vein thrombosis, you are not treating the pulmonary embolism, and you are not treating the deep vein thrombosis. You are using heparin as a prophylaxis in the hope that you will stop new or further thrombosis and the complications that it will produce. You certainly don't stop pulmonary embolism if there is thrombus present in the limbs which is in a situation where it can break up and embolize, and you don't do anything in the immediate short-term to the cardiopulmonary effects of the pulmonary embolism. I think it is a wrong word to use. It we sit back, after having given some heparin and we think we have treated the patient, we haven't.

DR. STANFORD WESSLER: I will be very brief. I would like to make two points. One is a guess for the future about heparin, and the other is data on warfarin. As several people have pointed out, when confronted with active thrombosis, we need more heparin than later on. We are trying to study this in an animal; we have not studied it in man. I wondered if some of the answer to the problem would be if we could give a large dose of heparin, let's say 60,000 units as a sweep for 1 day. I go back to the British experience with massive pulmonary embolism where for a day, 36 hours, they have given 60,000 to 100,000 units without monitoring. Those high numbers make me nervous, but the concept behind it would be that the sweep would wipe out the thrombus, and then we could go to the lower dose, which is all we would need to block activated factor X. It is conceivable that some experimental work in man could be done to validate or invalidate this.

It is rather unfair to say that warfarin is not an effective antithrombotic agent. One of the things that we found recently is that, if you compare low dose heparin studies to warfarin studies, they are equipotential in preventing large pulmonary embolism. We have now confirmed the equipotentiality of these two drugs. Heparin is obviously a better antithrombotic agent in larger doses in an animal, and most recently we have correlated this with the activated factor X inhibitory activity. Patients on warfarin have an increase in activated factor X inhibitory activity comparable to the increase induced by heparin.

One of the reasons we are in trouble in anticoagulation therapy is we have never had the assay that the hypertensive therapists have had. Even before modest hypertension was proven to be a hazard, physicians always had a blood pressure measurement. They knew that they were getting effective treatment.

Some of the new assays may be among the first handles of the antithrombotic potential of the anticoagulant drugs. They may be a way of using what is needed at the particular stage in the disease.

So, I would close by saying that I think warfarin is an effective drug, but if somebody is actively clotting, there is no point in using warfarin any more than there is any point in using low dose heparin.

DR. SIMON SEVITT: I would just like to say a brief word on the question of thrombolysis. It is believed that use of thrombolytic agents experimentally in animals or streptokinase or urokinase in man is a removal process. We have believed that in the past, and it is based upon the models of rising clots. Recent examinations of the lysis in deep vein thrombosis show differences as postmortem indicates. There is another process and that process is at least partly one of fragmentation of the thrombus or the embolus — this through the invasion by the endothelium from the vein into the thrombus or embolus. This spontaneous mechanism of lysis is accelerated by the use of streptokinase or urokinase.

19 / Methodology in Diagnosis of Pulmonary Embolization

ARTHUR A. SASAHARA, M.D., G.V.R.K. SHARMA, M.D., DONALD E. TOW, M.D., RICHARD J. ARMENIA, B.S., AND JOHN S. BELKO, M.S.

Medical, Research and Nuclear Medicine Services, Veterans Administration Hospital, West Roxbury, Massachusetts and the Departments of Medicine and Radiology, Peter Bent Brigham Hospital and Harvard Medical School, Boston, Massachusetts

DURING THE PAST DECADE, a great deal of progress has been made in the development of techniques to diagnose pulmonary thromboembolism: selective pulmonary angiography, perfusion and ventilation lung scanning, objective assessment of the deep venous circulation and the proper interpretation of arterial blood gas values in the appropriate clinical setting. All of these techniques have served to underscore one fact—that pulmonary thromboembolism (PE) is a very common medical and surgical disease.

The true incidence of PE, on a clinical basis, is not known. Despite many published reports, there is great variation in the incidence of PE, depending upon the vigor and intensity of the diagnostic screening process. In our 2-year study, the incidence was 23 patients among 1000 inpatients, or 2.3%.[1] All patients admitted to the Medical and Surgical Services during this period were placed on a common protocol in which all suspected patients were studied by perfusion lung scanning. When the scan was abnormal, pulmonary angiography was performed to confirm or exclude the diagnosis. It seems reasonable, therefore, to expect nonfatal PE to occur in about 20 patients per 1000 inpatients and fatal PE to occur in about 5 patients per 1000 inpatients in a general medical-surgical hospital.[2] On these bases, approximately 568,000 patients suffer nonfatal PE and 142,000 suffer fatal PE in the United States each year. In addition, there is evidence to suggest that the frequency of PE is increasing.

309

The mortality of untreated PE is high, ranging from 18–38%, but once recognized and treated, it becomes a low-mortality disease.[3, 4] In the National Heart and Lung Institute Urokinase-Pulmonary Embolism Trial, the mortality of treated PE was 8.3%.[5] Therefore, early diagnosis and early treatment should be the principal objective in the attempt to reduce mortality. This objective can be achieved only by the aggressive use of lung scanning and/or pulmonary angiography. There are, however, several factors which hinder early diagnosis: (1) variability of the clinical picture, (2) lack of a specific laboratory test and (3) inability to obtain the appropriate graphic diagnostic procedure when needed.

Clinical Presentation

SYMPTOMS AND SIGNS

When PE occurs, a number of symptoms may develop which are relatively nonspecific. The latest such tabulations, obtained from the NHLI Urokinase-Pulmonary Embolism Trial (UPET), a national cooperative study involving 14 institutions, indicate: dyspnea (81%), pleural pain (72%), apprehension (59%), cough (54%) and hemoptysis (34%).[5] Some of these symptoms were related to the size of the embolic occlusion (Table 19–1). In this analysis, massive PE indicated occlusion of two or more lobar arteries or equivalent and submassive PE indicated less than this amount. Only two symptoms were related statistically to embolic size: pleural pain (more in submassive PE) and syncope (more in massive PE). No other symptoms such as apprehen-

TABLE 19–1.—UPET:
PRESENTING SYMPTOMS*

| | | PREVALENCE (%) | |
SYMPTOM	ALL	MASSIVE	SUBMASSIVE
Dyspnea	81	79	83
Pleural pain	72	62	84†
Apprehension	59	61	56
Cough	54	50	60
Hemoptysis	34	27	44
Sweats	26	27	24
Syncope	14	22†	4

*Massive indicates occlusion of two or more lobar arteries or equivalent. Submassive indicates occlusion of less than two lobar arteries.
†Related statistically to embolic size.

TABLE 19-2.—UPET:
PRESENTING SIGNS*

SIGN	PREVALENCE (%)		
	ALL	MASSIVE	SUBMASSIVE
Rales	53	50	57
↑ P$_2$	53	60†	44
Phlebitis	33	42	21
S$_3$, S$_4$	34	47†	17
Sweating	34	41	24
Cyanosis	18	28†	6
↑ Resp (> 16)	87		
↑ Pulse (> 100)	44		
Fever (≥ 37.8)	42		

*Massive indicates occlusion of two or more lobar arteries or equivalent. Submassive indicates occlusion of less than two lobar arteries.
†Related statistically to embolic size.

sion, cough, dyspnea, hemoptysis or sweating could be related to embolic size.

The signs which occur in response to PE are similarly nonspecific in the majority of patients: tachypnea (87%), rales (54%), accentuated pulmonary second sound (53%), tachycardia (44%), fever (42%), S$_3$ and S$_4$ gallop heart sounds (34%) and sweating (34%) (Table 19-2). When similarly analyzed to determine the influence of emboli size on the clinical signs, only three were found: S$_3$ and S$_4$ gallop heart sounds, accentuation of the pulmonary second sound and cyanosis. All three are manifestations of the cardiopulmonary response to PE and relate to the sudden impact of occlusion of the pulmonary arterial tree; hence, they were associated more with massive than with submassive PE.

Clinical Diagnosis

Although a number of abnormalities may occur, the *laboratory tests,* similar to the clinical presentation, are essentially nonspecific. The once promising elevation of the serum LDH and bilirubin in the presence of a normal glutamic oxaloacetic transaminase (considered "specific" for PE) has not proved to be helpful. Our experience has shown only 20% of patients with proved PE have this "biochemical triad" while another 21% with proved PE had no alterations of these tests. In fact, when the bilirubin was elevated in PE, there was a better correlation with the presence of right atrial pressure elevation, suggesting that the bilirubin rise was related to hepatic congestion.

TABLE 19-3.—UPET: FREQUENCY OF
ELECTROCARDIOGRAM ABNORMALITIES

	%	PATIENTS
Rhythm disturbances		11
Atrial premature beat	3	
Ventricular premature beat	9	
Atrial fibrillation	3	
P pulmonale		4
QRS abnormalities		65
Right axis deviation	5	
Left axis deviation	12	
Incomplete right bundle branch block	5	
Right bundle branch block	11	
$S_1 - Q_3 - T_3$	11	
ST Segment		44
T Wave ↓		40

The *plain chest radiograph,* valuable in all cardiopulmonary disorders, was found to be particularly useful when a pulmonary infiltrate or consolidation with elevation of the hemidiaphragm on the involved side was present.

Like the plain chest radiograph, a number of abnormalities on the *electrocardiogram* have been recorded in patients with PE (Table 19-3). However, many of the findings are nonspecific: arrhythmias (11%), QRS changes (65%) and ST-T wave abnormalities (44%). Only 11% of the patients in the UPET study showed the pattern of acute cor pulmonale ($S_1 - Q_3 - T_3$ pattern), the only recognizable pattern specific for massive pulmonary embolism. However, because it is most useful in excluding myocardial infarction, it remains a valuable ancillary study to be performed in all patients with suspected pulmonary embolism.

Currently, one of the most popular tests used in the evaluation of patients with suspected PE is the measurement of arterial oxygen tension.[6] Its usefulness is derived from the fact that virtually all patients with PE have some degree of hypoxemia. In fact, there is a significant inverse relationship between level of arterial oxygen tension and massivity of the embolic occlusion. Since there are very few patients with PE in whom the arterial oxygen tension is 90 mm Hg or above, it can be stated that in a patient with suspected PE, if the arterial oxygen tension is 90 mm or more, the likelihood of PE is quite remote. However, the use of this test on a quantitative basis requires that the oxygen electrode (highly unstable) be recalibrated with standard gas prior to each determination.

Graphic Diagnostic Studies

Following completion of the studies previously discussed, the patient with suspected PE should have multiple-view perfusion lung scanning performed. Currently, this relatively noninvasive procedure to assess regional distribution of pulmonary blood flow is the primary or central screening procedure for diagnosing PE. It may even be stated that a diagnostic evaluation for PE without perfusion lung scanning is incomplete.

When a multiple-view scan is normal, clinical PE can be excluded.[7] When the scan is abnormal, a probability estimate of the observed lesions having been caused by PE should be made. High probability lesions are those which assume the configuration of the pattern of vascular distribution: concave lesions along the lateral edge of the lung, segmental or wedge-shaped lesions and especially multiple lesions. Medium to low probability lesions are those which are not clearly interpreted as vascular in origin—long or round lesions which appear to cross lung segments—most commonly seen in patients with chronic obstructive lung disease. Such lesions generally require angiography for confirmation of PE. However, in younger patients without history or findings of prior cardiopulmonary disease, a compatible story, physical examination and high probability lesions on the lung scan may be all that are required to begin treatment.

Recently, the value of ventilation scanning has been emphasized in the diagnosis of PE.[8] Typically, an abnormal perfusion defect in an area of normal ventilation can be said to be due to pulmonary embolism. However, it is not known whether these findings are altered during the course of PE or how useful they may be in patients with underlying lung disease. Currently, there is no concensus regarding optimal techniques to perform ventilation scans. Until further data are available, pulmonary angiography is still the only positive means to identify pulmonary embolism.

Pulmonary angiography is most useful in patients with suspected PE who have underlying heart or lung disease. The clinical picture is frequently nonspecific, the arterial oxygen tension is lowered (just on the basis of the underlying disease) and the perfusion lung scan often shows medium-low probability lesions. It is also useful in patients without prior cardiopulmonary disease because of the ability to measure pressures in the right side of the heart and pulmonary arterial pressures, in addition to demonstrating the emboli. Since there is a close correlation between the size of the embolic occlusion and the severity of the hemodynamic response to PE, measurement of the pressures yields valuable diagnostic and therapeutic information. However, since many institutions do not have angiographic facilities or a trained team necessary to perform studies of good quality with safety, less invasive means now are being investigated as an aid to diagnosis.

Electrical Impedance Plethysmography

Our own efforts have centered around the problem of deep vein thrombosis and its causal relationship to PE, an observation made by Sevitt and Gallagher many years ago. We chose to investigate the usefulness of the electrical impedance plethysmograph (IPG) because of its simplicity, reproducibility and its excellent correlation with contrast venography.[9] In our series of patients with PE, documented by angiography, 95% had an abnormal IPG indicative of deep vein thrombosis (Table 19–4). None of these patients had evidence or history of recent major pelvic surgery, pelvic disease or pelvic manipulation. Our analysis also showed that in patients with suspected PE, if the IPG were abnormal, 90% had a positive pulmonary angiogram showing either an intravascular filling defect or a vessel cutoff or both, whereas if the IPG were normal, indicative of a patent deep venous system, 90% of the patients did not have a confirmatory pulmonary angiogram (Table 19–5). The results of these studies are very promis-

TABLE 19–4.—SUSPECTED PULMONARY EMBOLISM: CORRELATION BETWEEN PULMONARY ANGIOGRAPHY AND IMPEDANCE PLETHYSMOGRAPHY (IPG)

	NO. OF PATIENTS	IPG POSITIVE	IPG NEGATIVE
With pulmonary embolism	36	34 (95%)	2 (5%)
Without pulmonary embolism	22	4 (18%)	18 (82%)

ing for they do make the same strong relationship between deep vein thrombosis and pulmonary embolism. If these results are confirmed by further investigation, the invasive procedures such as pulmonary

TABLE 19–5.—SUSPECTED PULMONARY EMBOLISM: PULMONARY ANGIOGRAPHIC CONFIRMATION IN PATIENTS WITH AND WITHOUT DEEP VEIN THROMBOSIS

	NO. OF PATIENTS	PE POSITIVE	PE NEGATIVE
With deep vein thrombosis (IPG positive)	38	34 (90%)	4 (10%)
Without deep vein thrombosis (IPG negative)	20	2 (10%)	18 (90%)

angiography may not be required in the majority of patients with suspected PE.

A Diagnostic Approach (Fig 19–1)

Once the possibility of PE is recognized, the clinician is faced with the task of appropriate investigation commensurate with the facilities available. A careful history and physical examination with intelligent selection and interpretation of laboratory results still permits discrimination among differential diagnostic entities. Helpful in this area is the plain chest radiograph, the electrocardiogram, a well-performed arterial oxygen tension measurement and an impedance plethysmographic determination. If the latter is not available, a Doppler or con-

Fig 19–1.—A diagnostic approach to pulmonary embolism.

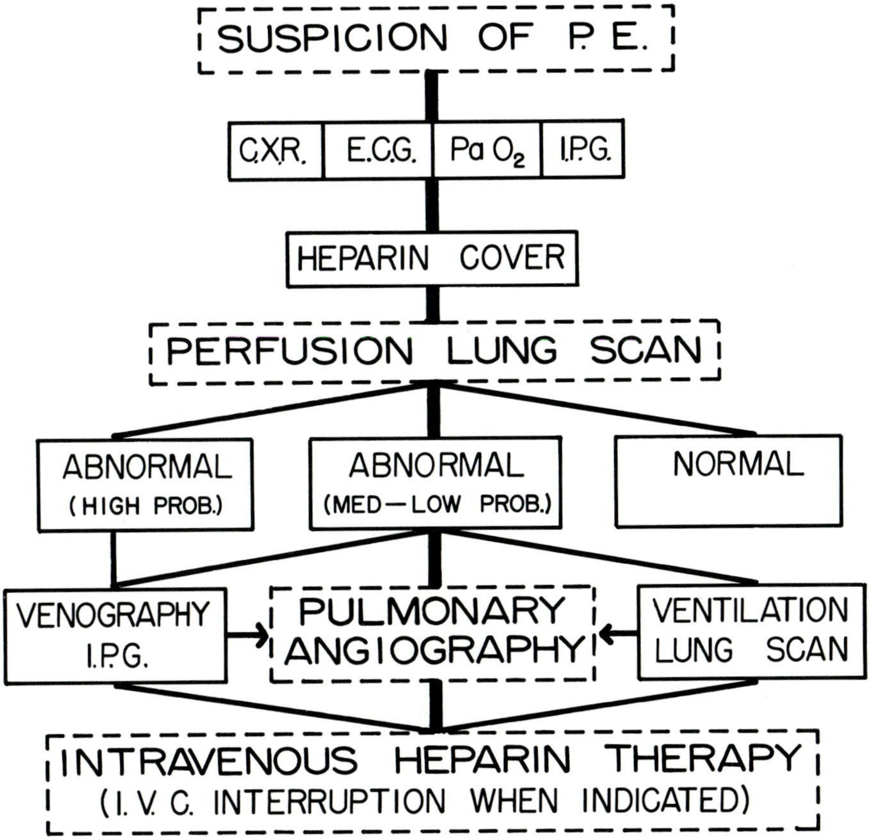

trast venography to assess the deep venous system is satisfactory. If the arterial oxygen tension is 90 mm Hg or more or if the IPG is normal, the likelihood of PE is very remote. However, until further confirmatory data are available concerning the accuracy of these predictive tests, perfusion lung scanning should be performed in all instances. It should be stated that during the diagnostic evaluation, an intravenous dose of heparin (5,000 – 10,000 units) should be administered as a "covering" dose(s). If the multiple-view perfusion scan is normal, the diagnostic evaluation may be terminated. If the perfusion scan shows multiple high probability lesions, further investigation depends upon the individual patient. If the patient is young without prior heart or lung disease, heparin therapy may be instituted without further study. However, if IPG, Doppler or venography is available, the finding of deep venous obstruction greatly strengthens the diagnosis of PE. Another permutation which may be helpful is the finding of a normal ventilation scan in the region of the perfusion defect.

If the perfusion scan shows medium-low probability lesions, pulmonary angiography is generally required to confirm the diagnosis. Again, an assessment of the deep venous system may be helpful. If xenon ventilation scanning is available, the finding of normal ventilation in the area of abnormal perfusion indicates PE. However, in older patients with chronic obstructive lung disease, the ventilation may already be abnormal, thereby requiring angiography as the definitive study.

It is encouraging to note that present vigorous investigation into the value of noninvasive studies has minimized the use of invasive pulmonary angiography which is still only available in the larger institutions.

REFERENCES

1. Sasahara, A. A., and Sharma, G. V. R. K.: Unpublished data.
2. Hume, M., Sevitt, S., and Thomas, D. P.: *Venous Thrombosis and Pulmonary Embolism* (Cambridge, Mass.: Harvard University Press, 1970), p. 4.
3. Coon, W. W., Willis, P. W., and Symous, M. J.: Assessment of anticoagulant treatment of venous thromboembolism, Ann. Surg. 170:559, 1969.
4. Barritt, D. W., and Jordan, S. C.: Anticoagulant drugs in treatment of pulmonary embolism: controlled trial, Lancet 1:1309, 1960.
5. The Urokinase Pulmonary Embolism Trial: A National Cooperative Study, Circulation 47 (Suppl. II):70, 1973.
6. Szucs, M. M., Brooks, H. L., Grossman, W., Dexter, L., and Dalen, J. E.: Diagnostic sensitivity of laboratory findings in acute pulmonary embolism, Ann. Intern. Med. 74:161, 1971.
7. Tow, D. E., and Simon, A.: Comparison of Lung Scanning and Pulmonary Angiograph in the Detection and Follow-up of Pulmonary Embolism: The Urokinase Pulmonary Embolism Trial Experience, in Sasahara, A. A., Sonnenblick, E. H., and Lesch, M. (eds.): *Pulmonary Emboli* (New York: Grune & Stratton, 1975), p. 57.

8. Wagner, H. N., Jr., Lopez-Majano, V., Langan, J. K., and Joshi, J. K.: Radioactive xenon in the differential diagnosis of pulmonary embolism, Radiology 91:1168, 1968.
9. Wheeler, H. B., O'Donnell, J. A., Anderson, F. A., and Benedict, K.: Occlusive impedance phlebography. A diagnostic procedure for venous thrombosis and pulmonary embolism, Prog. Cardiovasc. Dis. 17:119, 1974.

20 / Vena Caval Surgery to Prevent Recurrent Pulmonary Embolism

Marian F. McNamara, M.D., James K. Creasy, M.D., Harvey Takaki, M.D., Julius Conn, Jr., M.D., James S. T. Yao, M.D., Ph.D. and John J. Bergan, M.D.

Blood Flow Laboratory of the Department of Surgery, Northwestern University Medical School, Chicago, Illinois

This operation should be done only as a life-saving procedure and when it is done, it is life-saving. (Alton Ochsner,[1] 1965)

PRIORITY FOR VENOUS ligation has been ascribed to John Hunter,[2] but actual vena cava ligation was not performed successfully until Trendelenberg accomplished this in 1910. Later, John Homans (1934) established this operation on a physiologically sound basis and gave it proper emphasis in treatment of pulmonary embolism.[3] The rationale for Homans' idea was that the proximal interruption would prevent migration of distal thrombus.

Despite the fundamental wisdom of Homans' suggestion, distal venous ligation at the femoral level was still being advocated many years later.[4] However, the literature of the next 5 years terminated interest in distal venous ligature and returned attention to the cava as Homans had suggested.[5-7] The reasons for abandonment of femoral venous interruption included the fact that the operation failed to lower mortality rates of patients in whom it was performed, and it did not succeed in prevention of nonfatal pulmonary embolization.[1]

As the vena cava became accepted as the proper level for venous interruption, a philosophy grew that cava ligation was life-saving and

Supported in part by Grant No. HL 16253-61, National Heart and Lung Institute, and the Northwestern University Vascular Research Fund.

319

TABLE 20-1.—TYPES OF PARTIAL VENA
CAVA OCCLUSION

DATE	METHOD	AUTHORS
1952	Cat gut ligature	Streuter and Paine[17]
1954	Metal clip, removable	Moretz et al.[33]
1958	Filter (harp string grid)	DeWeese and Hunter[34]
1959	Teflon clip	Moretz et al.[16]
1960	Plication	Spencer[35]
1964	Serrated clip	Miles et al.[36]
1965	Staple plication	Sensenig et al.[37]
1967	Plastic filter	Eichelter and Schenk[38]
1969	Intracaval umbrella	Mobin-Uddin et al.[39]
1969	Channeling prosthesis	Barkett et al.[40]
1969	Intravascular spring	Pate et al.[41]
1970	Intracaval balloon	Hunter et al.[42]
1973	Intracaval wire cone	Greenfield et al.[43]

that undesirable sequelae were uncommon or inconsequential.[8, 9] Ochsner, in particular, and Collins described favorable experiences and pointed to serious consequences in a very few patients.[1, 10] More recent reports have admitted to serious stasis sequelae following caval ligation but have suggested that these are due to the phlebitic condition prior to cava interruption.[8, 11] Some reports have even indicated that no serious consequences were to be expected after cava occlusion in treatment of pulmonary embolization.[12, 13]

Ultimately, a realization grew that at least some undesirable effects followed operations on the vena cava in patients with venous thromboembolism. Shea and Robertson, reporting from Grady Hospital in Atlanta, indicated that only one patient in 25 evaluated up to 7 years after cava ligation was entirely free from adverse results of the surgery.[14] Writing some 15 years later, Wheeler et al. stated, "For two decades vena cava ligation has been the accepted surgical measure for control of pulmonary emboli, but many patients develop chronic stasis disease of their lower extremities after vena caval ligation."[15] It has become accepted that approximately 30% of cava ligation survivors develop serious leg sequelae and, therefore, methods of preventing these have emerged.[16]

Perhaps dissatisfaction with cava ligation was not justified. Nevertheless, as early as 1952, explorations were under way to find methods which could prevent recurrent pulmonary embolism and also avoid undesirable postoperative sequelae by preserving caval patency.[17] Within 20 years, 13 different methods of cava control had been advocated (Table 20-1). Now, sufficient experience with these has accumulated so that advantages and disadvantages of each technique can be defined.

The focus of this report is upon vena cava operations. Intracaval umbrella and wire filter are described elsewhere in this volume. The other intracaval procedures are still in the development stage and are not receiving significant general support.

Indications for Vena Cava Interruption

Well-defined indications for vena cava interruption exist[18] and are summarized in Table 20–2. These are strict and conservative. When indications are broadened, such as to include thrombus progression during anticoagulation, needless operations result. The first and most reliable line of defense in treatment of pulmonary embolization is intravenous heparin administered by continuous infusion. If heparin cannot be administered to a patient who has sustained a nonfatal herald pulmonary embolus, cava control must be instituted. Similarly, if a patient who is being maintained on constant heparin infusion sustains a recurrent pulmonary embolus of such magnitude that arterial blood oxygen content is lowered and tachycardia and tachypnea result, vena cava interruption is mandatory. Methods of diagnosis of pulmonary embolization are sufficiently sensitive today that many recurrent pulmonary emboli may be detected in patients receiving adequate anticoagulation. These should not, of themselves, call for cava interruption; only if cardiopulmonary compromise is produced is cava control required.

Occasionally, patients being treated by anticoagulation for pulmonary embolization will sustain an hemorrhagic complication such as gastrointestinal hemorrhage, hematuria or spontaneous hematoma. In such situations, if anticoagulation must be stopped, vena cava interruption must be done to prevent recurrent, possibly fatal, pulmonary emboli.

Finally, some patients may experience multiple, discontinuous epi-

TABLE 20–2.—INDICATIONS FOR VENA CAVA INTERRUPTION

When significant pulmonary embolization occurs
   After adequate anticoagulation
   When anticoagulants are contraindicated
   Chronically on multiple occasions
When anticoagulants given to prevent recurrent pulmonary embolism must be discontinued
When septic thrombophlebitis is uncontrolled
When pulmonary embolectomy is required

sodes of pulmonary embolization. Each of these may be treated with anticoagulation successfully, only to be followed by recurrent embolization once anticoagulation is withdrawn. Pulmonary hypertension with its sequelae of dyspnea, easy fatigability and tachycardia, may have developed. In such patients, an elective vena cava interruption is preferable to a lifetime of anticoagulants.

At the Northwestern University Medical Center, conservative indications for caval interruption have been utilized. Thus, in an 18-year period ending in 1976, only 129 patients were operated upon, an average of six to seven patients each year in an adult medical center of 1,500 to 2,000 beds. This population of patients requiring caval surgery was similar in many respects to that reported from this country and abroad. There were 83 men, 46 women ranging in age from 18 to 86 years. The male predominance of patients reflects an influence of a veterans' hospital cohort of individuals requiring this type of surgical intervention.

When indications for caval surgery were evaluated, it was found that failure of anticoagulation occurred in 88, contraindication to anticoagulation in 17, hemorrhage during anticoagulation in another 17. The operation was performed in conjunction with pulmonary embolectomy in seven patients.

Surgical Technique

Surgical exposure of the vena cava is similar regardless of the operation to be done on this structure. Usually, an extraperitoneal approach is employed and this is entirely satisfactory. Sometimes, especially when the procedure is used in connection with intra-abdominal surgery, or when the postpartum state dictates the need for concomitant ovarian vein ligation, the transperitoneal approach is utilized.

Local anesthesia for cava surgery is unsatisfactory. Spinal anesthesia is usually contraindicated because of the systemic anticoagulation used preoperatively to treat prior phlebitis or pulmonary embolism. Therefore, general anesthesia is usually given despite the fact that severe cardiopulmonary insufficiency is regularly present in these patients.

The skin incision is placed directly transversely in the right flank at the level of the umbilicus. The incision is not made obliquely but is placed from just lateral to the anterior axillary line to the lateral edge of the rectus sheath. As the incision is deepened through the subcutaneous fat, the medial and lateral wound edges are undermined to allow splitting of the fibers of the subjacent external oblique muscle.

When this muscle is incised from the rib margin to the rectus sheath, its undersurface is widely freed from the internal oblique. Later adequate deep exposure is dependent upon early wide mobilization of each anatomical layer.

Careful splitting of the fibers of the internal oblique muscle prevents inadvertent entering of the peritoneal cavity. Protection of the peritoneum is offered by the transversus abdominis muscle and properitoneal fat. The iliac crest and rectus sheath define the margins of the internal oblique muscle incision.

An attenuated transversus abdominis muscle usually is encountered at this midabdominal level. Its fibers initially are separated laterally in order to avoid the underlying peritoneum. This is adherent to the transversus abdominis muscle medially. The muscle split then is enlarged medially to the rectus sheath and laterally as far as exposure allows.

The retroperitoneal space is exposed next. Now, adequate muscle relaxation is mandatory. Exposure of the cava will be hazardous if coughing and straining are allowed to occur.

A hand is inserted into the incision and the peritoneum is mobilized widely superiorly and inferiorly. The iliac fossa serves as a natural guide to this blind development of the peritoneum. A conscious effort is made to avoid the retropsoas space since it is tempting to drop behind the psoas as the peritoneum is being mobilized medially. The blunt areolar tissue dissection is complete when the spine and sympathetic chain can be palpated easily in the depths of the wound.

At this point, placement of retractors exposes the cava. A broad retractor is placed anteriorly and held strongly in a medial direction against the peritoneum. Narrow curved retractors are then placed to retract pericaval fat superiorly and inferiorly. These retractors are essential to a continuous unobstructed view deep in the wound.

Easy dissection of the vena cava is dependent upon development of the proper adventitial plane. A lipoareolar layer envelops the vessel and must be split for 6 to 8 cm on its lateral surface. When this is done, a cotton-tipped dissector can be used to free the entire anterior and posterior surface of the vessel.

Often one small cotton dissecting sponge can be used to hold the cava while a second wipes away the areolar investing tissues so that the lumbar veins can be identified. These thin-walled vessels tear easily at their caval attachment and bleed ferociously. Direct-vision dissection of the vena cava insures against accidental tearing of tributary veins. A 6-cm length of cava is exposed and then a curved clamp is passed medially and posteriorly to encircle this vessel for positive control. This clamp catches an atraumatic rubber sling which aids further mobilization by allowing appropriate traction. At no time is blind dissection used. The clamp tip is watched at all times while passing behind the cava so that lumbar veins can be avoided. Even the medial caval attachments near the aorta are divided under direct vision.

Vena Cava Ligation

Cava ligation can be done swiftly, expeditiously and with minimum caval dissection. Once the curved clamp passes behind the cava and catches the ligature, the procedure is nearly over. Dacron umbilical tape is the ideal material for cava ligation. Its breadth prevents accidental cutting through as the first and subsequent knots are tied down.

In the present series, vena caval ligation was performed in 60 patients with eight operative deaths. Death occurred with cardiopulmonary failure in the early postoperative period in four patients. Hypotension following vena caval occlusion occurred in one of these. This resulted in death from renal failure. Three deaths occurred after 14 days and seemed unrelated to the operative procedure or to preoperative pulmonary embolization. Autopsy showed organized thrombus above the ligation site in two patients, neither of whom showed evidence of new emboli.

There were three recurrent emboli in the 52 operative survivors. This caused one death at 1 year following caval ligation.

Edema developed or increased in the lower extremities during the hospital course in 14 patients (27%). This edema was severe enough to complicate the postoperative management in six patients (12%). During the follow-up period, a comparison of lower extremity findings with the patients' preoperative status revealed new or increased edema in nine (17%). Three patients (6%) developed extremity ulcers and had edema which significantly altered their life style.

Although a syndrome of hypotension, oliguria and renal failure has been said to occur in one third of patients within 24 hr of cava ligation,[19] the Northwestern experience did not confirm such an observation. On the other hand, three patients were observed in the entire series of 131 who experienced acute hypotension with tachycardia or bradycardia during induction of anesthesia. These had abrupt cyanosis despite ventilation with 100% oxygen. Such patients should be suspected of having sustained acute, massive pulmonary embolization, possibly associated with nonsynchronous muscular fibrillation due to induced muscular relaxation.

The single death due to recurrent pulmonary embolization despite cava ligation and subsequent careful management of anticoagulation was tragic. Aggressive attempts were made to identify the offending site of thrombosis and the collateral pathways which allowed passage of the eventually fatal emboli. Neither thrombus nor significant treatable collaterals were found. Even autopsy examination failed to show a left-sided vena cava,[20] duplication of the cava,[21] or other significant anomalies.[22]

Collateral venous circulation studies have been performed in patients after cava ligation.[23, 24] Thrombi have been identified in the ascending lumbar vein, and huge ovarian veins have also been visualized. It is not unusual in cases of cava ligation to find the ovarian veins enlarged to the size of a normal vena cava. Because of these observations and experimental studies, DeWeese's group has said, ". . . we conclude that ligation of the inferior vena cava is seldom, if ever, indicated in the treatment of thromboembolic disease."[25] This observation assumes greater importance as newer procedures are introduced, such as the caval umbrella which occludes the vena cava in an intracaval fashion.

Vena Cava Plication and Suture Filtration

An early interest in cava interruption by methods which would favor cava patency allowed a large experience to accumulate over the years at Northwestern University. An analysis of the results of an early experience with these techniques was reported.[26, 27] The studies showed that techniques of suture placement which violated caval intimal integrity led to cava occlusion, especially if the cava was narrowed as in cava plication.

In the Northwestern experience, vena cava interruption was performed by suture plication or filter construction in 42 patients with three operative deaths. One patient with a massive pulmonary embolism died in the early postoperative period and might have been saved with pulmonary embolectomy. The other deaths resulted from myocardial infarction at 3 weeks and metastatic carcinoma, also at 3 weeks postoperatively.

Vena cavograms in nine patients with cava plication showed complete cava occlusion in six, only three of whom were symptomatic. A review of various forms of cava interruption at the Johns Hopkins Hospital revealed 40% to be occluded. "No correlation existed between the method of suture plication, clip, or staple, and the demonstration of plication thrombosis."[28] When the caval operative site occluded due to trapped embolus or thrombus, significant ileofemoral thrombosis developed and large collateral venous channels around the area of obstruction could be seen on cavograms. In the Hopkins series, there were three patients with proven recurrent pulmonary emboli in the group of 56 reviewed. Three patients died. At Northwestern, in the 39 survivors of the operation, there were two with recurrent emboli. One of these died early, following a second cava ligation done to prevent recurrent emboli.

Edema developed or increased during the hospital course in seven patients (17.5%). This was increased from the preoperative level in the follow-up period in 10 (34%). Edema altered the patient's life style in four instances. Two of these patients developed venous ulcers.

Vena cava plication and suture filtering operations are now of historic interest. Simpler methods of cava interruption are available which eliminate the need to pass suture through the vena cava.

Comparison of Ligation and Plication

Two diametrically opposing reports have compared cava plication and ligation. Wheeler et al.[15] conclude that, "Both ligation and plication prevent lethal pulmonary emboli. Patients with plication do not develop stasis disease of the lower extremities." On the other hand, the experience of Ochsner et al. was summarized in a single sentence from their report, "Our experience however demonstrates that the sequelae are less when a cava ligation is done which is certainly a simpler procedure than when the cava is plicated."[29]

Vena Cava Clipping

Although vena cava ligation never achieved unanimous support from surgeons, the cava clipping operation has attracted a large number of adherents. Part of the reason for this is the straightforward logic which holds that, assuming equal efficacy in prevention of recurrent pulmonary embolization, an open vena cava is better than an occluded vena cava.

At Northwestern, cava clipping has been done utilizing the suggestion of Flege,[30] who passes a silastic tubing around the cava and uses this as a guide for placement of the clip. In all, clips have been used for partial vena caval interruption in 31 patients with three operative deaths (10%). Death occurred from cardiopulmonary failure in the immediate postoperative period in one patient. The other two deaths were due to myocardial infarction in one patient at 4 days and congestive heart failure in another at 2 weeks.

There were two recurrent emboli in 29 of the patients. One embolus occurring in the immediate postoperative period was treated by vena caval ligation. The second, small embolus was found incidentally at autopsy.

New or increased edema occurred in the postoperative hospital course in nine (31%) with occurrence on follow-up in seven (29%). There were three patients with moderate to severe edema and one of these developed venous ulceration.

Couch, in reporting the Brigham experience with cava clipping, noted seven deaths within 30 days of operation in 112 patients (6%). In the 105 survivors, recurrent pulmonary embolism was proved in four patients. Several of the comments from this report are noteworthy: ". . . its [the serrated clip] almost perfect record in preventing fatal pulmonary embolism seems established by the present study as well as by others . . . . the act of applying the serrated clip, by whatever approach, entails a minimal hazard."[31]

Comment

Failure of anticoagulation to control recurrent emboli has been the major indication for vena cava interruption in the Northwestern experience. It necessitated 65% of the procedures. Introduction of new techniques for partial caval interruption influenced the type of procedures done on our service as elsewhere. Of 60 ligations performed, 55 were done before 1969 and since that time, patency procedures (74) have predominated. Caval clipping became dominant after 1969.

Consecutive data analysis reveals the gradual change in method of vena caval interruption and a salutory decline in the number of vena caval procedures in recent years. The single factor which influenced this decline most was the maintenance of adequate anticoagulation in the initial management. This was achieved by almost universal adoption of the constant infusion method of heparin administration.

The administration of anticoagulants in the postoperative period has been limited to those patients with evidence of active lower extremity venous thrombosis. Such anticoagulation correlates with development of wound and retroperitoneal hematomas in the postoperative period. This complication occurred in 10% of the patients receiving postoperative anticoagulants.

Frequency of postoperative stasis sequelae following caval interruption has varied in reported series from 10 to 50%.[32] Ambulatory venous hypertension is the common denominator in production of edema or ulceration. Such hypertension may result from vena caval obstruction from thrombosis or entrapped embolus. New thrombosis may be due to coagulation abnormalities such as antithrombin III deficiency, which predisposes the patient to recurrent peripheral thrombosis. In a clinical setting, it is difficult to determine the weighted significance of components of caval obstruction, venous thrombosis and predisposition to thrombosis as they singly and in concert produce stasis sequelae. In this series, 52 patients (40%) had edema of the lower extremities prior to vena caval interruption. This was due to acute thrombophlebitis in most instances. New or increased edema developed in 24% of these patients during the postoperative period. Subsequently, 31.3% of the group had new or increased edema in the remote follow-up period. The edema which occurred was easily controlled in nearly all cases and resulted in a change of life style in only a small number of people.

Doppler ultrasound and impedance plethysmography were utilized in an attempt to quantify the degree of venous obstruction in the lower extremities following vena caval interruption. These studies revealed a remarkable venous adaptability in those patients with known caval occlusion. Of the 10 studied patients with ligation, six had normal Doppler respiratory variations and impedance plethysmography, which indicated the formation of adequate collateral circulation. Normal Doppler respiratory variation with abnormal impedance plethysmography, which was found in five patients, indicated the presence of large collaterals with coexisting venous hypertension. The presence of abnormal Doppler respiratory variation with normal impedance plethysmography in two patients can best be explained on the basis of formation of multiple, small collaterals which failed to transmit respiratory variation but which adequately decompressed the venous system.

Recurrent pulmonary emboli after cava interruption presents a vexing problem. Because of prior unfortunate experience, vena caval ligation was performed promptly in two patients with recurrent pulmonary emboli which occurred soon after partial vena caval interruption. In retrospect, less prompt reoperation may have proved satisfactory.

Embolization following vena caval interruption may originate in thrombosis at the operative site or thrombi may traverse patent dilated collateral vessels. The right atrium or upper extremity may harbor thrombi. Rarely, vena caval anomalies cause failure of caval surgery. If recurrent embolization occurs following cava interruption, an inferior vena cavogram should be performed to study the venous anatomy and the status of the operative site. It should be remembered that the occurrence of pleuritic chest pain in the postoperative period may not be caused by pulmonary embolization. The majority of patients in this series who developed pulmonary embolic symptoms had perfusion lung scans which were unchanged in appearance from the preoperative status. Possibly, symptoms were caused by pulmonary infarction due to the initial pulmonary embolus.

Conclusions

Although intracaval devices for control of recurrent pulmonary embolization may find increased utility in the future, vena cava operations remain the standard of therapy to prevent pulmonary embolization when anticoagulation cannot be used or when it has failed. The mortality of such operations depends upon the physiologic status of the patient at the time of the surgical event and not upon the magnitude of the operative procedure. Stasis sequelae are apparently not affected by the type of operation performed. On the other hand, a closed cava engenders collateral venous circulation which can grow to enormous proportions. Such collaterals can transmit significant pulmonary emboli which, by their cumulative effect, may prove lethal. The vena cava clipping procedure performed with the serrated device has emerged as the technique of choice. The future will tell whether this operation can compete successfully with intracaval devices which do not produce total caval occlusion.

Summary

During the past 20 years, 134 vena cava operations have been performed on 131 patients at the Northwestern University Medical Center Hospitals. Indications for these operations have included recurrent pulmonary embolization while the patient was adequately anticoagulated, pulmonary embolization in a patient who could not be anticoagulated, multiple discontinuous episodes of pulmonary embolization occurring over long periods of time, and massive pulmonary embolization requiring pulmonary embolectomy.

The diagnosis of both venous thrombosis and pulmonary embolization was largely clinical before 1971. The confirmation of pulmonary embolization and its recurrence was initially obtained by evaluation of serum enzyme changes, electrocardiogram and chest radiographs but lung scanning and pulmonary angiography quickly added an element of objectivity to such diagnosis after 1966. Similarly, the diagnosis of venous thrombosis itself has become objective in recent years.

Although 60 vena cava ligations were done, 55 were performed before 1969 and since then, patency procedures have predominated.

Vena cava clipping (31 operations) has been the procedure of choice since 1969. Over the 20-year period, surgical mortality has remained 10.5% and long-term postoperative sequelae in the form of edema and venous ulceration (14%) have not seemed to be altered by changing indications and techniques of the operation. Recurrent pulmonary embolization has remained at a 5% level. Using Doppler ultrasound and impedance plethysmography as well as clinical evaluation in long-term follow-up to 12.5 years, remarkable venous adaptability has been seen in those patients with known caval occlusion. Major physiologic change seems to be more directly correlated with recurrent thrombotic events than with type of vena caval interruption done to prevent recurrent pulmonary embolus.

REFERENCES

1. Ochsner, A.: Discussion of Spencer, F. C., Jude, J., Rienhoff, W. F., and Stonesifer, G.: Plication of the vena cava for pulmonary embolism, Ann. Surg. 161:788, 1965.
2. Hunter, J.: Observations on inflammation of internal coat of veins, Trans. Soc. Improvement Med. Chir. Knowledge (London) 1:18, 1793.
3. Homans, J.: Thrombosis of the deep veins of the lower leg causing pulmonary embolism, N. Engl. J. Med. 211:993, 1934.
4. Allen, A. W.: Interruption of the deep veins of the lower extremities in the prevention and treatment of thrombosis and embolism, Surg. Gynecol. Obstet. 84:519, 1947.
5. Ravdin, I. S., and Kirby, C. K.: Experiences with ligation and heparin in thromboembolic disease, Surgery 29:334, 1951.
6. McLachlin, J., and Paterson, J. C.: Some basic observations on venous thrombosis and pulmonary embolism, Surg. Gynecol. Obstet. 93:1, 1951.
7. Erb, W. H., and Schumann, F.: An appraisal of bilateral superficial femoral vein ligation in preventing pulmonary embolism, Surgery 29:819, 1951.
8. Palumbo, L. T., and Paul R. E.: Effects of ligation of major veins, Angiology 4:337, 1953.
9. Mozes, M., Adar, R., Bogokowsky, H., and Abmon, M.: Vein ligation in the treatment of pulmonary embolism, Surgery 55:621, 1964.
10. Collins, C. G., MacCallu, E. A., Nelson, E. W., Weinstein, B. B., and Collins, J. H.: Suppurative pelvic thrombophlebitis, Surgery 30:298, 1951.
11. Annetts, D. L., Hoy, R., Ludbrook, J., and Tracy, G. D.: The effects of inferior vena cava plication and ligation on the lower limbs, Med. J. Aust. 2:703, 1968.
12. Krause, R. J., Cranley, J. J., Hallaba, M. A. S., Strasser, E. S., and Hafner, C. D.: Caval ligation in thromboembolic disease, Arch. Surg. 87:184, 1963.
13. Dale, W. A.: Ligation of the inferior vena cava for thromboembolism, Surgery 43:24, 1958.
14. Shea, P. C., Jr., and Robertson, R. L.: Late sequelae of inferior vena cava ligation, Surg. Gynecol. Obstet. 93:153, 1951.
15. Wheeler, C. G., Thompson, J. E., Austin, D. J., Patman, R. D., and Stockton, R. L.: Interruption of the inferior vena cava for thromboembolism: Comparison of ligation and plication, Ann. Surg. 163:199, 1966.
16. Moretz, W. H., Rhode, C. M., and Shepherd, M. H.: Prevention of pulmonary emboli by partial occlusion of the inferior vena cava, Am. Surg. 25:617, 1959.
17. Streuter, M. A., and Paine, J. R.: Temporary occlusion of the inferior vena cava suggested as a means of treatment in thromboembolism requiring cava ligation, Surgery 34:20, 1953.

18. Bergan, J. J., and Trippel, O. H.: Vena cava operations for prevention of pulmonary embolism, Surg. Clin. North Am. 46:195, 1966.
19. Gazzaniga, A. B., Cahill, J. L., Replogle, R. L., and Tilney, N. L.: Changes in blood volume and renal function following ligation of the inferior vena cava, Surgery 62: 417, 1967.
20. Agram, M. R., and Kratzman, E. A.: Inferior vena cava on the left side, J. Urol. 101: 149, 1969.
21. Wagner, M., and Mark, L.: Duplication of the inferior vena cava and its role in recurrent pulmonary emboli, JAMA 209:108, 1969.
22. Capdevila, J. M., Farre, J., Bongera, F., Curria, J. M., and Samaniego, E.: Situacion anomala de la vena cava inferior. A proposito de tres observaciones personales (Anomaly of the inferior vena cava. Three case presentations.), Angiologia 20:11, 1968.
23. Ferris, E. J., Vittimberga, F. J., Byrne, J. J., Nabseth, D. C., and Shapiro, J. H.: The inferior vena cava after ligation and plication. A study of collateral routes, Radiology 89:1, 1967.
24. Surington, C. T., and Jonas, A. F., Jr.: Intra-abdominal venography following inferior vena cava ligation, Arch. Surg. 65:605, 1952.
25. Parrish, E. H., Adams, J. T., Pories, W. J., Burget, D. E., and DeWeese, J. A.: Pulmonary emboli following vena caval ligation, Arch. Surg. 97:899, 1968.
26. Anlyan, W. G., Campbell, F. H., Shingleton, W. W., and Gardner, C. E., Jr.: Pulmonary embolism following venous ligation, Arch. Surg. 64:200, 1952.
27. Bergan, J. J., Kaupp, H. A., and Trippel, O. H.: Critical evaluation of vena cava plication. Prevention of pulmonary embolism, Arch. Surg. 88:1016, 1964.
28. DeMeester, T. R., Rutherford, R. B., Blazek, J. V., and Zuidema, G. D.: Plication of the inferior vena cava for thromboembolism, Surgery 62:56, 1967.
29. Ochsner, A., Ochsner, J. L., and Sanders, H. S.: Prevention of pulmonary embolism by caval ligation, Ann. Surg. 171:923, 1970.
30. Flege, J. B., Jr.: Application of inferior vena cava clip, Surgery 61:823, 1967.
31. Couch, N. P., Baldwin, S. S., and Crane, C.: Mortality and morbidity rates after inferior vena caval clipping, Surgery 77:106, 1975.
32. Silver, D., and Sabiston, D. C., Jr.: The role of vena caval interruption in the management of pulmonary embolism, Surgery 77:1, 1975.
33. Moretz, W. H., Naisbitt, P. F., and Stevenson, G. P.: Experimental studies on temporary occlusion of the inferior vena cava, Surgery 36:384, 1954.
34. DeWeese, M. S., and Hunter, D. C., Jr.: A vena cava filter for the prevention of pulmonary emboli, Bull. Soc. Int. Chir. 17:17, 1958.
35. Spencer, F. C.: Experimental evaluation of partitioning of the inferior vena cava to prevent pulmonary embolism, Surg. Forum 10:680, 1960.
36. Miles, R. M., Chappell, F., and Renner, O.: A partially occluding vena caval clip for the prevention of pulmonary embolism, Am. Surg. 30:40, 1964.
37. Sensenig, D. M., Achar, B. G., and Serlin, O.: Plication of the inferior vena cava with staples, Am. J. Surg. 109:679, 1965.
38. Eichelter, P., and Schenk, W. G., Jr.: A new experimental approach to prophylaxis of pulmonary embolism, Rev. Surg. 24:455, 1967.
39. Mobin-Uddin, K., McLean, R., and Jude, J. R.: A new catheter technique of interruption of inferior vena cava for prevention of pulmonary embolism, Am. Surg. 35: 889, 1969.
40. Barkett, V. M., Wright, R., and Greenfield, L. J.: Plication of the inferior vena cava by a new channeling prosthesis, Am. J. Surg. 118:981, 1969.
41. Pate, J. W., Melvin, D., and Cheek, R. C.: A new form of vena caval interruption, Ann. Surg. 169:873, 1969.
42. Hunter, J. A., Sessions, R., and Buenger, R.: Experimental balloon obstruction of inferior vena cava, Ann. Surg. 171:315, 1970.
43. Greenfield, L. J., McCurdy, J. R., Brown, P. P., and Elkins, R. C.: A new intracaval filter permitting continued flow and resolution of emboli, Surgery 73:599, 1973.

21 / The Intracaval Umbrella in Prevention of Pulmonary Embolism

KAZI MOBIN-UDDIN, M.B., B.S.

The Frederick C. Smith Clinic, Marion, Ohio

VENOUS THROMBOEMBOLIC disease continues to be a major cause of morbidity and mortality in hospitalized patients. It is estimated that pulmonary embolism causes approximately 200,000 deaths per year in the United States. Pulmonary embolism is the sole cause of death in 100,000 and is a major contributing cause of another 100,000.[1]

Anticoagulant therapy, initially with intravenous heparin followed by oral coumarin compounds, has become the standard treatment for patients with thromboembolic disease. Heparin in adequate doses blocks the coagulation mechanism and thus prevents further thrombus formation. Its use is prophylactic and it has no effect on preformed thrombi, except to prevent distal propagation. The clinical improvement following heparin therapy in deep venous thrombosis (DVT) is not due to anatomical lysis of thrombi as repeat radiographic findings are practically unchanged. The fate of venous thrombi is primarily dependent on the endogenous mechanisms—thrombolysis, thrombus fragmentation, organization and recanalization—rather than direct action of heparin. The results of uncontrolled studies[2] report fatal recurrent embolization rates ranging from 0 to 18.6%. The Urokinase Pulmonary Embolism Trial Phase I, National Cooperative Study,[3] reported 18% recurrence rate (fatal 9%) in 60 patients with proved pulmonary embolism and treated with adequate anticoagulation.

Ligation of the inferior vena cava (IVC) is a most effective procedure for preventing pulmonary embolism. However, operative ligation of IVC under general anesthesia is accompanied by an operative mortality rate that varies from 5%[5] to 40%,[6] depending upon the se-

verity of underlying disease and the extent of obstruction to pulmonary blood flow.

Transvenous insertion of the IVC umbrella filter (UF)[7-12] is performed under local anesthesia, avoids a major operation and can be
performed with minimal risk even in critically ill patients with acute
pulmonary embolism.

The present report includes the author's experience with the IVC-
UF as well as the results reported by other physicians.

Operative Technique for Umbrella Insertion

The IVC-UF (Figs 21–1 and 21–2) consists of six spokes of stainless steel alloy radiating from a central hub and covered on both sides

Fig 21–1.—**A,** *right,* 28-mm filter now recommended for use in all adult
patients. The 23-mm filter (*left*) may have application in patients weighing
less than 125 lb. **B,** catheter used for umbrella filter implantation.

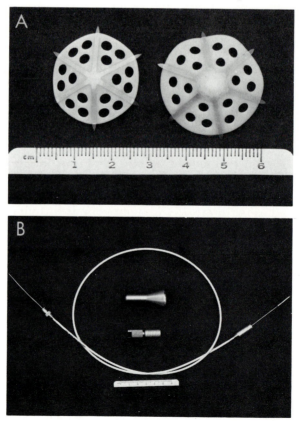

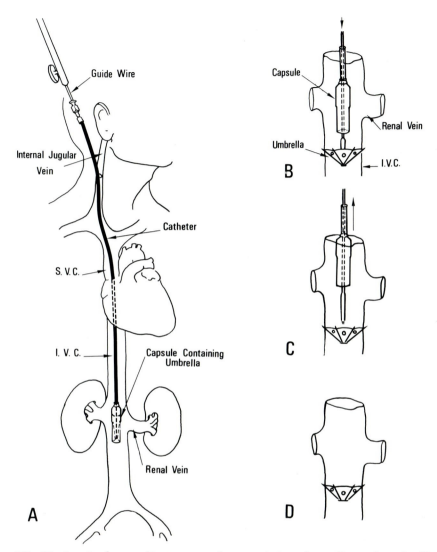

Fig 21–2.— A, the applicator-capsule containing the collapsed umbrella filter has been inserted via the right internal jugular vein into the inferior vena cava below the renal veins. **B,** the filter has been ejected from the capsule into the inferior vena cava. **C,** the stylet has been unscrewed from the filter and **D,** the applicator has been withdrawn.

by a circular thin sheet of silicone. The spokes extend 2 mm beyond the silicone webbing, which has 18 perforations 3 mm in diameter. The original umbrella was 23 mm in diameter, but episodes of filter migration led to the development of a 28-mm device. The catheter used for UF implantation has a metal capsule at the end, 7 mm in diameter and 32 mm in length. A threaded stylet fits inside the catheter and capsule.

The IVC-UF is folded into the catheter-capsule with the help of a loading cone. Under local anesthesia, through a small incision in the neck, the catheter is inserted via a venotomy in the right internal jugular vein and advanced under fluoroscopic control into the infrarenal IVC.

Fig 21–3.—Angiogram of inferior vena cava made by injecting radiopaque dye through the applicator, just prior to filter insertion.

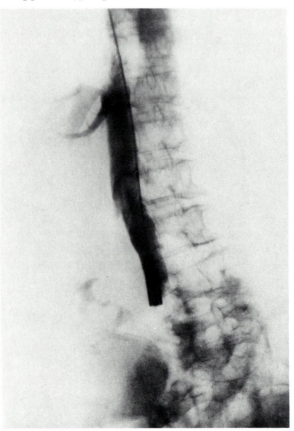

The new angiographic applicator is provided with a side injection port and several circumferential openings at the base of the applicator capsule for the injection of radiopaque dye through the applicator. The angiographic applicator capsule is positioned in the right iliac vein or in the lower portion of IVC if the iliac vein is obstructed with thrombus and IVC angiogram is obtained in each patient in order to identify the caval anatomy prior to filter insertion (Fig 21–3).

A vena cavogram made before IVC-UF insertion is a very valuable adjunct. It demonstrates the level of renal veins and the size of the IVC and it may reveal any unsuspected abnormalities of the IVC or of the renal veins. Any thrombus in the IVC that may interfere with placement of the UF can also be detected.

Selection of Patients for Umbrella Insertion

MASSIVE PULMONARY EMBOLISM

Patients with massive pulmonary embolism who have survived the acute insult can die from (1) arrhythmias, (2) low cardiac output and (3) recurrent pulmonary embolism. IVC ligation is usually recommended in these patients, as reliance on anticoagulant therapy alone is not justified since any additional embolization can be fatal. In acute massive pulmonary embolism, a direct operative approach for IVC ligation under general anesthesia carries a prohibitive risk. Berger[13] reported seven patients with massive embolism, five of whom developed circulatory collapse during operative ligation of IVC. Two patients died, and three were saved by pulmonary embolectomy. Six pulmonary embolectomies reported by Sautter et al.[14] were precipitated by rapid deterioration of the patient's condition during or just after the induction of anesthesia for caval ligation.

Transvenous insertion of the IVC-UF is the method of choice in these acutely ill patients, as the procedure is done under local anesthesia and avoids a major operation. Bloomfield[15] reported IVC-UF insertion in patients who had survived massive pulmonary embolism by 1 to 2 hr. Of the 12 patients, 8 made uncomplicated complete recovery. Bloomfield noted marked improvement within 2–12 hr after the IVC-UF insertion, as documented by symptomatic relief, objective increase in arterial oxygen partial pressure, and systemic blood pressure maintenance without vasopressor agents. Similar improvement was also noted previously by us.[8]

CONTRAINDICATIONS TO ANTICOAGULANTS

Contraindications to heparin therapy may be absolute or relative; treatment for each patient should be individualized and the need for therapy verified against the probable risk of hemorrhage. Usually heparin is not given to patients with recent cerebral vascular accident, operation or severe trauma or to those patients with actively bleeding lesions. Women over 60 years of age have a 50% risk of bleeding complications.[16]

FAILURE OF ANTICOAGULANTS

The main indication for the IVC-UF insertion has been in those patients in whom adequate heparinization (Lee-White clotting greater than 20 min) has failed to prevent recurrent embolic episodes. Recurrent pulmonary embolism is common in patients who have a basic predisposing cause for continued thromboembolism, such as chronic congestive heart failure and recurrent thrombophlebitis.

PRESENCE OF POTENTIALLY FATAL THROMBI IN ILIOFEMORAL VEINS OR IVC

Potentially fatal thromboemboli frequently arise in iliofemoral veins[17] and can be readily demonstrated by phlebography.[9, 18] A fresh, nonadherent thrombus appears as a radiolucent defect within the vein, with a thin white line representing contrast medium between the thrombus and the vein wall on each side. We perform phlebograms in all patients with pulmonary embolism to determine the location, extent and nature of residual venous thrombi. IVC-UF insertion is recommended if large, nonadherent thrombi are demonstrated in iliofemoral veins or IVC.

INDICATIONS FOR INFERIOR VENA CAVA UMBRELLA FILTER INSERTION IN PATIENTS WITH DEEP VENOUS THROMBOSIS

Insertion of IVC-UF is indicated in patients with deep venous thrombosis when anticoagulant therapy is contraindicated or when recurrent thrombophlebitis requires repeated hospitalization, especially if long-term adequate anticoagulant therapy is difficult to maintain.

Fullen and associates[19] reported the prophylactic use of the IVC-UF in hip fracture patients, with a controlled study group, Fifty-nine patients were in the control group. Of 70 patients offered the IVC-UF, 22 refused the procedure, and in 7 patients the IVC-UF could not be inserted because of technical reasons. The two groups were similar in regard to age, associated disease, type of fractures and the time delay between admission and fracture fixation. They reported no clinically detectable pulmonary emboli in the treated group versus a 20% incidence in the controls. The mortality rate in the treated group was 10% as compared to 24% in the control group. No patient in the treated group died from pulmonary embolism. In the control group, pulmonary embolism was considered to be the cause of death in 8 (13.5%).

Prophylactic IVC-UF insertion was performed at the University of Kentucky Medical Center in five patients who had developed deep venous thrombosis, confirmed by venography, while awaiting hip operation. These patients were considered to be at great risk of developing fatal pulmonary embolism following hip operation. All patients recovered without clinical evidence of pulmonary embolism.

Contraindications to IVC-UF Insertion

Insertion of the IVC-UF is not recommended in patients with septic emboli or in those with septicemia. We have advised removal of the IVC-UF and ligation of IVC in one patient with postoperative septicemia. The organisms cultured from the blood and from the clot on the proximal surface of the filter were identical.

Management after Umbrella Insertion

Following IVC-UF implantation, systemic anticoagulant therapy is withheld for 12 hr to minimize the possibility of bleeding in the neck incision or into the retroperitoneal space. Thereafter, intravenous heparin is resumed, if there is no contraindication to its use, for 7–10 days, preferably by continuous infusion, to maintain partial thromboplastin time for the Lee-White clotting time at two times the control value. Oral anticoagulation with warfarin sodium is started on the third postoperative day and continued for 3 months. Postoperative systemic anticoagulation plays an important part in the prevention of formation or propagation of peripheral thrombi. In patients with a continuing predisposition for recurrent emboli, long-term anticoagulant therapy is advised.

In an attempt to resist or prevent thrombus formation on the proxi-

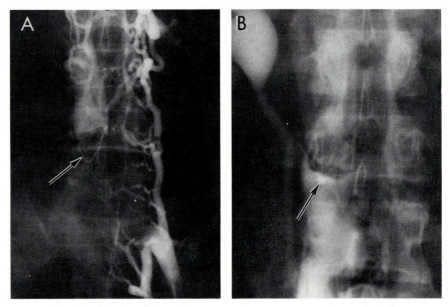

Fig 21–4. – **A,** angiogram of inferior vena cava in a patient five days after umbrella (*arrow*) implantation. Note complete thrombotic occlusion of IVC and development of collateral circulation. **B,** angiogram of IVC, 3 months after implantation of heparin-impregnated umbrella filter (*arrow*). Note free flow of blood through the filter.

mal surface of the IVC-UF, preoperative heparin impregnation[20] of the filter with TDMAC/heparin complex* is recommended. There is considerable experimental evidence to suggest that the filters preoperatively impregnated with heparin are less thrombogenic.[7] Local along with systemic anticoagulation can prevent or resist thrombus formation and allow for endothelium to grow in between the fenestrations of the IVC-UF (Fig 21–4). How long the heparin bonding is effective is not known. Once the IVC-UF is endothelialized, a process usually complete within 3 months, local or systemic anticoagulation is no longer necessary to maintain patency of the IVC. Our objective is to maintain patency of the ostia of the IVC-UF, except when they entrap emboli.

Author's Experience

Insertion of the IVC-UF was performed in 168 patients between July 1968 and November 1976. One hundred filter implants (July 1968

---

*Polysciences, Inc., Paul Valley Industrial Park, Warrington, PA 18976.

TABLE 21–1.—INFERIOR VENA CAVA
UMBRELLA FILTER–AUTHOR'S EXPERIENCE
(JULY 1968–NOVEMBER 1976)

Total no. of patients	168
Filter migration	0
Retroperitoneal bleeding	1
Recurrent emboli	3
Recurrent phlebitis	11

to June 1970) were done at the University of Miami Hospitals; 51 filter implants (July 1970 to June 1974) were done at the University of Kentucky Medical Center at Lexington, Kentucky; and 19 filter implants (July 1974 to November 1976) were done at the Community Med-Center Hospital in Marion, Ohio. The results are summarized in Table 21–1.

Mortality and Recurrent Embolism

Significant retroperitoneal bleeding following IVC-UF insertion may have contributed to the death of a 75-year-old man with chronic congestive heart failure who died on the fifth postoperative day. The bleeding was not recognized clinically. A 25-year-old markedly obese woman had sudden cardiac arrest 12 hr after IVC-UF insertion and could not be resuscitated. At autopsy, recent thrombosis of the right and left main pulmonary arteries was found; there was also an old resolving thrombus in the right main pulmonary artery. The IVC-UF was securely fixed in the IVC and had no evidence of thrombus formation. No source of emboli could be found. This may well have been a case of hypercoagulable state with primary thrombosis of the pulmonary arteries. Fatal recurrent pulmonary embolism occurred in a markedly obese patient 8 months after IVC-UF insertion. The filter was inadvertently placed at the junction of the left common iliac vein with the IVC. Thrombosis in the opposite iliac vein appeared to be the source of the pulmonary embolus. Recurrent pulmonary embolism with areas of infarction in lower lobe segments was documented at autopsy in two patients who died of heart disease 2 months after IVC-UF insertion. The embolization probably occurred via collateral veins.

Filter Migration

Filter migration has not occurred in our own experience. In one patient, tilting of the device was noted immediately after insertion. Another IVC-UF was implanted just above the dislodged filter to prevent migration.

IVC Patency

Of the first 50 patients in whom the IVC-UF impregnated with the TDMAC/heparin complex was used, 16 had IVC angiograms performed within 6 weeks after the filter insertion. Patency of the filter was demonstrated in 5 patients and occlusion of the IVC in the remaining 11 patients. Repeat angiograms in two of the five patients in whom the filter was patent, done at 6 months after the filter insertion in one and at 1 year 3 months in the other, demonstrated free flow of blood through the IVC. IVC angiograms done in patients in whom unheparinized IVC-UF were used demonstrated occlusion of IVC within 1 to 2 weeks.

Physicians' Experiences

The IVC-UF was released for general clinical use in January 1970. According to the estimates made by the Edwards Laboratories (Santa Anna, CA), 12,000 filters were implanted in the United States between January 1970 and November 1976. However, complete data, as reported by the evaluating physician, have been accumulated for 4,699 filter implants during the first 6 years of their use; these form the basis of the report. The results are summarized in Table 21–2.

Mortality and Recurrent Embolism

Recurrent pulmonary embolism has occurred in 2.2% of patients (fatal, 0.5%). For three patients, blood clots from the proximal surface of the IVC-UF were implicated as the source of recurrent embolus.

TABLE 21–2.—INFERIOR VENA CAVA UMBRELLA
FILTER—PHYSICIAN EXPERIENCE
(JANUARY 1970–NOVEMBER 1976)

	23 mm	28 mm	TOTAL
No. filter implants	2,848	1,851	4,699
Proximal migration	27	8	25
Distal migration	7	1	8
Dislodgement without migration	25	2	27
Misplacements			46
Renal vein (18)			
Iliac vein (26)			
Suprarenal IVC (2)			
Filter inversion	9	2	11
Recurrent embolism (26 fatal)		(26F)	106

FILTER MIGRATION

The clinical data for patients in whom filters migrated are given in Tables 21–3 and 21–4. The original caval umbrella was 23 mm in diameter, but episodes of migration (0.9%) led to the development of the 28-mm device. With the introduction of the 28-mm filter, the incidence of migration has been reduced to 0.4%. The main causes of filter migration have been (1) inadequate seating of the filter in the IVC, (2) exceptionally large IVC and (3) sudden embolic obstruction of the filter by a large thrombus, resulting in dilation of IVC and permitting

TABLE 21–3.—INFERIOR VENA CAVA
UMBRELLA FILTER MIGRATION—
PHYSICIAN EXPERIENCE (JANUARY
1970–NOVEMBER 1976)

SITE OF FILTER MIGRATION	23 MM	28 MM	TOTAL
Pulmonary artery	16	5	21
Right ventricle	2	1	3
Right atrium	4	1	5
Suprarenal IVC	5	1	6
Total	27	8	35

dislodgement and migration of the filter along with the embolus. Distal migration of the IVC-UF into the right iliac vein following closed cardiac massage within 4 weeks after filter insertion has been reported in eight patients.

Partial dislodgement of the IVC-UF without migration has occurred

TABLE 21–4.—CLINICAL DATA ON PATIENTS
WITH UMBRELLA FILTER MIGRATION

NO. OF PATIENTS	CLINICAL DATA
21	Pulmonary artery 3 fatal—Embolized with massive thrombus 13 removed—3 died postoperatively 5 left in place—4 died, death unrelated
3	Right ventricle 2 removed on cardiopulmonary bypass 1 died 6 days later, no autopsy
5	Right atrium 1 fatal—Embolized along with massive thrombus 1 found at autopsy, death unrelated 3 removed—1 died postoperatively
6	Suprarenal inferior vena cava All left in place 2 died, death unrelated

in 27 patients. To prevent migration, the larger 28-mm filter was implanted just above the dislodged filter in eight patients. In the remaining patients, either nothing was done or the IVC was ligated operatively with or without removal of the filter.

MISPLACEMENT OF THE FILTER

The IVC-UF was misplaced in the suprarenal IVC in two patients. The filters were pushed down by the applicator capsule into the infrarenal IVC. The IVC-UF was misplaced in the right renal vein in 18 patients. In five of these, the filter was removed by a direct operative approach. The IVC-UF was mistakenly placed in the iliac vein in 26 patients. These patients have been treated either by implanting another filter in the IVC or by ligation of IVC with or without removal of the filter.

FILTER INVERSION

Eleven cases of filter inversion due to excessive upward traction applied to the applicator stylet during the seating of the filter have been reported. In four patients, the umbrella was reinverted. One of these migrated to the pulmonary artery on the eighth postoperative day. In three patients the umbrella was removed transvenously and another filter was inserted. The inverted umbrella was left in place in three patients without any further complications. In one patient the IVC was surgically ligated proximal and distal to the umbrella.

MISCELLANEOUS COMPLICATIONS

Significant retroperitoneal bleeding has occurred in five patients, right recurrent laryngeal nerve injury in two, air embolism in two, perforation of duodenum in one and perforation of ureter in one. Postoperative septicemia led to removal of the filter in two patients.

STASIS SEQUELAE

Significant edema developed in 115 patients (5.1%), and phlebitis of the lower extremities, not previously present, developed in 35 (1.5%). The majority of these patients improved with standard medical treatment.

Gradual occlusion of the IVC-UF allows for the progressive development of the collateral circulation, thereby avoiding acute venous pooling of blood in the lower extremities. Edema of the lower extremities following IVC-UF insertion is less of a problem. The majority of patients with severe venous stasis problems had a history of preexisting venous disease. Occlusion of the cava with peripheral edema can result from sudden thromboembolic obstruction of the IVC-UF.

Summary

Anticoagulant therapy continues to be the standard treatment for thromboembolic disease. Transvenous caval interruption by the umbrella filter has provided an effective means for prevention of recurrent pulmonary embolism with minimal risk to the patient. Most investigators report satisfaction with the simplicity of the procedure and the results achieved and are now using the procedure as a method of choice for caval interruption.

New forthcoming developments include (1) angiographic applicator to perform IVC angiograms to identify the caval anatomy prior to filter insertion, (2) availability of heparin bonded umbrella filters to reduce or prevent thrombogenicity of the filter and (3) development of barbed umbrella filters to eliminate filter migration.

REFERENCES

1. Dalen, J. E., and Alpert, J. S.: Natural history of pulmonary embolism, Prog. Cardiovasc. Dis. 17:257, 1975.
2. Aggeler, P. M., and Kosmin, M.: Anticoagulant Prophylaxis and Treatment of Venous Thromboembolic Disease, in Sherry, S., Brinkhous, K. M., Genton, E., and Stengle, J. E. (eds.): *Conference on Thrombosis* (Washington, D. C.: National Academy of Sciences, 1969).
3. Urokinase Pulmonary Embolism Trial Phase I Results: A Cooperative Study, JAMA 214:2163, 1970.
4. Crane, C.: Femoral vs. caval interruption for venous thromboembolism, N. Engl. J. Med. 270:819, 1964.
5. Krause, R. J., Cranley, J. J., Hallaba, M. A. S., Strasser, E. S., and Hafner, C. D.: Caval ligation in thromboembolic disease, Arch. Surg. 87:184, 1963.
6. Amador, E., Li, T. K., and Crane, C.: Ligation of inferior vena cava for thromboembolism, JAMA 206:1758, 1968.
7. Mobin-Uddin, K., McLean, R., and Jude, J. R.: A new catheter technique of interruption of inferior vena cava for prevention of pulmonary embolism, Am. Surg. 35:889, 1969.
8. Mobin-Uddin, K., McLean, R., Bolooki, H., and Jude, J. R.: Caval interruption for prevention of pulmonary embolism, Arch. Surg. 99:711, 1969.
9. Mobin-Uddin, K., Bolooki, J., and Jude, J. R.: Intravenous caval interruption for pulmonary embolism in cardiac disease, Circulation (Suppl. 2) 41:152, 1970.
10. Mobin-Uddin, K., Trinkle, J. K., and Bryant, L. R.: Present status of the inferior vena cava umbrella filter, Surgery 70:914, 1971.
11. Mobin-Uddin, K., Callard, G. M., Bolooki, H., Rubinson, R., Michie, D., and Jude, J. R.: Transvenous caval interruption with umbrella filter, N. Engl. J. Med. 286:55, 1972.

12. Mobin-Uddin, K., Utley, J. R., and Bryant, L. R.: The inferior vena cava umbrella filter, Progr. Cardiovasc. Dis. 17:391, 1975.
13. Berger, R. L.: Pulmonary embolectomy for massive embolization, Am. J. Surg. 121: 437, 1971.
14. Sautter, R. D., Myers, W. O., and Wenzel, F. J.: Implications of the urokinase study concerning the surgical treatment of pulmonary embolism, J. Thorac. Cardiovasc. Surg. 63:54, 1972.
15. Bloomfield, D. A.: The Use of Intracaval Umbrella Filters in Massive Pulmonary Embolism, in Mobin-Uddin, K. (ed.): *Pulmonary Thromboembolism* (Springfield, Ill.: Charles C Thomas, Publisher, 1975).
16. Jick, H., Slone, D., Bold, I. T., and Shapiro, S.: Efficacy and toxicity of heparin in relation to age and sex, N. Engl. J. Med. 279:284, 1968.
17. Browse, N. L., Thomas, M. L., and Solan, M. J.: Management of source of pulmonary emboli; value of phlebography, Br. Med. J. 4:596, 1967.
18. Thomas, M. L., Andress, M. R., Browse, M. L., Fletcher, E. W. L., Phillips, J. D., Pim, H. P., McAllister, N., Stephenson, R. H., and Tonge, K.: Phlebography in the prevention of recurrent pulmonary embolism — Technique and value, Am. J. Roentgenol. Radium Ther. Nucl. Med. 110:725, 1970.
19. Fullen, W. D., Miller, E. H., Steele, W. F., and McDonough, J. J.: Prophylactic vena cava interruption in hip fractures, J. Trauma 13:403, 1973.

Discussion: Chapters 19 through 21

DR. WILEY BARKER: I agree with the general tenets of the excellent diagnostic and therapeutic protocol outlined by Doctor Sasahara. We are relying more and more on the pulmonary angiogram for the diagnosis of pulmonary embolism, and are putting less reliance on lung scans unless they are completely negative. A positive perfusion scan is of value in identifying an area for selective angiography rather than subjecting the entire lung to the full load of contrast medium.

The philosophic approach to caval interruption described by Doctor McNamara and her associates is substantially identical to ours.

Doctor Mobin-Uddin's presentation of the unilateral operation is unusual, but we too have had occasion to utilize unilateral external iliac interruption in similar circumstances. In order to do this one must have excellent modern diagnostic methods to prove that the disease is indeed limited to one side so that it will truly be segregated below the clip, ligature or umbrella.

We have published a retrospective summary of over 500 cases of pulmonary embolism from three major UCLA hospitals.[1] I have some misgivings about the diagnostic accuracy and the adequacy of anticoagulant therapy in some of these patients, but I believe this is a representative series treated by a group of competent physicians.

The importance of treatment of *some* kind is brought out by Table 1 which shows that in 19 patients in whom it was believed anticoagulation was contraindicated and no surgical therapy was offered, there

TABLE 1.—MEDICAL CONTRAINDICATION
FOR ANTICOAGULATION

Total patients	19
Recurrent pulmonary emboli	9
Deaths	
Initial pulmonary emboli	3
Recurrent pulmonary emboli	5
Total deaths (42%)	8

were recurrent emboli, five of which were lethal; three patients died from the initial embolism. One must be very sure of his ground before he denies a patient with embolism the right to some form of treatment.

In those patients in whom only anticoagulant therapy was used the death rate from embolization was 4 or 5%. The death rate from further embolization and the operation itself was identical: but it must be recognized that patients treated surgically are those who could not be managed by anticoagulants, or who were failures of anticoagulant therapy or who were believed to have a continuing process which would perpetuate their risk of further embolization.

Table 2 shows the operations performed to interrupt the cava and the outcome. Today most patients would be treated by interruption of the immediately infrarenal cava by a Miles clip through a midline transperitoneal incision. Most of these patients, especially parous women, would have a large Weck clip placed across the left gonadal vein where it enters the renal vein. An increasingly large percentage of patients are being treated by the umbrella; surgical interruption is reserved for the patients less critically ill.

Interruption of the cava has long been damned for its causative role in the development of later postphlebitic complications. Doctor de Takats recognized long ago that it was the severity of the thrombotic process rather than the caval interruption that caused the trouble. On this basis we have used anticoagulants as soon as possible after interruption and maintained chronic anticoagulant therapy for at least a year after operation.

Justification of this policy is provided by a survey recently completed by Dr. Sergio Mandiola. He was able to evaluate carefully 80 extremities done 2 to 15 years after caval interruption. Table 3 indicates our criteria for grading the status of the extremities.[2]

Table 4 summarizes the outcome. Of the patients who had never had, preoperatively or postoperatively, a serious, red-hot inflammatory thrombophlebitis, 38 were described as normal, and only 2 were severely afflicted. Indeed even when thrombophlebitis in its severe form had occurred only half of the extremities showed moderate to severe disease.

It would appear, then, that anticoagulant therapy is the basic form of management, but that caval interruption has an important life-saving role, and that the late complications of caval interruption have been seriously overrated. The quotation from Doctor Ochsner's work is most appropriate.

DR. ALTON OCHSNER: I am very much interested in this presentation. My interest in pulmonary embolism dates back 52 years to when

TABLE 2.–INFERIOR VENA CAVA INTERRUPTION

PROCEDURE	NO. PATIENTS	RECURRENT PULMONARY EMBOLI	DEATHS
Ligation	57	3	1
Clipping	10	3	0
Plication	1	1	1
Umbrella	2	1	1
Total	70	8	3 (4%)

TABLE 3.–GRADING OF SYMPTOM SEVERITY

Normal: Normal or minor abnormality but better than preoperative.
Minimal: Minor edema; varicose veins persist from preoperative status.
Moderate: Worse than preoperative assessment.
Severe: Ulcers; major edema; true disability; frequent recurrent disability.

TABLE 4.–RELATIONSHIP BETWEEN PRE- AND/OR POSTOPERATIVE PHLEBITIS AND LATER SYMPTOMS

STATUS AT 2 YR	NO PREOPERATIVE PHLEBITIS		PREOPERATIVE PHLEBITIS		UNCERTAIN	TOTAL
	NO POSTOPERATIVE PHLEBITIS	POSTOPERATIVE PHLEBITIS	NO POSTOPERATIVE PHLEBITIS	POSTOPERATIVE PHLEBITIS		
Normal	38	0	6	0	4	48
Minimal	3	5	3	0	2	13
Moderate	2	3	5	1	2	13
Severe	1	2	1	2	0	6

I was an exchange surgical resident in Frankfurt, Germany. I went to Munich in March 1924, to attend the German Surgical Congress, and at this Congress the first successful pulmonary embolectomy was presented by Kirchner. Although the operation had been described by Trendelenburg in 1908 and had been done rather sporadically by the German and Scandinavian surgeons, it wasn't until 1924 that Kirchner, then in Danzig, was able to do the operation successfully. The patient was presented to the German Surgical Congress and, I can assure you, ladies and gentlemen, that no case could have electrified a group of surgeons more than that case did. To see this young woman who was presented to the Congress who had been brought back from death was a thrill.

This immediately gave great impetus to pulmonary embolectomy on the Continent, particularly among the German clinics and in Scandinavia. In our institution in Frankfurt am Main, because of the very short time available in which one can do the pulmonary embolectomy in an individual who has a massive pulmonary embolism, they moved into the patient's room a so-called Trendelenburg set, all of the instruments that would be used in doing a pulmonary embolectomy. There was a skeleton crew who sat by the patient's bedside waiting for the patient to die. All of this was for any individual who had had a pulmonary embolism and who was a candidate for pulmonary embolectomy. Being the youngest individual on the totem pole, it was my job to sit there night after night in these cases. Most times, they didn't die, fortunately. When they did develop a massive pulmonary embolism, a call was sent out. The crew was mobilized, and we were successful in a relatively high percentage of cases. Sitting there night after night as I did, it was like a wake, and I thought, there must be a better way to do this.

Early on, we did superficial femoral vein ligation bilaterally, but because we had 11 cases of fatal pulmonary embolism at the Charity Hospital in New Orleans after superficial vein ligation, we went to caval ligation.

In our experience, in a study made 4 years ago, there were 315 caval interruptions, most of which were ligation. There were only 28 partial interruptions. In these patients, 1.5% died at the time of the operation; 7.6% died within 2 weeks postoperatively, usually of the condition that produced the phlebothrombosis; 8.5% died from 2 weeks to a year; 10.8% died after 1 year up to a follow-up of now over 25 years.

We had 28 cases in which an incomplete interruption was done. My son John said, "Dad, we ought to be doing these." I had not done them because, as I had said, this should be done as a life-saving procedure, and I thought the simplest way in which it could be done would be to put a ligature on the cava. This takes about 10 min, and is the least risk to the patient.

In patients with partial interruption, most had clips, few of them had plication, all had cavograms immediately afterward, and all were patent. In this group, there were two lost to follow-up and two hospital deaths. Although all cavas were patent immediately after the operation, 12 were obstructed within a week, 8 more occluded after that. There were only four in which the cava remained open permanently. Not only did many occlude, but the two worst cases that we have seen of venous thrombosis occurred after partial caval interruption.

We had two cases of phlegmasia cerulea dolens after cava clipping. These needed thrombectomy as a life-saving procedure. We have never observed this after caval ligation.

I think the reason why the sequelae following partial interruption are worse than those following caval ligation is that, when one interrupts the cava, one increases the venous pressure distal to the ligature. This does two things. It is a stimulus to the development of the collaterals, and it acts as a deterrent to the detachment of any clot that may be remaining. If one does not interrupt the cava completely, venous pressure in the cava is not increased. There is no stimulus for the development of collaterals. More importantly, there is no deterrent to the detachment of the clot.

If the remaining clot does break off, it is stopped by the grid and prevents the death of the individual. But because of the fact that there are no collaterals, they get massive thrombosis. I would emphasize the paucity of symptoms after caval ligation if the patient is treated carefully at the time.

A minimum number of those that had ligation had recurrent phlebitis. We have never had a recurrent pulmonary embolism in our series of cases in which we have done caval ligation, and one of 24 with the clip.

DR. LAZAR GREENFIELD: My comments will be limited to the excellent presentations of Doctors McNamara and Mobin-Uddin. Early in our catheter embolectomy experience we lost two patients because of recurrent massive pulmonary embolism following successful embolectomy and before a clip could be applied to the vena cava. It was obvious that a vena cava filter should be inserted immediately following embolectomy and we approached the problem from an engineering standpoint. The cone shape (Fig 1) was selected because of its unique geometry which permits trapping of embolus for 80% of its depth before a hemodynamic pressure gradient occurs. Therefore

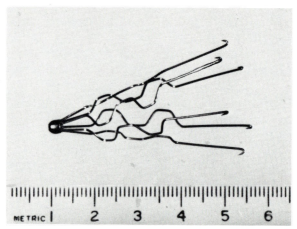

Fig 1. — Kim-Ray Greenfield filter for prevention of pulmonary embolism.

continued flow and filtration are possible and as an unexpected benefit the experimental studies in dogs showed subsequent lysis of the
trapped autologous emboli. Fixation of the device by recurved hooks
provides security against migration because of the "fishhook" principle and avoids major penetration of the vena caval wall. Our clinical
experience over the past 4 years consists of 76 patients followed for a
minimum of 6 months at the University of Oklahoma and the Medical
College of Virginia. The incidence of recurrent embolism is two episodes or 2.6%, neither of which was fatal. The hospital mortality rate
is 4% and the incidence of late edema and recurrent phlebitis has
been comparable to other series. However, a major difference was
seen in 44 vena cavograms in 31 patients after an average of 11 months
postoperative which showed patency in 97% of them. In addition,
sequential studies in four patients showed trapping and subsequent
resolution of large thromboemboli. The Kim-Ray Greenfield filter
usually has been inserted via the jugular vein reserving the femoral
approach for patients who have had catheter embolectomy or failure
of the jugular approach. On the basis of this experience and the fact
that no filter has migrated, I feel that the device has significant advantages over other available methods of mechanical interruption of
the vena cava.

DR. ELIAS HUSNI: We'd like to raise the issue of prophylactic clipping of the inferior vena cava (IVC). During the last 3 years we
clipped the IVC in all high-risk patients undergoing vascular reconstruction in the abdominal cavity. This adds an average of 5 min to the

TABLE 5.—PULMONARY EMBOLISM—
CAVAL INTERRUPTION

PATIENT SELECTION	PROCEDURE	NO. OF CASES	NEW EMBOLISM
Recurrent embolism	Ligation	9	2
	Plication	128	4
Prophylactic	Plication	38	0

operative time and is probably worthwhile as we have seen no adverse complications in over 38 patients (Table 5). All patients undergoing prophylactic plication were entirely free of edema or stasis of their legs.

REFERENCES

1. Pollak, E. W., Sparks, F. C., and Barker, W. F.: Pulmonary thromboembolism—an appraisal of therapy in 516 cases, Arch. Surg. 107:66, 1973.
2. Mandiola, S., and Barker, W. F.: Unpublished data.

22 / Surgery for Pulmonary Embolism

LAZAR J. GREENFIELD, M.D.

Professor and Chairman, Department of Surgery, Medical College of Virginia, Virginia Commonwealth University, Richmond, Virginia

THE SURGICAL TREATMENT of acute massive pulmonary embolism was attempted originally by Trendelenburg[1] who proposed thoracotomy for unilateral pulmonary embolectomy. The procedure fell into disrepute, however, because of a low survival rate,[2] which would be anticipated in these critically ill patients. Following the perfection and widespread use of techniques of cardiopulmonary bypass, a new era of surgical intervention began heralded by the successful case report of Sharp.[3] The improved access to the entire pulmonary vascular bed increased the potential of the embolectomy and permitted more extensive removal of emboli, but this was not accompanied by an improvement in mortality rate.[4] In fact the extreme variability in mortality rates for pulmonary embolectomy on cardiopulmonary bypass ranging from 24%[5] to 93%[6] suggests that patient selection is the primary determinant of outcome. The effect of time in excluding nonsurvivors was well demonstrated in the most favorable series reported where the average interval between embolization and operation exceeded 7 hr.[5] It seems likely that these patients had passed the most critical period of hemodynamic imbalance from the embolus and were more likely to survive.

Since patient selection is the most critical factor, certain guidelines are essential to permit discrimination between patients who are likely to survive after massive embolism and those destined to die without surgical intervention. The observations of Del Guercio et al.[7] suggested the importance of right-sided heart overload as reflected by elevation of mean right ventricular pressure above 22 mm Hg to predict a fatal outcome. Other experience, however, did not confirm the cor-

TABLE 22-1.—CLASSIFICATION OF PULMONARY EMBOLIC DISEASE*

	CLASS				
	I	II	III	IV	V
Symptoms	None	Hyperventilation Anxiety	Dyspnea Collapse	Shock Dyspnea	Dyspnea Syncope
Arterial PO$_2$	80–90 mm Hg	<80 mm Hg	<65 mm Hg	<50 mm Hg	<50 mm Hg
Arterial PCO$_2$	35–40 mm Hg	<35 mm Hg	<30 mm Hg	<30 mm Hg	30–40 mm Hg
Arterial pH	Normal	Alkalosis	Acidosis	Acidosis	Normal
Hemodynamics	Normal	Tachycardia	Central venous pressure ↑ Pulmonary artery pressure > 20 mm Hg	Central venous pressure ↑ Pulmonary artery pressure > 30 mm Hg BA↓	Central venous pressure ↑ Pulmonary artery pressure > 40 mm Hg No shock, CI ↓
Pulmonary artery occlusion	< 20%	20–30%	30–50%	> 50%	> 50%

*From Greenfield.[10]

relation between pressures of the right side of the heart and survival.[8] Since the net effect of increased pulmonary vascular resistance is a reduction in output of the left side of the heart, the most widely accepted criteria for operative intervention have been those proposed by Sasahara[9] which include systolic blood pressure less than 90 mm Hg, urine output less than 20 ml/hr and Pa_{O_2} less than 60 mm Hg after 1 hour of nonoperative management. A more comprehensive assessment is possible at the time of initial evaluation based on arteriographic findings, blood gases and hemodynamic measurements as we have proposed[10] (Table 22–1). Using these guidelines, it seems clear that the outlook for patients who show persistent hypotension (class IV) is so poor that some form of surgical intervention is required. However, there often is reluctance to proceed to open embolectomy on cardiopulmonary bypass because of the high mortality rate quoted previously and a morbidity that includes intra-alveolar bleeding[11] and pulmonary infarction.[12] These latter complications also have been observed following delayed thrombectomy for pulmonary hypertension. Consequently, management by nonoperative means usually is pursued including positive pressure ventilation with high FI_{O_2}, isoproterenol infusion and systemic heparinization (150 μ/kg).

Other alternatives to open embolectomy have been attempted including closed-chest massage, prolonged partial cardiopulmonary bypass and embolectomy at thoracotomy or under inflow circulatory occlusion. Of these methods, partial venoarterial bypass provides the most consistent hemodynamic support and may be essential after cardiac arrest to permit pulmonary arteriography to be performed to confirm the diagnosis. No procedure for massive pulmonary embolism should be undertaken until the diagnosis is confirmed by arteriogram, preferably accompanied by pressure measurements. Partial bypass support also is essential for induction of general anesthesia for open embolectomy as proposed originally by Beall and Cooley.[13] Following median sternotomy and conversion to total cardiopulmonary bypass, a pulmonary arteriotomy allows extraction of emboli by forceps and suction. Care must be taken to avoid embolectomy in regions of the lung which are infarcted to avoid serious intrapulmonary hemorrhage. Although a thorough embolectomy often can be performed, the magnitude of the procedure has limited survival rates and its application is restricted to large hospital centers where standby pump teams are available. As another alternative, we have investigated the possibility of embolectomy under local anesthesia from a peripheral vein using a catheter technique. The feasibility of this approach was demonstrated initially in dogs[14] and in patients in 1970.[15]

Catheter Embolectomy Technique

Access in the animal or in a patient is obtained through the right common femoral vein exposed under local anesthesia. The catheter is filled with heparinized saline through an extension tube and a guide-wire may be used during introduction to prevent buckling of the tip. The cup is radiopaque and can be seen readily under fluoroscopy as it is guided up the vena cava with the right hand while the left hand holds the control unit to provide tip deflection. Passage into the right ventricle is aided by medial angulation and then anterior deflection to enter the pulmonary artery. Oscilloscopic monitoring should be maintained to detect premature ventricular contractions or other arrhythmias which usually will respond to withdrawal of the catheter from that area. The left main pulmonary artery (PA) usually is entered most readily and the cup then can be positioned according to the angiographic location of the major embolus on that side, usually in the left lower lobe. Entry into the right main PA requires deflection of the cup in that direction as it reaches the superior edge of the heart shadow, which still is within the main PA. Rotational movement of the tip also assists in making the catheter advance. Again, the cup is positioned according to the angiogram and usually will come to rest against the embolus. This can be confirmed by injection of 6–8 ml of contrast medium to exclude the possibility of wedging in a patent branch of the PA.

A 30-ml lubricated glass syringe then is attached to the control handle via the intravenous extension tubing that has been used to flush the catheter and inject contrast medium. After the cup is positioned, the barrel of the syringe is pulled back sharply by the assistant and will produce either a vacuum if the embolus is suctioned into the cup or a sustained jet of blood if the cup is not in approximation. Aspirated blood can be returned to the patient. It is possible to suction the wall of the PA but this can be avoided by contrast injection as described. When the embolus is aspirated, it is held in the cup by sustained suction by the assistant while the catheter is withdrawn slowly through the right side of the heart, down the inferior vena cava and then out the femoral venotomy.

Dislodgement can occur if the embolus is captured on its side and withdrawn in a folded position. If this occurs it may be retrieved by the same process and usually will not fragment. The Teflon cup should be cleaned and the catheter tip checked for free passage of fluid and effective suctioning prior to each attempted retrieval. Arrhythmias are uncommon during removal and significant hemodynamic improvement usually occurs as soon as the embolus is dis-impacted from the pulmonary vascular bed. Reduction in pulmonary arterial pressure is rapid and the improved cardiac output allows the vasopressor infusion to be discontinued. The procedure is com-pleted by transvenous insertion of a cone-shaped stainless steel filter through the same femoral venotomy.[10]

Clinical Results

The initial series of patients who underwent catheter embolectomy at the University of Oklahoma Health Science Center has been reported[16] and consisted of 10 patients who were treated using a non-directional stiff cardiac catheter to which a stainless steel angled cup had been affixed. Emboli were extracted in nine of the 10 patients but one patient 78 years of age who sustained cardiac arrest and cerebral infarction during angiography died after the procedure. Catheter per-foration of the myocardium occurred as an agonal event in this patient and was the only instance of this complication. The rigid catheter has

Fig 22–1.—The directional cup catheter is shown without the control handle, which attaches to the four guide wires. Attached to the black flexible end of the catheter is the standard 7-mm radiopaque cup. Adjacent to it is the optional 4-mm cup for retrieval of more distal emboli.

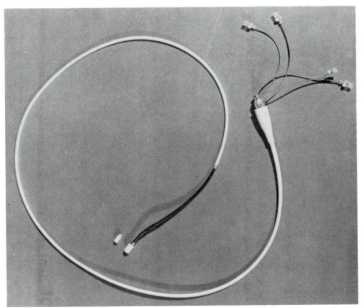

not been used since that time. Emboli could not be extracted from one patient with a 5-day history of embolization presumably because of fixation to the wall of the pulmonary artery. Early death from recurrent emboli occurred in two patients prior to routine insertion of a vena caval filter and these deaths should be regarded as preventable. One additional patient died of sepsis 1 month after embolectomy.

This group therefore showed a high percentage of retrievable emboli (90% of patients) and the importance of early extraction of emboli prior to fixation to the pulmonary artery. In addition, the need for immediate protection against recurrent embolism was well demonstrated. Delay in placement of a vena caval clip was responsible for two early deaths (20%). In this initial experience there was a high early mortality rate (40%) followed by the one additional late death to limit overall survival to 50% of the patients.

On the basis of this experience, a directional catheter cup device (Fig 22–1) has been used since 1974 at the Medical College of Virginia in eight additional patients. Emboli were removed in six of these patients and vena caval filters were inserted in all of them. The two patients in whom emboli were not extracted had long-standing pul-

Fig 22–2. — Pulmonary arteriogram of the 76-year-old male patient showing bilateral acute massive embolic occlusion. Minimal pulmonary blood flow remains only to the right upper lobe and a portion of the lower lobe.

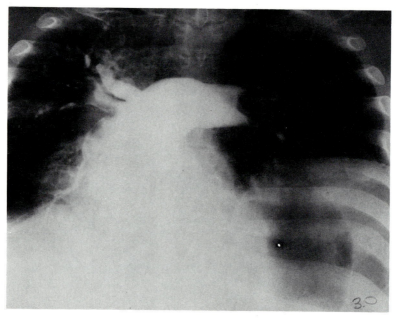

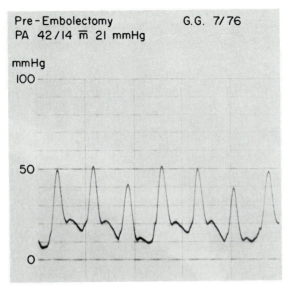

Fig 22–3.—Pulmonary arterial pressure tracing of patient in Figure 22–2 showing pulmonary hypertension with phasic pressure of 42/14 mm Hg prior to embolectomy.

Fig 22–4.—Pulmonary arterial pressure tracing following removal of a single large embolus without significant change from preoperative tracing in Figure 22–3.

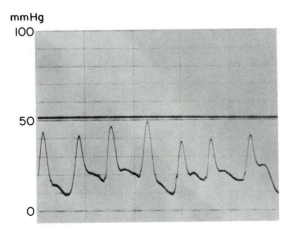

monary hypertension secondary to chronic recurrent pulmonary emboli. It was thought that a more recent embolus was responsible for their hemodynamic deterioration and that extraction would permit cessation of vasopressor support. Only one of them survived after extensive catheter manipulation and extraction of fragments of thrombi. The remaining six patients were on vasopressor support or had been resuscitated from cardiac arrest. All but one of them survived and three have been reported previously.[10]

The patient who died after removal of multiple large emboli was a 76-year-old male hospitalized 1 month earlier in congestive heart failure and was known to have chronic lung disease. He was recovering from a myocardial infarction which occurred 2 weeks earlier. There was a 6-hr history of sudden collapse, dyspnea and hypotension requiring vasopressor support. His arterial blood during oxygen ventilation showed Pa_{O_2} of 50 mm Hg and Pa_{CO_2} of 28 mm Hg with pH 7.24. Despite intensive ventilatory and circulatory support he was deteriorating rapidly and emergency pulmonary arteriography showed bilateral massive embolic occlusion (Fig 22–2). Pulmonary arterial catheterization showed a pressure of 42/14 mm Hg with mean 21 mm Hg (Fig 22–3). The directional cup catheter was inserted under local

Fig 22–5.—Pulmonary arterial pressure tracing following removal of two large emboli and markedly improved cardiac output. The effects of the vasopressor are shown by elevated pulmonary arterial pressure, which indicated ability to discontinue vasopressor infusion.

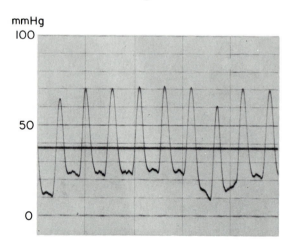

Post – Embolectomy # 2   G.G. 7/76
PA 70/21 m̄ 33 mmHg

Post-Embolectomy #3   G.G. 7/76
PA 42/12 m̄ 22 mmHg

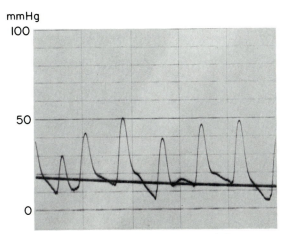

Fig 22–6.—Pulmonary arterial pressure tracing following removal of three emboli showing reduction of phasic pressure to levels seen previously under vasopressor support.

anesthesia from the right femoral vein and a single large embolus was removed which did not change the pulmonary arterial pressure (Fig 22–4). An additional large embolus was removed and there was a dramatic increase in systemic and pulmonary arterial pressures under the influence of the steady infusion of vasopressor (dopamine) (Fig 22–5). With this evidence of increased cardiac output, the vasopressor infusion was discontinued and a third embolus removed which resulted in the same pulmonary arterial pressure seen with previous vasopressor support (Fig 22–6). Finally, a fourth large embolus was removed along with additional fragments (Fig 22–7) which resulted in a decrease in pulmonary arterial pressure to normal mean levels (15 mm Hg, Fig 22–8), a slowing of heart rate and restoration of responsiveness of the patient. At this point the cup catheter was withdrawn and a Swan-Ganz catheter was positioned in an embolectomized segment of pulmonary artery for pressure and cardiac output measurements. Suddenly the patient had a massive hemoptysis and cardiac arrest. Tracheostomy and bilateral thoracotomies for resuscitation were unsuccessful and he expired. The middle lobe was found to be grossly hemorrhagic at thoracotomy and a clamp at the hilum seemed to control the hemorrhage but the recent myocardial infarction had rendered the myocardium incapable of resuscitation.

It is not possible to be certain of the cause of the pulmonary hemorrhage which has been a frequent cause of death after open embolectomy on cardiopulmonary bypass.[11, 12] Of obvious concern is the balloon inflation of the Swan-Ganz catheter in the region which was found to be hemorrhagic, although the entire vascular bed must be considered vulnerable to reperfusion after prolonged ischemia.

Other complications have occurred in use of the cup catheter including loss of captured emboli during passage through the right ventricle and transient arrhythmias which respond to altering catheter position. Hemorrhagic pleural effusions occurred in two patients early in our experience when heparin administration was not regulated by continuous infusion. Groin wound hematomas have occurred in six of the 18 patients treated, for an incidence of 33%. The latter complication can

Fig 22–7.—Pulmonary emboli removed by multiple catheter extraction in the patient presented in Figures 22–2 through 22–6 and 22–8.

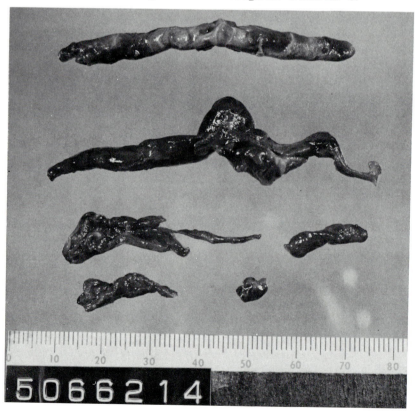

Post - Embolectomy #4   G.G. 7/ 76
PA 36/9 m̄ 15 mmHg

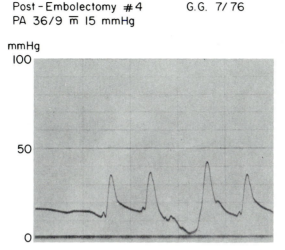

Fig 22–8. – Final pulmonary arterial tracing after removal of emboli shown in Figure 22–7. There is some residual systolic hypertension but the mean pressure is within normal limits.

be related to the routine resumption of heparin anticoagulation within 8–12 hr postoperative.

Summary

The accumulated experience with transvenous catheter embolectomy in 18 patients has been reviewed (Table 22–2). Extraction of emboli has been possible in 15 of them (83%). The initial high mortality rate of 50% has been reduced to 25% by use of a directional cup catheter and the routine insertion of a vena caval filter at the conclusion of the embolectomy. This procedure under local anesthesia avoids thoracotomy and cardiopulmonary bypass in these critically ill

TABLE 22–2.–CLINICAL EXPERIENCE WITH
TRANSVENOUS CATHETER PULMONARY EMBOLECTOMY

DATE	NO. PATIENTS	EMBOLI REMOVED	DIED EARLY	LATE	% SURVIVAL
1970–1974	10	9	4	1	50
1974–1976	8	6	2	0	75
Total	18	15	6	1	61

patients and offers the possibility of a higher rate of patient survival in all hospitals.

REFERENCES

1. Trendelenburg, F.: Uber die operative Behandlung der Embolie der Lungenarterie, Arch. Klin. Chir. 86:686, 1908.
2. Benichoux, R.: Surgical treatment of massive pulmonary embolism: Report of 22 cases of Trendelenburg's operation, J. Int. Chir. 11:464, 1951.
3. Sharp, E. H.: Pulmonary embolectomy: Successful removal of a massive pulmonary embolus with the support of cardiopulmonary bypass: A case report, Ann. Surg. 156:1, 1962.
4. Cross, F. S., and Mowlem, A.: A survey of the current status of pulmonary embolectomy for massive pulmonary embolism, Circulation 35 (Suppl. 1):86, 1967.
5. Berger, R. L.: Pulmonary embolectomy with preoperative circulatory support, Ann. Thorac. Surg. 16:217, 1973.
6. Scannell, J. G.: The surgical management of acute massive pulmonary embolism, Prog. Cardiovasc. Dis. 9:488, 1967.
7. Del Guercio, L. R. M., Cohn, J. D., Feins, N. R., Coomaraswamy, R. P., and Montle, L.: Pulmonary embolism shock: Physiologic basis of a bedside screening test, JAMA 196:71, 1966.
8. Wechsler, B. M., Karlson, K. E., Summers, D. N., Krasmow, N., Garson, A. A., and Chait, A.: Pulmonary embolism: Influence of cardiac hemodynamics and natural history on selection of patients for embolectomy and inferior vena cava ligation, Surgery 65:182, 1969.
9. Sasahara, A. A.: Pulmonary vascular responses to thromboembolism, Mod. Concepts Cardiovasc. Dis. 36:55, 1967.
10. Greenfield, L. J.: Pulmonary Embolism: Diagnosis and Management, in Ravitch, M. M. (ed.): *Current Problems in Surgery* (Chicago: Year Book Medical Publishers, Inc., April 1976).
11. Makey, A. R., Bliss, B. P., Ikram, H., Sutcliffe, M. M. L., and Emery, E. R. J.: Fatal intra-alveolar pulmonary bleeding complicating pulmonary embolectomy, Thorax 26:466, 1971.
12. Brown, S., Mulder, D., and Buckberg, G.: Massive pulmonary hemorrhagic infarction following revascularization of ischemic lungs, Arch. Surg. 108:795, 1974.
13. Beall, A. C., Jr., and Cooley, D. A.: Surgical treatment of pulmonary embolism, Heart Bull. 13:41, 1964.
14. Greenfield, L. J., Kimmel, G. O., and McCurdy, W. C., 3d: Transvenous removal of pulmonary emboli by vacuum-cup catheter technique, J. Surg. Res. 9:347, 1969.
15. Greenfield, L. J., Bruce, T. A., and Nichols, N. B.: Transvenous pulmonary embolectomy by catheter device, Ann. Surg. 174:881, 1971.
16. Greenfield, L. J., Peyton, M. D., Brown, P. P., and Elkins, R. C.: Transvenous management of pulmonary embolic disease, Ann. Surg. 180:461, 1974.

THE POSTPHLEBITIC SYNDROME

Introduction

IN DEALING WITH the postphlebitic syndrome, one can only be impressed with its chronicity. Despite the positive advocacy of various surgical and nonoperative maneuvers, it is acknowledged, as indicated in the discussion that follows, that no treatment is fully effective.

Standard, well agreed-to methods of care of the postphlebitic patient are detailed in the chapters that follow. Also, a fresh thought on the subject is provided by one of England's foremost-thinking surgeons. His observations and new ideas are consistent with evidence of cyclic recurrence of postphlebitic ulcers.

It may be that surgeons now stand on the threshold of direct venous repair. Diagnostic techniques for patient screening are appearing and definitive venography has been available for some time. Experiments in autogenous reconstruction have been done and evaluated. Such results are detailed in this section. Even valve repair is beautifully illustrated here.

What is necessary, however, is a valve-containing venous prosthesis which may allow direct vein replacement. It is curious that so much information attends arterial replacement and so little has been accumulated about the veins.

This section of this Symposium gathers together a summary of available knowledge about venous reconstruction and suggests application to the postphlebitic state.

23 / The Postphlebitic Syndrome: Management by Conservative Means

J. CUTHBERT OWENS, M.D.
University of Colorado Medical Center, Denver, Colorado

THE MANAGEMENT OF A postphlebitic syndrome is primarily an ambulatory problem, no matter what caused the condition from the onset. Untreated patients are plagued with chronic edema, pigmentation and ulceration, pain, venous congestion and recurrent episodes of venous thromboses. Until recent wide acceptance of the aggressive use of anticoagulant (heparin) and specific anti-inflammatory therapy for thrombophlebitis, few patients escaped the sequelae of chronic venous insufficiency of the lower extremities and many ultimately developed leg ulcers. Its occurrence is far less common today for it is considered preventable when treatment for thrombophlebitis is prompt and adequate.

In the postphlebitic syndrome, the patient's demolished deep veins are beyond repair; therefore, the management of this condition is aimed at preventing more disfigurement, eliminating the discomfort and halting the disease.

Etiology

Even though the name postphlebitic implies that there is a previous history of deep venous thrombosis, approximately one out of five patients has no history of thrombophlebitis or the usual conditions where it may have escaped identification (e.g., cardiac disease, extremity injury, previous operation or pregnancy).[1] The development and severity of postphlebitic sequelae depends on the extent to which the deep venous valves are destroyed from the venous thrombosis, the amount of inflammation present and how adequate the acute attack of thrombophlebitis was managed. The damage is due to the phlebitic or inflammatory reaction of the vein wall and the surrounding tissues, while the thrombosis occludes the venous tube totally or partially. If a small segment of vein is involved or the vein is simply ligated, there is little likelihood for chronic edema to result, especially if the extremity is elevated, placed at rest and an elastic support is applied. Collateral venous channels are capable of compensating for the localized occlusion, even without anticoagulant (heparin) and/or anti-inflammatory therapy. However, if the venous thrombosis is extensive and involves more than the iliac or calf veins the extent of demolished valves in the deep veins is the important factor. This factor is critical, for recanalization and/or collateral venous channels then are unable to handle the load of venous return efficiently, at least, not until time for recovery without additional physiologic changes is permitted. Treatment therefore is directed toward reversing as much of the complicating symptomatology as possible. In this way, injury to the venous system is reduced, but not eliminated.[2, 3]

Diagnosis

Diagnosis of the postphlebitic syndrome is based on a history of deep vein thrombophlebitis followed by edema and any combination of skin pigmentation, dermatitis, subcutaneous fibrosis, chronic ulceration, varicose veins, recurrent infection and such disabling subjective symptoms as heaviness, fatigue and pain. In some cases without a history of thrombophlebitis, the typical findings of the syndrome are present, but no other known cause (e.g., cardiac disease, primary lymphatic obstruction or simple varicose veins) can be found; these are considered nonthrombotic.[2, 3]

Women outnumber male patients approximately 2:1, but the disability occurs at an earlier age in women than men: 55–61 years. This can possibly be explained on the higher incidence of obesity in women, monthly occurrence of the menstrual cycle producing intermittent water retention, the use of oral contraceptive drugs, the infrequent exposure to an exercise program in women and the higher incidence of cardiac failure in men shortly after middle age.[1]

Admission of patients is required in a little more than 10% of the cases. They are most commonly admitted for recurrent thrombophlebitis, cardiac failure, marked cellulitis to the extremity, large unresponsive ulcers, necessity for excision and ligation of varicose veins, or necessity for grafting of ulcers.

Duration of the syndrome may be any length of time but usually averages 10 years while the average appearance of an ulcer is 7 years and seldom less than 2 years. Ulcers may occur as late as several decades after the initial acute episode.

Lower extremity edema is essential for the diagnosis and occurs especially in the morning hours but is seldom the subjective and objective complaint. It may be unilateral or bilateral. Trauma is often the initiating cause of the ulcer and may be the major factor for reappearance of the syndrome with or without ulcer. Other common causes for the reappearance of the syndrome are pregnancy, cardiac failure or recurrent thrombophlebitis. Malignant ulcers do occur but are very rare unless the ulcer has been present and unhealed for 15–30 years.[8] Achilles tendon fibrosis may occur when ulcers have developed close to the tendon and are left untreated for a prolonged period.[1]

Varicose veins are a common factor with their presence prior to the syndrome or developing after its onset.

Allied disorders noted on history or examination are present in the majority of patients. These, as stated, may cause a flare-up of the syndrome or hamper therapy. The most frequent of these are obesity, cardiovascular conditions including cardiac therapy, cor pulmonale, hypertensive cardiovascular disease, arteriosclerosis obliterans, mental or emotional problems and recurrent thrombophlebitis due to a hypercoagulable state. Multiple disorders are frequently present. In recent years the use of oral contraceptive drugs has replaced sclerosing therapy for varicose veins as the leading iatrogenic factor causing or contributory to the condition. The "pill" today is widely used for contraception while sclerosing therapy for varicose veins has recently become a much less popular procedure.[4] Other situations in this area are removal of varicose veins while the extremity is in an edematous phase, "hardware" being present from open reduction of a fracture and placement of a "screen" or ligation of the inferior vena cava following extensive venous thrombosis in the iliac and femoral vein area with ineffective treatment of the acute thrombophlebitis in the postoperative period.

Venography on occasion may be necessary to establish a diagnosis, though reliance on reading of the study may often be questioned, especially when pelvic venography is not included. Since there is a higher incidence of left lower extremity involvement the initiating or contributory factor may be due to iliac vein pathology which occurs spontaneously or from partial occlusion of the iliac vein by the right common iliac artery which may or may not be atherosclerotic. The same area may be partially occluded on the right from the right iliac artery and/or an intimal web may be present in either iliac vein where the artery crosses over the vessel(s). Venous injury during pelvic or groin surgery such as inguinal hernia repair should be considered, especially if prominent superficial veins are present in the groin area. Use of a Doppler flowmeter, impedance plethysmography, venous pressures or labeled isotopes may be beneficial in screening certain patients and special coagulation studies may be ordered in centers interested in clotting problems. Coagulation studies are essential in all patients having recurrent episodes of thrombophlebitis.[4]

Treatment

Treatment is established principally on an outpatient basis, following a complete general medical examination. Optimally, where possible, vascular clinics should be staffed by a team consisting of an internist, a surgeon and a podiatrist. Interpreters, clinic or visiting nurses and members of the family are often needed to aid in the education of the patient.

The internist and the surgeon see every patient jointly to evaluate the extremity involved and the patient's overall problem. The team first initiates a conservative treatment program, consisting of (1) patient cooperation, (2) treatment of allied disorders, (3) control of infection and (4) elevation, compression and exercise of the extremity. Special studies such as the use of a Doppler flowmeter, venography (pelvic and thigh veins) and coagulation studies may be required in patients who present unusual or diagnostic problems.

Patient cooperation is demanded for thorough education in the physiopathology of the condition, both for immediate care and for continuing prophylaxis. Mimeographed instruction sheets are issued and the patient is repeatedly "quizzed" on this material.[4] Cooperation implies not only compliance with instructions for lower limb care but also willingness to assist in caring for allied disorders.

Allied disorders are present in over 75% of cases, emphasizing the importance of "total" treatment.[1] Those with cardiac failure may require digitalization, diuretics and salt-poor diets. Obesity, of course, necessitates weight reduction. Thrombophlebitis, when still active or recurrent, is treated on an inpatient anticoagulant (heparin) basis until there is complete subsidence of symptoms. When superficial, an anti-inflammatory agent such as Butazolidin is used for 3–5 days (100 mg three times daily after meals). No effort is spared in obtaining successful treatment of the allied disorder, since this is a prerequisite to successful primary treatment of the postphlebitic syndrome.

Elimination of infection, whether it be dermatitis, epidermophytosis or infected ulcer, is approached with the concept that the majority are due to fungi. Therefore, treatment is initiated by means of potassium permanganate soaks of 1:10,000 dilution including the foot at home three times daily for 30-min periods for three days. This not only eliminates or decreases the fungus present and tends to dry the ulcer but also demonstrates the patient's interest in the care, for the toenails will be black when instructions are properly followed. When an ulcer appears to be infected by bacteria, or fungicidal treatment is not adequate, antibiotic ointments such as bacitracin or neomycin are applied to the ulcer twice a day. However, this is rarely necessary when attention has been directed toward fungicidal therapy. When cellulitis is not present, an Unna boot is used for intervals of 3 weeks until the ulcer is completely healed. Often it is reapplied one or two times after the ulcer heals to allow the new skin to mature. No medication, gauze or other material should ever be applied on the ulcer beneath the boot. The Unna paste impregnated in the gauze of the boot must be in direct contact with the bed of the ulcer. In those patients where the ulcer is too deep to comply with this policy, an attempt should be made first to stimulate granulation and fill in the defect before a series of Unna boot applications are begun. Often, these ulcers will have much less depth when there is a reduction of the surrounding edema and inflammation by elevation, diuretics and an anti-inflammatory agent. Parenteral antibiotics are not used unless the patient has a widespread cellulitis. Admission to the hospital may be advisable in these cases.

The edema is initially cleared by elevation. This is usually accomplished overnight, but some patients require 2 weeks or more of continuous elevation to reach the edema-free state. A daily diuretic is administered in most patients. Active and passive exercise during elevation is encouraged, especially when ulcers are slow in subsiding. Progressive ambulation is begun, using elastic compression support, only after the edema has disappeared or lessened significantly.

Four types of *elastic compression* support have been used. If the leg is markedly swollen and edema returns on ambulation in less than 1 hr, or if previous therapy with cloth-rubber support has failed, pure rubber (Esmarch) bandages are advised; a cotton stocking may be worn beneath this to avoid skin reaction to the rubber. Elastoplast, as advised by Linton, is used with similar indications.[3] Most cases, however, require only cloth-rubber compression bandages or elastic stockings from the beginning. Following an increase to 2 or more hours of edema-free ambulation, elastic stockings are substituted for the cloth-rubber or pure rubber bandages. Elastic stockings should be tailored, or well-fitted for the patient's edema problem. It should be recognized that elastic stockings, unlike pneumatic compression, do not force fluid from the limb; they only delay the progress of the edema. The amount of time involved in the delay is directly related to the quality of the compression or elasticity provided by the stocking. Thin or sheer "elastic" stockings are not advised for they are worn more for modesty than therapy. In *no* case is the elastic support worn above the knee. Objections to the use of full-length elastic stockings or a leotard are: (1) they produce a garter effect at the knee and/or groin during flexion of the extremity, (2) an edematous thigh cannot be optimally controlled by compression, (3) they are expensive to replace every 2–4 months and (4) patients are prone not to use them regularly since they are difficult and time-consuming to apply. Few patients will have thigh edema after proper treatment. Therefore, edema below the knee becomes the primary problem which needs to be controlled. Occasionally, Unna boots are utilized permanently with changes made monthly for patients who develop recurrent ulcers in spite of adequate measures. Patients who require this approach are: (1) those who are aged and seldom if ever ambulate, (2) those whose occupation requires prolonged periods of standing or sitting, (3) those who are uncooperative in spite of an intense educational program and (4) those who have a fixed ankle and/or knee joint and are unable to utilize the "venous heart" muscles of the involved extremity.

Active ambulatory, standing or sitting time is stopped 15 to 30 min prior to the appearance of fullness, heaviness, fatigue or edema in the extremity, and the patient returns to extremity elevation above the heart level for at least a 15-min period. Each week the period of ambulation is increased, short of the expected appearance of the fullness or edema if a trial period demonstrates a lengthening of the previous symptom index. These periods may fluctuate with the type of exercise and the patient is so informed. In general, each week finds improvement; if not, the patient's habits and daily activities are reviewed to find the reason for failure. When he has reached a 2-hr edema-free period (usually in less than 2 weeks) the patient is allowed to return to work, provided he may elevate the extremity (above heart level) for 15 min at the end of each 2-hr edema-free period. This is then extended to 4 hr (if edema-free), then 6, and finally is left to the patient's discretion. During the day, he always wears an elastic stocking until there is no leg edema present. Most patients may then go without support most of the time, except when it is necessary for their legs to be dependent with little or any movement, for a prolonged period. Similarly, sitting or standing for long periods is discouraged during early therapy unless active movement of the extremity is undertaken—an attempt to utilize the "venous heart."

In summary, the patient is instructed that he must "never be ambulatory when fullness or swelling is present, or without his elastic support" and each case is individualized throughout the treatment. Foot care is stressed and prophylactic medications are prescribed: talcum and fungicidal powder for the moist foot or leg wearing an elastic support; lanolin or an ointment with a methyl cellulose base for the dry, scarred or indurated extremity. The maxim for foot hygiene is "never wash your face without washing your feet." Corns, callouses, thickened toenails, and the like, are managed by a podiatrist.

Certain *operative conditions* which appear early in the program need correction to bring about a successful outcome. Indolent ulcers may need grafting, or immediate healing is sometimes required for economic reasons. Seldom does the latter present a problem, for most ulcers heal within 6 weeks to 3 months when Unna boots are routinely used, providing the fungus infection is cleared and the edema is controlled. However, wide excision and grafting are advised if this healing is unduly delayed or if the ulcer has been present for several years and malignant degeneration could possibly be present. When malignant lesions do develop, it will be necessary to do wide excision and grafting, and possibly even amputation.

In recent years we have rarely found it necessary to excise and graft postphlebitic ulcers. Possibly we have become too conservative. However, we are influenced by our past experience of seeing too many patients who were surgical failures or had recurrent ulcers after previous "successful" excision and grafting. The morbidity and cost to these patients seemed excessive. One of our referred patients had experienced 16 unsuccessful attempts to excise and graft his leg ulcer at a cost of more than $50,000! Adherence to the nonoperative regimen described here resulted in healing of the ulcer in 4 months. In the past 14 years he has had no recurrence (Fig 23–1).

Two factors are important in treatment to prevent the complication of Achilles' tendon shortening causing an *equinus deformity,* which may occur: (1) when an ulcer is present, it is inadvisable for the patient to walk with the heel off the ground or to wear high-heeled shoes for relief of pain; (2) prompt healing is imperative for such an ulcer

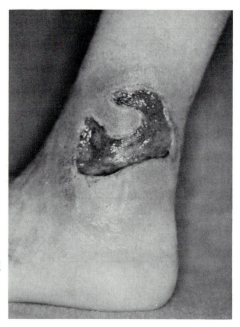

Fig 23–1.—Postphlebitic ulcer healing by nonoperative approach after multiple attempts to excise and graft area. Ulcer has remained healed for past 14 years.

overlying the tendon presents a problem on grafting. It may be necessary for these patients to sleep with posterior ankle splints. Delay in therapy may require future tenoplasty (Fig 23–2).

Large brawny ulcers with surrounding induration and edema failing to respond to the aforementioned regimen after several months may

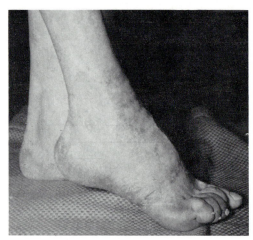

Fig 23–2.—Healed postphlebitic ulcer with equinus deformity from shortening of Achilles tendon.

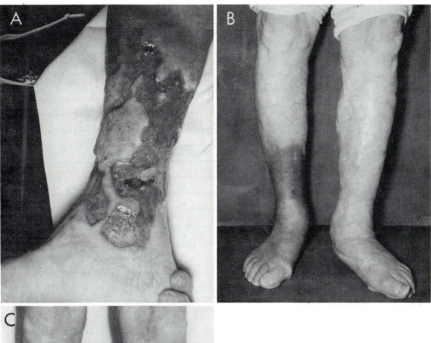

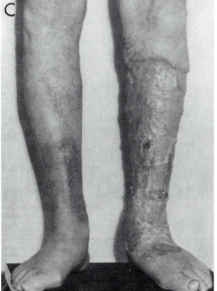

Fig 23–3. – **A,** large brawny post-phlebitic ulcer treated by wide excision and grafting (modified Kondoleon procedure). **B,** appearance 6 months postoperative. **C,** extremity 4 years later with beginning of recurrent ulcer.

be considered for a subfascial vein ligation, radical excision of the ulcer and skin grafting. A modified Kondoleon or Linton procedure may be indicated in a rare case.[3, 5, 6] It should be recognized that this radical approach is not a definitive operation. Therefore, following recovery it is essential that the patient follow a rigid postphlebitic syndrome program. Otherwise, in a few years some if not all of his previous problems may have recurred (Fig 23–3).

The patient presenting with a cold, sweating, cyanotic or pale foot and markedly painful hyperesthesia about the leg ulcer is given an intra-arterial sympatholytic drug (Priscoline, 25 mg). This not only establishes the diagnosis of *causalgic type* pain but also may sometimes give permanent relief of the intolerable pain. This is followed, when indicated, by an oral sympatholytic drug, paravertebral lumbar sympathetic block(s) or, if no permanent relief occurs, by a lumbar sympathectomy. We do not believe that postphlebitic syndrome without the above signs and symptoms is an indication for sympathectomy. These patients are most resistant to treatment for they are unable to withstand topical medications, especially an Unna boot. Relief of this type of pain is therefore an essential factor in their therapy.[7] *Somatic pain* is controlled by means of an anti-inflammatory agent and/or a mild sedative.

Varicose veins are not approached surgically until the patient has had 3–6 months of conservative therapy. Even then, this is delayed until the morning and early afternoon edema has been controlled (Fig 23–4). The patient is instructed to walk a few minutes out of every waking hour for several days following operation, with elastic support to the knee, and to follow the postphlebitic syndrome routine. The afternoon swelling which may have been present before surgery usually disappears and the patient wears an elastic stocking for at least 3 months. When no swelling appears during the day, the patient may ambulate without support. A warning is given that any trauma or infection to the extremity or prolonged standing or sitting may result in return of the syndrome and necessitate reinstituting the elevation-exercise routine as well as the daily use of an elastic support.

Excision of varicose veins in patients with a postphlebitic syndrome should not be considered lightly. The procedure is contraindicated in any patient with morning edema of the leg(s). When indicated, the major benefit derived by the patient is prophylactic; the operation greatly reduces the possibility of recurrent acute superficial thrombophlebitis and eliminates the burdensome chronically inflamed subcutaneous veins. Their presence is a potential hazard while their removal is often very rewarding.[1]

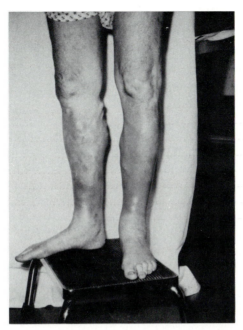

Fig 23–4.—Varicose veins secondary to chronic deep thrombophlebitis. Ligation and excision of varicosities indicated only when morning and afternoon edema controlled by postphlebitic syndrome regimen.

Discussion

The regimen of managing a majority of patients with a postphlebitic syndrome on an outpatient basis obviates the expense of inpatient care, and the 2-hr edema-free rule for return to work decreases the number of man hours lost to industry. Every effort is made to fit the therapy into the patient's daily routine by means of the type of elastic compression and utilization of the American custom of "coffee breaks" and the lunch hour—the 2-hr intervals between the beginning of the workday, coffee break, lunch hour, coffee break and the end of the day, each interspersed with 15-min periods of elevation of the limb above the heart level.

Insistence that the extremity be edema-free before ambulation is started is a sound and well-established principle, allowing nature to develop collaterals without hinderance. Major veins recanalize and until this occurs there conceivably is a delay in the initial phase of the recovery period, but this recanalization may only cause additional harm when collaterals have not been protected during and after their development. Choking of these vessels from beneath the integument by edematous fluid can only cause harm in this process.

Clearing of ulcers should not generally be a problem, once edema and fungus contamination are removed. Large ulcers on a brawny indurated extremity and the rare malignant ulcers are definitely the biggest problem in this group; here radical therapy may be required (Fig 23–5).[1]

Varicosities frequently bring out complaints which appear exaggerated, even in patients without the postphlebitic syndrome. Afternoon and evening swelling is not uncommon in these patients. The postphlebitic patient with varicose veins should be spared this potential source of edema, which is frequently resistant to therapy after morning edema has cleared. Removal of these damaged veins almost invariably brings clearance of this residual. Sclerosing therapy is strongly discouraged, especially when a concomitant postphlebitic syndrome exists.[1]

Fig 23–5. – Rare example of squamous carcinoma arising in chronic postphlebitic ulcer. Ulceration had been present for 27 years and finally underwent malignant degeneration.

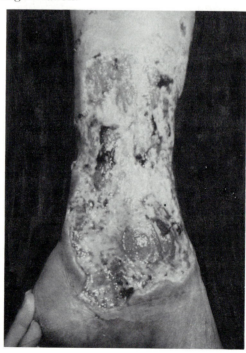

Resistant edema, especially in the thigh, frequently can be relieved by means of oral diuretics. When thigh edema remains, the patient should be ordered to bed for elevation exercise until edema free. It is an absolute sign of severe iliac vein involvement and often denotes inadequate inpatient therapy.

There is general agreement regarding the initial treatment of acute thrombophlebitis by means of rest, elevation, anticoagulants (heparin), antibiotics with infection, anti-inflammatory agents and possibly major vein ligation or screening when pulmonary emboli occur. In addition, attention is directed toward establishing a diagnosis and etiology and toward prophylaxis of deep vein thrombosis. The postphlebitic syndrome should be treated with the same broad viewpoint as advised for the acute disease. Interestingly, the progressive ambulatory regimen described above was originally recommended by John Homans in 1937 when he wrote on the convalescent treatment of deep vein thrombophlebitis: "There should be urged, when the leg appears normal, the application of a semi-elastic bandage and guarded exercise in the standing position. First, a few become cyanotic. If no recurrence follows, you can call the patient cured. Otherwise, the femoral vein is divided distal to the profunda."[9] Excluding the latter surgical recommendation, his convalescent treatment has been extended to include those patients who develop the chronic phase of the deep vein thrombosis.

The program described herein follows what Luke identified in 1949 as the "new way of life" concept, to a degree, but the restrictions should not necessitate any radical change in the patient's activity for the future.[10] It is true that an occasional case will be more complicated than average and such a patient may find it necessary to change his occupation, restrict his daily activity, and/or receive ambulatory anticoagulant (subcutaneous heparin) therapy.

Summary

Outpatient treatment gives 85% excellent to good results in the postphlebitic syndrome. The program requires careful patient education and patient cooperation, vigorous treatment of allied disorders, control of local infection and elevation, compression and exercise, followed by progressive edema-free ambulation with compression. Unsatisfactory results occur in the failure or inability of the patient to adhere to an established program. Failures are in patients with incurable diseases such as malignancies, pulmonary or cardiac failure, cir-

rhosis, ankylosed lower extremity joints, mental diseases, hypercoagulable states and obesity resistant to treatment.

REFERENCES

1. Owens, J. C., and Anderson, L. L.: Indications for surgical treatment of the post-phlebitic syndrome, Surgery 1:81, 1957.
2. Bauer, G.: Rationale and results of popliteal vein division, Angiology 169:189, 1955.
3. Linton, R. B.: The post-thrombotic ulceration of the lower extremity: its etiology and surgical treatment, Ann. Surg. 138:415, 1953.
4. Owens, J. C.: Peripheral Blood Vessels—Vascular Surgery, in Hill, G. J., II (ed.): *Outpatient Surgery* (Philadelphia: W. B. Saunders Company, 1973).
5. Kondoleon, E.: Die chirurgische Behandlung der elefantiastichen Oedeme durch eine neue Methode der Lymphableitung, Munch. Med. Wochenschr. 59:276, 1912.
6. Homans, J.: Exploration and division of the femoral and iliac veins in the treatment of thrombophlebitis of the leg, N. Engl. J. Med. 224:179, 1941.
7. Owens, J. C.: Indications for Lumbar Sympathectomy, in Dale, W. A. (ed.): *Management of Arterial Occlusive Disease* (Chicago: Year Book Medical Publishers, Inc., 1971).
8. Martorell, F.: *Ulceres des Jambes d'Origine Neuro-vasculaire* (Paris: Masson et Cie, 1953), p. 5.
9. Homans, J.: Venous thrombosis in the lower limbs: Its relation to pulmonary embolism, Am. J. Surg. 38:316, 1937.
10. Luke, J. C.: The pathology and treatment of the post-phlebitic leg and its complications, Can. Med. Assoc. J. 61:270, 1949.

24 / The Postphlebitic Syndrome: Management by Surgical Means

WILEY F. BARKER, M.D.

Chief, Division of General Surgery and Professor of Surgery, School of Medicine, University of California, Los Angeles, California

THE POSTPHLEBITIC SYNDROME represents a complicated series of processes resulting from several components of the original disease. Although it may seem obvious to say that these processes were generated by an onset of venous thrombosis, there are instances in which the postphlebitic syndrome appears to occur without an antecedent recognizable episode of venous thrombosis. This syndrome is often modified by iatrogenic intervention; indeed, the use of venous interruption in the management of pulmonary embolism is often credited with causing the syndrome, but Doctor de Takats[1] indicated his understanding of this process many years ago when he noted that it was the venous thrombosis and not the ligation that caused the major symptoms.

Mandiola and Barker[2] have surveyed the postphlebitic status of 84 patients whose limbs were subjected to venous interruption in the treatment of potential pulmonary embolism. In these cases the main factor contributing to late edema was the existence of serious phlebitis occurring at the time of the original interruption or at a later date.

Just as venous interruption may be deemed necessary in treating venous thrombosis which is actually or potentially complicated by pulmonary embolism, the administration of heparin during the active phase of venous thrombosis may alter the disease process by restricting propagation of clot, by preventing damage to valves and by allowing recanalization.

We can gain an understanding of the postphlebitic syndrome by studying its component parts and recognizing that each component can exist alone. However, it is more likely that two or even all five major components coexist, and moreover, some of these components serve to aggravate the others.

Edema stems from increased venous pressure in the extremities, brought about by venous obstruction, which may occur because of anatomical or physiologic obstruction. The latter condition exists when inadequately valved venous systems fail to pass blood toward the heart. A variant of this situation occurs when, despite the fact that many venous channels *are* competent, a large system which does not have competent veins serves as a spillway, causing recirculation of blood within the limb, e.g., down through a large incompetent saphenous system. When the recirculating volume increases beyond the capacity of the remaining competent veins, local venous hypertension leads to edema.

The same phenomena may lead to the development of recurring varicose veins. The mechanism is simple: venous collaterals distend as an increased demand is placed upon them because of mainline obstruction or incompetence accompanied by reversal of flow. As these veins (especially those in a subcutaneous position) distend, their previously functioning valves may cease to function and regurgitant flow occurs, adding the newly devalvulated system to the overall venous burden of the extremity.

Recurrent venous thrombosis may develop as a result of the stagnation, hypoxia, and metabolic injury to the venous endothelium. It may also be an extension of the original clotting aberration that led to the initial venous thrombosis—polycythemia, cardiopulmonary disease, hypoxia, etc. In other words, it would appear that one episode of venous thrombosis begets another.

Pigmentation and ulceration tend to supervene when large venous channels exist near the skin. Minor but multiple microscopic hemorrhages occur; in the earliest form these appear as perifollicular petechiae. When present, edema as well as deposition of blood pigment lead to a brownish pigmentation with cutaneous fibrosis, which in turn leads to cutaneous atrophy, and the stage is thus set for an episode of minor trauma to establish a chronic ulceration. Moreover, extreme pruritus and subsequent excoriation may initiate or aggravate the initial injury. The skin of the lower leg develops a remarkable allergic ability, and may respond unfavorably to almost any local medication. Indeed, a serious dermatitis medicamentosa is commonly found in the presence of chronic venous ulceration.

It should be emphasized that chronic infection is always present, with a variety of infecting bacteria from diphtheroids to staphylococci.

Cockett[3] has recently stressed the importance of *Staphylococcus aureus.*

Coexisting arterial insufficiency is a serious but infrequent complication. Ankle pressure measurements are of great value, especially when edema and induration preclude evaluation of palpable pulses.

Pain is described variously by these patients; for example, heaviness and fullness are equated with pain by some individuals. On the other hand, ulcerations are rarely seriously painful. In fact, the presence of pain in an ulcer should alert concern for infection or arterial insufficiency. Bauer[4] describes a type of bursting pain in the calf related to femoropopliteal venous insufficiency. A more serious type is described by Homans[5] as a pain of causalgic pattern, in which there is often some sympathetic hyperactivity, but the full-blown causalgia occurs infrequently. Nonetheless, some patients with this complaint are dramatically relieved by sympathetic interruption.

On the basis of the foregoing observations with respect to the pathophysiologic aspects of the postphlebitic syndrome, the following treatment scheme has been adhered to by the author for 20 years.

Edema is controlled by classical conservative means, as outlined by Doctor Owens earlier. Intermittent elevation, snug pressure bandages or even intermittent pneumatic compression are the recommended procedures. Occasional circumstances exist in which the crossover vein graft popularized by Dale and Allen,[6] direct reconstruction of the valves as done by Kistner,[7] or decompression of a left iliac vein at its site of compression by the right iliac artery may likewise be useful measures.

Varicose veins secondary to chronic obstruction are treated by excision (rarely by injection in our hands) only when it is clear by physical examination that flow is centrifugal and not toward the heart. The Doppler velocity sensor is helpful in this determination.

Patients who suffer recurrent thromboses are maintained on long-term anticoagulant management with Coumadin. Initiation of such a course of therapy or treatment of intercurrent thrombotic episodes with heparin is often effective. Some patients who fail to respond to chronic anticoagulation with Coumadin have been managed by antiplatelet therapy with aspirin and Persantine (dipyridamole).

The major thrust of this section is, however, directed at the management of ulceration, although the modalities described in the preceding paragraphs are also used when necessary. First in importance is healing of the ulcer, and for this purpose bed rest with the legs elevated and frequently changed dressings have been the most effective measures. Modifications of the wet dressing technique may vary with the individual surgeon. A medicated gelatin case (Unna paste boot) can be applied to attempt healing on an ambulatory patient, but bed rest has proved more effective. Treatment of skin inflammation stemming from sensitivity to medications is best accomplished by withdrawing all medication, except for a bland lotion or cream containing a topical steroid.

Once the ulcer is clean and proved by culture to be free of serious pathogens such as *S. aureus*, small ulcers will epithelialize quickly. Larger ones are better treated by split-thickness skin grafts. In these cases, failure of a graft to take suggests the presence of unrecognized major pathogenic bacteria.

When the ulcer is healed, large hypertensive venous channels in the vicinity of the ulcer are removed. This may entail stripping of an

Fig 24–1.—A, Linton's subfascial approach to the division of communicating veins in the medial compartment of the leg. The incision is carried directly down to the deep fascia which is then incised and widely undermined. The largest number of communicating veins are found near the attachment of the fascia to the edge of the tibia. These are divided as shown in **B.** (From Barker, W. F. [ed.]: *Surgical Treatment of Peripheral Vascular Disease* [New York: McGraw-Hill Book Co., 1962].)

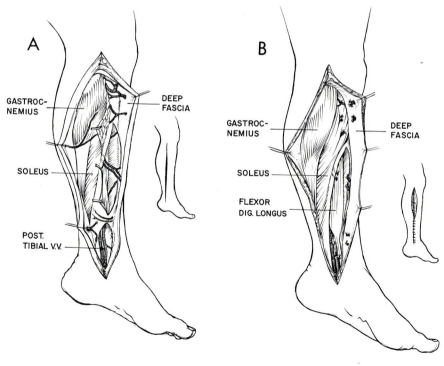

incompetent long saphenous system with excision of associated vari-
ceal masses in the subcutaneous compartment and interruption of
such communicating veins as are identified. Even if prior superficial
venous surgery has been extensive, one may still find incompetent
venous channels, either longitudinal or communicating, and these
must be removed. The use of the subfascial ligation of perforators as
described by Linton[8] has been the author's preference for more than
two decades. Most commonly, the medial incision (Fig 24-1) is
applicable, although the other anatomical approaches are used. Less
favored is the midline posterior approach, which deviates from the
midline of the back of the calf either to the medial or lateral post-
malleolar areas below the junction of the middle and lower thirds
of the calf (Figs 24-2 and 24-3).

Fig 24-2.—Communicating veins are divided and ligated beneath the
fascia. The fascia is split in the midline posteriorly, and if the lesser saphenous vein is diseased, it may be removed at this time through this incision.
The posterior fascial defect is left unsutured, but the anterior fascia is closed
to support the skin closure. (From Barker, W. F. [ed.]: *Surgical Treatment
of Peripheral Vascular Disease* [New York: McGraw-Hill Book Co., 1962].)

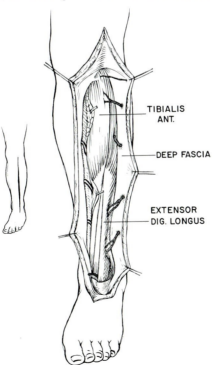

TIBIALIS
ANT.

DEEP FASCIA

EXTENSOR
DIG. LONGUS

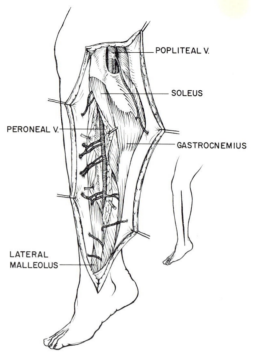

Fig 24–3.—The surgical approach to the posterolateral group of perforating veins draining primarily from the peroneal veins. (From Barker, W. F. [ed.]: *Surgical Treatment of Peripheral Vascular Disease* [New York: McGraw-Hill Book Co., 1962].)

All identifiable communicating veins are divided beneath the level of the fascia. The lesser saphenous vein is removed if it is diseased. If the medial or one of the lateral incisions is used, the fascia is closed under the skin incision, but it is split and left open at the posterior limit of the wound. Such a closure supports the skin repair when the skin is fibrous and edematous. Closure by a running nylon subcuticular suture or by interrupted skin sutures of nylon should be performed carefully.

In several patients the full procedure was modified by using shorter incisions than those described above. Although Linton has advocated concomitant ligation of the superficial femoral vein, this procedure has not been a part of our regimen.

Postoperatively, the patient is cautiously allowed ambulation for limited but infrequent periods after 48 hr. Snug elastic support is used whenever the patient is vertical. Small doses of heparin (5,000 units

TABLE 24–1.—BASIC PATIENT DATA

PATIENT NO.	SEX	AGE (YR)	YRS WITH SYNDROME	ORIGIN OF SYNDROME†	EDEMA	RECURRENT VARICOSE VEINS	RECURRENT THROMBOSIS	PIGMENTATION ULCER	PAIN
1	F	72	4	Trauma	+			+	
2	M	35	5	Fractured thigh	++°			+	
3	F	35	5	Postpartum	+	+	+		
4	M	40	2	Postoperative	+				
5	F	75	15	Fractured foot		+		+++	++
6	F	46	20	Spontaneous	+	+		++	
7	M	50	5	Spontaneous	+			+	
8	F	53	35	Postpartum	+	++			
9	F	55	35	Postpartum	+	++	+		
10	F	52	32	Injections for varicose veins	+	+		+	
11	M	55	2	Postphlebography	+				
12	F	61	30	Spontaneous	++		++	+++	
13	M	65	10	Spontaneous	++			++	+
14	F	73	20	Postoperative	++		+		
15	M	35	5	Retroperitoneal tumor	++				
16	M	62	13	Fractured thigh	++			+	
17	M	40	5	Head injury	++				+
18	M	60	25	Injections for varicose veins	+				
19	M	52	1	Trauma	++				
20	F	47	10	Postsaphenous stripping	+				
21	M	66	40	Trauma	++	+	+		+
22	F	45	2	Trauma	+				

°Massive.
†"Spontaneous" indicates no specific recognizable cause.

TABLE 24-2.—RESULTS OF THERAPY FOR INDIVIDUAL COMPONENTS OF SYNDROME

PATIENT NO.	YRS OF FOLLOWUP	EDEMA	RECURRENT VEINS	RECURRENT THROMBOSIS	PIGMENTATION ULCER	PAIN
1	2	Elastic support, good			Unilateral modified Linton flap (too early for evaluation)	
2	1	Elastic support, good				
3	1/2	Elastic support, fair	Saphenous stripping			
4	3	Elastic support, fair		Coumadin, good	Bilateral Linton flap	
5	4		Two local excisions, fair		Unilateral modified Linton flap, good	
6	20	Elastic support, good			Unilateral Linton flap, good	Sympathectomy, cordotomy, fair
7	5	Elastic support, good	Fair		Bilateral stripping, unilateral modified Linton flap, fair	
8	10	Elastic support, good		Coumadin, good	Bilateral modified Linton flap, good	
9	1		Saphenous stripping, good			
10	5	Elastic support, good	Bilateral saphenous stripping, good		Bilateral saphenous stripping, poor	
11	1	Elastic support, fair		Coumadin, good	Unilateral Linton flap, good	
12	25	Elastic support, fair		Coumadin, poor		
13	1/4	Elastic support, fair			Stripping of lesser saphenous, too early for evaluation	
14	10	Elastic support, poor			Unilateral modified Linton flap, poor	No treatment, poor
15	4	Elastic support, fair		Coumadin, good		
16	5	Aeropulse boot, good			Unilateral Linton flap, good	
17	2	Elastic support, poor		Coumadin intermittent, poor		No treatment, poor
18	2	Elastic support, good				
19	1	Elastic support, good				
20	1	Elastic support, good				
21	1	Elastic support, fair	Crossover vein, poor	Coumadin, good		Poor

subcutaneously or intravenously every 6 hr) are administered as prophylaxis against further deep venous thrombosis for a period of 7–10 days.

In patients who are particularly subject to recurrent thrombosis, Coumadin is substituted for heparin and is maintained for 6 months or as indicated. In all cases, firm elastic support is mandatory as long as edema persists.

Data

Twenty-two private patients who had been treated during the last five years constituted the patient population discussed in this report. Follow-up data regarding patient self-care were good in this group but were not considered reliable with respect to the larger clinic population.

Table 24–1 presents the basic patient data and the spectrum of components as distinctly as possible. In Table 24–2 data are summarized regarding therapy for the separate components and the results obtained, notably for patients 14 and 17, who failed to cooperate and follow careful regimens. Sex distribution was even. The current ages are listed, since the time of onset of the syndrome was not always definable. The average age of the women was about 5 years older than that of the men.

Table 24–3 lists the causes of the syndromes, summarized from Table 24–1. The puzzling lack of recognized onset during medical illnesses may be explained by possible inclusion in the category labeled "spontaneous." It should be pointed out that none of the 22 patients had Buerger's disease or cancer.

At times the true origin of the syndrome was difficult to identify on the basis of a long history. However, a profile of the syndrome can be extracted from Table 24–1. All but two of the 22 patients had edema, and in six it was massive. Six suffered from significant and recurrent

TABLE 24–3.—FREQUENCY OF CAUSES OF THE
POSTPHLEBITIC SYNDROME

CONDITION	NO. OF PATIENTS
Trauma (diffuse) or ipsilateral fracture	8
Postpartum or postoperative thrombophlebitis	5
Postinjection (varicose veins)	2
Post-saphenous stripping	1
Post-femoral vein catheterization and phlebography	1
Spontaneous or unidentified causes	4

varicose veins; six others had a significant component of recurrent thromboses. Half (11) exhibited ulceration or preulcerative pigmentation demanding treatment. Pain was a major complaint in four patients, one of whom manifested a true causalgia which at first responded to sympathectomy but later required a cervical cordotomy. It has been apparent that edema and ulceration or pigmentation are major components of this syndrome. Recurrent varicose veins, recurrent thromboses and serious pain patterns are also important but less frequent symptoms.

The results of treatment as presented in Table 24–3 can be condensed as follows. In the management of edema, use of elastic support ranged from fair to good, except for two patients whose cooperation was minimal. Protection against edema produced by elastic support, however, did not protect against ulceration. In 11 extremities (nine patients), a subfascial excision of communicating veins was carried out. Eight extremities were good (i.e., the ulceration has healed and the thin pigmented skin has become softer and more pliable). One patient who has been unwilling either to use elastic support or to follow a proper hygienic regimen has had repeated recurrences of the ulceration. Another has experienced a minor recurrence which healed promptly. Still another patient was operated on too recently to know the final result.

As a rule, the subfascial excision of communicating veins has been carried out only after excision or stripping of the diseased superficial veins. Excessive cutaneous dissection accompanied by subfascial dissection has lead to wound breakdown. However, no significant problems related to wound healing have been encountered among this group (see Figs 24–1 through 24–3).

Although Linton's operative approach (utilized for some patients) involves division of the superficial femoral vein, no superficial femoral vein interruptions were done. If significant reflux occurred down a diseased femoral vein, either ligation or plication (Kistner) was considered the appropriate procedure.

Recurrent varicosities generally have responded well to saphenous stripping and excision without exacerbating the edema. Nevertheless, one patient has had recurrent pigmentation in spite of stripping and may eventually require subfascial excision of communicating veins.

Recurrent thromboses generally have responded well to Coumadin for protracted periods during periods of several years or longer. One uncooperative patient has not responded well, but dosage and prothrombin content have been variable. While no patients in this series have been controlled by aspirin or persantin, others at UCLA who have had difficulty with Coumadin have responded well.

The serious pain manifested by four patients represents the most uncommon problem in the syndrome. In three patients, reassurance and the use of minimal nonnarcotic analgesics have been barely acceptable. However, one patient suffered pain patterns representing the classical picture of a true causalgia. She was treated initially by sympathectomy which provided relief for a year, but when severe pain returned, she attempted suicide. Eventually she underwent cervical cordotomy with good success for many years, but the pain recently returned at the margin of the degenerated area and now requires narcotics for relief. We do not consider these four patients to have been successfully treated.

Summary

A useful profile of the postphlebitic syndrome and the efficiency of its treatment has been revealed by a review of the components exhibited by a group of 22 patients. We have concluded that if a patient is willing and able to cooperate with rigid instructions, edema can be effectively managed by methods utilizing external support. However, such methods do not totally control the other components. Recurrent varicose disease was handled fairly well by excision of the appropriate veins. Recurrent venous thrombosis responded favorably to anticoagulant or antiplatelet therapy. However, pigmentation and ulceration developed despite elastic support, yet responded well to surgical removal of large hypertensive venous channels from the involved area. Pain cannot be effectively diminished when it appears in serious causalgia-like patterns.

REFERENCES

1. de Takats, G.: *Thromboembolic Disease* (Springfield, Ill.: Charles C Thomas, Publisher, 1955).
2. Mandiola, S., and Barker, W. F.: The late status of the extremity following major vein interruption (in preparation).
3. Cockett, F. B.: Post-phlebitic ulceration — the intricacy of management. Presented at the Fourth Annual Symposium on Vascular Surgery, March 19, 1976, Palm Springs, California.
4. Bauer, G.: Rationale and results of popliteal vein division, Angiology 6:169, 1955.
5. Homans, J.: The late results of femoral thrombophlebitis and their treatment, N. Engl. J. Med. 235: 249, 1946.
6. Dale, W. A., and Allen, T. R.: Unusual problems of venous thrombosis, Surgery 78: 707, 1975.
7. Kistner, R. L.: Surgical repair of the incompetent femoral vein valve, Arch. Surg. 110:1336, 1975.
8. Linton, R. R.: The communicating veins of the lower leg and the operative technique for their ligation, Ann. Surg. 107:582, 1938.

25 / The Postphlebitic Syndrome: A New Look

NORMAN L. BROWSE, M.D., F.R.C.S.

Professor of Vascular Surgery, St. Thomas' Hospital Medical School, London, England

AND

K. G. BURNAND, F.R.C.S.

Department of Surgery, St. Thomas' Hospital Medical School, London, England

Introduction

THE CHANGES THAT OCCUR in the skin and subcutaneous tissues of the lower leg associated with varicose veins or following a deep vein thrombosis—commonly called the postphlebitic syndrome—affect 0.5% of the population of Great Britain and the United States[1] and cause an estimated loss of 500,000 working days each year in England and Wales and 2,000,000 in the United States.

The problem is conspicuous but the solution avoids us because there is a large gap in our knowledge of the etiology of venous ulceration. The prime cause is an abnormality of the venous side of the circulation which usually is obvious and easy to demonstrate with simple physiologic tests of the efficacy of the calf muscle venous pump. However the way in which this abnormality of the circulation ultimately causes death of the skin of the leg has never been explained satisfactorily.

The final event which leads to a venous ulcer must be the death of the cells of the skin but the common causes of cell death such as trauma, ischemia or infection are conspicuously absent. When the edge of a venous ulcer is cut it bleeds vigorously and normally, its base usually forms healthy granulation tissue and there is no apparent serious insufficiency of arterial blood flow.

It has been postulated that the blood flow in the region of a venous ulcer is abnormal in that much of it is shunted past the nutritional vessels, thus starving the tissues of nutriments[2] and causing the high oxygen content in the venous blood draining an ulcer which has been observed by numerous workers[3]. We find this explanation unsatisfactory because these shunts never have been demonstrated satisfactorily by physiologic,[4] radiologic[5] or pathologic[6] techniques.

Because of our ignorance of the mechanism by which a disordered calf muscle pump gives rise to venous ulcers, most surgeons have directed their therapeutic efforts solely toward correcting the pump abnormality with various surgical procedures. However, surgical treatment often fails to prevent recurrent ulceration. When we recently reviewed 41 patients with ulcers who had been treated by carefully planned surgery we found that 23 of the ulcers had recurred within 2 or 3 years[7] and that all of the recurrences were in patients with extensive phlebographic evidence of deep vein damage. There may be two reasons for such failures. Either the calf muscle pump may be so damaged by previous thrombosis that it is irreparable, or there may be other unrecognized abnormalities affecting the microcirculation which must be corrected before treatment can be successful.

Two years ago when we were reviewing this problem two observations seemed to be unexplained.

1. Many patients appear to have recurrent, even persistent, venous thrombosis in the tissues, which precedes the appearance of their ulcer, making the skin and subcutaneous tissue thick, hard and tender. This condition is commonly called "the postphlebitic syndrome" or "fat necrosis" but as there is often no evidence of a previous thrombosis and the skin and subcutaneous fat is not dead, simply thick and fibrous, we think this condition should be called lipodermatosclerosis, or simply _liposclerosis._

2. There is often extensive pigmentation with hemosiderin on the medial aspect of the lower leg in patients with venous disease. This is often claimed to be due to bleeding into the tissues following the rupture of small venules but this explanation seemed unlikely and we wondered if the capillaries were abnormally permeable. This hypothesis was supported by the observations of one of our colleagues, Dr. I. Whimster, who had seen an increased number of capillaries within the dermis and around venous ulcers.

In the light of these observations we decided to investigate the fibrinolytic status of our patients to see if there was any abnormality which might explain their apparent recurrent thrombophlebitis, to see if there was capillary proliferation in the skin on the medial side of their lower limbs and to test the permeability of these new capillaries. To achieve the last aim we have had to develop an experimental model of venous hypertension.

By chance the two main lines of investigation — fibrinolysis and capillary permeability — gelled to produce what we believe is a possible explanation of the cause of venous ulceration, a rational approach to treatment and a new concept of the physiologic function of tissue fibrinolysis.

Blood Fibrinolytic Activity in Patients with Liposclerosis

The blood fibrinolytic activity has been measured by estimating the dilute blood clot lysis time[8] and the fibrin plate lysis area.[9] The fibrinolytic activator activity in tissue has been estimated in sections of hand vein using the Todd technique[10] modified by Browse et al.[11]

Thirty-nine patients with extensive liposclerosis have been studied. They have been compared with 32 normal patients and with 50 patients with varicose veins but without associated liposclerosis. The results are shown in Table 25–1. The patients with liposclerosis have a significantly reduced blood and tissue fibrinolytic activity. The patients with varicose veins but normal skin have normal blood fibrinolytic activity.

Are these changes in the blood a primary or a secondary phenomenon? At first sight it would seem a little unlikely that the systemic blood and the walls of the veins in the hands could be altered or affected by disease in one or both legs and we do not know if the defect in fibrinolytic activity predated the development of the venous disease because it had not been previously measured. In a review of 88 patients with a history of deep vein thrombosis we found the blood and tissue fibrinolytic activity to be significantly reduced, but not as depressed as in the patients with liposclerosis. As some of these 88 patients are quite likely to develop the postphlebitic leg in future years, at least part of the fibrinolytic defects observed in those with liposclerosis may be a primary abnormality.

The only way to prove if the blood changes are primary or secondary is by investigating the fibrinolytic status of all patients undergoing operation and observing them for many years to see whether those who develop a postoperative deep vein thrombosis and ultimately the postphlebitic syndrome had an abnormality before their operation, a formidable task. Regardless of whether the blood changes are primary

TABLE 25-1.—BLOOD AND TISSUE FIBRINOLYTIC ACTIVITY IN NORMAL SUBJECTS, PATIENTS WITH VARICOSE VEINS AND PATIENTS WITH LIPOSCLEROSIS

	NORMAL SUBJECTS (N = 32)		SUBJECTS WITH VARICOSE VEINS (N = 50)		SUBJECTS WITH LIPOSCLEROSIS (N = 39)	
	BEFORE 10 MIN VENOUS CONGESTION	AFTER 10 MIN VENOUS CONGESTION	BEFORE 10 MIN VENOUS CONGESTION	AFTER 10 MIN VENOUS CONGESTION	BEFORE 10 MIN VENOUS CONGESTION	AFTER 10 MIN VENOUS CONGESTION
Dilute blood clot lysis time (min)	256 (SE = 18)	153 (SE = 35)	271 (SE = 27)	174 (SE = 27)	627* (SE = 73)	335* (SE = 49)
Fibrin plate lysis area (sq mm)	453 (SE = 37)	568 (SE = 68)	394 (SE = 33)	518 (SE = 51)	291* (SE = 23)	410* (SE = 30)
Plasma fibrinogen (mg/100 ml)	275 (SE = 7.2)		312 (SE = 8.0)		419* (SE = 18)	
Hand vein activity (units)	24 (SE = 2.2)		19.4 (SE = 1.4)		12.5* (SE = 2)	

*Significantly different from normal subjects.

TABLE 25-2.—RELATIONSHIP BETWEEN THE EFFICIENCY OF
THE CALF MUSCLE PUMP AND SKIN CAPILLARY
PROLIFERATION

NO. OF LEGS STUDIED (TOTAL = 121)	CAPILLARY PROLIFERATION SCORE	MEAN FALL OF FOOT VEIN PRESSURE DURING EXERCISE (% OF RESTING LEVEL)
57	0	43
28	1	37
8	2	16
14	3	9
14	4	21

or secondary, the findings of an abnormality in fibrinolysis suggest that the fibrinolytic system may play an important part in the etiology of the liposclerosis.

Capillary Proliferation in Patients with Liposclerosis

In 66 patients with venous disease the changes in foot vein pressure during a standard exercise test have been correlated with the degree of capillary proliferation found in a biopsy of the affected skin. The biopsy was taken from a point 7.5 cm above the medial malleolus and was examined by an independent pathologist (Dr. I. Whimster) who assessed the number of capillaries visible in the dermis and allocated each specimen to one of four grades. Table 25-2 shows the relationship between the fall of foot vein pressure during exercise, which is an indication of the efficiency of the calf muscle pump, and the degree of capillary proliferation. It can be seen that the less effective the calf muscle pump the greater the degree of capillary proliferation. These studies therefore suggest that prolonged high pressure in the veins of the lower limb due to an abnormal muscle pump stimulates, or is associated with, the growth of new capillaries in the skin and subcutaneous tissues. Similar capillary proliferation was produced in 16 dogs in whom prolonged venous hypertension was induced by making an arteriovenous fistula in the groin.

Capillary Permeability in Liposclerosis

At present there is no ethically acceptable, accurate method of measuring capillary permeability in the skin around a venous ulcer in man. When we found an abnormality of fibrinolysis in the patients with liposclerosis we stained further sections with phosphotungstic

TABLE 25-3.—RELATIONSHIP BETWEEN EFFICIENCY OF THE
CALF MUSCLE PUMP AND EXTRAVASCULAR FIBRIN
DEPOSITION*

	NO EXTRAVASCULAR FIBRIN (15 PATIENTS)	EXTRAVASCULAR FIBRIN (26 PATIENTS)
Mean fall of foot vein pressure during exercise (% of resting level)	55% (±20%)	7% (±18%)

* $t = 6.006$; $p < 10^{-6}$.

acid hematoxylin (PTAH) which stains fibrin, as well as myofibrils and neurofibrils, to see if there was any extravascular fibrin. Many of the biopsies with grade IV capillary proliferation had blue-staining extravascular fibrillary material extremely suggestive of fibrin. To confirm this a number of sections were incubated with fluorescent rabbit antifibrin and examined under ultraviolet light. This immuno-fluorescent technique confirmed the presence of a cuff of fibrin around many of the small capillaries in the dermis corresponding to the blue-staining material seen using PTAH.

A study was, therefore, undertaken to correlate the presence of extravascular fibrin (using the PTAH stain) with the degree of capillary proliferation and the efficiency of the calf muscle pump. Table 25-3 shows the mean reduction in venous pressure during exercise in 26 patients with extravascular fibrin deposition and 15 patients without extravascular fibrin deposition and confirms an association between the failure of the calf muscle pump and the deposition of extravascular fibrin. Table 25-4 shows the relationship between the degree of capillary proliferation and fibrin deposition. Almost all of those with extravascular fibrin had severe capillary proliferation. Thus prolonged venous hypertension appears to stimulate the development of new but abnormally permeable capillaries. We think

TABLE 25-4.—RELATIONSHIP BETWEEN EXTRAVASCULAR
FIBRIN DEPOSITION AND DERMAL CAPILLARY PROLIFERATION*

	NO EXTRAVASCULAR FIBRIN (15 PATIENTS)	EXTRAVASCULAR FIBRIN (26 PATIENTS)
Absent or minimal capillary proliferation	13	2
Moderate or severe capillary proliferation	2	24

*($\chi^2 = 25.57$; $p < 0.001$).

that the fibrinogen which leaks out of these capillaries is then converted to fibrin, probably by the extrinsic coagulation mechanism, to form an impermeable cuff in the extravascular space around the capillary.

Capillary Permeability in Experimental Venous Hypertension

To study the permeability of the capillaries that form in response to venous hypertension we implanted Guyton capsules in the hind limbs of dogs after making an arteriovenous fistula in one groin. Once the fistula had produced sustained chronic venous hypertension, various radioactively labeled molecules were injected intravenously and their rate of appearance in the capsule fluid of the affected and control legs was compared. Sodium-24 and ^{125}I-human serum albumin accumulated at the same rate and reached the same concentration in both normal and venous hypertensive legs, but radioactive fibrinogen appeared more rapidly in the capsules buried beneath the dermis of the legs with prolonged venous hypertension. By 48 hr there was a significantly higher concentration of fibrinogen in the capsule fluid of the abnormal leg. This suggests that an increased quantity of fibrinogen passes through the capillary wall in chronic venous hypertension.

The Cause of Venous Ulceration

The findings described above, namely a failure to reduce venous pressure during exercise, capillary proliferation, extravascular fibrin deposition and a reduced systemic and blood and tissue fibrinolytic activity, have led us to postulate the following hypothesis. In the first instance the normal calf pump mechanism fails because the veins are damaged by thrombosis or are congenitally abnormal. The normal reduction of superficial venous pressure during exercise is lost and the small veins and venules are repeatedly subjected to abnormally high pressures. This high pressure causes the development of multiple small new capillaries in the dermis with wide intercellular "pores" at their venular end, which allow an increased loss of large molecules from the blood into the extravascular space. Most important among these large molecules are fibrinogen and other clotting factors. Once the fibrinogen has passed through the vessel wall it comes into contact with tissue factors and is converted to fibrin.

It is highly likely that this process occurs in normal venular capillaries but the quantity of fibrin deposited outside the vessel is probably very small and it is degraded by normal tissue fibrinolytic activity and reabsorbed into the circulation directly or via the lymphatics.

In the patients with liposclerosis there is not only a high venous pressure and excessive fibrinogen loss but also *inadequate blood and tissue fibrinolysis.* Whether this is simply due to an exhaustion of fibrinolytic activity by excessive consumption of fibrin or a primary defect remains unknown. Ultimately, because the tissue fibrinolysis fails, fibrin is deposited around most of the dermal capillaries. This cuff of mature polymerized fibrin forms a barrier to the diffusion of oxygen and other nutriments into the tissues, and leads to the death of the tissues, clinically apparent as ulceration. This diffusion barrier also explains the high oxygen content found in the venous blood of the postphlebitic leg.[3]

The Treatment of the Postphlebitic Leg

If the hypothesis above is correct, the logical treatment of liposclerosis and venous ulceration is to correct the high venous pressure in order to reduce the leak of fibrinogen into the tissues and to correct any defect of fibrinolysis in order to hasten the reabsorption of extravascular fibrin. To test the relative importance of the fibrinolytic defect we treated 14 patients who had had extensive liposclerosis for many years with fibrinolytic enhancement alone. They all had a rapid and marked reduction in their area of liposclerosis during 3 months of treatment (stanozolol, 5 mg twice daily) together with a return to normal limits of their blood fibrinolytic activity. In a double-blind crossover trial currently in progress the results available to date show that the use of fibrinolytic enhancement is more effective than good elastic support, and the best improvement occurs in the second 3 months of treatment. We would suggest that good elastic stockings are effective (hardly a new observation!) because by reducing the transmural pressure in the small vessels they decrease the amount of fibrinogen leaking into the tissues. In some patients this may be all that is required, but others appear to need fibrinolytic enhancement. Six of the patients treated for 9–12 months by fibrinolytic enhancement alone have been cured. The pain, redness and thickening have completely disappeared, the tissues have become soft and even the pigmentation has slowly faded.

In our view the treatment of venous ulceration should begin by an assessment of the state of the venous pump. In particular the deep veins should be assessed by phlebography and pressure measurements to discover whether the pump can be returned to normal by surgical means. In our experience the only situation in which this can be done is when *the deep veins are normal* and the prime abnormality is incompetence of the "perforating" veins which connect the superficial and deep systems.

When the calf muscle pump can be corrected, no other treatment is required but when the valves and vessels within the deep fascia are damaged no form of surgery will produce prolonged relief. In this situation good counterpressure with elastic stockings to reduce the transmural pressure and the extravazation of fibrinogen, together with stimulation of the fibrinolytic system with drugs which enhance fibrinolysis, such as stanozolol 5 mg twice daily, will produce a worthwhile symptomatic improvement. This treatment will not increase the rate of healing of an ulcer because once the skin is lost the defect must either heal in the normal way by epithelialization from the edges of the ulcer or be covered by skin grafting, but it will produce a dramatic improvement in the state of the tissues of the lower legs and many grateful patients.

A New Physiologic Concept: "Perivascular Tissue Clearance"

These studies have led us to reconsider the role of the fibrinolytic activity that we can observe in the blood and the tissues. It is always assumed that the fibrinolytic activity in blood exists to counterbalance the coagulation mechanism. However, one only sees fibrinolysis fully activated during "flight and fright" and there is very little hard evidence to support the concept that there are multiple minor episodes of coagulation and fibrinolysis occurring within the circulation. Our studies of fibrinolysis and venous disease suggest that the blood fibrinolytic activity may be nothing more than a spillover from tissue fibrinolytic activity and that the important role of fibrinolysis is in the tissues where it keeps the pericapillary spaces clear of unwanted fibrin and perhaps other proteins. There is always a small but continuous leak of large molecules out of the venular end of the capillaries.[12] The majority of these molecules pass on into the lymphatics, but if fibrinogen is converted to fibrin it may become bound to the surrounding tissues and block diffusion through the perivascular space. Our hypothesis is that the principal physiologic function of tissue fibrinolysis is to keep the pericapillary spaces clear, therefore acting as a *perivascular tissue clearing mechanism*.

Summary

Changes that occur in skin and subcutaneous tissues of the lower leg associated with varicose veins or deep venous thrombosis are caused by an abnormality of the venous side of the circulation which is easy to demonstrate with simple physiologic tests of the calf muscle venous pump. The final event which leads to venous ulcer has never been satisfactorily explained. Although the thickened subcutaneous tissues are hard and tender and this condition is commonly termed the postphlebitic syndrome, we think this condition should be called liposclerosis. This has been investigated by us, emphasizing studies of the fibrinolytic status of the patients and capillary permeability. These studies have led to the conclusion that, when the calf muscle mechanism fails, normal reduction of venous pressure during exercise is lost. The subsequent high pressure causes development of multiple small new capillaries in the dermis. These have wide intracellular pores which allow loss of large molecules from the blood into the intravascular space. Among these molecules is fibrinogen, which is then converted to fibrin in contact with tissue factors. In patients with liposclerosis, there is inadequate blood and tissue fibrinolysis and the tough, mature, polymerized fibrin is a barrier to diffusion of oxygen and other nutrients into the tissue, thus leading to death of these tissues.

REFERENCES

1. Boyd, A. M., Jepson, R. P., Ratcliff, A. H., and Rose, S. S.: The logical management of chronic ulcers of the legs, Angiology 3:207, 1952.
2. Piulachs, P., and Vidal-Barraquer, F.: Pathogenic study of varicose veins, Angiology 4:59, 1953.
3. Fontaine, R.: Du role physiopathologique des conceux de deviation arterioveneuse ditres de sucquet dans certaines affections vasculaires, Lyon Chir. 49:506, 1952.
4. Lindmeyer, W., Lofterer, O., Mostbeck, A., and Partsch, H.: Arteriovenous shunts in primary varicosis, Vasc. Surg. 6:9, 1972.
5. Haimovici, H., Steinmann, C., and Caplan, L. G.: Role of arteriovenous anastomoses in vascular disorders of the lower extremity, Ann. Surg. 164:990, 1966.
6. Gius, J. A.: Arteriovenous anastomoses and varicose veins, Arch. Surg. 81:299, 1960.
7. Burnand, K. G., O'Donnell, T. F., Thomas, M. L., and Browse, N. L.: The relationship between post-phlebitic changes in the deep veins and results of surgical treatment of venous ulcers, Lancet 1:937, 1976.
8. Fearnley, G. R., Balmforth, G. V., and Fearnley, E.: Evidence of a diurnal fibrinolytic rhythm, with a simple method of measuring natural fibrinolysis, Clin. Sci. 16:645, 1957.
9. Astrup, T., and Mullertz, S.: The fibrin plate method for estimating fibrinolytic activity, Arch. Biochem. Biophys. 40:346, 1952.
10. Todd, A. S.: The histological localization of fibrinolysin activator, J. Pathol. Bacteriol. 78:281, 1959.
11. Browse, N. L., Gray, L., Morland, M., and Jarrett, P. E. M.: Blood and vein wall fibrinolytic activity in health and vascular disease, Br. Med. J. 1:478, 1977.
12. Landis, C. M., and Pappenheiner, J. R.: *Handbook of Physiology* (Baltimore: Williams and Wilkins, 1963).

Discussion: Chapters 23 through 25

DR. GEZA DE TAKATS: In the early thirties at Northwestern University, we tried to show, mostly with histologic methods, the enormous amount of protein and fibrin which appears in a postphlebitic leg. We also measured the protein in the experimental animal and in man. We found that this is not a simple transudate due to increase in venous pressure, but is a true exudate. We then proposed to try to get rid of the acute edema as fast as possible by maximal elevation, by bandaging and by early and massive heparinization. I am not talking only of the post-thrombotic limb. Heparinization seems to hasten the disappearance of all edema.

How this works, I don't know even today. Certainly, it is not an effect on the clot itself, not an effect on the existing fibrin. The mechanism is entirely unclear. About 6 or 8 years ago, I became very much interested in the fibrinolytic mechanism, and described a simple test which we thought measured the fibrinolytic potential of the individual.

As is perfectly well known, venous constriction, something like 60 mm of pressure held for 10 minutes, will increase fibrinolysis in the constricted extremity, and you can measure that. We have found in a certain percentage of patients, particularly postpartum and postoperative, that the line remains flat or, certainly, diminished. This is something that has to be put on a statistical basis, which I am unable to do at the age of 84.

I would like to talk about Doctor Barker's excellent presentation. We have followed his regimen, more or less. This is an ambulatory disciplinary regimen, such as Doctor Owens has described. Then, we excise perforators, which we have tried to identify not by any phlebographic method, but simply by clinical examination. We excise the large ulcers, grafting them but realizing that they do break down. There is no question that the incidence of recurrent ulceration is high. I cannot quote an exact figure, but we can always say to the patient, "It is because you didn't follow our instructions."

I would like to say a word about the causalgic state which has been of great interest to us, not only in the postphlebitic field, but elsewhere. There is no question that there is a certain group of women, many of them doctors' wives, nurses or people who have been on long-term anticoagulants, who develop a thrombophobia. This is a definite syndrome. Each time they have a little twinge in the leg, they have another clot. This is the type of individual who develops hot, burning pain which is very sensitive to heat and relieved by cold and supposed to be due to demyelinization of peripheral nerve fibers. Our results from sympathectomy have been excellent. Of course, like in any other causalgic state, you don't do an L2–L4 sympathectomy; you do an L1–L4. You have to start at T10. The reason we found this out is in two of the patients on whom we have operated, we got recurrence and continuance of pain. Paravertebral blocks and added sympathectomy stopped the pain. That occurs very, very infrequently, but when it does occur, it is a real problem.

Finally, I would like to comment on Doctor Owens' paper. He really has shown us the basis of how to take care of these patients. It is true, though, that the type of discipline which he is trying to use cannot be enforced on certain types of people. It takes a dominant personality, such as his, to tell patients how to behave and see that they really do.

It is exceedingly difficult to get patient compliance just like it is difficult to get them to use a hypertensive medication. What he is saying is that, with extensive deep valvular damage, none of our present surgical methods except those we are going to hear about very shortly show lasting improvement. The fact of the matter is that a deep valvular insufficiency with four valves gone, with high deep venous pressure which is not lowered by ambulation or by the muscle pump, is really not influenced by our present surgical methods.

DR. JOHN CRANLEY: In our experience, about 25% of the ulcers of the leg due to venous disease are considered to be due to varicose veins or superficial venous incompetence. The superficial variety is considered to be curable. After the ulcer has healed, operation is recommended. The incompetent superficial veins are extirpated as radically as possible. Following the recovery period of 2–4 weeks, the patient is discharged without the use of elastic stockings. There is no permanent swelling and the recurrence rate in this group is about 4%.

On the other hand, if the patient has chronic deep venous disease, he is told from the beginning that this is an incurable condition although it is controllable. In our experience, the postphlebitic syndrome is preventable. If the patient will wear a stocking heavy enough to prevent edema following deep venous thrombosis, the postphlebitic syndrome will not develop. If the patient has an ulcer when first examined, he is treated on an ambulatory basis with pressure bandages. After the ulcer has healed, a heavyweight elastic stocking is prescribed. The vast majority of patients can be controlled in this way. Some will stop wearing the stocking and will develop another ulcer. But this can be healed in the same way and the patient is readvised to wear elastic stockings. Approximately 10% of the patients cannot be controlled at all by this regimen and for these operation is recommended. The Linton-type operation is performed. This includes subfascial ligation of communicating veins and complete stripping of the long and short saphenous veins. Although the results are satisfactory, if the patients are followed long enough, the recurrence rate gradually rises. After approximately 15 years, the recurrence rate in our experience approaches 33%. Thus, in contrast to ulcers due to superficial venous disease, ulcers due to deep venous disease must be considered incurable, and require life-long attention.

DR. JOHN HOBBS: I fell into a trap during the last 10 years by operating on the major proximal veins in these people, often with not very good results. Looking at the postphlebitic syndrome in more detail, it is really a big problem in bad management. Inadequate methods by nurses and junior doctors and bad bandages, bad elastic stockings. The postphlebitic syndrome has two separate parts. It has the proximal venous outflow disease with obstruction or valvular damage, and it has the peripheral problem of incompetent perforating veins. They may occur together or they may occur separately. What we have heard about so far is the problem of incompetent perforating veins; later, we will hear about the proximal veins.

With true venous ulcers, there are superficial and deep vein problems. As we heard from Doctor Owens and Doctor de Takats, it is really common sense to treat these conservatively, and they do not need very clever treatment. They just need simple cleaning. Most of the agents that people put on do more harm than good. You really can spit on the ulcers and then just put on a piece of paper and a tight bandage. The essential thing is a tight bandage.

I enjoyed everything that Doctor Owens said, until he said he was against injection. Having gotten these people healed, you can find one or two veins that are the source of potential trouble. We use injection in these patients in a very restricted way. Two or three injections will keep a leg in very good shape with quite light stockings for anywhere up to 5 years. Then, we repeat injections and have lots of people that are returning every 5 years, as you saw in the random trial. One of the great things the random trial did for me was to stop me operating on the postphlebitic syndrome in the lower leg.

The most exciting thing was what you heard from Professor Browse. Two years ago, I heard of his new ideas and managed to corner one of his juniors at a surgical meeting in England. I learned about stanozolol, and could not believe what he said. Soon afterwards, I had a colleague's mother with subcutaneous fat necrosis, which goes on to scar tissue. Liposclerosis is really what it is, and she had exactly this. In the past, I treated these with firm bandaging, which may have to be on for months and months. Eventually, they do get better. This lady was going on holiday to the south of France and refused to be heavily bandaged. So, I gave her 5 mg of stanozolol, twice daily. She came back from holiday and was much better. Then she got worse, and we started the drug again, and the condition again improved.

DR. VICTOR BERNHARD: We for a long time have advised our patients to put their feet up in the air. The trouble is that they always find it is inconvenient, and they are uncooperative. So, we decided to do an end run on them and found out how to make them cooperate. One of the physical therapists who had bad venous disease joined with her husband, who is a good artist, and drew up what they thought would be a proper leg elevator. We got a commercial concern to produce it, and have given it to about 150 patients. It is convenient. It is easy. It is cleanable. You can take the cover off of it, and it can go into any kind of a bed, and it doesn't offend the individual's sleeping partner, and it does the job. It gets the feet above the head, and most people like it.

DR. J. CUTHBERT OWENS: Many of these patients are different, and that is why they fall into the causalgic group. They have wet hands, wet feet and you have to be an amateur psychiatrist with them.

The thing that Doctor Barker thought up needs emphasis. This is that failure occurs because of failure to get the patient's cooperation. A number of years ago, when I first talked on this, one of my mentors said, "Don't be like a psychiatrist and blame it on the patient."

One last thing. I would certainly look into the use of stanozolol. Not only for the postphlebitic syndrome, but also in patients who have steroid ulcers. I use heavy doses of heparin, and it clears them up. It looks to me like the stanozolol might have a possibility in that group, too.

DR. WILEY BARKER: I want to thank everyone for that which has been said. In case you think that surgical therapy is ideal and the last way to go in treating these patients, I don't. I think it works remarkably well in a few patients, considering that it is really a destructive procedure. Yet, I would like to find a way that I could count on as being consistently successful.

Maybe, in southern California, where people wear shorts and sit by the swimming pool a lot, it is a little harder to get them to wear proper elastic support. I have not been able to enlist the cooperation of patients in the way that I would like to, and in some people who seem to cooperate, I have still had failures which I have been able to treat surgically. I hope that there is some other answer to this, however, and I hope that it will come out of this program.

DR. NORMAN BROWSE: Doctor de Takats raised the $64,000 question. Is the abnormality of thrombolysis the cause or the effect? I don't know the answer to that. I find it rather difficult to imagine how a change in one leg of a person will produce changes in blood removed from an arm vein or in the tissues of a hand. I just have a feeling that, perhaps, it is a primary effect. It may also be part of the cause of the thrombosis. There is a fair bit of evidence that people who get extensive deep vein thrombosis have a deficient fibrinolytic system. The only way we will find out is to study all patients who develop thrombosis and follow them for a long time to see who gets the postphlebitic leg and who does not.

Thank you very much, Doctor Hobbs, for that unsolicited support. One is always worried when one finds something that works. For those of you who might want to think a little more, it is called stanozolol. It is an anabolic steroid. The dose is 5 mg twice daily. There are other drugs which will stimulate fibrinolysis. Many have been described, but this is one drug that is easier to administer. It is slightly androgenic. Most people put on the odd pound in weight. You have to tell them to be careful. Some women find they have a little infrequency of their periods, or occasional amenorrhea. If they have had migraine before, they may find their attacks recurring. So, it is not a drug without any complications and clearly should be used only when the patient has a serious problem in his leg. It does not have an effect on the blood before 3–4 weeks. So, the treatment must last for at least 3 months. We have a number of patients now who have been treated for between 6 and 9 months.

26 / Crossover Grafts for Iliofemoral Venous Occlusion

W. Andrew Dale, M.D.

Department of Surgery, Vanderbilt University School of Medicine, St. Thomas Hospital, and Baptist Hospital, Nashville, Tennessee

Chronic obstruction of the iliac or femoral veins may produce severe swelling of the lower extremity and even of the lower abdomen; the pain associated with this distension is often severe. The striking appearance of the syndrome is matched by the coexisting disability. Extrinsic pressure by malignant tumors account for almost half of the cases while the remainder are due to intrinsic obstruction following venous thrombosis.

Crossover shunt grafting to bypass the venous obstruction is not a frequently required surgical procedure and many physicians and surgeons are not aware of its usefulness to relieve this congestive edema and pain. Experience with 42 patients indicates that the operation is simple, does not involve great risk and offers relief in a high percentage of cases.

Experimental and Clinical Background

Grafting in the venous system dates back to the animal experiments of Carrel and Guthrie soon after the turn of the century, for which Carrel was awarded the Nobel Prize in 1912. Approximately 50 years of inactivity in this field was followed by rapid progress in vascular surgery after World War II.

Our interest was attracted to the poorly understood and chaotic field of venous grafting in 1960 and in 1962 a report was made to the Society for Vascular Surgery of 100 completed animal experiments and seven clinical cases of grafts placed in various portions of the venous system.[2] This experience was correlated with that of others and led to the proposal of four conclusions that appear applicable to venous grafting: (1) recanalization of some autogenous vein grafts following initial thrombosis, (2) dependence of graft patency upon internal pressure and flow rather than upon graft rigidity and external pressure, (3) the continued long-term patency of grafts once they remain open for several weeks and (4) the importance of delicate, precise and refined surgical technique and of practical experience in the placement of venous grafts.

The natural development of crossing collaterals in patients whose iliac veins are obstructed suggests the surgical creation of such a shunt (Fig 26–1). Palma and Esperon of Montevideo in 1958 first used a saphenous vein crossover graft to avoid dissection within the abdomen or extraperitoneal space.[10] Flores Izquierdo summarized his experience in Mexico City in 1965, indicating satisfactory results in

Fig 26–1.—Stenosis or occlusion of the iliac vein produces crossing collateral of considerable size such as these which suggested crossover grafting. This patient has pressure from the crossing iliac artery and has not been operated upon yet.

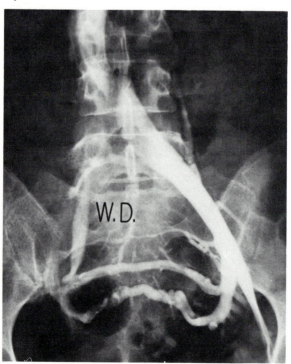

TABLE 26-1.—CAUSES OF ILIOFEMORAL VENOUS
OBSTRUCTION AMONG 42 PATIENTS

Postphlebitic	23
Extrinsic pressure of crossing iliac artery	1
Malignant tumor	
Cervix	7
Lymphoma	4
Bladder	3
Rectum	2
Prostate	1
Pancreas	1
Total	42

Fig 26–2.— Four examples of severe edema of the lower extremity treated successfully by crossover vein grafts.

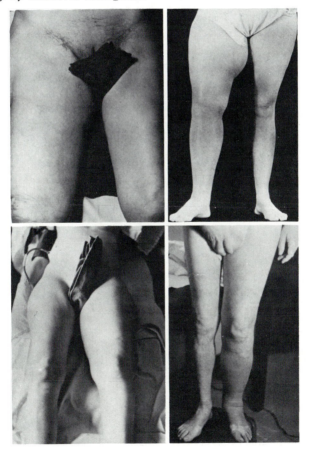

11 crossover transplants.[6] Other scattered case reports have followed.[5, 9, 11] Husni in 1971 reported his success with 30 crossover and 21 saphenous grafts to the popliteal vein, commenting upon the successful reduction of ambulatory venous hypertension.[7]

The present series was updated in 1968,[1] in 1969[4] and again in 1973.[3] Total experience has now, in 1976, reached 42 cases.

Etiology

The variety of malignant tumors which have occurred in these patients is shown in Table 26–1 and indicates a careful search for such whenever an elderly individual develops a massively swollen extremity without an immediately evident cause (Fig 26–2). Among all patients there were 18 (43%) with malignant tumors, but if patients over 50 years only are considered, the incidence of malignant tumors was 65%.

Plan of Management

The general plan of diagnosis and therapy outlined in Table 26–2 was followed with necessary individual modifications. The search for tumor may even require laparotomy or retroperitoneal exploration to establish a diagnosis and obtain tissue for microscopic analysis. Such exploration can be done as an immediate preliminary to a crossover venous shunt.

Phlebography

A variety of methods of opacification of the iliofemoral venous system and of the inferior vena cava are now available (Fig 26–3) and

TABLE 26–2.—PLAN OF MANAGEMENT OF CHRONIC
ILIOFEMORAL VENOUS OCCLUSION

1. Diagnosis: tumor or phlebitis? Examination—includes
   pelvic and rectal
   Visceral x-ray—intravenous pyelogram, barium enema
   Cystoscopy, sigmoidoscopy
   Exploration—laparotomy or retroperitoneal
2. Delineation of venous block by phlebography:
   Site and extent
   Contralateral patency
3. Treatment: Crossover vein graft if:
   a. Venous thrombosis is stable and nonrecanalized
   b. Tumor with life expectancy over 6 months

PHLEBOGRAPHY

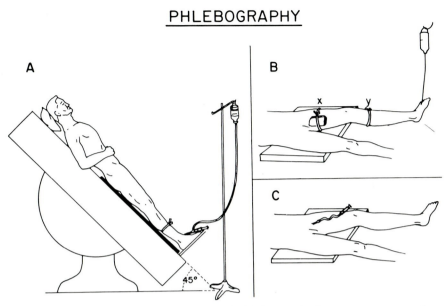

Fig 26–3. – **A,** the standard method of phlebography by injection into a foot or ankle vein may not visualize the proximal veins within the pelvis. **B,** with the patient lying flat across the x-ray changer the radiopaque material may be pooled in the thigh distal to a very tight tourniquet at *x* until its sudden release allows it to fill the iliofemoral system as the films are rapidly changed. **C,** direct needle or catheter injection into the femoral vein should be proceeded by distal injection to ascertain that there is not fresh clot lying at the intended point of injection.

details are not discussed again here.[8] The entire venous system of the involved extremity must be opacified to delineate areas of patency versus occlusion (Fig 26–4). This is often possible by injection at the ankle or foot level if the dye is pooled distal to a tourniquet prior to sudden release or if it is pooled in the dependent extremity which is later elevated. A more direct way of opacification of the iliofemoral system is by needle or catheter injection directly into the common femoral vein. This is not always possible because this vein may be occluded. It also may have some risk if there should be a fresh thrombus in the area so that it is generally preferable to place the radiopaque material more distally.

A contralateral phlebogram is also made to determine the suitability of the saphenous vein on the other side as well as the patency of that iliofemoral venous system.

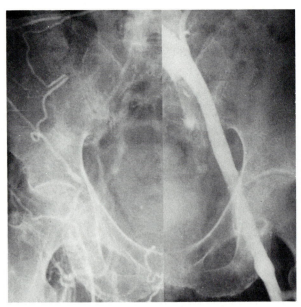

Fig 26–4.—Phlebogram demonstrating completely occluded right ilio-femoral venous system due to direct extension of carcinoma of the rectum. The left iliofemoral venous system was patent so that a successful crossover graft was possible. The patient who had been completely incapacitated by severe edema was immediately relieved and able to walk.

Technique of Operation

The crossover saphenous vein graft is a simple operation confined to the subcutaneous tissues of the upper thighs and suprapubic region (Fig 26 – 5) and can ordinarily be done under low spinal anesthesia in 1.5 – 2 hr. If laparotomy or retroperitoneal exploration is required for diagnosis or to obtain tissue for examination, this should be completed first. Instruments and gloves should be discarded to prevent tumor implantations into the thigh wounds; the wound is covered and new drapes are applied.

Initially the symptomatic thigh is explored through a longitudinal femoral approach so that the patent femoral vein peripheral to the obstructed segment may be exposed. Dissection of the edematous thigh first permits oozing to subside and firm clotting to occur.

The contralateral saphenous vein is carefully dissected and its tributaries are tied with 4-0 silk to a distal point where measurement indicates that sufficient length for the crossover graft has been obtained. The vein is cut across caudally, flushed and forcibly distended from that end with heparinized saline. A bulldog serrefine clamp is placed

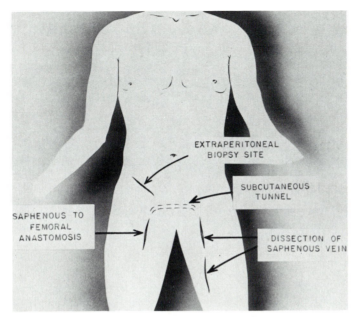

Fig 26–5. — Sites of the incisions for tumor biopsy as well as for the crossover vein graft.

at the saphenofemoral junction to prevent reflux during subsequent manipulation. A second bulldog clamp is placed at the cut end of the vein to keep it distended with heparin solution. This helps prevent accidental rotation of the graft when it is placed in its subcutaneous tunnel.

A sterile sigmoidoscope or vascular tunneler is pushed across the suprapubic space in the fatty subcutaneous tissue to connect the two thigh incisions, and through this tunnel is led a long clamp to seize the end of the saphenous vein for transplantation across the suprapubic region.

When all oozing has been controlled and the dissection is finished, 5,000 units of aqueous heparin is administered intravenously to discourage clotting during the period of venous occlusion.

In the earliest operations vascular clamps were placed completely across the femoral vein during the anastomosis. More recently a U-shaped clamp (Fig 26–6) has been obtained so that the femoral vein does not require elevation from its bed, and it has been only side-clamped during the anastomosis. The handle of this U-shaped clamp is angled sharply away from the jaw to allow it to lie flat on the skin and out of the way during subsequent anastomosis.

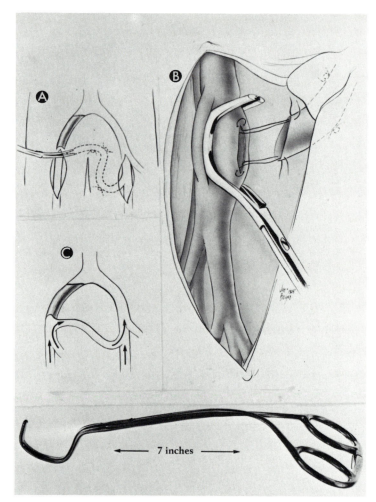

7 inches

Fig 26–6. — Crossover vein grafting is performed by dissecting the saphenous vein from the normal side and passing it across the tunnel and suprapubic fat. A special vascular clamp occludes the common femoral vein during the anastomosis. Postoperatively blood flows through the graft across into the patent iliac vein and bypasses the obstruction.

An end-to-side venous anastomosis emphasizing an opening about 3 times the diameter of the saphenous vein is constructed with continuous 6-0 Dacron. It has not ordinarily been necessary to use the heparin antidote protamine following clamp removal. The wounds have been closed primarily. No anticoagulant therapy has been used in the postoperative period.

Technical points for emphasis include prevention of axial twisting of the vein transplant, insuring that the anastomotic sutures do not narrow the attached orifice of the saphenous vein and creation of a large anastomotic stoma. After anastomosis the low-pressure venous blood does not balloon the graft in the same way as when an autogenous vein is placed in the arterial system. Blood flow is not ordinarily visible without temporary occlusion of portions of the graft.

Results

Only 6 of the 42 total patients failed to obtain any relief at all from the crossover graft. The overall results are shown in Table 26–3.

The longest follow-up in the series is a man recently seen 11 years following operation whose crossover vein graft was dilated and obviously carrying much blood because it was easily palpable throughout its entire length across the suprapubic space. The patient had been completely rehabilitated by the operation. The shortest follow-up is a patient at 6 months.

Some of the postphlebitic patients did retain some degree of edema which required stocking support but the operation appeared to relieve pressure to the extent that they no longer felt tightness and pain due to venous hypertension in the groin and thigh.

The cancer patients were particularly benefited and their relief was often dramatic, even to the extent that patients who were essentially bedridden by severe thigh edema with pain became ambulatory within 24 hr.

There were no deaths due to the operation. The only complications were a single hematoma and a seroma of the donor thigh site.

Conclusions

Crossover saphenous shunt grafting is a simple, safe and usually effective operation designed to relieve the edema and pain of chronic

TABLE 26–3.—RESULTS OF 42 CROSSOVER
VEIN GRAFTS

	TUMOR	POST-PHLEBITIC	TOTAL NO.
Complete relief	12	10	22
Partial relief	4	10	14
No relief	3	3	6
Total	19	23	42

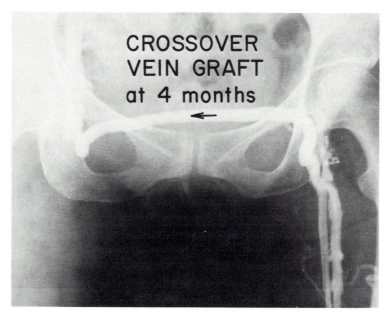

Fig 26–7. — Patent crossover vein graft 4 months after operation.

iliac and/or femoral venous obstruction due to tumor or venous thrombosis. Twenty-two of our 42 patients were afforded complete relief and 14 others partial relief of symptoms with minimal operative complications and no deaths. Wider use of this procedure by other surgeons is merited.

REFERENCES

1. Dale, W. A., and Harris, J.: Cross-over vein grafts for venous occlusion, Ann. Surg. 168:319, 1968.
2. Dale, W. A.: *Graft Replacement of the Venous System: Fundamentals of Vascular Grafting* (New York: McGraw-Hill Book Company, Inc., 1963).
3. Dale, W. A.: The Swollen Leg, in Ravitch, M. M. (ed.): *Current Problems in Surgery* (Chicago: Year Book Medical Publishers, Inc., Sept. 1973).
4. Dale, W. A., and Harris, J.: Cross-over vein grafts for iliac and femoral venous occlusion, J. Cardiovasc. Surg. 10:458, 1969.
5. DeWeese, J. A.: Discussion, Arch. Surg. 95:833, 1967.
6. Izquierdo, G. Flores: Homologous vein transplants, surgical treatment of the post-phlebitic sequelae, J. Cardiovasc. Surg. 6:188, 1965.
7. Husni, E. A.: The post-phlebitic limb, Hosp. Med. 7:73, 1971.
8. Lewis, M. R., and Dale, W. A.: Phlebography as a clinical tool, Surg. Gynecol. Obstet. 133:301, 1971.
9. Nolan, T. R.: Discussion, Arch. Surg. 95:833, 1967.
10. Palma, E. C., and Esperon, R.: Vein transplants and grafts in the surgical treatment of the post-phlebitic syndrome, J. Cardiovasc. Surg. 1:94, 1960.
11. Taylor, R. S.: Personal communication, 1965.

27 / Iliofemoral Venous Thrombectomy

JAMES A. DEWEESE, M.D.

The University of Rochester Medical Center, Division of Cardiothoracic Surgery, Rochester, New York

THROMBOSIS OF THE ILIAC and femoral veins results in a striking clinical picture. The immediate effect is a massive painful swelling of the entire leg. If the leg is pale the condition may be called phlegmasia alba dolens. If there is a reddish blue appearance the term phlegmasia cerulea dolens very appropriately describes the massively swollen, cyanotic painful extremity.

The swelling is secondary to the thrombotic occlusion of the iliac vein with marked increases in the distal venous pressures which have been observed as high as 115 cm of H_2O or approximately 10 times normal.[9] The waxy appearance of alba dolens can best be attributed to the distention of the skin by the marked edema. Vasospasm may be present and could also explain pallor in some patients. The bluish discoloration of cerulea dolens is secondary to distention of the veins and venules. The extremity may be pale in the horizontal position but become cyanotic in the dependent position when the venous pressure increases.

The thrombus in the iliac vein could ascend from distal veins or originate in the pelvis. Thrombi occur most frequently in the calf veins, which has been documented in pathologic studies and more recently by radioactive iodinated fibrinogen scans.[20] On the basis of phlebographic observations of propagation of thrombosis from calf to femoral vein in one patient, Bauer postulated that iliac vein thrombosis routinely began in the calf.[2, 29] It should be noted, however, that Bauer's technique of phlebography was precisely designed to visualize the calf and femoral vein and not the iliac vein. Studies which include iliac phlebograms and observation of thrombectomy operations indicate that iliofemoral venous thrombosis most frequently begins proximally and then propagates distally (Fig 27 – 1).[9, 29]

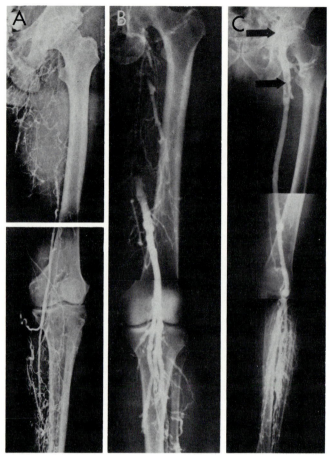

Fig 27–1.—Patterns of iliofemoral venous thrombosis. **A,** phlebogram demonstrating extensive thrombosis of calf and iliac veins. All major veins are occluded and only collateral veins are visualized. **B,** phlebogram demonstrating thrombosis of iliac and femoral veins with only collateral veins seen in thigh and pelvis. The popliteal and calf veins appear normal. **C,** phlebogram showing thrombosis of iliac veins, large thrombi in common femoral veins *(lower arrow)*, and normal femoral, popliteal and calf veins. (From Haimovici, H. [ed.]: *Vascular Surgery Principles and Techniques* [New York: McGraw-Hill Book Co., 1976], Chapter 51. Used by permission.)

There are several reasons for thrombi to originate proximally. The most common cause is probably the presence of congenital or acquired stenotic lesions of the left common iliac vein where it is crossed by the right common iliac artery.[3, 30] The importance of these lesions as a cause of iliofemoral venous thrombosis is supported by the fact that in almost all reports the left leg is affected two to three times as often as the right. Compression of the common femoral vein by the inguinal ligament or the femoral vein by the adductor magnus tendon may explain why thrombosis has been observed to originate from these sites.[31] Pelvic venous thrombosis may easily spread directly to the internal and common iliac veins. Thrombi may also propagate from the greater saphenous to the femoral veins.[9, 16]

Thrombi may embolize from the iliofemoral venous segment to the pulmonary arteries. Since a massive fatal embolus usually requires at least a 50% occlusion of the pulmonary arteries, it is easily understood that the iliofemoral venous segment is more frequently the site of a fatal embolus than the smaller calf veins. For example, Mavor and Galloway observed that of 113 patients with pulmonary emboli originating in the iliofemoral venous segment, 7 died whereas of 33 patients with emboli from the calf veins none died.[29]

Patients with iliofemoral venous thrombosis may have such extensive distal propagation of thrombi that gangrene results. Although arterial spasm has been suggested as the reason for the gangrene, the cause is undoubtedly thrombotic venous occlusion sufficient to present arterial inflow to the periphery. Once gangrene is established the outcome is a loss of limb or life.

Veins occluded by thrombi may remain occluded with fibrous tissue invasion and microscopic recanalization or the clot may contract and become adherent to the wall of the vein. The pathologic changes have been documented by phlebography.[2, 25] During the healing phase swelling and pain may be disabling for several weeks until collaterals or restitution of venous patency occurs. There is good evidence that unless restoration of patency occurs within the first several days that occlusion of the vein persists and that functional "recanalization does not occur".[29] Either form of healing results in veins without valves.[11] Venous valvular insufficiency results in the post-thrombotic syndrome of edema, secondary varicosities, brawny induration, brownish discoloration and ulceration. These changes develop slowly. Bauer followed a group of patients with proven deep venous thrombosis for several years. Ulcers developed in 20% of the patients within 5 years, in 52% within 10 years and in 79% at a later date.[2]

Since the thrombus is the reason for all of the possible consequences of iliofemoral venous thrombosis, a successful thrombectomy would be of great advantage to the patient. The early morbidity of pain and swelling could be relieved. Pulmonary embolism and venous gangrene could be avoided. The late morbidity of the post-thrombotic syndrome could be prevented.

Historical Background

Lawen in 1938 described the "ideal" venous thrombectomy.[24] He stressed the importance of suturing the venotomy without ligation of any major veins to restore normal venous circulation. de Takats in 1940 described an iliac thrombectomy performed through the greater saphenous vein which was then ligated flush with the femoral vein.[5] More extensive experiences with thrombectomies were reported by Mahorner et al. and by Fontaine in 1957[14, 26] who emphasized the advantage of postoperative anticoagulants. Mavor introduced us to the procedure in 1956 and our early experiences were reported in 1960.[9] Haller enthusiastically reported a good experience with 45 procedures in 1963[17]; Lansing et al. reported discouraging 5-year follow-up on many of Haller's patients.[23] These and other reports dampened the enthusiasm of many for performing thrombectomy. Subsequent reports by Edwards, Mavor and ourselves, however, indicate that thrombectomy has a place in the management of some patients with iliofemoral venous thrombosis.[7, 8, 12, 29]

Preoperative Management

The diagnosis and extent of thrombosis should be confirmed by a phlebogram prior to thrombectomy[10] (see Fig 27–1). An acute lymphedema or cellulitis can mimic an iliofemoral venous thrombosis and negative explorations of the femoral veins because of mistaken diagnoses have been reported.[32] Femoral thrombectomies as opposed to iliofemoral venous thrombectomies have rarely been successful in our and others' experiences and thrombectomy should be avoided if the iliac vein is not involved.[19] A knowledge of the amount of thrombus in the calf and popliteal arteries can be demonstrated by phlebography and dictates how aggressive one must be in exploring these distal veins.

A central venous pressure line or Swan-Ganz catheter and urinary catheter should be inserted for monitoring of fluid balance. Patients with sudden onset of their venous occlusion and resultant edema may sequester large amounts of fluid in their extremity and require considerable amounts of fluid.

The foot of the bed should be elevated to at least 20 degrees from the horizontal to increase venous drainage from the legs.

Intravenous heparin should be administered in doses of 5,000 to 10,000 units every 4 hr until the operation is performed.

Blood which has been cross-matched must be available. Average blood losses of 1,000 to 1,500 ml have been reported.[19, 23]

Operative Technique

The entire leg, lower abdomen and opposite groin are prepared. Local anesthesia is preferred. The leg is draped with a sterile stockinette so it can be manipulated during the operation.

The incision is a hockey-stick incision beginning superior and parallel to the inguinal ligament with its midpoint one finger-breadth lateral to the pubic tubercle and extended distally along the course of the vessels. Heparin is administered intravenous in a 5,000-unit amount.

The common femoral, superficial femoral and deep femoral veins are completely visualized. All branches are controlled with tapes. It is the author's observation that the posterior branches are most frequently neglected and are the source of unnecessary blood loss.[7]

A longitudinal venotomy is made and stay sutures are placed in the side of the venotomy to avoid repeated handling of the vein edges with forceps (Fig 27–2, A). Thrombus present in the vein is gently extracted with ring forceps.

A large Fogarty catheter is inserted carefully into the iliac vein until its tip is in the vena cava. Fogarty recommends that a second catheter be introduced into the vena cava from the opposite femoral vein to prevent the clot from being pushed into the vena cava by the catheter. We share others' feelings that this is unnecessary and traumatic to the opposite vein.[12, 13] The balloon on the tip of the catheter is inflated and withdrawn resulting in thrombus being extruded from the venotomy (Fig 27–2, B).

The completeness of the iliac thrombectomy cannot be determined by backflow. Approximately 80% of patients have a competent valve in the iliac vein above the inguinal ligament preventing backflow. Conversely, patients with continual obstruction of the common iliac vein may still have excellent backflow from the internal iliac or iliolumbar veins. The only reliable way of determining patency of the thrombectomy is a phlebogram performed by injecting a contrast ma-

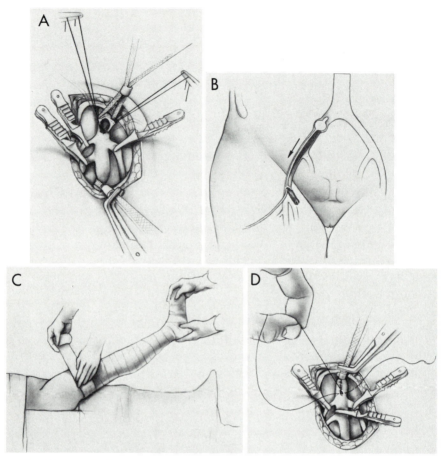

Fig 27–2.—Technique of iliofemoral venous thrombectomy. **A,** common femoral, deep femoral and greater saphenous veins are occluded with tapes and a longitudinal venotomy is performed. **B,** a Fogarty catheter is passed into the vena cava, the balloon is inflated and the catheter is withdrawn. **C,** the leg is elevated and a tight elastic bandage is wound around the foot, calf and thigh to extrude clot from the venotomy. **D,** patency of the iliac vein is determined by a phlebogram and the venotomy is closed. (From Haimovici, H. [ed.]: *Vascular Surgery Principles and Techniques* [New York: McGraw-Hill Book Co., 1976], Chapter 51. Used by permission.)

terial directly into the femoral vein through a soft catheter (Fig 27–3, B). If it is not possible to remove the older thrombus from the iliac vein a direct exploration of the vein is not advised.[9]

Clots in the calf and thigh are best removed by elevating the leg and wrapping an elastic bandage snugly around the leg from the foot to the

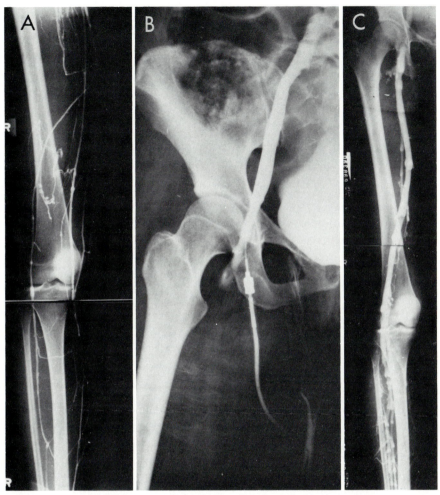

Fig 27–3.–Phlebographic control of venous thrombectomy. **A,** preoperative phlebogram demonstrates extensive thrombosis with occlusion of all major veins. **B,** operative phlebogram after thrombectomy demonstrates patent iliac vein. **C,** postoperative phlebogram demonstrates patency of femoral, popliteal and calf veins. Valves are visible in all veins. (From Haimovici, H. [ed.]: *Vascular Surgery Principles and Techniques* [New York: McGraw-Hill Book Co., 1976], Chapter 51. Used by permission.)

groin to extrude clot from the femoral venotomy (see Fig 27–2, C). It is also occasionally possible to thread a Fogarty catheter through the valves in the femoral vein to remove clots from the thigh and calf veins.

The venotomy is then closed with fine vascular sutures (see Fig 27–2, D). The patient is given 5,000 units of concentrated aqueous heparin (20,000 units/ml) into the deep fat of the abdominal wall every 12 hr for 2 days and then heparin is administered intravenously to maintain partial thromboplastin times or whole blood clotting time about two times normal for 7 days. Warfarin is begun on the 4th day and prothrombin times 2–2.5 times normal are maintained for at least 6 weeks.

The patient is ambulated to walk but not to sit in snug elastic stockings beginning the first postoperative day.

Ascending phlebograms are obtained prior to discharge from the hospital. (see Fig 27–3, C).

Results

There is general agreement that the initial results of the operative management of venous thrombectomy achieve their goal of rapidly relieving the early morbidity of swelling and pain in patients with iliofemoral venous thrombosis. It must be admitted, however, that bed rest with the marked elevation of the legs and heparin anticoagulation may also provide rapid improvement. Objective evaluation of thrombectomy requires the performance of phlebograms within the first few weeks after operation. Preferably these films should be compared with preoperative and operative studies. Mavor and Galloway obtained iliac phlebograms immediately after and within 14 days following 67 thrombectomies performed with Fogarty catheters.[29] It was possible to remove all of the thrombus from iliac vein in 42 of 67 extremities (62%) as demonstrated by an immediate phlebogram showing complete clearance. Complete clearance was again demonstrated within 14 days in 36 of 42 extremities (85%). The 25 phlebograms which demonstrated partial clearance intraoperatively remained unchanged in 17 extremities (68%) when restudied within 14 days.[29] Unfortunately, phlebography of the femoral, popliteal and calf veins were not reported. Harris and Brown reported restoration of patency in early postoperative phlebograms in 15 of 17 patients following thrombectomy.[18] Although some residual nonobstructing thrombi are visible in their phlebograms, patency of the major veins of the iliac, femoral and calf veins and some valves are well demonstrated. They attribute their success to persistence in clearing iliac, femoral and popliteal veins with Fogarty catheters. Barner et al.[1] performed phlebograms within three weeks following thrombectomy in seven patients and noted extensive thrombosis in five of seven extremities. Karp and Wylie found phlebographic evidence of extensive thrombosis in eight of eight extremities prior to discharge from the hospital.[21] No mention of preoperative or intraoperative phlebograms is made in either of these reports and only elastic compression was used to clear the distal veins of thrombi. We have had the opportunity to perform phlebograms on 21 extremities within 6 weeks following thrombectomy. The phlebograms demonstrated patent veins with visible valves in the major veins of three extremities, patency of most veins known to be clotted preoperatively in six extremities, patency of some veins but with residual or new thrombosis in seven extremities and thrombosis equal or greater than that seen preoperatively in five extremities.[8]

Thrombectomy has been advocated most frequently for the prevention of the late morbidity of the post-thrombotic syndrome. There are several clinical reports including late follow-up but there are only a few which include objective evaluation with phlebograms. Mavor and Galloway evaluated 23 extremities 3 months to 5 years following Fogarty catheter thrombectomies. The iliac vein appeared normal in 11 or 48% of the cases. There were eight of these extremities which were asymptomatic and appeared normal. There were three patients who had minimal symptoms of leg discomfort but no swelling. Phlebograms demonstrated obstruction of a portion of the iliac vein with direct collaterals such as ascending lumbar veins or venae comitantes. Three of these extremities were normal and four produced minimal symptoms. The iliac vein remained occluded in another five extremities and there were large crossover collaterals to the opposite iliac vein. One extremity produced minimal symptoms and four demonstrated persistent swelling and symptoms. Eighteen of the 23 (78%) produced minimal or no symptoms and were asymptomatic. Unfortunately, phlebograms of the thigh and calf veins were not reported.[29] Barner et al. obtained phlebograms on 10 extremities 16 to 102 months following thrombectomy. One extremity demonstrated normal calf, femoral and iliac veins and the patient was asymptomatic. There were six extremities with at least one of the distal venous segments (calf, popliteal or femoral) patent. These extremities demonstrated minimal edema with or without elastic support and were considered to have a good result. Preoperative or intraoperative films were not available for comparison so the degree of improvement cannot be evaluated. Seven of the 10 (70%) did have good or excellent results.[1] Johansson et al.

performed phlebograms on 14 extremities 6–24 months following Fogarty catheter thrombectomies without intraoperative phlebograms. Three of the 14 extremities demonstrated patent iliofemoral segments but more peripheral valvular damage was observed.[19] Lansing and Davis performed phlebograms on 15 patients 5 years after thrombectomy of which 14 demonstrated significant edema and wore elastic support. Only popliteal and femoral veins were visualized and their published phlebograms show patency of the femoral vein in three of five extremities. Valves were not demonstrated but the films were taken with the patient supine. The radiopaque contrast materials are heavier than blood and valve cusps may not be demonstrated unless the patient is in the semierect position.[23] We have performed late phlebograms on 12 extremities 2 months to 5 years after thrombectomy. Five of these were performed on patients with ideal results who were asymptomatic and had normal appearing limbs. The phlebograms demonstrated patent veins with visible valves (Fig 27–4). Four of the patients with minimal edema demonstrated patency of most major veins with some valves present. Three of the patients had significant symptoms and edema and occluded or recanalized veins were seen. Evaluation of 50 patients by clinical criteria and phlebograms in 27 of them indicated that about one third had a very good to excellent result with minimal or no edema, another third were significantly improved but demonstrated some edema and one third were not improved by the operation.[6, 8]

There is a paucity of reports comparing operative and nonoperative management of iliofemoral venous thrombosis. Matsubara et al. did compare the results 6 months or more following thrombectomy operations in 18 extremities with 82 extremities treated with elevation and heparin. Thirty-four per cent of the patients treated without operation as compared to 67% of the patients operated upon were either asymptomatic or experienced slight edema on prolonged standing or walking.[28] Results of operative treatment of 13 extremities were compared to the nonoperative management of 14 extremities during our early experience with thrombectomy. Early morbidity but not late morbidity was decreased by thrombectomy in that group of patients and was related to the selection of cases for thrombectomy.[9]

There are several factors which may influence the result of the operation other than the actual surgical technique. These include age of the thrombosis, associated pelvic disease and ability of the patients to ambulate. Several reports have emphasized that the results of thrombectomy are better the earlier the operation is performed following onset of symptoms. Results have been compared between thrombec-

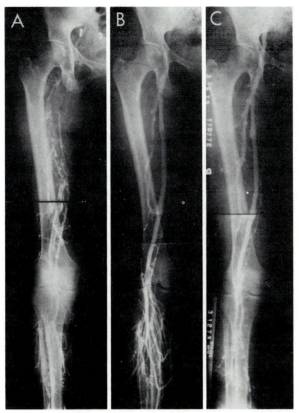

Fig 27–4.—Late phlebographic result of venous thrombectomy. **A,** pre-operative phlebogram demonstrating extensive iliofemoral venous thrombosis; large clots are visible in the popliteal vein. **B,** phlebogram 5 months after venous thrombectomy showing all major veins to be present with valves clearly seen. **C,** phlebogram 8 years later demonstrated continued patency of veins with visible valves.

tomies performed after and before 5 days, 10 days, 2 weeks and 4 weeks.[12, 17, 27, 28, 32] These results unfortunately do not provide the answer to the often asked question, "When is it too late to do a thrombectomy?" Pathologic studies indicate that thrombi become quite organized and adherent to the intima within 1 week. These observations and our own experiences have led us to not recommend thrombectomy if the symptoms have been present for more than 7 days. Pelvic disease may be responsible for the onset of the venous thrombosis and may also be responsible for rethrombosis following successful thrombectomy. Mahorner observed poor results following operations in patients with pelvic malignancies.[27] We observed rethrombosis in patients with pelvic inflammatory processes and feel that pelvic diseases are contraindication to thrombectomy.[9] Patients immobilized in bed or in casts are prone to development of venous thrombosis and continued immobilization following thrombectomy leaves them prone to rethrombosis. Harris and Brown observed rethrombosis in two patients unable to ambulate and we would agree with them that thrombectomy best not be performed unless the patient is able to actively ambulate following operation.[18]

Thrombectomy has been combined with interruption of the vena cava or femoral veins. Mahorner observed that in eight patients with associated ligation of the inferior vena cava the clinical results were excellent in three, good in two and poor in three. He compared these results with those seen in seven patients without ligation where six were excellent and one was good.[27] Mahorner cites similar observations by Fogarty who observed excellent immediate results in 19 of 21 extremities following primary venous thrombectomy as compared to excellent results in seven of 12 extremities following thrombectomy and vena caval plication.[27] Edwards et al. performed thrombectomy and vena cava ligation on three patients who developed venous thrombosis in their opposite leg within 11 months. Fontaine compared the clinical results of 48 pure thrombectomies with 48 thrombectomies plus phlebectomies and concluded that thrombectomy alone gave the best short- and long-term results.[15] Cranley et al. compared thrombectomy and vena caval ligation to vena caval ligation alone and found little difference in the long-term results of the two procedures.[4] Mavor and Galloway observed better long-term results in 83 extremities following thrombectomy alone than those in 76 extremities in which the femoral vein was also ligated.[29]

Complications

Despite a frequently expressed fear, pulmonary embolism rarely occurs during thrombectomy. Mavor observed two positive fatal pulmonary emboli during operations in 228 patients.[29] Kitainik reported two intraoperative pulmonary emboli of which one was fatal.[22] Operative manipulation did not result in pulmonary embolism in several reported series including 70 cases of Barner et al., 45 cases of Smith, 50 cases of DeWeese et al. and 106 cases of Mahorner.[2, 8, 27, 32]

Pulmonary embolism in the postoperative period has usually been reported to occur following 2–8% of thrombectomies.[1, 8, 22, 23, 27, 32]

Mavor observed a 5% incidence of pulmonary embolism following thrombectomy if the iliac phlebogram demonstrated complete clearance and a 23% incidence of emboli if there was only partial clearance. These studies suggest that emboli can be attributed to either an incomplete thrombectomy or rethrombosis. Mavor observed postoperative recurrent nonfatal embolism in 19% and fatal embolism in 6% of 109 patients who had pulmonary embolism prior to thrombectomy. Nonfatal emboli occurred in 3% and no fatal emboli occurred in 119 patients without preoperative embolism.[29]

Death following thrombectomy usually was related to the condition for which the patient was admitted to the hospital and was also responsible for the complication of venous thrombosis. Mahorner observed seven deaths in 106 patients only two of which were attributable to pulmonary emboli, with death occurring 7 days and 25 days after operation.[27] Mavor observed 9 deaths in 228 patients. Two deaths occurred from pulmonary emboli related to operation and five deaths from pulmonary emboli occurred following an incomplete or failed thrombectomy.[29] Barner observed 12 deaths within 30 days following thrombectomy in 70 patients, only one of which was due to pulmonary embolism.[1] Lansing reported five deaths following operations on 39 patients, two of which were from pulmonary embolism.[23]

Summary

Since thrombosis of the iliac and femoral veins is responsible for consequences of such venous occlusion, a successful thrombectomy could prevent the early morbidity of pain and swelling, prevent pulmonary embolism, and the late morbidity of post-thrombotic venous stasis disease. The diagnosis should be confirmed by phlebography prior to thrombectomy. The operation is performed through a longitudinal venotomy with the patient anticoagulated with intravenous heparin. Large Fogarty catheter manipulations and intraoperative phlebography confirms the adequacy of proximal thrombectomy. Distal clots are best removed by elevating the leg and wrapping an elastic bandage snugly from foot to groin. Subcutaneous heparinization is used for the first 48 hr postoperatively, when intravenous heparin is begun and this is continued for 7 days. Warfarin is begun on the fourth day and the prothrombin time is maintained at 2 to 2.5 times normal for 6 weeks. Objective evaluation of thrombectomy requires performance of phlebograms within the first few weeks after operation. Late evaluation of patients by clinical criteria and phlebography indicates that one third have very good to excellent results, another third are significantly improved, and one third are not improved by the operation.

REFERENCES

1. Barner, H. B., Willman, V. L., Kaiser, G. C., and Hanlon, C. R.: Thrombectomy for iliofemoral venous thrombosis, JAMA 208:2442, 1969.
2. Bauer, G.: A roentgenological and clinical study of the sequels of thrombosis, Acta Chir. Scand. 86:Suppl.74:104, 1942.
3. Cockett, F. B., Thomas, M. L., and Negus, D.: Iliac vein compression—Its relation to iliofemoral thrombosis and the post-thrombotic syndrome, Br. Med. J. 2:14, 1967.
4. Cranley, J. J., Krause, R. J., Strasser, E. S., and Hafner, C. D.: Femoroiliac thrombophlebitis: Immediate and late results after thrombectomy, caval ligation and conservative management, J. Cardiovasc. Surg. 10:463, 1969.
5. de Takats, G., and Jesser, J. H.: Pulmonary embolism suggestions for its diagnosis, prevention and management, JAMA 114:1415, 1940.
6. DeWeese, J. A.: Thrombectomy for acute iliofemoral venous thrombosis, J. Cardiovasc. Surg. 5:703, 1964.
7. DeWeese, J. A., and Adams, J. T.: Iliofemoral Venous Thrombectomy, in Haimovici, H. (ed.): Vascular Surgery Principles and Techniques (New York: McGraw-Hill Book Co., 1976).
8. DeWeese, J.A., Adams, J.T., and Rogoff, S.M.: Restoration and maintenance of venous patency in venous thrombosis: Anticoagulation, thrombectomy and venous interruption, Pac. Med. Surg. 75:77, 1967.
9. DeWeese, J. A., Jones, T. I., Lyon, J., and Dale, W. A.: Evaluation of thrombectomy in the management of iliofemoral venous thrombosis, Surgery 47:140, 1960.
10. DeWeese, J. A., and Rogoff, S. M.: Phlebographic patterns of acute deep venous thrombosis of the leg, Surgery 53:99, 1963.
11. Edwards, E. A., and Edwards, J. E.: The effect of thrombophlebitis on the venous valve, Surg. Gynecol. Obstet. 65:310, 1937.
12. Edwards, W. H., Sawyers, J. L., and Foster, J. L.: Iliofemoral venous thrombosis: Reappraisal of thrombectomy, Ann. Surg. 171:961, 1970.
13. Fogarty, T. J., Dennis, D., and Krippaehne, W. W.: Surgical management of iliofemoral venous thrombosis, Am. J. Surg. 112:211, 1966.
14. Fontaine, R.: Remarks concerning venous thrombosis and its sequelae, Surgery 41:6, 1957.
15. Fontaine, R., Tuchmann, L., and Suhler, A.: Surgical treatment of deep and recent venous thromboses. Its role, methods and results, J. Cardiovasc. Surg., Spec. Suppl.:174, 1966.
16. Glover, W. J., Vaughn, A. M., and Caserta, J. A.: Venous thrombectomy in the management of acute venous thrombosis of the saphenous system, Am. J. Surg. 93:798, 1957.
17. Haller, J. A., and Abrams, B. L.: Use of thrombectomy in the treatment of acute iliofemoral venous thrombosis in forty-five patients, Ann. Surg. 158:561, 1963.
18. Harris, E. J., and Brown, W. H.: Patency after thrombectomy for iliofemoral thrombosis, Ann. Surg. 167:91, 1968.
19. Johansson, E., Nordlander, S., and Zetterquist, S.: Venous thrombectomy in the lower extremity—Clinical, phlebographic and plethysmographic evaluation of early and late results, Acta Chir. Scand. 139:511, 1973.
20. Kakkar, V.: The diagnosis of deep vein thrombosis using the ^{125}I-fibrinogen test, Arch. Surg. 104:152, 1972.
21. Karp, R. B., and Wylie, E. J.: Recurrent thrombosis after iliofemoral venous thrombectomy, Surg. Forum 17:147, 1966.

22. Kitainik, E., and Quiros, R. S.: Thrombectomy and caval interruption. Indications and results, J. Cardiovasc. Surg. 13:440, 1972.
23. Lansing, A. M., and Davis, W. M.: Five-year follow-up study of iliofemoral venous thrombectomy, Ann. Surg. 168:620, 1968.
24. Lawen, A.: Weitere Erfahrungen über operativ Thrombenentfernung bei Venenthrombose, Arch. Klin. Chir. 193:723, 1938.
25. Lipchik, E. O., DeWeese, J. A., and Rogoff, S. M.: Serial long-term phlebography after documented lower leg thrombosis, Radiology 120:563, 1976.
26. Mahorner, H., Castleberry, J. W., and Coleman, W. O.: Attempts to restore function in major veins which are the site of massive thrombosis, Ann. Surg. 146:510, 1957.
27. Mahorner, H.: Results of surgical operations for venous thrombosis, Surg. Gynecol. Obstet. 129:66, 1969.
28. Matsubara, J., Ban, I., Nakata, Y., Shinjo, K., Hirai, M., Miyazaki, H., Kawai, S., and Shionoya, S.: Long-term follow-up results of the iliofemoral venous thrombosis, J. Cardiovasc. Surg. 17:234, 1976.
29. Mavor, G. E., and Galloway, J. M. D.: Iliofemoral venous thrombosis. Pathological considerations and surgical management, Br. J. Surg. 56:45, 1969.
30. May, R., and Thurner, J.: The cause of the predominantly sinistral occurrence of thrombosis of the pelvic veins, Angiology 8:419, 1957.
31. Sevitt, S.: Venous thrombosis and pulmonary embolism. Their prevention by oral anticoagulants, Am. J. Med. 33:703, 1962.
32. Smith, G. W.: Iliofemoral venous thrombectomy indications, technique and results in forty-five cases, Circulation 37:847, 1968.

Discussion: Chapters 26 and 27

DR. VICTOR BERNHARD: Doctor Dale, I have done the crossover graft on one occasion with good results, in a lady with pelvic cancer. Until she died, she had a leg she could walk on. I found the Doppler was useful in determining patency of the graft. Doctor Dale, did you make some comments about the character of your immediate postoperative anticoagulation therapy and how long you carried it on?

Regarding Doctor DeWeese's presentation, I wondered whether or not there was any difference between results in patients who had calf origin of their deep venous thrombosis progressing up to the iliofemoral region, as opposed to those who had primary origin in the iliac vein with essentially normal distal flow? In a dog study, we tried to evaluate this. We were able to determine that by standard methods clot was left behind. However, if we subjected the dog to an intensive period of arteriovenous perfusion of the isolated limb, we could clean out all thrombi. We haven't tried this in the human.

DR. JULIUS JACOBSON: I would like to talk about a variant of what Doctor Dale has presented. This is an operation we conceived of for cases of so-called effort thrombosis. It is an operation that does not have to be done frequently, but it can be done on occasion when the patient cannot earn a normal livelihood because of arm swelling.

Three of our cases will be reported in *Surgery*. The operation detaches the jugular vein as it comes out of the head and then swings it down beneath the clavicle to be attached to the axillary vein (Fig 1). These patients have done very well with no recurrence of symptoms. This is the same operation that Doctor Dale has talked about, but in another anatomical situation.

In regard to Dr. DeWeese's paper, we have developed a bidirectional embolectomy catheter, a modification of the Fogarty catheter (Fig 2). With the bidirectional catheter, you can pull out the balloon in the same direction that it was inserted. This means that you can go

436

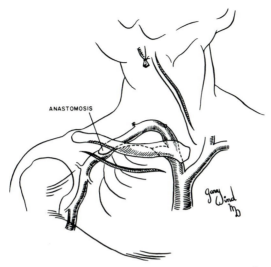

Fig 1.—This diagram illustrates the autogenous venous bypass performed for effort thrombosis. Note detachment of the internal jugular vein and the performance of a single peripheral anastomosis.

into a vein in the foot and pass the catheter up and take it out through the femoral vein, pulling all of the clot with it (Figs 3 and 4).

DR. J. CUTHBERT OWENS: Doctor Bernhard, you mentioned something about the dog experiments you had done at the Medical College of Wisconsin. I did this on one patient. I had taken one arterial embolus out, then raised the pressure on the venous side and another embolus came out. I think there is a possibility of getting additional clots by this or some other modality. I just wonder whether your work was ever published.

Fig 2.—The Fogarty catheter modified for bidirectional use.

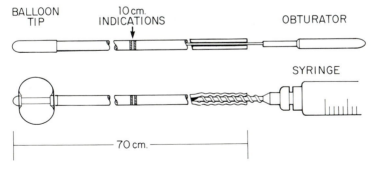

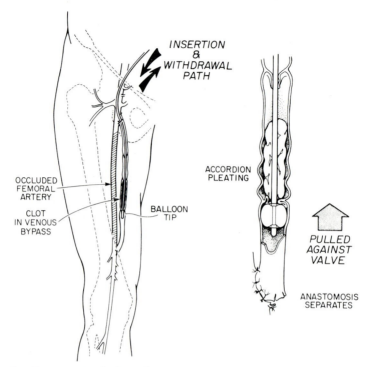

INSERTION
&
WITHDRAWAL
PATH

ACCORDION
PLEATING

OCCLUDED
FEMORAL
ARTERY

CLOT
IN VENOUS
BYPASS

BALLOON
TIP

PULLED
AGAINST
VALVE

ANASTOMOSIS
SEPARATES

Fig 3.—Conventional thrombectomy of a saphenous vein arterial bypass using a Fogarty catheter.

Dr. Victor Bernhard: Yes, it was published in *Current Topics in Surgical Research* (2:513, 1970).

Dr. John Hobbs: I would like to ask both speakers the same question. About 10 years ago, I did a series of saphenous crossover grafts, and all but one failed because of primary thrombosis. Some of them did recanalize during the subsequent year and functioned.

Professor Vollmar, working in Ulm, Germany, recently described the use of distal arteriovenous fistula with his venous reconstruction. Later, I visited Doctor Petrovski in Moscow and learned that he is shortly to report 562 deep vein reconstructions. He also insists that an arteriovenous fistula is essential.

Doctor Dale, you mentioned the importance of internal pressure and flow in reconstructive venous surgery. This is obviously what the European workers are thinking.

We now use the arteriovenous fistula and close it in 3 months. However, Doctor Vollmar and the Russians recommend closure of the fis-

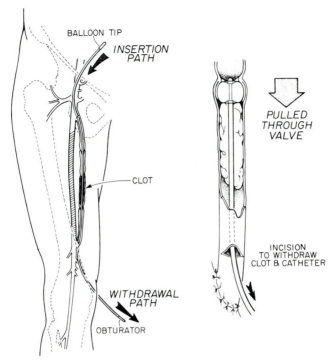

Fig 4.—Thrombectomy of a closed saphenous vein arterial bypass using the new bidirectional catheter. This technique could have application to venous thrombectomy also.

tula after 6 months. I have successfully used it with the saphenous crossover and closed the fistula at 6 weeks because it was easier technically.

DR. W. ANDREW DALE: In answer to the anticoagulation question, we heparinize with 5,000 units of heparin during the operation and not at all postoperatively. Doctor Jacobson's ingenious jugular vein transplant is certainly a splendid application of the crossover principle. I would also record under discussion our first use of a long vein graft dissected out of the arm and anastomosed to the saphenous vein in the thigh, running up along the abdominal wall and chest wall to bypass the inferior vena cava obstructed by retroperitoneal fibrosis. The operation was done only 7 days ago, and we do not yet know the long-term results.

Doctor Hobbs, thank you for your discussion of the arteriovenous fistula. We are aware of that and used it in experimental dog series before we began the clinical series. We have not used it in any patients.

DR. JAMES DeWEESE: First, in regard to Doctor Bernhard's question about whether we differentiated between the results of thrombi that started in the calf veins and those that started in the iliac system, I have not differentiated. I do know that, if they start in the iliac system because of pelvic phlebitis or because of cancer, it is unlikely that we can get them cleaned out. As far as comparison of a group with and without thrombectomy, we did do it on a small group of patients. When we first started, we found that about the same results were obtained in the first 13 patients. But with experience, the technique improved, and we felt that the thrombectomy results were better.

I can tell you that, in late phlebograms on patients who had iliac venous thrombosis, we never find a patent iliac vein, whereas after thrombectomy we do find patent iliac veins.

I would like to compliment Doctor Jacobson on his ingenious modification of the Fogarty catheter. I think this is a real contribution and one that may be of value in both venous and arterial embolectomies.

We are aware of Doctor Vollmar's work, also. We have tried to keep thrombectomy a simple operation, feeling that we can get a good result under local anesthesia with a simple operation. If we don't get a good result, or find we cannot get all of the clot out, then we treat the patient in nonoperative fashion and have not hurt him.

28 / Historical Aspects of Direct Venous Reconstruction

NORMAN M. RICH, M.D., COL., M.C., U.S. ARMY

Chief, Peripheral Vascular Surgery Service, Walter Reed Army Medical Center and Professor and Chairman of Surgery, Uniformed Military Medical Services School of Medicine, Washington, D.C.

ROBERT W. HOBSON, II, M.D.

Chief, Surgical Service, Veterans Administration Hospital, East Orange, New Jersey and Associate Professor of Surgery, College of Medicine and Dentistry of New Jersey, Newark, New Jersey

CREIGHTON B. WRIGHT, M.D.

Associate Professor of Surgery, Division of Thoracic and Cardiovascular Surgery, University of Iowa and Veterans Administration Hospital, Iowa City, Iowa

Initially, when we started the Vietnam Vascular Registry we felt that the greatest interest would come from management of arterial injuries. We more or less pushed venous injuries to the background. But in the last year we have become more interested in the repair of venous injuries and feel that this area needs to be pursued with greater vigor. (Rich,[6] 1969)

Introductory Remarks

THROUGHOUT HISTORY, it has been repeatedly recognized and documented that important surgical progress has occurred during periods of armed conflict when surgeons were required to treat large numbers of injured patients within a relatively short period of time. This corol-

441

lary has been particularly noteworthy between vascular surgery and military surgery in the twentieth century. The introductory quote emphasizes the recent stimulation for a more aggressive approach to repair of peripheral venous injuries which resulted from the recent experience of hundreds of well-trained American surgeons treating thousands of combat casualties in Southeast Asia.

The challenge remains in obtaining successful direct venous reconstruction, whether it is the repair of an injured vein or the elective reconstruction of the venous system compromised by thrombus or tumor. There has not been as much success in venous reconstruction during the past 25 years as there has been with arterial reconstruction. A major obstacle remains in identifying the "ideal conduit" which will have a high degree of success with long-term patency in the venous system, where pressure and flow are frequently lower than in the arterial system. Also, differences exist in various anatomical areas of the venous system ranging from the superior vena cava and inferior vena cava through the portal system to the peripheral veins. Etiology of the venous compromise ranging from trauma through thrombophlebitis to anomalies and direct tumor involvement must be considered. Nevertheless, some of the most recent controversy has centered around the question of whether or not injured veins should be repaired. There has been concern on the part of some that venous repair would be associated with a higher incidence of thrombophlebitis and pulmonary embolism.[9]

Although many of the principles and techniques associated with surgical repair of injured veins were known and practiced at the turn of this century, it is possible to historically emphasize that the greatest impetus in reconstruction of venous injuries has occurred within the past 10 years.[4, 6-10, 13, 14] In the early development of vascular surgery, venous as well as arterial reconstruction was utilized by pioneers in surgery including Kümmel, Murphy, Dörfler, Clermont, Jensen, Goyanes, Lexer, Carrel and Guthrie.[1-3, 5, 7-9, 11, 12] For these pioneers, success in venous surgery paralleled that of arterial surgery in both the clinical and experimental setting. It appears that, partially due to the lack of antibiotics and readily accessible blood for transfusion, there was a hiatus for both the development and application of venous and arterial repair during the period of World War I and World War II.[7] Nevertheless, there has been a disproportionate delay in accepting venous repair compared to arterial repair since the experience during the Korean Conflict in the early 1950s. As previously noted, the Korean Conflict and the Vietnam War have stimulated additional interest in venous surgery; however, civilian trauma, caused in part by a high speed, mechanized society and by increased urban violence with the use of more sophisticated weaponry, has also been associated with a recent increase in the number of traumatized patients who have sustained venous trauma.

The dichotomy involving the development of venous repair of injured veins is emphasized by the following quotes:

". . . closure of wounds in the veins by suture is now an acceptable surgical practice." (Murphy, 1897[5])

"Most vein injuries were treated by ligation, resulting in various degrees of venous stasis. Some patients with major vein ligations were asymptomatic, but severe venous stasis resulted in instances of limb loss. To eliminate these complications, two investigators began to repair major veins. . . . some were known to have thrombosed later but without complications." (Hughes, 1959[8])

"Simple ligation of injured veins is the classic method of management. . . . Lateral suture repair is preferred to ligation. . . . Grafts to bridge venous defects are not advocated." (Gaspar and Treiman, 1960[8])

"Whether or not concomitant venous injuries should be repaired remains a point of contention." (Morton, Southgate and DeWeese, 1966[8])

"An effort to repair major venous injuries should be made. . . . initial follow-up indicates a low incidence of complications associated with venous repairs and emphasizes the benefit, particularly in the lower extremity. The initial impression is that the majority of lateral vein repairs remains patent. Autogenous vein grafts in the venous system provide time for collateral circulation even if the graft thromboses early. Recanalization of this thrombosis is possible." (Rich, Hughes and Baugh, 1970[6])

"Though recanalization of the venous system, especially in the peripheral portion, is not necessarily required, an occasional need arises for re-establishment of the great vein such as the superior or inferior vena cava." (Hasegawa, et al., 1973[9])

Despite remaining controversy, documented clinical and experimental results in the past 10 years have refuted many of the concerns expressed by those who favored ligation of injured veins over venous repair.[9] The fear of an increased incidence of thrombophlebitis and pulmonary embolism following venous repair has not been substantiated. Conversely, the increased morbidity associated with acute venous hypertension and chronic venous insufficiency has been well-documented. Recent clinical experience, supported by experimental corroboration, has provided encouragement for continued application of venous repair. This has been stimulated in part by the necessity of managing large numbers of combat casualties during the fighting in Vietnam (1965–1972).[6, 9] Physicians in the United States Army Medical Department have been able to evaluate thousands of vascular injuries, including relatively large numbers of patients with venous trauma. Documentation and continued evaluation has been accomplished through the Vietnam Vascular Registry at Walter Reed Army Medical Center. The most intensive investigative efforts ever undertaken to evaluate the pathophysiologic changes associated with acute venous interruption and with various modalities of venous repair, with the added study of the role of numerous adjunctive measures to increase the patency rate of venous repairs, have been carried out between 1969 and 1976 at Walter Reed Army Institute of Research.[4, 9, 10, 13, 14]

Historical Notes

Table 28–1 outlines numerous contributions of surgeons during the latter part of the 19th and early 20th century. In the early 19th century, Travers and Guthrie were successful in closing small venous lacerations. An important contribution in experimental vascular surgery was made in 1877 by the Russian surgeon, Eck, who performed the first successful anastomosis of two vessels with a lateral communication between the portal vein and the inferior vena cava.

It is ironic that Murphy in his report of 1897 described and advocated lateral suture repair of venous injuries stating that this approach was accepted practice.[5] However, his approach remains in question in the minds of some surgeons approximately 75 years later. There is historical interest in a number of individual reports of venous repair during the early and mid-19th century which described closure of small lacerations in veins. Schede, nevertheless, in Germany, is generally given credit for performing the first successful lateral suture repair of a laceration of a vein in 1882.[1] This accomplishment prompted Schede to advocate lateral closure of wounds of femoral veins in man by vascular suture. Billroth, Braun of Koenigsberg and Schmidt are among a number of other surgeons who successfully sutured wounds in veins in the late 19th century.[8] Kümmel is given credit for performing the first clinical end-to-end anastomosis of a femoral vein in 1889.

In an historical review, Haimovici noted that Dörfler recommended in 1899 the same method for repairing veins and arteries emphasizing that there were general improvements in vascular surgery.

The essential features of his method consisted of the use of fine, round needles and fine silk and his suture was continuous, embracing all of the coats of the vessel. From his experience, although limited to 16 cases, he concluded that aseptic silk thread in the lumen of the vessel does not necessarily lead to thrombosis and, therefore, the penetration of the intima was not contra-indicated.[2]

TABLE 28-1.–DIRECT VENOUS RECONSTRUCTION, SELECTED
CONTRIBUTIONS BY PIONEER VASCULAR SURGEONS[1-3, 5, 8-11]

YEAR	CONTRIBUTOR	ACHIEVEMENT
1816	Travers	Closed a small wound in a femoral vein.
1830	Guthrie	Closed a laceration of the internal jugular vein by placing a tenaculum through the cut edges with a suture around the tenaculum.
1877	Eck	First permanent union of two blood vessels establishing a lateral communication between the portal vein and vena cava.
1878	Agnew	Used lateral suture in closure of venous wounds.
1881	Hirsch	Sutured divided veins successfully in dogs.
1882	Schede	Performed the first successful lateral suture repair of a femoral vein in man and advocated this procedure in the clinical situation.
1889	Kümmel	First clinical end-to-end anastomosis of a femoral vein.
1897	Murphy	Advocated successful application of venous repair at a time when he described the first successful end-to-end anastomosis of an artery in man.
1899	Dörfler	Recommended fine, round needles, fine sutures and inclusion of all layers of the vessel in venous as well as arterial anastomoses.
1901	Clermont	Successful end-to-end anastomosis of a divided inferior vena cava with continuous fine silk sutures.
1903	Jensen	Reunited the ends of divided veins by continuous suture through all layers. Four of seven operations were successful. When prostheses were used, only two of 10 remained patent.
1903	Exner	First attempt at grafting. Transplanted autogenous segments of the jugular vein 4 cm long into the opposite side in two dogs with the magnesium prosthesis of Payr.
1904	Payr	Attempted his technique of uniting divided vessels by invaginating the ends over cylinders of magnesium (first described in 1901) in a human femoral vein.
1912	Carrel and Guthrie	Confirmed and established many of the basic principles of vascular surgery.

Carrel and Guthrie are recognized for their many outstanding contributions to establishing the basic principles of vascular surgery.[1] Although many surgeons know the details of the controversy in the earlier part of this century regarding the concept of elective ligation of the accompanying vein when an injured artery was ligated, there is a startling concept in managing vascular trauma that is not generally remembered. In the mid-19th century the approach to the management of venous injuries included ligation of the concomitant artery! Gensoul in 1833 was supposedly the first to describe venous engorgement as a dangerous problem that would result if only the femoral vein was ligated in an extremity.[12] Because of this finding, it was recommended that ligation of the femoral artery should be carried out for injuries of the femoral vein. This concept was repeatedly ascribed to by numerous other surgeons for the ensuing 50 years. When this concept was finally disproved, many felt that the accompanying vein should be ligated with arterial injuries. This, however, was refuted in turn by the World War II experience reviewed by DeBakey and Simeone.[9]

TABLE 28-2.—DIRECT VENOUS RECONSTRUCTION, SELECTED EXPERIMENTAL STUDIES[3, 4, 10, 11, 13, 14]

YEAR	CONTRIBUTORS	ACHIEVEMENT
1947	Johns	Reestablished experimental studies on suture and nonsuture methods of venous anastomosis.
1949	Gerbode Yee Rundle	Produced good results with the azygos-caval shunt. Results were less successful with atrioazygos and atriocaval anastomoses.
1955	Deterling Bhonslay	Replaced segments of superior vena cava in dogs with various grafts and prostheses.
1958	Bryant Lipton Miyagishima Labrosse	Utilized autogenous venous grafts, freeze-dried arterial homografts and various prostheses in the inferior vena cava.
1958	Bryant Lazenby Howard	Combined arteriovenous fistulas with prostheses in the femoral vein to improve patency.
1959	Schauble Anlyan Postlethwait	Studied the fate of various grafts in the jugular vein and femoral vein.
1960	DeWeese Niguidula	Replaced segments of femoral vein with autogenous venous grafts.
1960	Earle Horsley Villavicencio Warren	Compiled autogenous venous grafts from segments of either femoral or jugular veins. These compilation grafts were used to replace defects in the inferior vena cava.
1961	Silver Analyan	Evaluated various grafts, suture materials and suture techniques in jugular veins with poor results.
1961	Symbas Foster Scott	Performed portal vein grafts with various conduits and compared the patency of these grafts with portal-caval shunt grafts.
1962	Carter	Demonstrated that suture methods of anastomosing jugular veins was superior to nonsuture Vitallium cuff anastomoses.
1963	Dale Scott	Emphasized that autogenous veins and prostheses were both successful in superior vena caval replacement. They also achieved a 100% patency rate inserting autogenous jugular venous grafts into the femoral vein of seven dogs.
1964	Collins Douglass	Applied the operative microscope to improve techniques of small vein anastomoses.

Experimental Contributions

After a hiatus of nearly 40 years, following the experimental and clinical experience established around the beginning of the 20th century, Johns re-established experimental studies on suture and nonsuture methods of venous anastomosis in 1947.[3] Table 28–2 provides a few selected experimental studies from the numerous studies that have been performed in the last 30 years. As might be anticipated, some of the best early results were obtained in reconstruction of the superior vena cava. Results were favorable in reconstruction of the portal system. However, results were less successful in the abdominal inferior vena cava and the peripheral venous system.

A vast number of conduits have been used; however, no uniform degree of success has been established with any of them. A variety of techniques and adjunctive measures have also been utilized without being able to establish any as uniformly associated with a high degree of patency in direct venous reconstruction.[3, 9, 13, 14]

Clinical Progress

Table 28–3 outlines a few of the selected clinical contributions to direct venous reconstruction. There has generally been more limited success in the clinical situation compared to some of the previously outlined experimental work.

As previously stated, the best early results have occurred in direct venous reconstruction of the superior vena cava. There have also been

TABLE 28–3.—DIRECT VENOUS RECONSTRUCTION, SELECTED CLINICAL CONTRIBUTIONS[3, 9, 14]

YEAR	CONTRIBUTORS	ACHIEVEMENT
1951	Reynolds Southwick	Used azygos vein segments to create portacaval shunts.
1952	Rousselot	Autogenous venous grafts utilized in splenorenal and mesocaval shunts.
1954	Warren Thayer	Transplanted the long saphenous vein in 14 patients with postphlebitic venous stasis.
1958	Allansmith Richards	Clinical success in 21 patients with a variety of superior vena caval reconstructions.
1959	Palma Esperon	Crossover saphenofemoral bypass in eight patients with the postphlebitic syndrome.
1962	Hardin	Saphenous vein bypass used successfully in five patients with venous obstruction to an extremity.
1966	Dale	Further experience with the crossover vein grafts treating chronic iliofemoral venous occlusion.

improved results in the portal system. The crossover saphenofemoral bypass of Palma has been demonstrated to be of value by Dale in the United States in treating patients with chronic iliofemoral venous occlusion.[3, 10]

Discussion

Obviously, many of the historical aspects of direct venous reconstruction are current. The symposium on venous problems in honor of Dr. Geza de Takats is an historical event of its own honoring a world-renowned surgeon who has made many contributions to vascular surgery.

Again, to emphasize that much of the history of direct venous reconstruction has taken place in the last 10 years, one must do little more than review the topics and the names of the surgeons contributing to the present symposium. The significance of the many important current developments concerning venous reconstruction will be apparent to those fortunate enough to attend this symposium. Obviously, the international exchange with many surgeons from other nations who are making important contributions in this field is important to further progress.

Experience at Walter Reed Army Medical Center and Walter Reed Army Institute of Research has been professionally stimulating to those who have participated in the evaluation of the problems of direct venous reconstruction. It could be recorded in history that outstanding contributions based on experience of managing Vietnam casualties by American military surgeons did as much to stimulate and direct interest and success in repair of venous injuries as was established during the Korean Conflict with the repair of arterial injuries.

Summary

Throughout history, it has been repeatedly recognized that important surgical progress has occurred during periods of armed conflict. Experience with the Vietnam Vascular Registry has indicated that repair of venous injuries is a subject which needs to be pursued with greater vigor. A major obstacle remains in identifying the ideal conduit which will have success with long-term patency in the venous system. In fact, the question of whether or not venous injuries should be repaired has remained a point of contention, despite the clinical and experimental results in the past 10 years which have refuted many of the concerns expressed by those who formerly favored ligation of injured veins.

Although clinically, there has been a more limited success in venous repair than in the experimental laboratory, the best early results have occurred in direct venous reconstruction of the superior vena cava. There have been improved results in the portal system and the crossover saphenofemoral bypass has been demonstrated to be of value.

REFERENCES

Due to the potentially extensive bibliography, only selected review material is cited where original references can be found.

1. Guthrie, C. G.: *Blood Vessel Surgery and Its Application* (London: Edward Arnold & Co., 1912).
2. Haimovici, H.: History of arterial grafting, J. Cardiovasc. Surg. 4:152, 1963.
3. Haimovici, H., Hoffert, P. W., Zinicola, N., and Steinman, C.: An experimental and clinical evaluation of grafts in the venous system, Surg. Gynecol. Obstet. 131:1173, 1970.
4. Hobson, R. W., II, Wright, C. B., and Rich, N. M.: Investigative Aspects of Venous Reconstruction, in Witkin, E., et al. (eds.): *Venous Diseases, Medical and Surgical Management*, American European Symposium on Venous Diseases, Mouton, The Hague, Netherlands (Montreux, Switzerland: Foundation International Cooperation in the Medical Sciences, 1974).
5. Murphy, J. B.: Resection of arteries and veins injured in continuity: End-to-end suture. Experimental and clinical research, Med. Rec. 51:73, 1897.
6. Rich, N. M., Hughes, C. W., and Baugh, J. H.: Management of venous injuries, Ann. Surg. 171:724, 1970.
7. Rich, N. M.: Vascular trauma, Surg. Clin. North Am. 53:1367, 1973.
8. Rich, N. M., and Hobson, R. W., II: Historical Background of Repair of Venous Injuries, in Witkin, E., et al. (eds.): *Venous Diseases, Medical and Surgical Management*, American European Symposium on Venous Diseases, Mouton, The Hague, Netherlands (Montreux, Switzerland: Foundation International Cooperation in the Medical Sciences, 1974).
9. Rich, N. M., Hobson, R. W., II, Wright, C. B., and Fedde, C. W.: Repair of lower extremity venous trauma: A more aggressive approach required, J. Trauma 14:639, 1974.
10. Rich, N. M., Hobson, R. W., II, Wright, C. B., and Swan, K. G.: Techniques of Venous Repair, in Swan, K. G., et al. (eds.): *Venous Surgery in the Lower Extremities* (St. Louis: Warren H. Green, Inc., 1975).
11. Shumacker, H. B., Jr.: Arterial suture techniques and grafts: Past, present and future, Surgery 66:419, 1969.
12. Simeone, F. A., Grillo, H. C., and Rundle, F.: On the question of ligation of the concomitant vein when a major artery is interrupted, Surgery 29:932, 1951.
13. Swan, K. G., Hobson, R. W., II, Reynolds, D. G., Rich, N. M., and Wright, C. B. (eds.): *Venous Surgery in the Lower Extremities* (St. Louis: Warren H. Green, Inc., 1975).
14. Wright, C. B., Hobson, R. W., Swan, K. G., and Rich, N. M.: Extremity venous ligation: Clinical and hemodynamic correlation, Am. Surg. 41:203, 1975.

29 / The Pathophysiology of Extremity Venous Occlusion

CREIGHTON B. WRIGHT, M.D.

Associate Professor of Surgery, Division of Thoracic and Cardiovascular Surgery, University of Iowa and Veterans Administration Hospital, Iowa City, Iowa

ROBERT W. HOBSON, II, M.D.

Chief, Surgical Service, Veterans Administration Hospital, East Orange, New Jersey and Associate Professor of Surgery, College of Medicine and Dentistry of New Jersey, Newark, New Jersey

KENNETH G. SWAN, M.D.

Chief, Division of General and Vascular Surgery and Professor of Surgery, College of Medicine and Dentistry of New Jersey, Newark, New Jersey

NORMAN M. RICH, M.D., COL., M.C., U.S. ARMY

Chief, Peripheral Vascular Surgery, Walter Reed Army Medical Center and Professor and Chairman of Surgery, Uniformed Military Medical Services School of Medicine, Washington, D.C.

Introduction

THE HEMODYNAMICS of the venous circulation have intrigued physiologists, physicians and surgeons since the initial observations of Sir William Harvey confirmed the circulation and the valvular function in the veins of the extremity (Fig 29–1). The presence of double venous drainage systems, as well as the apparent abundance of collaterals found at an anatomic dissection or venography, have led investigators to feel that the venous collateralization was more than adequate in most circumstances. However, phlegmasia alba dolens and phlegma-

451

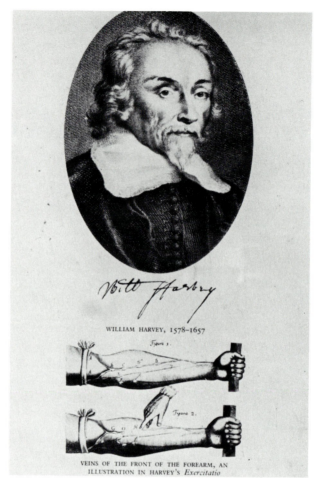

WILLIAM HARVEY, 1578–1657

VEINS OF THE FRONT OF THE FOREARM, AN
ILLUSTRATION IN HARVEY'S *Exercitatio*

Fig 29–1. – Sir William Harvey.

sia cerulea dolens (venous gangrene) have long been recognized to be
the result of inadequate venous outflow. From a clinical standpoint,
although the techniques for vascular anastomosis have been available
since the turn of the century through the efforts of Eck, Schede, Murphy, Dörfler, Jensen, Carrel and Guthrie,[4, 7, 12, 17, 20] enthusiasm for
reconstruction of the veins in the trauma setting was dampened by
fear of infection, occurrence of arteriovenous fistulas, and following
World War I by the teaching of Makins that limb survival was improved by venous ligation.[6, 14, 15, 19] DeBakey and Simeone later refuted the clinical observations of Makins on a statistical as well as a clini-

cal basis from World War II data.[6] In more recent times, failure of transplantation of kidneys and replantation of extremities has occasionally occurred due to inadequate venous outflow. Nevertheless, prior to the Vietnam conflict, injuries to major extremity veins were infrequently repaired.[3, 5, 6, 13, 20-24, 28] Clinical investigators, specifically Chandler, Cohen, Rich, and Sullivan, called attention to the occurrence of venous stasis in some limbs which were lost following satisfactory arterial repair.[2, 3, 5, 21-23] Hughes and Spencer and Grewe had seen similar problems during the Korean conflict; however, very few venous reconstructions were attempted,[13, 26] in spite of the major advances in surgical management of arterial injuries. Sullivan and his associates in 1971 reported an experience of 35 patients with popliteal vessel injury and noted severe venous insufficiency and morbidity in patients with major venous ligation.[28] They demonstrated patency of venous repair by postoperative venogram and noted that massive edema did not occur in any of the 21 patients who had had primary vein repair. This dramatic report set the stage for additional clinical and laboratory observations of the effects of acute venous ligation.

Experimental Data

Historically the relevant laboratory observation was that of Ney,[18] subsequently confirmed by Hooker in Halsted's laboratory, that the arterial pressure beyond a ligature was increased by ligation of the concomitant vein.[8] This also resulted in an increase in the backbleeding.[29] The interpretation was that more blood was supplied to the tissue distal by concomitant ligation of the normal vein in the presence of an arterial injury requiring ligation.

Following his review and experimental observations, Montgomery[16] presented a paper entitled "Therapeutic Venous Occlusion—Its Effect on the Blood Flow in the Extremity in Acute Arterial Obstruction." He concluded that, "The belief that ligation of the vein increases the flow of blood through the extremity must, therefore, be discarded and the cause of such benefits as accrue from its use must be sought for elsewhere." In addition he stated, "Because of the marked decrease in the flow of blood which follows obstruction of the venous return proximal to the point of arterial occlusion, and because of the possible danger of producing a serious venous stasis thereafter, it would appear that the use of this principle in the treatment of patients requiring ligation of the main artery of an extremity should be avoided."

In an infrequently quoted abstract Pritchard,[19] working in Gregg's laboratory, noted that in dogs, "During acute femoral vein occlusion, as the venous pressure rose, arterial flow at first decreased considerably and then later rose somewhat, but never regained the controlled value." They had been stimulated by an earlier report of Linton et al.[14] suggesting that peripheral venous occlusion increased arterial inflow. In the 1941 paper Linton et al. stated, "There is practically universal agreement that ligation of the concomitant vein is beneficial." The thermostromuhr used by Linton et al. apparently suffered from the inability to indicate directional changes in flow as noted by Pritchard. In 1951 Simeone et al.,[25] in a paper entitled "On the Question of Ligation of the Concomitant Vein, When a Major Artery is Interrupted," in addition to a superb review of the historical literature, reported that "papers suggesting that ligation of the satellite vein did not improve the residual circulation after interruption of the artery were in the minority." They addressed the issue in an experimental model which included sciatic nerve stimulation during and after femoral artery and vein individual and concomitant occlusions. Alterations in muscle function showed that occlusion of the femoral vein alone had an ischemic effect almost identical with that of occluding the femoral artery alone. There was also a rise in the base line of the muscle contractions which suggested an engorgement of the muscle. In conclusion, no evidence was obtained from any of this experiment that after interruption of the artery the function of the muscle is improved by occlusion of the concomitant vein. In this paper Simeone et al.[25] also called attention to the fact that the clinical figures upon which Makins had based his clinical suggestion for venous ligation were in fact not statistically significant. Their conclusions were:

(1) In a review of the clinical and experimental evidence favoring ligation of the concomitant vein, when a major artery has to be interrupted it is revealed that the conclusion drawn from previous data has been either unwarranted or subject to different interpretations; (2) in the cat acute obstruction of the femoral vein causes as much functional impairment of the gastrocnemius soleus group of muscles as obstruction of the femoral artery; and (3) ligation of the concomitant vein causes no improvement in muscle function although the artery is intact or interrupted or if the experiment is acute or chronic.

Following this report, enthusiasm for ligation of the concomitant normal vein diminished and the issue is hardly ever raised. During the Korean war and subsequently during the Vietnam conflict, attention was drawn again to the management of the veins in association with vascular injuries. This time the major question was the efficacy of venous repair in conjunction with an isolated venous injury or in conjunction with repair of a concomitantly injured artery.

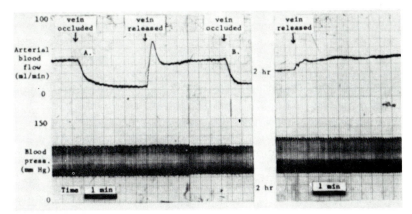

Fig 29–2.—Representative tracing from one animal demonstrating the effect of femoral vein occlusion on concomitant arterial flow. Venous occlusion (A) for 2 min reduced arterial flow from 46 ml/min to 13 ml/min. Upon release of occlusion, arterial flow returned to the baseline level within 30 sec after a brief "overshoot." A second occlusion (B) produced essentially the same initial effect. During a 2-hr period of venous occlusion arterial flow gradually rose from 16 ml/min to 32 ml/min and upon release, flow returned to the baseline level within minutes. (From Barcia et al.[2])

In 1972 Barcia et al.[2] demonstrated in the dog hind limb a significant reduction in the femoral arterial flow following femoral venous occlusion. In their initial observations the arterial flow reduced dramatically and there was a noticeable reactive hyperemia following release which suggested that in addition to engorgement there was, in fact, an ischemic component to the reaction (Fig 29–2). The longest duration of femoral venous occlusion in their experiments was 2 hr. Other flows, cardiac output and physiologic modifications of this response were not studied. Subsequently at the Walter Reed Army Institute of Research, Division of Surgery, additional investigations were undertaken (Table 29–1).[9-12, 32-39]

TABLE 29–1.—THE MAIN QUESTIONS

1. What are the effects of acute femoral venous occlusion on femoral flow (a) with artery obstructed, (b) with artery open or repaired?
2. What is the time course of these events?
3. What is the effect of venous reconstruction and/or stenosis on arterial flow?
4. Are the effects of femoral venous occlusion due to local or central alterations?
5. If major veins are ligated and cannot be repaired, what physiologic or pharmacologic manipulations can affect the adverse hemodynamics?
6. Are the observations in the canine hind limb reproducible in species phylogenetically closer to man?

The anatomy of the hind limb of the dog has often been misrepresented, but in the area of the femoral artery it most resembles the superficial femoral artery of man (Fig 29–3). The profunda artery originates above the inguinal ligament. The concomitant veins are similarly disposed. The hemodynamic responses to interruption of the femoral vein with and without occlusion of the other major collateral veins are shown in Figure 29–4. It was clear that the hemodynamic effects of the concomitant vein occlusion were dramatic and the effect of occlusion of the collateral veins was minimal. This results from the induced changes in peripheral venous pressure and peripheral resistance when the ipsilateral femoral venous outflow is obstructed (Fig 29–5).

In a separate series of experiments these responses were confirmed after end-to-end reconstruction or after interposition vein grafting with an autogenous jugular vein was performed. The arterial flow and venous pressure returned to control upon release of the temporary

Fig 29–3.–The femoral vascular anatomy of the dog (right leg extended). (From Wright, C. B., and Swan, K. G.[32])

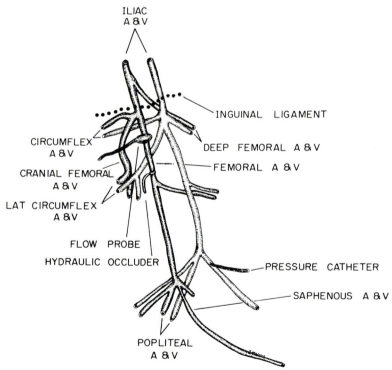

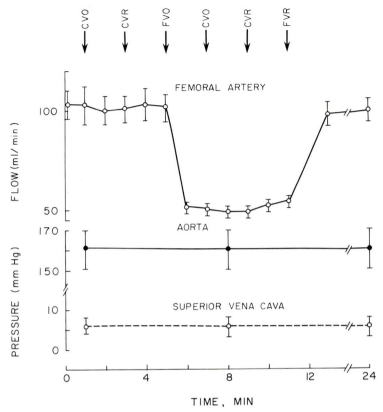

Fig 29–4.—The effects of short-term femoral venous occlusion and occlusion of the remaining branches of the femoral vein on femoral arterial blood flow and peripheral venous pressure. Each point on the graph represents mean ± SE of five experiments in five dogs. Abbreviations: *CVO*, collateral venous occlusion; *CVR*, collateral venous release; *FVO*, femoral venous occlusion; *FVR*, femoral venous release. (From Wright, C. B., and Swan, K. G.[32])

venous occlusion. It was noted, however, that any compromise of the venous outflow by a narrowing of the venous anastomosis resulted in an elevation of the distal venous pressure and led to a persistent decrease in the femoral arterial flow. This suggests that although flow may occur through a small or stenotic vein graft or lateral repair, the ideal hemodynamic situation is a return to homeostasis, as confirmed by return of distal venous pressure to normal.

In the clinical setting of phlegmasia alba dolens or in the period after vascular injury, a critical interval of 2–3 days followed by a few

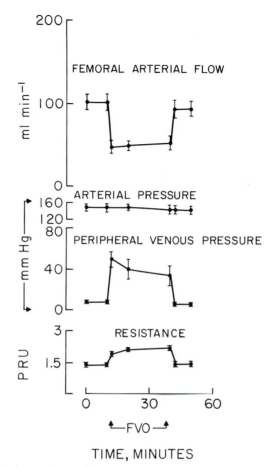

Fig 29–5. — The effects of femoral venous occlusion *(FVO)* on femoral arterial blood flow, arterial and venous pressure and peripheral resistance are presented graphically. Each point represents the mean ± SE of six experiments in six dogs. (From Wright et al.[35])

days of persistent swelling has been related to the inadequacy of venous outflow. In experiments in the dog and the baboon the hemodynamic alterations following chronic femoral venous occlusion have been demonstrated (Figs 29 – 6 and 29 – 7). In essence the baboon femoral arterial flow is reduced for 72 hr and returns to normal as the venous pressure declines. This corresponds with a return of the peripheral resistance to normal. Apparently although initial venograms after a femoral venous occlusion appear to show an abundance of collater-

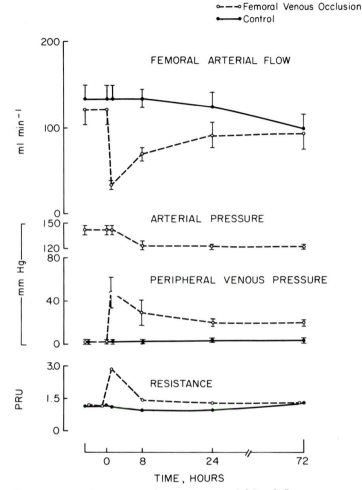

Fig 29–6.—The changes in femoral arterial blood flow, venous pressure and resistance are presented graphically. The data are presented as a mean ± SE and are the result of five experiments in five animals. (From Hobson et al.⁹)

als (Fig 29–8), these are hemodynamically inadequate to handle the arterial inflow which is reduced by the dramatic increase in peripheral resistance and does not return to normal until additional dilatation of collaterals has occurred.

Recently, other investigators have confirmed the hemodynamic alterations which occur following acute femoral venous occlusion with

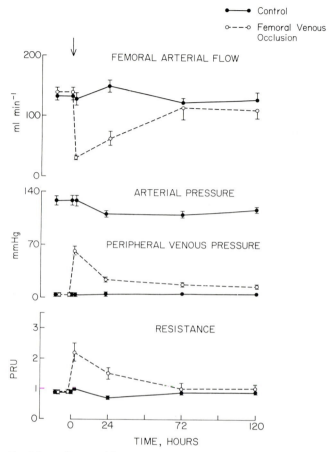

Fig 29–7.—The effects of femoral venous ligation on femoral hemodynamics are presented. Each point represents the mean ± SE of five experiments in five baboons. The *arrow* indicates point of unilateral femoral vein ligation. (From Wright, C. B., and Hobson, R. W.[38])

additional flowmeter studies as well as xenon washout radioisotope techniques.[1, 31] The observation (see Fig 29–6) that only unilateral femoral arterial flow is reduced by ipsilateral femoral venous occlusion supports the concept that these flow changes result primarily from local hemodynamic effects rather than from alterations of the cardiac output or some other reflex pathway.

In the course of discussions after obtaining the above data, it became clear that although the ideal clinical circumstance would be complete reconstitution of venous outflow, there were circumstances

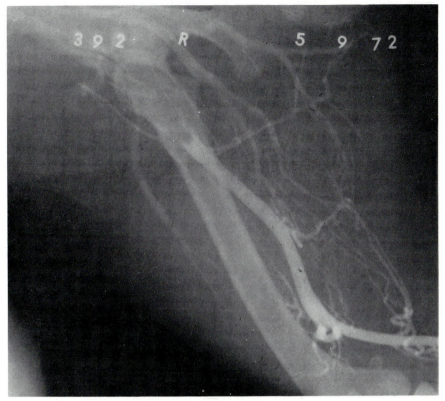

Fig 29–8. – Venogram. Occluded canine femoral vein.

when (1) disruption of the venous continuity would be such that no repair would be feasible or that only a smaller than ideal graft was available and (2) additional disruption of bone and soft tissues would further compromise collateral venous drainage. Therefore physiologic or pharmacologic improvement of the femoral arterial flow collateral bed and therefore reduction of peripheral resistance might be useful adjuvant techniques for limb salvage. At first the intra-arterial vasodilator isoproterenol was studied. Although femoral arterial flow during femoral venous occlusion could be transiently increased with injections of isoproterenol, the femoral venous pressure rose to 30–60 mm Hg in response to doses which raised arterial flow significantly. In a clinical setting this response, although transient, might lead to overwhelming edema. The dramatic rise in venous pressure probably results from opening of arteriovenous communications in the dog hind limb.

Since the initial study of beta-adrenergic stimulation with isoproterenol seemed unlikely to be of benefit clinically, a subsequent study of alpha-adrenergic blockade was started. In Figure 29–9, data are presented demonstrating the femoral flow responses to venous occlusion before and after systemic alpha-adrenergic blockade with phenoxybenzamine in the dog. It is noted that femoral arterial flow at the 30-min observation point returned nearly to normal levels. There was an apparent decline in peripheral resistance in response to this drug. Once again, however, systemic administration of this drug might not meet with wide acceptance in the clinical arena where shock and multiple injuries are likely to be involved. For this reason, lumbar sympathectomy was next considered as a means of reducing sympathetic tone and peripheral resistance unilaterally. Lumbar sympathectomy was subsequently performed before and during femoral venous occlu-

Fig 29–9.—The effects of femoral venous occlusion on canine femoral arterial flow, aortic pressure and saphenous venous pressure are presented before and after alpha-adrenergic blockade (phenoxybenzamine, 1.5 mg kg⁻¹, IV). Each point represents the mean ± SE of six experiments in six dogs. (From Wright et al.[34])

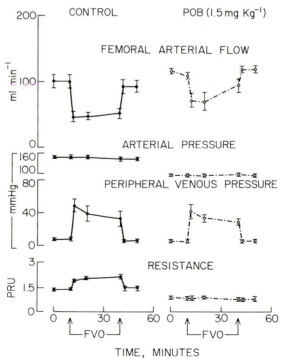

sion in canine and primate experiments. The findings included a significant increase in femoral arterial flow with no significant additional increase in the femoral venous pressure. This represents, therefore, a reduction in the peripheral resistance (Fig 29–10). Sympathetic denervation would appear to be a useful measure to increase arterial flow when venous outflow is partially compromised. Following sympathectomy, most reported arterial flow improvements have been through superficial arteriovenous anastomoses or the cutaneous bed. We were concerned that the decrease in peripheral resistance which

Fig 29–10. – The effects of lumbar sympathectomy of femoral hemodynamics are presented during sustained femoral venous occlusion. Each point represents the mean ± SE of five experiments in five baboons. (From Wright, C. B., and Hobson, R. W.[38])

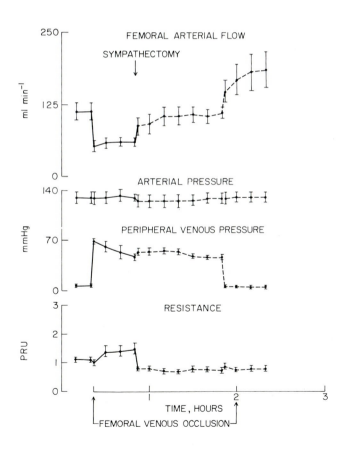

BABOON FEMORAL VENOUS OCCLUSION

we noted might be due to a similar phenomenon. In a subsequent experiment the entire skin and soft tissue down to the fascial layer of the hind limb was transected and all superficial venous branches were ligated. When femoral venous occlusion was performed, flow reduction occurred promptly as in our earlier experiments and following sympathectomy the femoral arterial flow once again increased to control levels. It is apparent then that the improvement in femoral arterial flow is not entirely based on superficial venous collaterals. Apparently the release of sympathetic tone allows further dilatation of patent deep venous collaterals, and thus improvement in overall limb hemodynamics.

It must be made clear in this discussion that previous investigators[27, 30] have shown in phlegmasia cerulea dolens where all venous outflow is obstructed that sympathectomy may cause worsening engorgement of the limb and either no or only minimal improvement in arterial flow. The present experimental and clinical situation seems to more closely resemble phlegmasia alba dolens—or partial venous compromise—rather than obstruction of all venous channels as in phlegmasia cerulea dolens. For this reason, it seems that pharmacologic or nerve block sympathectomy could be used in the venous trauma situation to improve ipsilateral femoral arterial blood flow by improvement of the venous collateral outflow.

Discussion

From a historical standpoint, although a great deal of time has passed since Harvey's initial observations, our knowledge of the circulatory system, particularly the venous side, remains incomplete. A variety of different clinical circumstances have encouraged investigators to return to the experimental laboratory to delve into the physiology of the venous circulation. Our studies were stimulated by clinical observations from the Vietnam war, made primarily by contributors to the Vietnam Vascular Registry. In spite of improved transportation, improved arterial reconstruction, improved antibiotic coverage and better management of associated soft tissue and bone injuries, a persistent high incidence of amputation following extremity vascular injuries, particularly if there was concomitant or isolated venous damage, was reported.[3, 5, 21-24] Additional reviews of the literature disclosed interesting physiologic observations and clinical notes which have furthered our progress in these investigations. From the present review of laboratory investigations the following conclusions have been derived.

1. Acute femoral venous occlusion in the presence of arterial obstruction:
   a. increases the distal arterial, capillary, and venous pressure,
   b. reduces the arterial inflow,
   c. renders the muscle more ischemic and congested.
2. Acute femoral venous occlusion in the presence of a patent or repaired patent femoral artery:
   a. reduces arterial flow,
   b. increases peripheral venous pressure,
   c. increases peripheral resistance,
   d. produces distal ischemia as judged by occurrence of postrelease reactive hyperemia.
3. Venous collaterals appear abundant on early venograms but are hemodynamically insufficient for 48–72 hr as demonstrated by venous pressure and femoral arterial flow measurements.
4. Normal hemodynamics occur promptly with release of venous occlusion or reconstitution of venous continuity by end-to-end anastomosis or adequate interposition grafting.
5. Persistent elevation of venous pressure due to narrowing of the femoral vein after a lateral repair, small grafts, or "purse-stringing" of an anastomosis may result in some residual decrease in arterial flow, but this is less than if the vein is totally occluded.
6. The hemodynamic effect of unilateral venous occlusion on femoral arterial flow seems to be primarily due to local pressure relationships and not alterations in cardiac output as estimated from simultaneous bilateral femoral flow measurements before and during femoral venous occlusion.
7. When major extremity venous injury cannot be repaired and the distal venous pressure is significantly elevated, sympathetic blockade—or sympathectomy—may improve the arterial inflow dramatically.
8. Occasionally the congenital variability of the venous circulation will allow ligation of a major vein with no untoward sequelae. The measurement of distal venous pressure is a simple, readily available hemodynamic tool to assess this during surgery.
9. The subhuman primate, an animal phylogenetically close to man, responds with the same hemodynamics as the dog to femoral venous occlusion.

Acknowledgments

The authors wish to recognize the contributions to this work made by their previous research associates at the Walter Reed Army Institute of Research: David G. Reynolds, Ph.D., James Sayre, M.D., Peter F. Casterline, M.D., George J. Collins, M.D., Robert Lamoy, B.S., and Ernest C. Alix, B.S.

REFERENCES

1. Abbott, W. M., Mione, P. S., and Austen, W. G.: Effect of venous interruption on arterial circulation, Surg. Forum 25:246, 1974.
2. Barcia, P. J., Nelson, T. G., and Whelan, T. J.: Importance of venous occlusion in arterial repair failure: An experimental study, Ann. Surg. 175:223, 1972.
3. Chandler, J. G., and Knapp, R. W.: Early definitive treatment of vascular injuries in the Vietnam Conflict, JAMA 202:960, 1967.
4. Child, C. G., III: Ecks fistula, Surg. Gynecol. Obstet. 96:375, 1953.
5. Cohen, A., Baldwin, J. N., and Grant, R. N.: Problems in the management of battlefield vascular injuries, Am. J. Surg. 118:526, 1969.
6. DeBakey, M. E., and Simeone, F. A.: Battle injuries of the arteries in World War II, Ann. Surg. 123:534, 1946.
7. Guthrie, C. G.: *Blood Vessel Surgery and Its Application* (London: Edward Arnold & Co., 1912).
8. Halsted, W. S.: Ligation of the left subclavian artery in its first portion, Johns Hopkins Hosp. Rep. 21:1, 1921.
9. Hobson, R. W., Howard, W. E., Wright, C. B., Collins, G. J., and Rich, N. M.: Hemodynamics of canine femoral venous ligation: Significance in combined arterial and venous injuries, Surgery 74:824, 1973.
10. Hobson, R. W., Rich, N. M., Wright, C. B.: Concepts in Venous Trauma and Reconstruction, in Hobbs, J. (ed.): *Treatment of Venous Disorders* (Lancaster: International Medical Publishers, 1976) pp. 351–382.
11. Hobson, R. W., Wright, C. B., and Rich, N. M.: Investigative Aspects of Venous Reconstruction, in Witkin, E., et al. (eds.): *Venous Disease, Medical and Surgical Management* (Montreux, Switzerland: Foundation International Cooperation in the Medical Sciences, 1974).
12. Holman, E.: Surgery of large arteries, Ann. Surg. 85:173, 1927.
13. Hughes, C. W.: Arterial repair during the Korean War, Ann. Surg. 147:555, 1958.
14. Linton, R. R., Morrison, P. J., Ulfelder, H., and Libly, A. L.: Therapeutic venous occlusion, Am. Heart J. 21:721, 1941.
15. Makins, G. H.: *On Gunshop Injuries to the Blood Vessels* (Bristol: John Wright and Sons, Ltd., 1919).
16. Montgomery, M. L.: Therapeutic venous occlusion, Arch. Surg. 24:1016, 1932.
17. Murphy, J. B.: Resection of arteries and veins injured in continuity end to end suture—experimental and clinical research, Med. Record 51:73, 1897.
18. Ney, E.: Du role des veines dans la circulation collaterale arterielle, Rev. Chir. 46:903, 1912.
19. Pritchard, W. H., Weiberger, A. S., Schroeder, E. F., Shipley, R. E., and Gregg, D. E.: The acute effects of peripheral venous occlusion on blood flow in the dog's leg, Fed. Proc. (abstract) 1:68, 1942.
20. Rich, N. M., and Hobson, R. W.: Historical Background of Repair of Venous Injuries, in Witkin, E., et al. (eds.): *Venous Diseases, Medical and Surgical Management* (Montreux, Switzerland: Foundation International Cooperation in the Medical Sciences, 1974).
21. Rich, N. M., and Sullivan, W. G.: Clinical recanalization of autogenous vein graft in the popliteal vein, J. Trauma 12:919, 1972.
22. Rich, N. M., Baugh, J. H., and Hughes, C. W.: Popliteal artery injuries in Vietnam, Am. J. Surg. 118:531, 1969.
23. Rich, N. M., Hughes, C. W., and Baugh, J. H.: Management of venous injuries, Ann. Surg. 171:724, 1970.

24. Rich, N. M., Hobson, R. W., Collins, G. J., and Andersen, C. A.: The effect of acute popliteal venous interruption, Ann. Surg. 183:365.

25. Simeone, F. A., Grillo, H. C., and Rundle, F.: On the question of ligation of the concomitant vein when a major artery is interrupted, Surgery 29:932, 1951.

26. Spencer, F. C., and Grewe, R. V.: The management of arterial injuries in battle casualties, Ann. Surg. 141:304, 1955.

27. Stallworth, J. M., Najib, A., Kletke, R. R., and Ramirez, A.: Phlegmasia cerulea dolens: An experimental study, Ann. Surg. 165:860, 1967.

28. Sullivan, W. G., Thornton, F. H., Baker, L. H., LaPlante, E. S., and Cohen, A.: Early influence of popliteal vein repair in the treatment of popliteal vessel injuries, Am. J. Surg. 122:528, 1971.

29. Theis, F. V.: Ligation of artery and concomitant vein in operations on large blood vessels, Arch. Surg. 17:244, 1928.

30. Veal, J. R., Dugan, T. J., Jamison, W. L., and Bauersfeld, R. S.: Acute massive venous occlusion of the lower extremities, Surgery 29:355, 1951.

31. Weber, T. R., Lindenauer, S. M., and Pazderac, R. V.: Venous occlusion and xenon[133] muscle clearance, Surg. Forum 25:260, 1974.

32. Wright, C. B., and Swan, K. G.: Hemodynamics of venous occlusion in the canine hindlimb, Surgery 73:141, 1973.

33. Wright, C. B., and Swan, K. G.: Hemodynamics of venous repair in the canine hindlimb, J. Thorac. Cardiovasc. Surg. 65:195, 1973.

34. Wright, C. B., Swan, K. G., Reynolds, D. G., and Nelson, T. G.: Venous occlusion in the canine hindlimb: Hemodynamic effects of adrenergic stimulation and blockade, Surgery 73:507, 1973.

35. Wright, C. B., Sayre, J. T., Casterline, P. F., and Swan, K. G.: Hemodynamic effects of sympathectomy on canine femoral venous occlusion, Surgery 74:405, 1973.

36. Wright, C. B., Casterline, P. F., Sayre, J. T., and Swan, K. G.: Management of Venous Ligation, in Swan, K. G. (ed.): Venous Surgery in the Lower Extremity (St. Louis: Warren H. Green, Inc., 1975).

37. Wright, C. B., Hobson, R. W., and Alix, E. C.: Results Following Reconstruction of the Canine Femoral Vein, in Swan, K. G. (ed.): Venous Surgery in the Lower Extremity (St. Louis: Warren H. Green, Inc., 1975).

38. Wright, C. B., and Hobson, R. W.: Hemodynamic effects of femoral venous occlusion in the subhuman primate, Surgery 75:453, 1974.

39. Wright, C. B., Hobson, R. W., Swan, K. G., and Rich, N. M.: Extremity venous ligation: Clinical and hemodynamic correlation, Am. Surgeon 41:203, 1975.

30 / Current Status of Venous Injury and Reconstruction in the Lower Extremity

ROBERT W. HOBSON, II, M.D.

Chief, Surgical Service, Veterans Administration Hospital, East Orange, New Jersey, and Associate Professor of Surgery, College of Medicine and Dentistry of New Jersey, New Jersey Medical School, Newark, New Jersey

CREIGHTON B. WRIGHT, M.D.

Associate Professor of Surgery, University of Iowa School of Medicine and Veterans Administration Hospital, Iowa City, Iowa

KENNETH G. SWAN, M.D.

Chief, Division of General and Vascular Surgery and Professor of Surgery, College of Medicine and Dentistry of New Jersey, New Jersey Medical School, Newark, New Jersey

NORMAN M. RICH, M.D., COL., M.C., U.S. ARMY

Chief, Peripheral Vascular Surgery Service, Walter Reed Army Medical Center and Professor and Chairman of Surgery, Uniformed Military Medical Services School of Medicine, Washington, D.C.

SURGICAL PRINCIPLES and technical considerations for successful vascular reconstructive procedures were developed in the late 19th and early 20th centuries by surgeons such as Murphy, Dörfler, Goyanes, Lexer, Carrel and Guthrie.[14, 15, 30, 34] Although successful application of these technical advances in the repair of arterial trauma awaited the availability of clinical blood transfusion and implementation of antibiotics therapy, improvements in limb salvage occurred

469

following repair of injuries to major arteries. The success of these techniques should have paved the way for more frequent reconstruction of injured major veins. However, recommendations concerning management of venous injuries have followed a more varied course.

Several important clinical studies as well as possible misinterpretations of experimental observations resulted in a tendency to favor venous ligation rather than repair following acute trauma. Early in the 20th century, experimental observations by Ney[31] suggested that the increase in distal femoral venous pressure which followed venous ligation would be beneficial in the presence of femoral arterial ligation. Propping[32] believed that venous ligation minimized the development of gangrene following arterial ligation by restoring the normal balance between inflow and outflow of blood within the extremity. Independent observations by Makins[27] resulted in similar recommendations on the basis of his extensive clinical experience during World War I. He reported an improvement in limb salvage attending acute venous ligation and major arterial injury treated by ligation. This report influenced the treatment of major concomitant venous injuries until the early 1940s as reflected by the statement by Linton et al.: "Following acute occlusion of the major artery to an extremity, there is practically universal agreement that ligation of the concomitant vein is beneficial."[26] However, subsequent analysis of clinical observations by DeBakey and Simeone[8] during World War II refuted the concept that venous ligation reduced the development of gangrene following arterial ligation.

Nevertheless, injury to major veins continued to be treated by ligation. Many surgeons were unaware that venous ligation could result in acute or subsequent chronic venous insufficiency. In addition, some were concerned that repair of venous injuries increased the likelihood of venous thrombosis and pulmonary embolization. Original concern[5] regarding an apparent increased incidence of thromboembolism after venous repair seems unwarranted.[10, 41] In a recent report comparing ligation and repair of injured popliteal veins, the incidence of thromboembolism was actually higher in the patients whose venous injuries were treated by ligation.[41] However, these potential hazards continued to deter many surgeons from recommending venous repair as opposed to venous ligation.

During the last 20 years, it has become increasingly apparent that repair of acute venous injuries in the lower extremity at the time of arterial repair is a valuable adjunct and may significantly improve limb survival.[3, 4, 10, 16, 23, 24, 35-37, 45, 47, 49, 50] Although ligation of injured major veins has been a common alternative form of treatment, these recent clinical and laboratory studies[2, 17, 21, 54-57] have emphasized the importance of venous repair rather than ligation. Venous ligation in the hindlimb of the dog[18, 21, 55] or subhuman primate[56] will result in acute venous insufficiency. Clinical reports of combined arterial and venous injuries in the lower extremity have documented occurrences of acute venous insufficiency in man, occasionally necessitating amputation when venous ligation has accompanied successful arterial repair. An additional number of patients who appear to tolerate initially acute major venous ligation may at some later date develop chronic venous insufficiency which may have been avoided by earlier repair.[39, 41]

Other reports in this symposium have reviewed the pathophysiology of venous ligation as well as the historical aspects of venous reconstruction. The purpose of this paper is to evaluate the current status of clinical venous reconstruction as applied to the lower extremity of man.

Etiology and Incidence of Venous Injury

The etiology of vascular injuries in casualties from the Vietnam War[37] included fragment wounds in 60.1% of patients. High velocity gunshot wounds accounted for 34.5% of vascular injuries.[37] In comparable civilian series,[10, 12] sharp instruments and lower velocity gunshot wounds have accounted for the majority of vascular injuries.

Reports of the incidence of venous injuries associated with major arterial injuries paralleled recognition of the importance of venous injury to patency of arterial repair as well as limb salvage. In a review of the U.S. experience during the Korean War, Hughes[24] noted that 63% of major arterial injuries were accompanied by major venous injuries. He advocated thorough exploration of war wounds and documented the frequency of venous injuries and described techniques for their repair. He also reported the incidence of venous ligation.

Injuries to minor veins are appropriately managed without complication by ligation; however, injured major veins at or above the level of the popliteal vein which are managed by ligation may result in significant alteration of regional hemodynamics and ultimately loss of limb. Hughes[24] was one of the first to document this phenomenon when he reported: "Most of these vein injuries were treated by ligation but in some, ligations resulted in various degrees of venostasis. On rare occasions, massive venostasis resulted in amputation of the extremity. To eliminate this complication, two investigators[23, 47] began the repair of major veins." He collected data on 20 major venous re-

TABLE 30–1.—VENOUS REPAIR,
KOREAN CONFLICT
EXPERIENCE*

TYPE OF REPAIR	NO.	%
Lateral suture	19	95
End-to-end anastomosis	1	5

*Modified from Hughes.[24]

pairs and documented the techniques for these repair as presented in Table 30–1.

In a preliminary report by Rich and Hughes,[36] approximately 25% of patients sustained venous trauma. These figures were reported at a time when the overall incidence of vascular trauma represented approximately 2% of major injuries in the Vietnam War. Five hundred patients sustained injuries to 718 major arteries and veins. This figure included 194 major venous injuries. Isolated injuries of major veins occurred in 28 patients. A majority of venous injuries had concomitant arterial injury. In an interim report by these authors,[35] the incidence of venous injuries accompanying major arterial injury was 37.7%. The high incidence of lower extremity venous injuries is documented in

TABLE 30–2.—LOCATION OF VENOUS INJURIES ASSOCIATED
WITH ARTERIAL TRAUMA, VIETNAM VASCULAR REGISTRY*

		ARTERIES	CON-COMITANT VEINS	LIGATION	REPAIR	% VEIN REPAIR
Neck	Carotid	50	14	10	4	28.6
Chest	Innominate	3	1	0	1	100.0
	Subclavian	8	4	1	3	75.0
Upper extremity	Axillary	59	20	18	2	10.0
	Brachial	283	54	42	12	22.2
Abdomen and pelvis	Abdominal aorta	3	1	0	1	100.0
	Common iliac	9	6	6	0	0.0
	External iliac	17	5	3	2	40.0
Lower extremity	Common femoral	46	17	8	9	52.9
	Superficial femoral	305	139	83	56	40.3
	Popliteal	217	116	82	34	29.3
Total		1000	377	253	124	

*Modified from Rich et al.[35]

Table 30-2 and this predominance of injuries in the extremities is consistent with recent military experience. The majority of popliteal arterial injuries (116 of the total 217) were associated with venous injuries (53.3%). The types of venous repair performed are outlined in Table 30-3. In a separate study devoted to popliteal arterial injuries with resultant amputation,[39] the incidence of concomitant venous injury was in excess of 80%. Although injury to bone and soft tissue contributed to a higher incidence of amputation, interruption of venous return from the extremity may have been a significant additional factor resulting in a higher amputation rate.

In an additional series of vascular injuries during the Vietnam conflict, Chandler and Knapp[3] reported a 62% incidence of concomitant major venous injury associated with arterial injuries. Although most of these injuries were treated by ligation, the authors were unable to determine the clinical significance of venous ligation in terms of limb salvage. However, in a separate series of 35 consecutive patients with wounds to the popliteal vessels, Sullivan and associates[49] suggested that popliteal venous reconstruction appeared to significantly improve limb salvage. Twenty-six patients had injury to the popliteal vein and in 21 instances repair was successfully accomplished, by lateral suture in nine patients, by interposition venous grafts in seven patients and by end-to-end anastomosis in another five cases. Failure to perform venous reconstruction in five patients resulted in significant complications. One patient required early amputation. Four patients developed massive edema and tense fascial compartments. Massive edema did not occur in any of the 21 patients who had venous repair. Early venograms showed patency of venous repairs in eight of eleven instances.

In a major appraisal of vascular injuries occurring in a civilian population, Drapanas and associates[10] reported a 41.1% incidence of adjacent venous injuries among 226 patients treated for arterial injury from 1942 to 1969. Fifty per cent of these venous injuries were re-

TABLE 30-3.—VENOUS REPAIR,
VIETNAM CONFLICT
EXPERIENCE*

TYPE OF REPAIR	NO.	%
Lateral suture	106	85.5
End-to-end anastomoses	10	8.1
Vein interpositional graft	5	4.0
Vein patch graft	3	2.4

*Modified from Rich et al.[35]

paired. In our own clinical experience[51] during the last year in Newark, 38 major vascular injuries were treated with twelve (32%) associated venous injuries. One third of these venous injuries were successfully repaired primarily. Although the subsequent patency of these repairs[10, 51] could not be evaluated accurately in all instances, we agree with these authors who suggested repair of injured major veins by primary anastomosis whenever practical, realizing that adequacy of venous return may be of major consideration in limb salvage.

Clinical Management

Although repair of major injured veins remains controversial as reflected by the number of clinical instances in which ligation of these injuries is performed, many authors recommend venous reconstruction by lateral suture repair, end-to-end anastomosis, venous patch graft or venous interposition grafting whenever possible. Meticulous surgical technique is of major importance in performing a venovenous anastomosis as has been emphasized from our laboratory experience.[18, 21, 22, 54, 57] The margin for error in completing the venous anastomosis is less than that for the arterial anastomosis. Tension must be minimized and anastomotic narrowing avoided if early and long-term patency is to be anticipated. Although interrupted sutures occasionally may be used, particularly in smaller venous reconstructive procedures, a continuous suture line is recommended clinically[40] and evidence from laboratory experience[18, 21, 57] has proved it to be a satisfactory technique. Figures 30–1 and 30–2 demonstrate venographic evidence of satisfactory venous repairs performed in the laboratory and clinical settings. One of the major problems in interposition venous grafting is the disparity in size that may occur between a major injured vein and an autologous saphenous vein. This discrepancy may be overcome by one of the techniques outlined in Figure 30–3 or as other authors have advocated by use of panelled saphenous vein grafts.[43] Autologous internal jugular vein has been utilized successfully in mesocaval shunting for the management of complicated portal hypertension[52] and use of this larger vein should be considered when interposition grafts are necessitated in the repair of common femoral venous injuries in man. Although not substantiated by experimental or clinical reports, the internal jugular vein may be superior to the panelled saphenous vein for femoral venous reconstructive procedures.

Preoperative use of venography has been recommended for the evaluation of potential venous injuries. Reynolds and Balsano[33] have

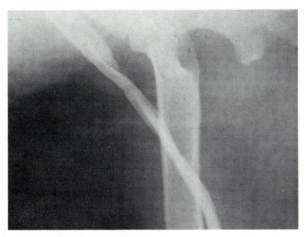

Fig 30–1.—Immediate postoperative venogram demonstrating a satisfactory repair of the canine femoral vein by interposition grafting. (From Hobson et al.[18] Used by permission.)

Fig 30–2.—A distal superficial venous injury was repaired by application of an autogenous vein patch. This postoperative venogram documents the satisfactory result. (From Rich et al.[35] Used by permission.)

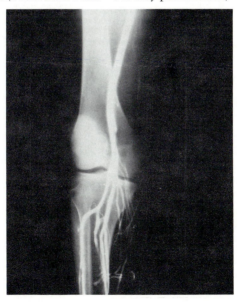

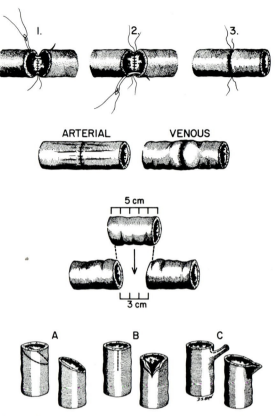

Fig 30–3.—These drawings demonstrate some of the basic principles in performing venous anastomoses. In an effort to prevent any constriction at the anastomosis, loops of a continuous suture are placed loosely in contrast to the usual technique for arterial anastomosis. Grafts in the venous system should be somewhat longer than the segment to be replaced and approximately of the same diameter. Diagonal cuts (A), 'fishmouthing' (B), and use of adjacent branches (C) can help prevent stenosis at the suture line, particularly when the graft is smaller than the recipient vein. (From Rich et al.[40] Used by permission.)

utilized this technique for identification of venous injuries accompanying pelvic fractures. Gerlock and associates[13] have recommended preoperative venography to identify venous injuries caused by penetrating wounds of the extremity, thereby facilitating their successful repair. In addition, Sullivan et al.[49] have used venography to evaluate postoperative results of venous repair and have documented patency of these repairs in the postoperative period. In addition, experimental data suggest the usefulness of operative venography[18, 21, 22] as well as distal pressure measurements[55] in the assessment of venous injuries. In the canine[17] and subhuman primate[56] vascular trauma models, venous collateralization was inadequate during the first 72 hr after femoral venous occlusion. Marked elevation in distal venous pressure or venographic evidence of major venous disruption or occlusion would indicate venous repair. On the other hand, absence of major distal venous hypertension as measured by saline manometry at the operating table or absence of demonstrable major venous injury radiographically would reduce the need for repair. This attractive use of venography during the preoperative period has been substantiated in a recent clinical report by Gerlock and associates.[13]

With regard to choice of graft materials for venous reconstruction, the autogenous vein remains the substitute of choice.[6, 7] The major drawback of the saphenous vein in venous reconstruction in the lower extremity is probable size disparity; however, this disadvantage can be overcome by use of panelled saphenous vein grafts or alternately by use of the autogenous internal jugular vein as discussed above. Our experience with a variety of graft materials in the venous system of the canine hindlimb has been reviewed in several recent reports.[21, 22, 57] This has emphasized the superiority of autografts as compared with homografts, collagen tubes, bovine heterografts and Dacron or Teflon grafts. As a generalization, synthetic grafts should be avoided in venous reconstruction in the lower extremities. Further clinical trial is suggested for fresh and frozen irradiated homografts.[54, 57] Modification of the immunogenicity of these homografts[53] may also provide improved patency in arterial and venous reconstructive procedures.

Although some authors have avoided use of interposition venous grafts[12, 29] because of their potential for thrombosis, others have suggested that use of these grafts to avoid venous ligation and thereby the adverse regional hemodynamics occurring during the first 72 hr postoperatively may be of value in improving limb salvage.

If graft occlusion does occur, the possibility of recanalization of the venous graft exists and has been documented in a clinical report by Rich and Sullivan.[38] Certainly, recanalization of interposition venous grafts has been carefully documented in the laboratory.[6, 9, 18, 57] Figures 30–4 and 30–5 show obvious recanalization in both clinical and experimental situations, respectively. Whether or not this ultimate recanalization would result in a reduction in chronic venous insufficiency is speculative and would be dependent upon competency of proximal and distal venous values.

Other adjuvant techniques following the performance of venous

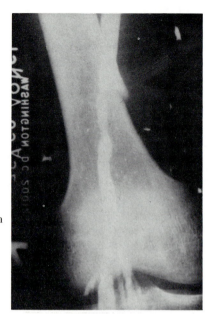

Fig 30–4.—This venogram shows recanalization of a 3-cm interposition autogenous vein graft used to repair a popliteal venous injury sustained 4½ months previously. (From Rich and Sullivan.[38] Used by permission.)

Fig 30–5.—Venogram 6 weeks after thrombosis of an autogenous vein graft in the canine femoral vein demonstrating early recanalization. (From Hobson et al.[18] Used by permission.)

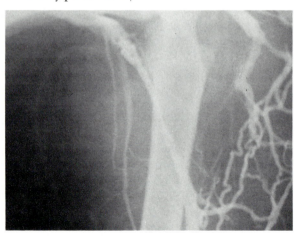

reconstruction have included recommendations for pharmacologic agents such as heparin or dextran and use of arteriovenous fistulas. A variety of experimental studies have demonstrated that heparin may improve initial patency, but probably has little influence on long-term patency.[1, 18] In one laboratory report,[28] clinical dextran was ineffective in improving patency of vein grafts in the venous system. In contrast, Eadie and de Takats[11] reported an improvement in patency of canine femoral venous reconstructions with use of clinical dextran. Low-molecular-weight dextran[18] may also be of value in venous reconstructive procedures because of its antithrombogenic effect as well as its capacity to increase femoral venous flow, as documented in normovolemic dogs.[44] Whether or not pharmacologic agents significantly influence ultimate patency of a venous reconstruction awaits further clinical confirmation.

Several reports have suggested use of distal arteriovenous fistulas to improve patency of either autogenous or synthetic grafts in the canine superior vena cava,[42] inferior vena cava[48] and femoral vein.[19, 25] Johnson and Eiseman[25] reported the first clinical use of a distal arteriovenous fistula in the management of femoral venous reconstruction. These authors concluded that this fistula might be a useful adjunct to venous reconstructive surgery following trauma or venous occlusion from neoplastic or inflammatory disease and in the management of the postphlebitic syndrome. In a recent report. Schramek and associates[43] described use of a distal arteriovenous fistula to support venous reconstruction following penetrating wounds of the extremity. Although use of distal arteriovenous fistulas remains controversial, these authors[43] adopted use of the fistula in repairs of the femoral vein in four patients citing better results in those cases where the fistula was used and remained functional as compared with those instances where the fistula was not used or occluded in the immediate postoperative period.

Although some investigators have described potentially detrimental hemodynamic effects of a fistula placed immediately distal to the venous reconstruction,[19, 46] other data have suggested its usefulness when placed in a more distal location, well away from the primary venous repair.[20] This more distal placement provided for improvements in flow through the reconstructed vein, thereby improving patency, and yet at the same time avoiding the potentially detrimental local and systemic hemodynamic effects of the more centrally located fistula. In addition, ultimate closure of the arteriovenous fistula can be accomplished without jeopardizing the venous repair if that fistula were located more distal.

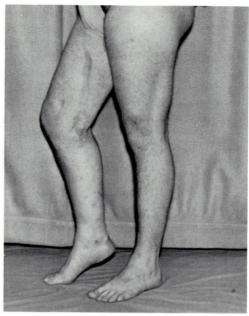

Fig 30–6. — This patient's right lower extremity demonstrates some of the physical findings characteristic of chronic venous insufficiency. The patient had an uneventful ligation of the right superficial femoral vein following multiple fragment wounds in Vietnam several years previously. He has developed edema and signs of venous insufficiency only in recent months. (Courtesy of Vietnam Vascular Registry.)

Analyses of clinical results following venous reconstruction or ligation are of limited number. Long-term statistics with regard to the ultimate fate of patients in whom venous ligation is performed without apparent immediate complications await further clinical evaluation. Although recent reports[22, 41] have suggested that venous ligation may ultimately result in the appearance of chronic venous insufficiency as is shown in Figure 30–6, further studies to evaluate patency of lymphatics as well as the influence of the magnitude of soft tissue injury are required before final conclusions can be made with regard to treatment of the isolated venous injury.[41] However, the desirability of repairing venous injuries in the presence of concomitant arterial injury is clear and every effort should be made to perform these reconstructions, particularly in the presence of distal venous hypertension. Further follow-up clinical evaluation of these reconstructions is needed, particularly with regard to application of diagnostic and adjuvant techniques and choice of graft materials.

Summary

Reconstruction is the treatment of choice for the management of venous injuries in the lower extremity of man. Venous repair by lateral suture, primary anastomosis or interposition venous grafting is superior to venous ligation, particularly in the presence of concomitant arterial injury.

Surgical techniques must be precise and completion of the venovenous anastomosis must be performed without undue tension or stenosis, if early and long-term patency is to be insured.

Preoperative and operative venography as well as operative venous pressure measurements are recommended to assess the extent of venous injury, the technical adequacy of venous repair, and the hemodynamic significance of the venous injury before and after repairs. In those instances where major venous injuries are identified and associated distal venous hypertension is documented, venous reconstruction is recommended and preferred over ligation.

Use of pharmacologic agents such as low molecular weight dextran or application of the distal arteriovenous fistulas in clinical venous reconstruction remains controversial. Observations from the laboratory as well as conclusions from some clinical studies suggest potential application of these adjuvants.

Autogenous venous grafts are superior for use in venous reconstruction in the lower extremity. Synthetic grafts are to be avoided. Results from laboratory investigations suggest the future possible clinical application of fresh or irradiated homologous veins. However, an acceptable substitute graft for the autogenous vein remains unavailable.

REFERENCES

1. Baird, R. J., Lipton, I. H., Mivagishima, R. T., and Labrosse, C. J.: Replacement of the deep veins of the leg, Arch. Surg. 89:797, 1964.
2. Barcia, P. J., Nelson, T. G., and Whelan, T. J.: Importance of venous occlusion in arterial repair failure: An experimental study, Ann. Surg. 175:223, 1972.
3. Chandler, J. G., and Knapp, R. W.: Early definitive treatment of vascular injuries in the Vietnam conflict, JAMA 202:960, 1967.
4. Cohen, A., Baldwin, J. N., and Grant, R. N.: Problems in the management of battlefield vascular injuries, Am. J. Surg. 118:526, 1969.
5. Cook, F. W., and Haller, J. A., Jr.: Penetrating injuries of the subclavian vessels with associated venous complications, Ann. Surg. 155:370, 1962.
6. Dale, W. A.: Thrombosis and recanalization of veins used as venous grafts, Angiology 12:603, 1961.

7. Dale, W. A., and Scott, H. W.: Grafts of the venous system, Surgery 53:52, 1963.
8. DeBakey, M. E., and Simeone, E. A.: Battle injuries of the arteries in World War II, Ann. Surg. 123:534, 1946.
9. DeWeese, J. A., and Niguidula, F.: The replacement of short segments of veins with functional autogenous venous grafts, Surg. Gynecol. Obstet. 110:303, 1960.
10. Drapanas, T., Hewitt, R. L., Weichert, R. F., and Smith, A. D.: Civilian vascular injuries: A critical appraisal of three decades of management, Ann. Surg. 172:351, 1970.
11. Eadie, D. G. A., and de Takats, G.: The early fate of autogenous grafts in the canine femoral vein, J. Cardiovasc. Surg. 7:148, 1966.
12. Gaspar, M. R., and Treiman, R. L.: The management of injuries to major veins, Am. J. Surg. 100:171, 1960.
13. Gerlock, A. J., Thal, E. R., and Snyder, W. H. III: Venography in penetrating injuries of the extremities, Am. J. Roentgenol. Radium Ther. Nucl. Med. 126:5, 1976.
14. Guthrie, G. C.: *Blood Vessel Surgery* (London: Edward Arnold & Co., 1912).
15. Haimovici, H.: History of arterial grafting, J. Cardiovasc. Surg. 4:152, 1963.
16. Haimovici, H., Hoffert, P. W., Zinicola, N., and Steinman, C.: An experimental and clinical evaluation of grafts in the venous system, Surg. Gynecol. Obstet. 131:1173, 1970.
17. Hobson, R. W., Howard, E. W., Wright, C. B., Collins, G. J., and Rich, N. M.: Hemodynamics of canine femoral venous ligation: Significance in combined arterial and venous injuries, Surgery 74:824, 1973.
18. Hobson, R. W., Croom, R. D., and Rich, N. M.: Influence of heparin and low molecular weight dextran on the patency of autogenous vein grafts in the venous system, Ann. Surg. 178:773, 1973.
19. Hobson, R. W., Croom, R. D., and Swan, K. G.: Hemodynamics of the distal arteriovenous fistula in venous reconstruction, J. Surg. Res. 14:483, 1973.
20. Hobson, R. W., and Wright, C. B.: Peripheral side to side arteriovenous fistula: Hemodynamics and application to venous reconstruction, Am. J. Surg. 126:411, 1973.
21. Hobson, R. W., Wright, C. B., and Rich, N. M.: Investigative Aspects of Venous Reconstruction, in: Witkin, E. et al. (eds.): *Venous Disease: Medical and Surgical Management* (Montreaux, Switzerland: Foundation International Cooperation in the Medical Sciences, Publ., 1974).
22. Hobson, R. W., Rich, N. M., and Wright, C. B.: Concept in Venous Trauma and Reconstruction, in Hobbs, J. (ed.): *Treatment of Venous Disorders* (Lancaster: International Medical Publishers, 1976) pp. 351–382.
23. Hughes, C. W.: Acute vascular trauma in Korean War casualties, Surg. Gynecol. Obstet. 99:91, 1954.
24. Hughes, C. W.: Arterial repair during the Korean War, Ann. Surg. 147:555, 1958.
25. Johnson, V., and Eiseman, B.: Evaluation of arteriovenous shunt to maintain patency of venous autograft, Am. J. Surg. 118:915, 1969.
26. Linton, R. R., Morrison, P. J., Ulfelder, H., and Libly, A. L.: Therapeutic venous occlusion, Am. Heart J. 21:721, 1941.
27. Makins, G. H.: *Gunshot Injuries to the Blood Vessels* (Bristol, England: John Wright and Sons, Ltd., 1919).
28. Moncrief, J. A., Darin, J. C., Canizaro, P. C., and Sayer, R. B.: Use of dextran to prevent arterial and venous thrombosis, Ann. Surg. 158:553, 1963.
29. Morton, J. H., Southgate, W. A., and DeWeese, J. A.: Arterial injuries of the extremities, Surg. Gynecol. Obstet. 123:611, 1966.
30. Murphy, J. B.: Resection of arteries and veins injured in continuity—end-to-end suture—experimental and clinical research, Med. Record 51:73, 1897.
31. Ney, E.: Du role des veines dans la circulation collaterale arterielle, Rev. Chir. 46:903, 1912.
32. Propping, K.: Ueber die Ursache der Gangrna nach Unterbindung grosser Arterien, Munchen Med. Wochenschr. 64:598, 1917.

33. Reynolds, B. M., and Balsano, N. A.: Venography in pelvic fractures: a clinical evaluation, Ann. Surg. 173:104, 1971.
34. Rich, N. M., and Hughes, C. W.: Fifty years progress in vascular surgery, Bull. Am. Coll. Surg. 57:35, 1972.
35. Rich, N. M., Hughes, C. W., and Baugh, J. H.: Management of venous injuries, Ann. Surg. 171:724, 1970.
36. Rich, N. M., and Hughes, C. W.: Vietnam vascular registry: A preliminary report, Surgery 65:218, 1969.
37. Rich, N. M., Baugh, J. H., and Hughes, C. W.: Acute arterial injuries in Vietnam: 1000 cases, J. Trauma 10:359, 1970.
38. Rich, N. M., and Sullivan, W. G.: Clinical recanalization of an autogenous vein graft in the popliteal vein, J. Trauma 12:919, 1972.
39. Rich, N. M., Jarstfer, B. S., and Geer, T. M.: Popliteal arterial repair failure: Causes and possible prevention, J. Cardiovasc. Surg. 15:340, 1974.
40. Rich, N. M., Hobson, R. W., Wright, C. B., and Swan, K. G.: Techniques of venous repair, Swan, K. G. (ed.): in *Venous Surgery in the Lower Extremity* (St. Louis: Warren H. Green Publ. Inc., 1974).
41. Rich, N. M., Hobson, R. W., Collins, G. J., and Andersen, C. A.: The effect of acute popliteal venous interruption, Ann. Surg. 183:365, 1976.
42. Scheinin, T. M., and Jude, J. R.: Experimental replacement of the superior vena cava: Effect of temporary increase in blood flow, J. Thorac. Cardiovasc. Surg. 48:781, 1964.
43. Schramek, A., Hashmonai, M., Farbstein, J., and Adler, O.: Reconstructive surgery in major vein injuries in the extremities, J. Trauma 15:9, 1975.
44. Schwartz, S. I., Shay, H. P., Beebe, H., and Rob, C.: Effects of low molecular weight dextran on venous flow, Surgery 55:106, 1964.
45. Simeone, F. A., Grillo, H. C., and Rundle, F.: On the question of ligation of the concomitant vein when a major artery is interrupted, Surgery 29:932, 1951.
46. Smith, C. A., and Schisgall, R. M.: The effects of a distal arteriovenous fistula upon an autogenous vein graft in the venous system, J. Surg. Res. 3:412, 1963.
47. Spencer, F. C., and Grewe, R. V.: The management of arterial injuries in battle casualties, Ann. Surg. 141:304, 1955.
48. Stansel, H. C.: Synthetic inferior vena cava graft, influence of increased flow, Arch. Surg. 89:1096, 1964.
49. Sullivan, W. G., Thornton, F. H., Baker, L. H., LaPlante, E. S., and Cohen, A.: Early influence of popliteal vein repair in the treatment of popliteal vessel injuries, Am. J. Surg. 122:528, 1971.
50. Swan, K. G., Hobson, R. W., Reynolds, D. G., Rich, N. M., and Wright, C. B.: *Venous Surgery in the Lower Extremity* (St. Louis: Warren H. Green, Publ. Inc., 1974).
51. Swan, K. G., and Hobson, R. W.: Unpublished data.
52. Thompson, B. W., Read, R. C., and Casali, R. E.: Interposition grafting for portal hypertension, Am. J. Surg. 130:1975.
53. Williams, G. M., ter Harr, A., Krajewski, C., Parks, L. C., and Roth, J.: Rejection and repair of endothelium in major vessel transplants, Surgery 78:694, 1975.
54. Wright, C. B., Hobson, R. W., and Swan, K. G.: Autografts and homografts in canine femoral venous reconstruction: A double-blind study, Surgery 74:654, 1973.
55. Wright, C. B., and Swan, K. G.: Hemodynamics of venous repair in the canine hindlimb, J. Thorac. Cardiovasc. Surg. 65:195, 1973.
56. Wright, C. B., and Hobson, R. W.: Hemodynamic effects of femoral venous occlusion in the subhuman primate, Surgery 75:453, 1974.
57. Wright, C. B., Hobson, R. W., Giordano, J. M., DeWitt, P. L., and Rich, N. M.: Acute femoral venous occlusion: Management by segmental venous replacement, J. Cardiovasc. Surg. (in press).

31 / Clinical Experience with Femoropopliteal Venous Reconstruction

E. A. HUSNI, M.D., F.A.C.S.

Department of Surgery, Huron Road Hospital, Cleveland, Ohio

THROMBOSIS OF THE FEMORAL vein is ordinarily attended by recanalization and destruction of functioning valves. These two pathologic changes produce both incompetence of the vein and high resistance to venous return from the limb against the pull of gravity. The result is ambulatory venous hypertension that may cause the classical postphlebitic skin changes in the dependent areas of the limb including edema, dermatitis, secondary varicose veins, pigmentation, ulceration and scar formation.

The degree of pathologic changes will depend upon the extent of the damaged venous segment. The bridging collaterals, notably from the popliteal to the deep femoral vein and via the long saphenous vein, are nature's attempt at bypassing an incompetent or occluded superficial femoral vein (Fig 31–1).

When these natural collaterals are absent, or when the deep femoral and/or popliteal veins are also involved in the pathologic process, the ipsilateral saphenous vein may be used as an in situ bypass by simply anastomosing it to the popliteal vein[1] as an imitation of a large natural collateral from the popliteal to the common femoral vein (Figs 31–2, 31–3 and 31–4).

Case Selection

Clinical evaluation of the postphlebitic limb is not enough for patient selection. Phlebography is the primary tool as it outlines the

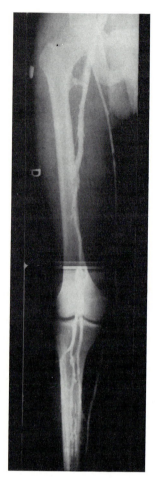

Fig 31–1. — Phlebogram demonstrating filling of the deep femoral vein from the popliteal with absence of the superficial femoral vein.

pathologic morphology of the veins (Fig 31 – 5). In general, three criteria should be fulfilled in order to promote a successful outcome of the bypass procedure:

1. The saphenous vein must be free of varicosities or acute phlebitis.

2. The popliteal and the common femoral veins must be free of acute phlebitis.

3. The disease must be limited to the femoral and popliteal veins. These findings, combined with a high ambulatory venous pressure of the limb, constitute the ideal prerequisites for an in situ saphenopopliteal venovenous bypass.

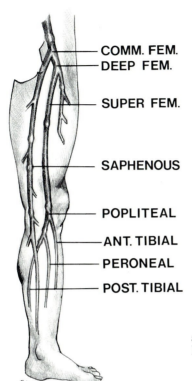

COMM. FEM.
DEEP FEM.

SUPER FEM.

SAPHENOUS

POPLITEAL

ANT. TIBIAL
PERONEAL
POST. TIBIAL

Fig 31–2. – Diagram illustrating anatomy of the veins in the lower limb.

Operative Procedure

The saphenous and popliteal veins are exposed through a vertical incision medial to the upper tibia. Tributaries to the saphenous vein are ligated and interrupted, yielding a free segment of vein long enough to effect a relaxed anastomosis to the popliteal vein. The fascia is opened and the popliteal vein is dissected away from the medial wall of the popliteal artery. A site that is relatively free of fibrosis and recanalization is selected. Anastomosis to the anterior tibial or posterior tibial veins may be undertaken as alternative sites to the popliteal veins when the latter is unsuitable (see Fig 31–4). Anastomosis is made in a routine fashion utilizing fine cardiovascular suture material and meticulous handling of the tissues.

In advanced cases, the removal of all varicose veins and the subfascial ligation of incompetent perforators will reduce the venous pool of the leg and will probably increase the rate of venous return through the bypass.

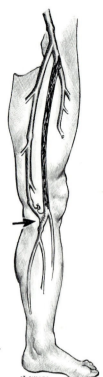

Fig 31–3.—Diagram illustrating a
saphenopopliteal anastomosis (*arrow*).

After completion, the leg is wrapped in elastic bandage from the
toes to the midcalf. Ambulation is started within 12–16 hr.

In well selected cases, this procedure has a great deal to offer in the
rehabilitation of the postphlebitic limb by alleviating ambulatory
venous hypertension and restoring health to the skin of the leg (Figs
31–6 and 31–7).

Results and Discussion

The clinical experience with venous reconstruction for the femoropopliteal veins, spanning a period of about 12 years, is summarized in
Table 31–1. It is noted that among the patients that were reevaluated
1–8 years postoperatively with phlebograms and hemodynamic
studies, the rate of success was highest (100%) in the direct repair of
veins where a short segment of vein, single or panelled, was utilized

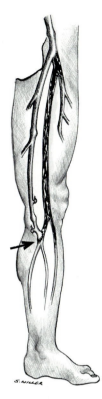

Fig 31–4. — Diagram illustrating anastomosis at the posterior tibial vein level (*arrow*).

with the end-to-end technique to restore venous continuity. The cross-pubis bypass grafts were also highly successful: 100% in cases of extraluminal compression and 83% in cases of post-thrombotic disease. In the case of the saphenopopliteal reconstruction there was a higher failure rate, 34%. It is worthwhile to mention at this point that in all cases where the graft had thrombosed, there was acute or subacute phlebitis encountered in the popliteal vein and/or its tributaries at the time of reconstruction and this particular fact should probably constitute a contraindication to this surgical procedure.

Anticoagulants were not employed in our venous reconstructions, but perhaps their judicial use may enhance the patency rate. Also, the creation of a distal arteriovenous fistula to the site of anastomosis has been undertaken by some investigators in an effort to maintain patency in the immediate postoperative period, after which time (3–4 weeks) it is interrupted. While this additional procedure will increase both the venous pressure and venous return from the limb and thereby possibly increase the chances of patency of venovenous bypass, it is not considered necessary in those cases where the peripheral ambulatory venous pressure is already close to arterial levels. In instances where the venous pressure is not significantly elevated, then this maneuver may indeed play a significant role in maintaining a patent

Fig 31–5 (left).—Phlebogram demonstrating postphlebitic disease of the popliteal and superficial femoral veins (*arrows*). (Inset from Fig 31–6.)

Fig 31–6 (center).—Phlebogram demonstrating femoropopliteal disease and a relatively healthy long saphenous vein. The ambulatory venous pressure was 133 cm saline.

Fig 31–7 (right).—Phlebogram demonstrating a functioning bypass 1 year postoperatively. The ambulatory venous pressure was 68 cm saline.

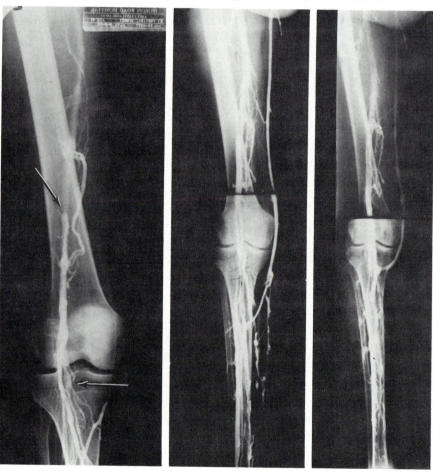

TABLE 31–1.—VENOUS RECONSTRUCTION (1965–1975)

CONDITION	NO. OF CASES	PROCEDURE	NO.	NO. PATENT/ NO. REEVALUATED	% PATENCY
Postphlebitic disease	85	Cross-pubis bypass	56	30/36	83
		Saphenopopliteal bypass	24	12/18	66
		Free graft	5	0/2	0
Trauma	37	Direct repair	28	10/12	83
		Free graft	8	4/6	66
		Saphenopopliteal	1	0	0
Extrinsic pathology with compression	7	Cross-pubis bypass	3	3/3	100
		Direct repair	3	3/3	100
		Iliac vein bypass	1	1/1	100

anastomosis. In doing this one must be aware that this artificial arteriovenous fistula may cause valvular damage and defeat the purpose of the bypass and may also add complications of its own. I am certain that long-term follow-up in these cases will shed light and offer direction in this endeavor.

Summary

Thrombosis of the femoral vein is attended by destruction of functioning valves as recanalization takes place. The resultant ambulatory venous hypertension may produce classical postphlebitic skin changes in dependent skin areas. The degree of pathologic change is dependent upon extent of autogenous collateralization or whether or not deep femoral and/or popliteal veins are involved in the pathologic process. This report deals with use of the ipsilateral saphenous vein as an in situ bypass to decrease postphlebitic changes in dependent skin. The operation is dependent upon anastomosis of the saphenous vein to the popliteal vein. Clinical evaluation is dependent upon phlebography and this should show the saphenous vein to be free of varicosities and phlebitis. Likewise, the popliteal and common femoral veins must be free of acute phlebitis and the pathologic process must be limited to the femoral and popliteal veins. When these findings are combined with high ambulatory venous pressure, the ideal requisites for in situ saphenopopliteal venovenous bypass are present.

REFERENCE

1. Husni, E. A.: In situ saphenopopliteal bypass graft for incompetence of the femoral and popliteal veins, Surg. Gynecol. Obstet. 130:279, 1970.

32 / Transvenous Repair of the Incompetent Femoral Vein Valve

Robert L. Kistner, M.D.

Department of Peripheral Vascular Surgery, Straub Clinic and Hospital, Inc. and Associate Professor of Surgery, John A. Burns School of Medicine, University of Hawaii, Honolulu, Hawaii

In the erect human, functional integrity of the valves in the veins of the lower extremity is known to be important for proper return of blood from the lower extremity to the heart. In spite of this, we know surprisingly little of the pathology or treatment of these valves. This report describes a specific valve defect found in patients with various degrees of deep vein insufficiency, and a method for diagnosis and repair of the defective valve.

The thesis presented here is that there is a condition of femoral valve incompetence that allows venous hypertension to occur in the thigh and calf, and that this can cause progressive, severe venous insufficiency. The exact relationship of this condition to thrombophlebitis is not clear. The femoral valve defect is probably not caused by thrombophlebitis, but it may be complicated by the occurrence of thrombophlebitis distally in the extremity.

This report describes the specific valve defect, the diagnostic steps in identifying it, the spectrum of clinical findings in these patients and a technique of transvenous repair of the valve defect.

Valves of the Femoral Vein

At least one valve, and usually more, is found in the normal femoral vein. A valve is found at the upper end of the superficial femoral vein near the junction with the profunda in over 85% of limbs. This is the most constant site for a valve in the femoral system.[1] Valves are found in the profunda veins in the majority of patients. A valve is also found high in the common femoral vein in most patients.

Femoral vein valves are bicuspid. The valve cusp is a gossamer-thin membrane which originates from the wall of the vein in a half-moon shape with the convex aspect directed downward and the straight free margin upward. As blood flows centrally, the cusp floats in the flowing stream or lies back against the vein wall and presents no obstacle to flow. When the blood is forced distally, the cusp acts as a cup or chamber which fills with blood and meets its fellow cusp in the midline to form an effective valve and prevent the backflow of blood down the leg.

In the normal state, the bicuspid valve is surprisingly strong. Under fluoroscopy, contrast material placed above the valve will not reflux through a competent femoral valve in the erect human. Even with the Valsalva maneuver, little or no blood will reflux through a competent valve. With the vein exposed at surgery, a fully competent valve entirely prevents the backflow of blood even with manual pressure applied above the valve. This is demonstrated by clamping the vein distally, then milking all distal blood through the valve, leaving a collapsed distal segment. When the valve is competent, no blood will seep back through the valve into the collapsed segment, and no blood will be forced through the valve by reasonable pressure applied from above.

It is not to be inferred that the normal human femoral valve is always totally competent. It has been shown repeatedly by others, and confirmed in our experience, that some degree of valve leakage may occur even in a patient who has apparently normal venous circulation in the lower extremity. This is discussed later in the paper.

The effect of thrombophlebitis on the venous valve has been shown to be thickening or destruction of the valve cusp. This has been clearly reported and documented.[2] The postphlebitic appearance of the vein is that of a thickened wall externally and a lumen traversed by irregular septa and random strands. This contrasts sharply with the pathology found in the patients described in this report.

The valve defect described here consists merely of elongation of the free margin of the valve cusp, producing a lip which prolapses when distended with blood. This prevents the formation of an effective cup, or chamber, by the distended valve, and results in a funnel effect of the edge of the cusp literally pouring blood down the distal vein. The valve structure itself is delicate and thin, and shows no evidence of ever having been involved by thrombophlebitis.

In a previous report, 14 patients with 17 involved extremities underwent surgical repair of the highest valve in the superficial femoral vein.[3] These patients had suffered severe venous complications prior to surgery, including ulcerations, swelling and stasis dermatitis. There were characteristics in these patients that seemed unusual in that most of them complained of a marked degree of aching in the legs and thighs and several had venous claudication.

The pathologic finding at surgery was unexpected and has not been described; yet the same defect has been found in each of these patients at surgery. When the vein was surgically exposed, it was found to be a thin-walled, normal-appearing vein, rather than the thick and obviously diseased postphlebitic type of vein. When the vein was opened, the lumen was clear and the endothelium was normal, in contrast to the scarred, septated appearance of the postphlebitic vein. The valve was delicate and thin, with soft, pliable cusps.

The only abnormality is elongation of the valve cusps to the point of having a floppy appearance. One or both cusps may be elongated. Because of its elongation, the cusp does not appose with the opposite cusp and leakage occurs.

This condition of the valve is reliably predicted by the findings at the time of descending phlebography, as detailed below. The cause of this condition of the valve is a matter of conjecture. There is no evidence to suggest the valve or the vein was ever involved with an inflammatory or thrombotic process. It is possible this is a developmental defect, because it has been found in several teenaged patients. Degenerative changes could account for loss of elasticity in the older patient, with subsequent stretching of the valve. Trauma might cause stretching or fatigue of the valve. Dilatation of the vein wall at the sinus of the valve might cause incompetence of the valve, as seen in one patient at surgery.

Diagnosis of the Incompetent Femoral Vein Valve

The diagnosis of incompetent femoral vein valves depends upon accurate phlebography, and requires both ascending and descending phlebography. The initial test is an ascending phlebogram performed in the conventional manner by injection of contrast material in a dorsal foot vein. We utilize a technique similar to that described by Rabinov and Paulin.[4] The essential finding is that of a patent superficial and common femoral system, with no trace of the linear septa that are seen in the recanalized postphlebitic limb. The calf may show evidence of previous phlebitis and may have dilated perforating veins, or it may appear normal. Valves in the superficial femoral vein may or may not be seen on the ascending phlebogram. The function of the valves cannot be ascertained by an ascending phlebogram.

When a patent femoral system is found in a patient with symptoms of swelling, pain or perforator vein disease, examination by descending phlebography can be done to test the integrity of the femoral valves. This is accomplished by placing a blunt needle or small catheter in the common femoral vein by percutaneous technique. On a tilting fluoroscopy table, the patient is elevated to a 60-degree foot-down position. Contrast material (Renografin-60) is injected into the common femoral vein in 20-ml aliquots under fluoroscopic observation, and the flow of the contrast material is observed.

Classification of the valve function as seen on descending phlebography has been simply outlined as:

1. *Competent valve:* No reflux of contrast material through the valve with the patient breathing normally in the 60-degree erect position.

2. *Mild incompetence:* Leakage of some of the contrast material through the valve, but flow of most of the contrast centrally.

3. *Moderate incompetence:* Leakage of much of the contrast material through the valve and down to the calf, but significant central flow of contrast still present.

4. *Severe incompetence:* Leakage of most, or all, of the contrast material through the valve, with little or no evidence of central flow. In this instance contrast should be followed all the way to the calf via the superficial femoral system.

In a patient whose femoral valves are completely competent, the contrast medium will all flow cephalad while it is being injected. The integrity of the valve can be further tested by having the patient do a Valsalva maneuver. In most instances this will cause some reflux of the contrast material, at least down as far as the valve. There are times, however, when all of the contrast material will flow cephalad even during the Valsalva maneuver.

In a patient with a severely incompetent valve, all of the contrast material will appear to flow retrograde down the leg with the patient breathing normally in a 60-degree foot-down position. As it flows down, it will clearly outline the femoral valves and will be seen to trickle through (more precisely, between) the valve cusps. The descending column of contrast material can be followed down the superficial femoral vein to the calf, outlining incompetent valves as it goes. It can also be seen in the system of profunda veins, where incompetent valves may also be outlined.

Between the extremes of total competence and severe incompetence lies a spectrum of relative degrees of valve leakage in which will be found some patients who have no symptoms and others who do have symptoms. Normal valve function appears to consist of a valve which is either completely competent or one which allows leakage of a minor proportion of the contrast material. These are categories defined above as "competent valve" and "mild incompetence." It appears that leakage of a small or even moderate amount of blood through a valve is a normal variant and causes no symptoms. Usually this amount of leakage is trapped by another valve lower in the thigh. This supports the findings of others[5] who report valve leakage as a normal variant.

Just how much valve leakage can be tolerated in a normal extremity is open to question. There appears to be a state of compensated valve leakage and a point of decompensation. This seems reasonable in view of the complex mechanism designed to force blood against gravity from the foot to the heart in the erect human. The pump is the exercising foot and calf musculature. The integrity of the system in the erect position depends upon functioning valves in the deep veins, the perforating veins and the superficial veins to prevent backflow and pressure buildup. Compensatory mechanisms of collateral flow complicate analysis of the system. Within this system lie multiple possibilities for failure and compensation, so that analysis of the cause of advanced venous insufficiency in the clinical situation requires knowledge of the functional behavior in each of three venous "systems," superficial, deep and perforator veins. This was pointed out by Linton in 1953.[6]

The degree of valve leakage defined as "moderate incompetence" has been found associated with more or less significant symptoms, especially the symptom of deep aching pain in the thigh or calf (bursting pain). In these patients, the larger proportion of contrast injected in the common femoral vein of the erect, normal breathing patient will be found to leak through the valve and descend in the superficial femoral system, and often in the profunda system. This descending column can be followed down the thigh. At times it will be caught by a lower femoral valve at the level of the adductor canal. In other cases, it will descend into the calf. An important aspect in these patients is that there is still a significant flow of contrast toward the heart at the femoral level. It is also likely that the perforating veins in the calf are still intact.

A third group of patients have been found in whom all, or nearly all, of the contrast material leaks through the valve and rapidly descends through the femoral and popliteal veins to the calf. This is the category of "severe incompetence." In these patients the findings at fluoroscopy are convincing and dramatic. A dark column of contrast material forms at the site of the injection and quickly descends the femoral system (Fig 32–1). In many instances none of the medium can be seen flowing centrally. The valves are clearly outlined (Figs 32–1 and 32–2) and the contrast medium is seen pouring through the valve as if it were being funneled down the leg (see Fig 32–2). The perforating veins in the calf are clearly diseased. It is in these patients that the clinical finding of severe venous insufficiency, with stasis pigmentation, severe edema, pain and ulceration has been correlated with the valve incompetence.

Frequently, the extremity with severe femoral valve incompetence is complicated by thrombophlebitis in the calf, and this combination may be the factor that leads to severe sequelae. Whether valve incompetence is the only cause, or is just one of the contributing causes of severe venous disease remains to be studied. Our experience is that once the condition of severe femoral valve incompetence exists along with severe disease in the leg, permanent control of the leg condition may only be achieved by correcting both conditions.

Regardless of the relationship between severe venous insufficiency in the calf and severe femoral valve incompetence, there is no doubt that patients who have deep aching and heaviness in the leg and thigh can be cured if their incompetent femoral system is repaired. This has been documented by Linton and Hardy[7] in discussing their experience with superficial femoral vein ligation, when he found dramatic

Fig 32–1.—Pre- and postoperative findings at time of descending phlebography, with line drawings. **A,** contrast material flows freely down the superficial femoral vein and less freely down the profunda system. **B,** after surgical repair of the superficial femoral vein valve, there is no reflux in this vessel while the reflux in the profunda vein is the same as preoperatively.

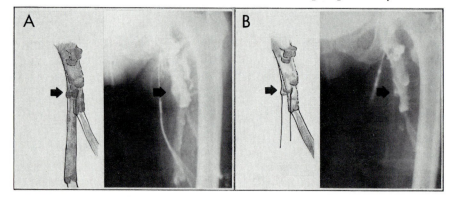

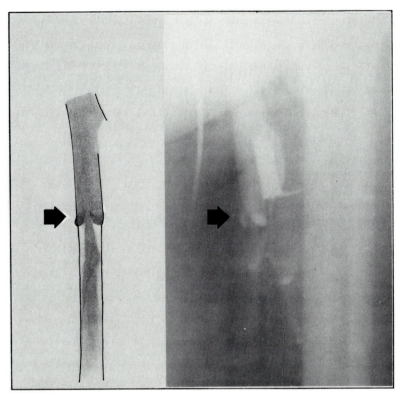

Fig 32–2. — Detail of leaking femoral valve (*arrow*) showing contrast medium pouring through the valve as if being poured through a funnel. Rendering at left accentuates photographic detail.

relief of this pain by these ligations. The same experience has been repeated in our patients who have had their valves repaired. Relief of this pain is an immediate effect of this operation.

Several case reports will illustrate some of the clinical problems correlated with phlebographic findings.

Case Reports

CASE 1. — A 17-year-old male athlete presented with bilateral varicose veins and a history of aching discomfort in the legs. Ascending phlebography revealed a normal deep system of veins and superficial varicosities. Reflux femoral phlebography revealed moderate to severe femoral valve reflux on both sides. Treatment at present is limited to symptomatic management of the varices. The course of his problem will be observed with the passage of time.

CASE 2. — A 21-year-old man presented with large unilateral varices and aching discomfort of the involved leg. His symptoms were aggravated in his occupation of musician because he was required to sit for long periods of time. The ascending phlebogram was normal except for superficial varices. Reflux femoral phlebogram showed "moderate incompetence," with leakage through femoral valves and down to the calf. Treatment at the present time is limited to symptomatic management of varicose veins and observation of the course of his problem. He has shown progressive symptoms during the past 12 months.

CASE 3. — A 26-year-old woman presented with unilateral severe aching discomfort. She was unable to sit at work more than 1 – 2 hr and was very uncomfortable. She had undergone ligation and stripping of varicose veins 2 years before, and was worse after the operation. There was a history consistent with venous claudication in the involved leg. Her symptoms had begun at age 15, and had been progressive since that time. Bilateral ascending phlebograms were normal. Bilateral reflux phlebograms showed completely normal valve function on the uninvolved side, and severe valve incompetence on the symptomatic side. The patient is being observed at present, but will probably come to valve repair in the near future.

CASE 4. — A 34-year-old woman presented with unilateral varicose veins and aching discomfort in the extremity. Multiple ligation therapy 3 years ago had been of no benefit. Her symptoms were progressive. Ascending phlebograms were normal. Bilateral reflux phlebograms showed moderate to severe valve incompetence on the symptomatic side, contrasted with completely normal valve function on the asymptomatic side. This patient is being observed for progression of symptoms.

CASE 5. — A 46-year-old woman was seen with varicose veins and an incipient ulcer of the right leg. She had a history of varicose veins on the left treated by ligation and stripping 15 years before, with a good permanent result. She presently complains of mild aching in the right leg. Bilateral ascending phlebograms showed patent deep veins on both sides, with perforator disease and varices on the right side. Bilateral reflux phlebograms revealed mild valve incompetence on the asymptomatic side and moderate reflux on the symptomatic side. Treatment at this time is correction of varices and perforator veins with plans to observe her future course.

CASE 6. — A 67-year-old woman presented with unilateral aching, mild swelling and incipient ulceration at the ankle. She gave a history of five operations for varicose veins. Her symptoms were progressive, though milder in the opposite leg. Ascending phlebograms showed a patent deep system and the presence of perforator disease. Bilateral reflux phlebograms showed moderate reflux in both femoral systems, with the more symptomatic side having significantly greater reflux. The present treatment is elastic support and observation of her course.

Discussion

These six cases demonstrate a variety of clinical pictures. None of them have a history of phlebitis or phlebographic evidence of old phlebitis. Two have perforator disease. All complain of aching pain, and in most of them this is a dominant symptom. Symptoms seem to be progressing over a long period of time. Vein stripping has been totally ineffective in one, and of no more than temporary benefit in others. There are three patients whose symptoms of aching began in puberty. Two showed strictly unilateral symptoms and in each instance the symptomatic side showed an advanced degree of valve incompetence, while the valves on the asymptomatic side were normal.

These case studies suggest that valve leakage is not associated with thrombophlebitis. The young age of several of the patients is compatible with a developmental defect in the valve, while the older age of others suggests the valve defect may be due to degenerative changes.

The full-blown clinical picture of severe venous insufficiency with ulceration, swelling and stasis dermatitis, in addition to aching and frequent venous claudication has been reported previously.[3] Two case reports from patients in that study will illustrate the type of problem encountered.

Case Reports

CASE 7. — A 51-year-old Hawaiian woman presented severe swelling of the left leg, severe stasis pigmentation, a 6 × 4 cm ulcer of the ankle and a typical story of venous claudication. Ascending phlebography revealed superficial varices and perforator vein incompetence. Reflux femoral phlebography showed severe incompetence of the femoral valves. Treatment consisted of ligation and stripping of varices, perforator interruption in the calf and repair of the valve located at the upper end of the superficial femoral vein in 1969. Surgery was followed by healing of the ulcer and complete relief of swelling.

At follow-up 6 years later she remained clinically cured, used no elastic support and had no swelling. Postoperative phlebography confirmed the integrity of the valve repair.

CASE 8. — A 65-year-old man presented with an incipient ulcer and recurrent cellulitis of the left leg, with severe stasis pigmentation. He had had deep aching pain in the leg for years. There was a past history of vein ligation and stripping in 1958 and 1963, with persistence of symptoms. He had clinical calf thrombophlebitis in 1963. An ascending phlebogram revealed abnormal calf and lower thigh veins and random varices, consistent with his history. Reflux femoral phlebography revealed severe valve incompetence in the superficial femoral vein with competent valves in the profunda vein. In July 1974 he underwent repair of the highest valve in the superficial femoral vein.

Immediately after surgery he was completely relieved of the pain in his legs. The cellulitis and incipient ulcer of the calf healed and have not recurred. He has no symptoms at all up to the present time. Postoperative phlebography confirmed the integrity of the valve repair.

Discussion

These case reports typify the severity of the problem found in all 14 cases in this study. All 14 patients who underwent valve repair had complete relief of their symptoms, including relief of aching in all, relief of swelling in all and healing of ulcers in all. At the time of valve repair, treatment of peripheral defects included vein stripping and perforator interruption when these systems were diseased.

A review of the clinical history in these 14 patients has uncovered five patients who had previously undergone vein stripping, and one who had previously had radical subfascial perforator vein interruption without control of symptoms. With a followup of 8, 7, 7, 4 and 2 years, respectively, and with continued control in all, it is thought these patients may be permanently cured now. These results suggest that femoral valve repair has added permanence to the good result obtained by appropriate distal venous corrective surgery.

Repair of the Femoral Vein Valve

The surgical technique for repair of the femoral vein valve was reported in detail in 1975.[3] An account of the technique of repair is repeated here, together with the illustrations from the previous report.

After intravenous heparinization, a longitudinal incision is made over the femoral vein to expose the common femoral vein, profunda

Fig 32–3. — Four steps in placing suture at commissure to shorten leading edge of cusp. **A,** needle passed from outside to inside of vein at level of commissure. **B,** needle passed through edge of cusp 2 mm away from commissure. **C,** needle brought back to original level at commissure and passed from inside of vein to the outside. **D,** suture tied outside vein, which results in a shortening of the edge of the valve cusp by 2 mm.

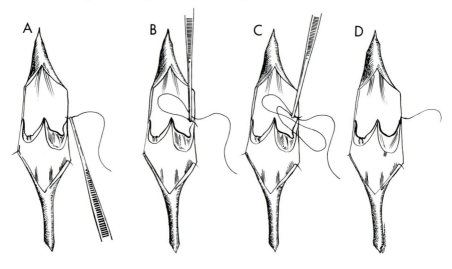

veins and the upper end of the superficial femoral vein. The highest valve in the superficial femoral vein has been chosen for repair because when it is competent the blood which drains into the common femoral from the profunda will be prevented from refluxing down the leg.

The valve is easily identified when the vein is exposed at surgery. Competence of the valve is checked in situ by clamping the vein distal to the valve, then milking all of the blood proximally through the valve. With all of the blood proximal to the valve and the vein collapsed distally, blood will reflux back through the incompetent valve and fill the distal segment.

The outline of the cusp insertion into the vein wall can be traced around the circumference of the intact vein, and the commissures can be precisely identified. A marking suture is placed at one of the commissures to guide the course of the venotomy between the valve cusps and through the commissure. The venotomy is begun 3 cm distal to the valve commissure and is carried proximally through the commissure, cutting right through the marking suture and extending proxi-

Fig 32–4 (left).—Method of placing suture through both cusps in midportion of opened vein. **A,** needle introduced from outside of vein to inside. **B,** needle passed through both cusps 2 mm away from commissure. The needle is then passed from inside the vein to the outside and tied on the outside, shortening both cusps by 2 mm.

Fig 32–5 (right).—Diagram of valve pre- (**A**) and postrepair (**B**). Note that there are multiple sutures in the valve commissures.

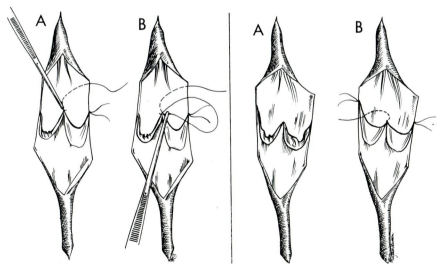

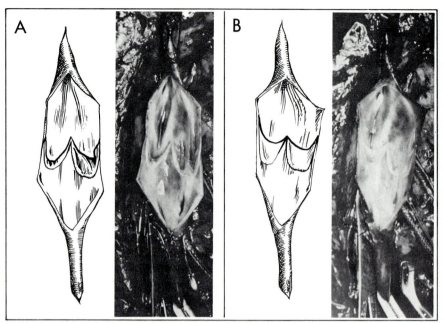

Fig 32‑6.—Photographs and line drawings of actual femoral valve pre‑ and postrepair. **A,** preoperative, showing the floppy valve cusps. **B,** post‑ repair, showing valve after the leading edge of the cusp was shortened.

mally into the common femoral vein. This step must be done carefully to avoid lacerating the valve cusp. Stay sutures are placed in the edges of the vein to minimize trauma. Inspection of the valve cusps will re‑ veal elongated, floppy margins on one or both cusps.

The valve repair involves placement of a series of interrupted su‑ tures designed to shorten the leading edge of the valve cusp. Figure 32–3 illustrates the method utilized to place each suture. Multiple sutures may be placed at each commissure. There are three sites to place sutures, i.e., at the commissure on each side of the opened vein and at the conjoint commissure on the posterior wall where the two cusps meet in the midline (Fig 32–4). Interrupted sutures are placed repeatedly until the leading edge of each cusp lies gently across the surface of the vein, and is neither taut nor lax. Figures 32–5 and 32–6 illustrate valve cusps pre‑ and postrepair. Before repair, the valve cusp was loose and floppy and severely incompetent. After repair, the valve was completely competent.

Repair of the venotomy is done with care to avoid injury to the valve cusp. Competence of the valve can be tested after closure of the venotomy, by the same maneuver as was done to show its incompetence.

Heparin is continued postoperatively for 2–3 weeks, and oral coumarin is continued for 3 months. There have been no thromboembolic complications. Postoperative bleeding in two patients has necessitated ligation of the superficial femoral vein.

Results of this operation on patients were reported in detail in 1975.[3] Suffice it to say that in the entire group of 15 successful surgical procedures there has been complete control of the venous insufficiency syndrome in every patient except for mild swelling in two patients. The universally good results have continued to hold up since the time of that report. The longest followup is now over 8 years.

Discussion

The importance of valve competence in the pathogenesis of severe venous insufficiency has been previously reported, and historical precedent for the existence of the problem discussed in this report is found in the literature. Homans in 1917[8] first related venous ulcers to destruction of valves by phlebitis and recanalization. Luke in 1941[9] described unilateral femoral valve insufficiency as a developmental defect in a 21-year-old woman with enlargement of the involved leg, dull aching pain and mild dependent swelling. The other leg was clinically normal and the valve function was normal in that leg. He found a similar circumstance in two other patients who had a previous history of phlebitis. This was probably the first description of valvular insufficiency producing symptomatic legs. In a subsequent report, Luke questioned the significance of femoral valve incompetence[10] because he found valve leakage in otherwise normal extremities.

Bauer[11] in 1948 described 30 cases with severe venous insufficiency due to thrombophlebitis. His detailed description is identical to the patients described in this report and there is no doubt they represent the same group of patients. His experience of immediate relief of bursting pain in his patients after popliteal vein ligation is exactly duplicated by the surgically treated patients in the present series.

Linton and Hardy in 1948[7] laid great stress on incompetence of the femoral system in the post-thrombotic syndrome and reported their favorable experience with division of the superficial femoral vein as an integral part of their management of this problem.

In 1951 Lockhart-Mummery and Smitham[12] described the syndrome of valve leakage in a paper devoted to their experience with retrograde venography. Their case 5 fits perfectly with the cases described in the present report. They state, as one of their important findings, that "in other cases showing induration and ulceration where previous thrombosis has not occurred, similar femoral vein insufficiency with back-pressure can be demonstrated and is probably the causative factor." They hypothesize that "valvular incompetence in the femoral vein is an important factor in the aetiology" of the venous ulcer in such patients. Furthermore, they state the cause of valvular incompetence is not known and suggest congenital valvular inadequacy as a possible explanation.

Dodd and Cockett[5] cite the frequency of deep venous thrombosis leading to serious sequelae, including pain, swelling, induration and ulceration. They ascribe the ulceration directly to incompetent valves in the ankle perforating veins, rather than to the femoral valve defects. They show that attention to the femoral system alone, i.e. by ligation of the superficial femoral vein, will not control the ulceration because the distal perforating veins are already diseased and must be treated. However, Burnand et al.[13] found control of the incompetent calf perforating vein alone will not control venous ulceration when the deep veins are damaged, since they found recurrence in all 23 patients with this combination within 5 years. They conclude that "incompetence of the superficial and communicating veins in patients who have had deep vein thrombosis is, like the development of venous ulcers, a result of deep vein malfunction and not in itself a cause of venous ulcers." They state that efforts to avoid recurrent ulceration should be directed toward curing the deep vein abnormality, and that as yet, there is no satisfactory treatment available.

It is our belief that control of the venous ulcer should be tailored to the veins involved in a given case. If perforators are diseased, they must be treated by subfascial interruption. If valve incompetence is aggravating, or perhaps causing, the problem, this requires separate treatment. When therapy is limited to only a part of the problem, recurrence will be seen too often.

Thrombophlebitis does not seem to cause the type of valve leakage described in this report because it destroys the valves, or at least shortens them. It is not clear whether thrombophlebitis in the calf is necessary to cause the incompetence of leg perforators or whether long-standing valve leakage in the deep system alone can cause this. In the patients who have been studied with severe venous insufficiency, there was a previous history of thrombophlebitis in only 30%, with a history that was indeterminate for phlebitis in another 30%, and 40% who had no history at all to suggest phlebitis. The phlebographic findings were of little help in determining previous thrombophlebitis in the calf, since by definition these patients had perforator vein disease coupled with patent, nonphlebitic superficial femoral systems. The conclusion at this time is that calf thrombosis will add further injury to an already compromised deep venous circulation in the face of severely incompetent femoral vein valves. Whether thrombophlebitis is necessary for the full-blown syndrome of recurrent venous ulceration is undetermined at this time.

A pattern has seemed to emerge from correlation of clinical findings with reflux femoral phlebogram findings. The completely normal valve is entirely competent and totally prevents reflux. Leakage of small amounts of contrast through the valve is a normal variant, and no symptoms are caused by this.

When a majority of the contrast material leaks through the femoral valve and passes down to the knee or calf, symptoms of deep aching and heaviness may occur. There will usually be no sign of advanced venous disease in the leg, such as pigmentation, brawny edema or ulceration, because the calf perforator valves are still intact. If varicose veins are present, vein stripping will provide only temporary or partial relief. The aching pain is relieved only by treatment of the deep veins, whether by valve repair, interruption of the superficial femoral vein or interruption of the popliteal vein.[11]

The ultimate stage is leakage of essentially all of the contrast through the valve and down the leg, coupled with incompetent leg perforators. These patients have the full-blown picture of edema, pigmentation and ulceration. In this situation, control of the problem requires treatment of the calf including vein stripping and perforator vein interruption when these systems are diseased, and control of the valve leakage at the femoral level if a permanent good result is to be achieved.

The indications for the femoral valve repair operation are presently limited to two groups of patients. The patient with severe venous insufficiency marked by pigmentation, edema and ulcer formation, who shows severe valve incompetence on descending phlebography, will be dramatically relieved by femoral valve repair coupled with appropriate vein stripping and perforator interruption. In this case, if surgery is limited to the calf alone, or to the femoral valve alone, results will be less than ideal and recurrence will be frequent. If both calf and femoral valve operations are done, the results are excellent and recurrence will be rare.

The second indication for femoral valve repair is in the patient with protracted and disabling bursting pain in the extremity. In this case, the perforator veins may be intact and surgery in the calf may not be needed. Femoral valve repair will provide immediate relief of the aching and heaviness and the patient will feel like he is walking on air. This symptom may be pathognomonic of deep vein incompetence. Other operations have been reported to give good results in this situation, such as interruption of the superficial femoral vein,[7] interruption of the popliteal vein[11] and transfer of the gracilis tendon to form a "substitute popliteal valve."[14] Which of these operations will prove to be the best remains to be seen. Our approach is to attempt femoral valve repair as the first effort since it is the most physiologic approach. If this fails, interruption of the superficial femoral vein can be done. From the results of superficial femoral vein interruption reported by Linton and Hardy[7] it seems likely that more swelling and a higher recurrence rate would follow this procedure than has been seen after valve repair.

The beneficial results from correction of the femoral valve malfunction have been striking when the indications for its use were carefully selected. It needs to be stressed that this procedure has no place in the management of the femoral segment that is deformed due to previous thrombophlebitis. It is believed that the benefit of femoral valve repair reported here is supportive to the concepts presented by others who have been struck by the important part played by an incompetent deep venous system in the pathogenesis of severe venous insufficiency. When this is due to a diseased postphlebitic vein, interruption of the vein is the procedure of choice. When it is due to valve deformity, the choice now exists between repair of the valve and interruption of the vein. When valve repair is chosen, the potential problems of thromboembolic complications from intravenous manipulation and the risks of anticoagulant therapy have to be weighed carefully.

Conclusion

Benefits derived from this experience with femoral valve surgery have been several. A new pathologic finding of the venous valve has been described. A spectrum of normal and abnormal valve function has been outlined. A concept of compensated versus decompensated venous drainage of the extremity has been suggested. Successful intravenous repair of the valve defect has been achieved and the newly competent valve has been shown to remain competent as long as 8 years. The return of competence to a single valve in the superficial femoral vein has been found to have profound effects on the venous dynamics of the leg.

REFERENCES

1. Mullarky, R. E.: Valves of the iliac and femoral veins, Northwest Med. 63:230, 1964.
2. Edwards, E. A., and Edwards, J. E.: The effect of thrombophlebitis on the venous valve, Surg. Gynecol. Obstet. 65:310, 1937.
3. Kistner, R. L.: Surgical repair of the incompetent femoral vein valve, Arch. Surg. 110:1336, 1975.
4. Rabinov, K., and Paulin, S.: Roentgen diagnosis of venous thrombosis in the leg, Arch. Surg. 104:134, 1972.
5. Dodd, H., and Cockett, F. B.: *The Pathology And Surgery Of The Veins Of The Lower Limb* (Edinburgh and London: E & S Livingston Ltd., 1956).
6. Linton, R. R.: The post-thrombotic ulceration of the lower extremity: Its etiology and surgical treatment, Ann. Surg. 138:415, 1953.
7. Linton, R. R., and Hardy, I. B.: Post-thrombotic syndrome of the lower extremity: Treatment by interruption of the superficial femoral vein and ligation and stripping of the long and short saphenous veins, Surgery 24:452, 1948.
8. Homans, J.: The etiology and treatment of varicose ulcer of the leg, Surg. Gynecol. Obstet. 24:300, 1917.
9. Luke, J. C.: The diagnosis of chronic enlargement of the leg with the description of a new syndrome, Surg. Gynecol. Obstet. 73:472, 1941.
10. Luke, J. C.: The deep vein valves: A venographic study in normal and postphlebitic states, Surgery 29:381, 1951.
11. Bauer, G.: The etiology of leg ulcers and their treatment by resection of the popliteal vein, J. Int. Chir. 8:937, 1948.
12. Lockhart-Mummery, H. E., and Smitham, J. H.: A study of the deep veins with special reference to retrograde venography, Br. J. Surg. 38:284, 1951.
13. Burnand, K., O'Donnell, T., Thomas, M. L., and Browse, N. L.: Relation between postphlebitic changes in the deep veins and results of surgical treatment of venous ulcers, Lancet 1:936, 1976.
14. Psathakis, N.: Has the "substitute valve" at the popliteal vein solved the problem of venous insufficiency of the lower extremity? J. Cardiovasc. Surg. 9(1):64, 1968.

Discussion: Chapters 28 through 32

COL. NORMAN RICH: I know all of you must feel as I do and as Doctor Dale has emphasized, that even with a diverse group of papers like this, the stimulation is fantastic. This makes it difficult to open a discussion and in a few brief moments bring it all together. There is one common denominator, though. Keeping with the historical theme, we must remember Hippocrates as we are trying to do these various procedures. We must make sure we don't do any ill to the patient.

The common denominator that goes along with all of these papers Doctor Hobson alluded to briefly at the end of his presentation, that of the development of thrombophlebitis and pulmonary embolism. Certainly, Doctor Husni as well as Doctor Dale have emphasized that this has not been a complication of their repairs, and Doctor Kistner has mentioned this.

In the acute venous injury repair area, it has been much more of a question. On the basis of one report of four patients, two of whom developed pulmonary embolism, many surgeons have developed a fear of any type of operative procedure on the venous system. In our long-term follow-up with 110 patients following ligation, there has been no significant incidence of thrombophlebitis. With repair, with similar numbers, there is no significant difference as far as incidence of thrombophlebitis or pulmonary embolism.

Doctor de Takats, the stimulus you have given to us and the challenge you have presented to us remain. I hope that you have some satisfaction in seeing the work that is being presented by Doctors Kistner, Husni and Dale with the new techniques. I think you recognize, as we do, that many challenges remain and, maybe, we should all go home and start working again.

DR. FUAD AL ASSAL: In Sao Paulo, Brasil, we have had operative experience with 24 cases of unilateral postphlebitic syndrome. The right limb was affected in 13; the left, in 11. There were 19 men and five women. Of these, 18 were white; 21 were married and three single. Fifteen were laborers and six were commercial tradesmen while three were maids. The age range of the population was between 20 and 40 years in 16; between 40 and 50 years in six. Only two patients were over 50.

Venography was by the ascending technique. Surgical treatment was selected for only those patients with widely recanalized deep veins of the lower extremities. In the study population, symptoms were pain and heaviness in all cases, as well as edema in all instances. Fifteen of the patients had internal maleolar and interomedial maleolar ulcers. Fourteen of these had severe pigmentation and 16 patients had severe varicose veins.

Since the basic abnormality in this syndrome is retrograde blood flow through valveless deep veins of the affected extremity, this is the condition to which treatment was directed. With this in mind, a free venous transplant containing valves is the foundation of treatment. In this study, two methods of free venous transplantation were used. The first was a short venous transplant used for the first 14 cases. In performing this operation, an oblique incision in the inguinofemoral region of the normal extremity was done. The saphenous vein was excised carefully for a distance of at least 12 cm and an attempt was made to obtain three competent valves. The venous segment to be grafted was then prepared. On the affected extremity, the popliteal vein from Hunter's canal to the midpopliteal level was dissected and this latter step is attended with great difficulty due to the tedious dissection through the strong adhesions accompanied by rich collateral venous supply. The popliteal vein was then resected, the ends fashioned obliquely so that the free venous transplant could be anastomosed end-to-end with the distal segment of the popliteal vein using monofilament nylon 5-0 sutures. At the proximal end, a similar oblique anastomosis was made with the same surgical technique. After the wounds were closed in layers, heparinization was not used postoperatively.

The second operation consisted of a long venous transplant, and this was used in 10 cases. Once again, the saphenous vein from the normal extremity was excised between the knee and the groin. The popliteal vein of the affected limb was then resected for approximately 5 cm above the knee and the proximal segment ligated. The saphenous transplant was then anastomosed by terminoterminal technique with continuous monofilament nylon 6-0 sutures. Thus, the distal venous segment was anastomosed to the graft and the graft was placed in a subsartorial plane so that the proximal anastomosis could be per-

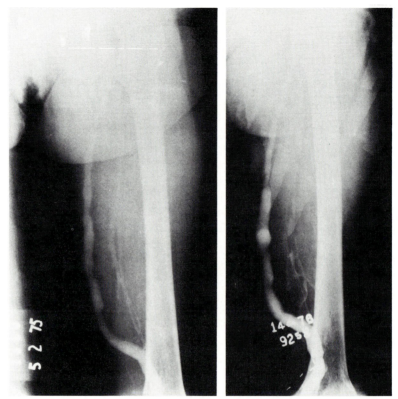

Fig 1 (left).—This venogram illustrates patency of a free transplant of an autogenous contralateral saphenous vein to bypass a superficial femoral venous occlusion.

Fig 2 (right).—An autogenous saphenous venous bypass is shown in this late postoperative phlebogram. Note functioning valves.

formed on the superficial femoral vein distal to the deep femoral vein. All venous sutures were performed according to the microsurgical principles proposed by Jacobson.

Venous pressures were obtained in the operating room prior to reconstruction and were 16–18 cm H_2O; after operation they were 10–12 cm H_2O. Phlebography was used before and after venous transplantation (Figs 1 and 2).

Because many of the patients had advanced venous stasis disease with stasis ulcers (16 cases) and incompetent saphenous communicating veins, a great many ancillary surgical procedures also were carried out. These included saphenectomy and subfascial ligations of incompetent veins. Results of venous reconstructive surgery were most gratifying. Ulcers healed in every case; pigmentation decreased in 80% of cases, and edema diminished in 70–90% of cases. I feel it is important to remember that edema may depend upon lymphatic disturbances of the leg.

The majority of our cases submitted to this treatment were invalids. After the surgical procedures, these returned to normal work and social life. Our follow-up in these cases is from 3 months to 4 years. The main complication of this type of surgery is hematoma formation in the popliteal space, and this was encountered twice. Four patients had thrombosis of the transplant and this was accompanied by acute clinical signs. Six patients had dehiscence of the skin incision. It is of some importance to note that transplant thrombosis occurred only in the first cases in this experience.

I would like to emphasize that with these results we are encouraged to continue with this research and think that new fields may be opened in venous reconstructive surgery.

Dr. Thomas Nolan: I would like to ask Doctor Kistner how he selects those patients on whom he does descending phlebography.

Dr. Creighton Wright: There was a question passed to me which is relevant to drug therapy rather than sympathectomy for alleviation of acute venous occlusion. We were led into the use of sympathectomy under our conditions following the administration of phenoxybenzamine. With regard to postphlebitic syndrome and the use of sympathectomy, we should go back historically to those who have shown that it did not increase blood flow in these limbs. I don't want everyone going out and trying sympathectomy again.

Dr. Robert Hobson: With regard to your comments on the saphenous vein in trauma, we would recommend that the opposite extremity be utilized. With regard to reimplantation, the general thought has been to do the venous reconstruction first. If we can get proximal and distal control of the artery and do a lateral venorrhaphy, I think that would be preferred. If an interposition graft were necessary, the arterial reconstruction should be done first, followed by a careful consideration of whether or not the venous reconstruction would be in order. The time required for the venous reconstruction would be an important factor. Intraoperative venography for measurement of venous pressure might guide one as to whether or not one might want to use an interposition graft in this circumstance.

One final question about the arteriovenous fistula. I think Doctor Husni indicated it was not required in the postphlebitic patient because of peripheral venous hypertension. However, in trauma, I think we should not yet rule out the use of arteriovenous fistula because there is very little peripheral venous hypertension. For the moment, I would suggest that we consider its use.

DR. W. ANDREW DALE: One more question. If a vein has been repaired either by lateral repair or by interposition graft and shown to be thrombosed by phlebography, do you have any figures on the chance of it reopening later on?

COL. NORMAN RICH: Most information on this is only anecdotal.

DR. ROBERT KISTNER: I congratulate Doctor Assal on his results. Doctor Nolan, thank you for the question because it is an important one. The people I evaluate with descending venography are those who have severe venous insufficiency in whom, when they are studied by an ascending venogram, we find a patent terminal segment. Now, we don't accept that terminal segment as being valveless unless we prove it with descending venography.

PREVENTION OF VENOUS THROMBOEMBOLISM

Introduction

IN THE Symposium on Venous Problems, no topic evoked more interest, no subject provoked more discussion than the problem of prevention of venous thromboembolism. The various techniques of miniheparinization, dextran, mechanical compression and full anticoagulation were presented in extenso. The curious paradox of lack of synergism between mechanical prophylaxis and subcutaneous heparinization was aired as was the fascinating fact that dextran failed to prevent deep venous thrombosis but did reduce the incidence of pulmonary embolization. These subjects form the last portion of this volume.

33 / The Current Status of Small-Dose Subcutaneous Heparin in the Prevention of Venous Thromboembolism

A. N. Nicolaides, M.S., F.R.C.S., F.R.C.S.E.

Senior Lecturer and Honorary Consultant Surgeon to the Cardiovascular Unit, Director of the Vascular Laboratory, St. Mary's Hospital Medical School, London, England

Soon after it was isolated, heparin was found to be valuable in preventing thromboembolism.[1, 2] However, difficulties of administration and control and the risk of bleeding prevented its widespread use in surgical patients. The suggestion that small doses of heparin should be used for the prevention of venous thromboembolism was first made in the 1960s by de Takats,[3] Bauer[4] and Lenggenhager.[5]

The observation that patients with shortened Lea-White coagulation times of 2.5–4 min (normal 5–10 min) submitted to operation were at risk of venous thrombosis[6] led Sharnoff et al. to suggest the minimum of anticoagulation to maintain normal coagulation as a means of preventing thrombosis without causing excessive bleeding.[7, 8] Ten thousand international units of sodium heparin were administered subcutaneously about 10 hr before operation and then 2,500–5,000 units every 6 hr depending on the Dale and Laidlaw coagulation time until the patient was fully active or discharged. There was one confirmed death from thromboembolism in 750 patients treated with the above regimen as compared to one in 90 cases among 18,729 without the prophylactic administration of heparin. There were only two instances where excessive bleeding at operation was attributed to heparin, this being traced to inadvertent incorrect administration of the anticoagulant. The main criticism of the work of Shar-

517

noff et al. has been that it was not a controlled trial and that somewhat less than 40% of the patients who died in each group had necropsies.[9]

Immediately after injury, factors IX, X, XI and XII are found circulating in the blood in an activated form as IXa, Xa, XIa and XIIa.[10, 11] The production of thrombi has been shown to depend on the presence of such activated factors in an area of stasis.[10, 11] However, thrombosis is not produced by stasis alone or by activated factors alone, but by a combination of the two.[10] The activated factors are serine esterases and can be neutralized by naturally occurring inhibitors.[12] Antithrombin III is such an inhibitor with broad specificity, but whose physiologic substrates are mainly factors Xa, IXa and XIa.[12] The activity of antithrombin III can be enhanced by heparin, and as little as 1 μg of activated antithrombin III by inhibiting 32 units of factor Xa can indirectly prevent the potential generation of 1,600 units of thrombin.[13] A relatively smaller amount of heparin is required to neutralize factor Xa irreversibly than is required to block the thrombin-fibrinogen reaction which emphasizes that the cascade coagulation mechanism functions as a biologic amplification system.[13] It therefore has been suggested that it would be reasonable to anticipate that, if hypercoagulability were treated before intravascular coagulation was initiated, less of the antithrombotic agent would be required than if therapy were begun after thrombin formation had occurred.

Bacterial endotoxin activates factor XI to produce a hypercoagulable state and thrombosis in areas of stasis. This hypercoagulable state can be prevented experimentally by as little as 10 units of heparin per kilogram injected intravenously, a dose insufficient to prolong the clotting time.[15]

Small-Dose Heparin

Kakkar and his colleagues[16, 17] and Williams[18] produced evidence that small doses of subcutaneous heparin reduce the incidence of postoperative venous thrombosis as detected by the ^{125}I-fibrinogen test. Gordon-Smith and his colleagues[19] in a controlled trial of two regimens of subcutaneous heparin, one administered for 24 hr and the other for 5 days, demonstrated that the incidence was reduced from 42% in the control group to 13.5% and 8.3% in the test groups, respectively.

The results of a larger trial demonstrated that small-dose subcutaneous heparin could safely prevent not only the early postoperative thrombi detected by the ^{125}I-fibrinogen test, but also their extensions proximal to the calf.[20]

TABLE 33-1.—THE INCIDENCE OF PROXIMAL THROMBI
DETECTED WITH THE ^{125}I-FIBRINOGEN TEST IN RANDOMIZED
TRIALS OF SMALL DOSE SUBCUTANEOUS HEPARIN IN
GENERAL SURGICAL PATIENTS

AUTHORS	NO. OF PATIENTS IN TRIALS	NO. OF PATIENTS WITH THROMBI EXTENDING INTO THE POPLITEAL AND MORE PROXIMAL VEINS°	
		CONTROL GROUP	HEPARIN GROUP
Williams, 1971[18]	56	1	0
Nicolaides et al., 1972[20]	244	9	0
Gordon-Smith, 1972[21]	100	3	0
Gallus et al., 1973[22]	209	4	0
Ballard et al., 1973[23]	110	0	0
Rem et al., 1975[24]	178	5	0
Rosenberg et al., 1975[25]	91	7	0
Joffe, 1976[26]	155	17	0
Total	1143	46 (7.4%)	0

°χ^2(with Yates correction) = 40.4, $p < 0.0005$.

Several other trials of small-dose subcutaneous heparin were reported subsequently.[22-26] In seven of the randomized trials in general surgical patients data is available about the incidence of thrombi extending into the popliteal and more proximal veins (Table 33-1). There were 46 thrombi proximal to the calf in 622 patients in the control groups and none in the 520 patients in the test groups ($\chi^2 = 40.4$; $p < 0.0005$). It has already been demonstrated that if thrombosis is limited to the calf the risk of large clinically detectable pulmonary emboli is for all practical purposes negligible, but if the popliteal and more proximal veins are involved the risk of clinical pulmonary embolism is increased to 50%.[27] Proximal extensions of the thrombi which start in the calf constitute approximately two thirds of all of the thrombi which involve the proximal veins.[28] It therefore could be argued that the reduction in the incidence of the proximal extensions by small-dose subcutaneous heparin would also result in the reduction of the incidence of pulmonary embolism. The results reported by Sharnoff and De Blasio[8] support this indirect inference. Direct evidence of the efficacy of small-dose subcutaneous heparin on the incidence of pulmonary embolism could not be obtained from trials in which the ^{125}I-fibrinogen was used because whenever proximal thrombosis was detected, conventional anticoagulation therapy was administered by most workers. It would have been unethical to do otherwise.

Direct evidence of the efficacy of small-dose subcutaneous heparin in the prevention of pulmonary embolism was first produced by Sagar et al. [29] in 1975 in a controlled prospective trial in patients over the age of 50 having major operations. In this study all patients who died came to necropsy. A dose of 5,000 units of sodium heparin was given subcutaneously 2 hr before operation and then every 12 hr for 5 days. Fatal pulmonary embolism did not occur in any of the 252 patients in the test group, whereas 8 (3.39%) patients of the 236 in the control group died of pulmonary embolism. At the same time, it was demonstrated by two independent teams that the number and size of postoperative pulmonary embolism detected by perfusion scans of the lungs was reduced by a similar regimen of heparin.[30, 31]

The results of the international multicenter trial[32] were published in July 1975. A total of 4,121 patients over the age of 40 having elective major abdominal and thoracic operations were included in this study; 2,076 of these were in the control group and 2,045 patients received heparin. Of these patients, 180 (4.4%) died during the postoperative period, 100 in the control and 80 in the heparin group. Necropsy examination was performed in 72% of deaths in the control and 66% in the heparin group. Sixteen patients in the control group and two in the heparin group were found at necropsy to have died from acute massive pulmonary embolism ($p < 0.005$). In addition emboli found at necropsy in six patients in the control group and three in the heparin group were considered either contributory to death or an incidental finding. Taking all pulmonary emboli together, the findings were also significant ($p < 0.005$). Though this study has certain design defects,[33] when it is taken in conjunction with previous work it provides the final link for the logical chain for establishing the efficacy of small-dose subcutaneous heparin in the prevention of pulmonary embolism.[33]

Problems with Small-Dose Heparin

Though we can now say that small-dose subcutaneous heparin can prevent deep venous thrombosis and pulmonary embolism in patients having general surgical and thoracic operations, problems remain concerning ineffective prophylaxis and bleeding.

Ineffective Prophylaxis

The 12-hr regimen is relatively ineffective in patients with fractured neck of femur (Table 33–2)[17] and for those undergoing total hip replacement,[17, 37] perhaps because the tissue trauma activates clotting factors before heparin can be administered.[34] The 8-hr regimen is superior (see Table 33–2) but deep venous thrombosis is by no means abolished. The results in patients with myocardial infarction are also

TABLE 33-2.—THE INCIDENCE OF DEEP VENOUS
THROMBOSIS DETECTED BY THE ^{125}I-FIBRINOGEN TEST IN
RANDOMIZED TRIALS OF SMALL-DOSE SUBCUTANEOUS
HEPARIN IN PATIENTS HAVING OPERATIONS ON THE HIP

| AUTHORS | FREQUENCY OF INJECTION OF 5,000 UNITS HEPARIN | INCIDENCE (%) | |
		CONTROL GROUP	TEST GROUP
Operations for fractured hips			
Kakkar et al., 1972[17]	12 hr	54	40
Gallus et al., 1973[22]	8 hr	56	23
Elective operations on the hip			
Kakkar et al., 1972[17]	12 hr	38	26
Morris et al., 1974[36]*	12 hr	50	11
Rosengarten et al., 1975[37]	12 hr	45	33
Gallus et al., 1973[35]	8 hr	42	9
Hampson et al., 1974[38]	8 hr	54	46
Nicolaides et al., 1975[39]	8 hr	40	4
Kakkar et al., 1975[40]	8 hr	34	11
Stamatakis et al., 1976[41]	8 hr	72	42

*Dextran-70 was used to replace blood loss.

conflicting (Table 33-3), but the 8-hr regimen can be used safely because of the absence of a wound.

BLEEDING

In one trial of 8-hr heparin there was a moderate and significant increase of blood requirements in those patients who required transfusion.[42] In many trials (see Tables 33-2 and 33-3) the number of hematomas has been greater in the heparin group, though the numbers were too small for any statistical significance. This with several anecdotal reports of wound hematomas[45-50] or fatal hemorrhages in patients

TABLE 33-3.—INCIDENCE OF DEEP VENOUS THROMBOSIS
DETECTED WITH THE ^{125}I-FIBRINOGEN TEST IN PATIENTS
WITH MYOCARDIAL INFARCTION REPORTED IN CONTROLLED
CLINICAL TRIALS OF SMALL-DOSE HEPARIN

| AUTHORS | FREQUENCY OF INJECTION OF 5,000 UNITS HEPARIN | INCIDENCE (%) | |
		CONTROL GROUP	TEST GROUP
Handley, 1972[43]	12 hr	29	23
Warlow et al., 1973[44]	12 hr	17.2	3.2
Gallus et al., 1973[22]	8 hr	22.5	2.6

receiving small-dose subcutaneous heparin[47-48] has been enough to make many surgeons cautious.

Direct evidence about the increased incidence of wound hematomas has been provided by the multicenter trial[39]; 117 patients in the control group and 158 in the heparin group developed a wound hematoma ($p < 0.01$).

The combination of dextran infusion with small-dose subcutaneous heparin in a small number of patients has led to excessive bleeding. Clearly such practice is dangerous.

In addition to the increased morbidity associated with the use of low-dose heparin, there is the ever-present risk of overdose which did occur.[39] However, methods such as the use of disposable cartridges or ampules containing the correct dose are now available and should eliminate human error.

Because of the suggested increased incidence of wound hematoma, a study now in progress at St. Mary's Hospital, London is designed to answer two questions. (1) What are the plasma levels of heparin in general surgical patients receiving 5,000 units of subcutaneous sodium heparin every 12 hr? (2) Is there any association between plasma levels of heparin and the incidence of wound hematoma?

This is a blind study in which patients over the age of 40 having elective general surgical operations are randomly allocated to a control and a test group. In the test group, subcutaneous heparin (5,000 units) is administered 2 hr before operation and then every 12 hr for 7 days. The patients in the control group receive the same regimen of isotonic saline. Blood is collected from each patient just before the preoperative subcutaneous injection and at 2, 4 and 6 hr subsequently on the day of operation. Blood is also collected just before and 2 hr after the morning injection on the 1st, 3d and 6th postoperative days. Plasma heparin levels are estimated using a sensitive assay based on the potentiating effect of heparin on the antifactor Xa.[51] The wounds are inspected on the 5th and 7th postoperative day by an observer who does not know the heparin levels. The patients are scanned with the ^{125}I-fibrinogen test for 10 days. So far, 92 patients have been admitted to the study (49 in the control and 43 in the heparin group). The mean heparin levels in the heparin group are shown in Figure 33–1, and varied markedly. In 15 (35%) patients plasma levels greater than 0.2 units/ml were detected. The patients receiving heparin were divided into two groups using the above arbitrary level of heparin (0.2 units/ml). There were thus 15 patients in whom plasma levels greater than 0.2 units/ml were detected on one or more occasions (group A), 28 patients in whom the plasma levels were always <0.2 units/ml (group B)

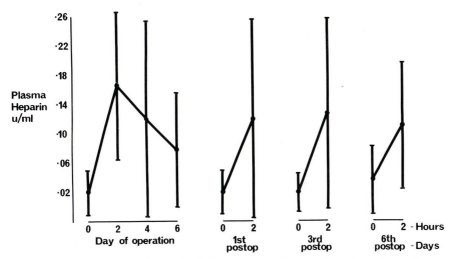

Fig 33–1.—Mean and standard deviation of heparin levels in the plasma of 43 patients before and after 5,000 units of subcutaneous heparin on the day of operation and morning of first, third and sixth postoperative days.

and 49 controls (Table 33–4). The increased incidence of wound hematoma in group A was significant ($p < 0.05$).

These results suggest that, if the increased incidence of wound hematoma is to be prevented, then the administration of heparin should be modified so as to avoid plasma heparin levels greater than 0.2 units/ml.

The plasma heparin level and antithrombotic effect of an intravenous bolus of heparin will depend on the amount of antiheparin activity in the blood, the antithrombin III and fibrinogen levels which bind it as inert carriers or substrates[52] and the rate of its elimination which includes not only renal excretion, but also its transport to the extravascular compartment, probably by the reticuloendothelial sys-

TABLE 33–4.—INCIDENCE OF POSTOPERATIVE WOUND HEMATOMAS IN RELATION TO HEPARIN LEVELS IN THE PLASMA

GROUP	NO HEMATOMA	HEMATOMA	TOTAL
A, heparin level > 0.2 units/ml	8	7 (47%)	15
B, heparin level < 0.2 units/ml	25	3 (11%)	28
C, saline	43	6 (12%)	49

Comparing groups A and B:$\chi^2 = 5.36$; $p < 0.05$ (with Yates correction)

tem.[53-54] The biologic activity will also depend on the level of heparin cofactors.[52] With subcutaneous injections, the rate of absorption is yet another variable. Therefore, it is hardly surprising that the plasma levels of heparin after a single dose of subcutaneous heparin will vary not only from patient to patient, but also from day to day in the same patient.

Conclusion

It will be obvious to all who have been familiar with the work on heparin in its early days in the 1940s that thinking has come full circle. Doctor de Takats has shown through several publications that the in vivo tolerance varied from patient to patient and that during surgical convalescence the patient went through certain phases of resistance followed by sensitivity to heparin.[55-59] "What is needed then is a simple, bedside screening test to determine the patient's heparin tolerance."[56] The question of which test should be adopted for the control of small-dose subcutaneous heparin has now to be answered. In the meantime many surgeons will avoid using this method of prophylaxis in patients in whom extensive dissection is anticipated.

We are now entering a period when it is not ethical to design trials with a control group consisting of patients without any form of prophylaxis. We shall witness a number of comparative trials in attempts to determine whether other methods of prevention such as dextran-70 and mechanical methods used singly or in combination are equally or more effective than small-dose heparin. The more effective these methods are, the larger the numbers that will be required to demonstrate a significant difference in their effect and safety. We predict that many of these trials will be inconclusive. What is really required is a method of determining the risk of pulmonary embolism for a patient, and the efficacy and morbidity of the various methods of prophylaxis when applied to the same patient.

Finally, what about the familiar question "Is there any difference between sodium and calcium heparin?" Most workers have, so far, used exclusively calcium heparin and others only sodium heparin. The sensitive heparin assays now available[60] have failed to demonstrate any difference in the plasma levels of healthy volunteers after the subcutaneous injection of 5,000 units of heparin.[53, 54] However, these studies involved small numbers only. Further work is required in a large number of patients in the postoperative period. In the meantime the only factor which determines which heparin is used is cost.

Summary

The suggestion that small doses of heparin should be used for the prevention of venous thromboembolism was first made in the 1950s by de Takats. Antithrombin III is a broadly specific inhibitor of thrombosis and can be enhanced by heparin. With as little as 1 μg of activated antithrombin III, which inhibits 32 units of factor Xa, the potential generation of 16,000 units of thrombin can be indirectly prevented. The ^{125}I-fibrinogen test provides an end point of clotting which can then be used to assess methods of prophylaxis. Such methods have been abundantly tried and it is now concluded that small-dose subcutaneous heparin can safely prevent early postoperative thrombi detected by ^{125}I-tagged fibrinogen and also their proximal extension in the calf. Direct evidence of efficacy of small dose subcutaneous heparin in prevention of pulmonary embolism has also been provided in small trials as well as a large, international multicentered trial.

REFERENCES

1. Wetterdall, P.: Use of heparin as a prophylactic following gynaecological operations, Acta Med. Scand. 107:123, 1941.
2. Bauer, G.: Thrombosis: Early diagnosis and abortive treatment with heparin, Lancet 1:447, 1946.
3. de Takats, G.: Anticoagulants in surgery, JAMA 142:527, 1950.
4. Bauer, S.: Proceedings of the first international conference on thrombosis and embolism (Basel: B. Schabe) p. 721.
5. Lenggenhager, K.: Genese und Prophylaxis der postoperativen Fernthrombose, Helv. Chir. Acta 24:316, 1957.
6. Sharnoff, J. G., Bagg, J. F., Breen, S. R., Rogliano, A. G., Walsh, A. G., and Scardino, V.: The possible indication of post-operative thromboembolism by platelet counts and blood coagulation studies in the patient undergoing extensive surgery, Surg. Gynecol. Obstet. 111:469, 1960.
7. Sharnoff, J. G.: Results in the prophylaxis of post-operative thromboembolism, Surg. Gynecol. Obstet. 123:303, 1966.
8. Sharnoff, J. G., and De Blasio, G.: Prevention of fatal post-operative thromboembolism by heparin prophylaxis, Lancet 2:1006, 1970.
9. Benson, E. A.: Prevention of fatal post-operative thromboembolism by heparin prophylaxis, Lancet 2:1135, 1970.
10. Wessler, S., and Yin, E. T.: On the mechanism of thrombosis, Progr. Haematol. 6:201, 1968.
11. Rosenberg, R. D.: Actions and interactions of antithrombin and heparin, N. Engl. J. Med. 292:146, 1975.
12. Damus, P. S., Hicks, M., and Rosenberg, R. R.: Anticoagulant action of heparin, Nature (Lond.) 246:355, 1973.
13. Yin, E. T., Wessler, S., and Stoll, P.: Biological properties of the naturally occurring plasma inhibitor to activated factor X, J. Biol. Chem. 246:3703, 1971.
14. Wessler, S.: The Issue of Hypercoagulability, in Kakkar, V. V., and Jouhar, A. J. (eds.): *Thromboembolism: Diagnosis and Treatment* (Edinburgh and London: Churchill & Livingstone, 1972).

15. Thomas, D., and Wessler, S.: Stasis thrombi induced by bacterial endotoxin, Circul. Res. 14:486, 1964.
16. Kakkar, V. V., Field, E. S., Nicolaides, A. N., Flute, P. T., Wessler, S., and Yin, E. T.: Low doses of heparin in prevention of deep vein thrombosis, Lancet 2:669, 1971.
17. Kakkar, V. V., Corrigan, T., Spindler, J., Fossard, D. P., Flute, P. T., Crellin, R. Q., Wessler, S., and Yin, E. T.: Efficacy of low doses of heparin in prevention of deep vein thrombosis after major surgery, Lancet 2:101, 1972.
18. Williams, H. T.: Prevention of post-operative deep vein thrombosis with peri-operative subcutaneous heparin, Lancet 2:950, 1971.
19. Gordon-Smith, I. C., Grundy, D. J., Le Quesne, L. P., Newcombe, J. F., and Bramble, F. J.: Controlled trial of two regimens of subcutaneous heparin in prevention of post-operative deep vein thrombosis, Lancet 1:1133, 1972.
20. Nicolaides, A. N., Dupont, P. A., Desai, S., Lewis, J. D., Douglas, J. N., Dodsworth, H., Fourides, G., Luck, R. J., and Jamieson, C. W.: Small doses of subcutaneous sodium heparin in preventing deep venous thrombosis after major surgery, Lancet 2: 890, 1972.
21. Gordon-Smith, I. C.: Personal communication, 1972.
22. Gallus, A. S., Hirsh, J., Tuttle, R. J., Trebilcock, R., O'Brien, S. E., Carroll, J. J., Minden, J. H., and Hudecki, S. M.: Small subcutaneous doses of heparin in prevention of venous thrombosis, N. Engl. J. Med. 288:545, 1973.
23. Ballard, R. M., Bradley-Watson, P. J., Johnstone, F. D., Kenney, A., McCarthy, T. G., Campbell, S., and Weston, J.: Low doses of subcutaneous heparin in the prevention of deep vein thrombosis after gynaecological surgery, J. Obstet. Gynecol. 80: 469, 1973.
24. Rem, J., Duckert, F., Fridrich, R. and Gruber, U. K.: Subkutane kleine Heparindosen zur Thromboseprophylaxe in der allgemeinen Chirurgie and Urologie (Subcutaneous small dose heparin in the thromboprophylaxis of general surgical and urological patients), Schweiz. Med. Wochenschr. 105:827, 1975.
25. Rosenberg, I. L., Evans, M., and Pollock, A. V.: Prophylaxis of postoperative leg vein thrombosis by low dose subcutaneous heparin or peroperative calf muscle stimulation: A controlled clinical trial, Br. Med. J. 1:649, 1975.
26. Joffe, S.: Drug prevention of post-operative deep vein thrombosis. A comparative study of calcium heparinate and sodium pentosan polysulphate, Arch. Surg. 111:37, 1976.
27. Kakkar, V. V., Howe, C. T., Flanc, C., and Clarke, M. B.: Natural history of deep vein thrombosis, Lancet 2:230, 1969.
28. Nicolaides, A. N., and O'Connell, J. D.: Origin and Distribution of Thrombi in Patients Presenting with Clinical Deep Venous Thrombosis, in Nicolaides, A. N. (ed.): *Thromboembolism—Aetiology, Advances in Prevention and Management* (Lancaster: Medical and Technical Publishing Co., 1975).
29. Sagar, S., Massey, J., and Sanderson, J. M.: Low-dose heparin prophylaxis against fatal post-operative pulmonary embolism, Br. Med. J. 4:257, 1975.
30. Anernethy, E. A., and Hartsuck, J. M.: Post-operative pulmonary embolism—A prospective study utilizing low dose heparin, Am. J. Surg. 128:739, 1974.
31. Lahnborg, G., Bergstrom, K., Friman, L., and Lagerglen, H.: Effect of low dose heparin on incidence of post-operative pulmonary embolism detected by photoscanning, Lancet 1:329, 1974.
32. Kakkar, V. V., Corrigan, T. P., and Fossard, D. P.: Prevention of fatal post-operative pulmonary embolism by low doses of heparin. An international multicentre trial, Lancet 2:45, 1975.
33. Sherry, S.: Low-dose heparin prophylaxis for post-operative venous thromboembolism, N. Engl. J. Med. 293:300, 1975.
34. Nicolaides, A. N.: The Prevention of Post-operative Deep Venous Thrombosis. Jacksonian Prize Essay, Royal College of Surgeons of England, 1972.

35. Gallus, A. S., Hirsh, J., Turpie, A. G. G., and Tuttle, R.: Prevention of venous thrombosis with small doses of subcutaneous heparin. Proc. IVth Int. Congr. Thrombosis and Hacmostasis, Vienna, Austria, 1973, p. 276.
36. Morris, G. K., Henry, A. P. J., and Preston, B. J.: Prevention of deep-vein thrombosis by low-dose heparin in patients undergoing total hip replacement, Lancet 2:797, 1974.
37. Rosengarten, D. S., and McNeur, J. C.: Prophylaxis of deep vein thrombosis after total hip replacement. Proc. Vth Int. Congr. Thrombosis and Haemostasis, Paris, 1975, p. 343.
38. Hampson, W. G. J., Harris, F. C., Keith Lucas, H., Roberts, P. H., McCall, I. V., Jackson, P. C., Powell, N. L., and Staddon, G. E.: Failure of low-dose heparin to prevent deep-vein thrombosis after hip-replacement arthroplasty, Lancet 2:795, 1974.
39. Nicolaides, A. N., Dupont, P. A., Parsons, D. C. S., Lewis, J. D., Desai, S., Appleberg, M., Horan, F. T., Walker, C. J., Benson, M. K. D., Jameson Evans, D. C. Miller, J., and Esah, K. M.: Small doses of subcutaneous sodium heparin in the prevention of deep vein thrombosis after elective hip operations, Br. J. Surg. 62:348, 1975.
40. Kakkar, V. V.: Low dose heparin in the prevention of venous thromboembolism. Rationale and results, Thrombos. Diath. Haemorrh. 33:87, 1975.
41. Stamatakis, J., Sagar, S., Higgins, A. F., Thomas, D. P., and Kakkar, V. V.: Heparin levels in patients undergoing hip surgery, Br. J. Surg. 63:158, 1976.
42. Gallus, A. S., and Hirsh, J.: Small Dose Subcutaneous Heparin in Preventing Deep Venous Thrombosis, in Nicolaides, A. N. (ed.): *Thromboembolism—Aetiology, Advances in Prevention and Management* (Lancaster: Medical and Technical Publishing Co., 1975).
43. Handley, A. J.: Low dose heparin after myocardial infarction, Lancet 2:623, 1972.
44. Warlow, C., Beattie, A. G., Terry, G., Ogston, D., Kenmure, A. C. F., and Douglas, A. S.: A double-blind trial of low doses of subcutaneous heparin in the prevention of deep-vein thrombosis after myocardial infarction, Lancet 2:934, 1973.
45. Vascilescu, C., and Ruckley, C. V.: Heparin venous Dextran in the prevention of deep venous thrombosis. A multi-unit controlled trial, Lancet 2:118, 1974.
46. Hume, M., Kuriakose, T. X., Zuch, L., and Turner, R. H.: [125]I Fibrinogen and the prevention of venous thrombosis, Arch. Surg. 107:803, 1973.
47. McWilliam, R., McCormick, J. St.C., and Aulaqi, A. I.: Bleeding and peri-operative heparin, Lancet 2:286, 1974.
48. Charnley, J.: Prophylaxis of post-operative thromboembolism, Lancet 2:134, 1972.
49. Le Vay, D.: Low dose heparin, Lancet 2:229, 1972.
50. Arden, G. P., Powell, H. D. W., and Fell, R. H.: Subcutaneous heparin treatment, Br. Med. J. 4:486, 1972.
51. Denson, K. W. E., and Bonnar, J.: The measurement of heparin. A method based on the potentiation of antifactor Xa, Thrombos. Diath. Haemorrh. 30:171, 1973.
52. Estes, J. W., and Poulin, P. F.: Pharmacokinetics of heparin. Distribution and Elimination, Thrombos. Diath. Haemorrh. 33:26, 1975.
53. Estes, J. W., Pelikan, E. W., and Kruger-Thiemer, E.: A retrospective study of the pharmacokinetics of heparin, Clin. Pharmacol. Therap. 10:329, 1969.
54. Monkhouse, F. C.: Physiological factors concerned with the removal of injected heparin from the circulating blood, Am. J. Phys. 178:223, 1954.
55. de Takats, G.: Heparin tolerance: A test of the clotting mechanism, Surg. Gynecol. Obstet. 77:31, 1943.
56. de Takats, G.: A sensitised clotting time, JAMA 146:370, 1951.
57. de Takats, G., and Marshall, M. H.: The response of the clotting equilibrium to post-operative stress, Surgery 31:13, 1952.
58. de Takats, G.: Heparin tolerance revisited, Surgery 70:318, 1971.

59. de Takats, G.: Heparin. The need for a flexible protocol, Am. J. Surg. 132:1, 1976.
60. Yin, E. T., Wessler, S., and Butler, J. V.: Plasma heparin. A unique submicrogram sensitive assay, J. Lab. Clin. Med. 81:298, 1973.
61. Wessler, S.: Personal communication, 1972.
62. Lahnborg, G., and Bergstrom, K.: Clinical and haemostatic parameters related to thromboembolism and low-dose heparin prophylaxis in major surgery, Acta Chir. Scand. 141:590, 1975.

34 / Dextran Prophylaxis of Venous Thromboembolism

SVEN-ERIK BERGENTZ, M.D.

Professor of Surgery, Malmö General Hospital, University of Lund, Malmö, Sweden

DEXTRAN, A POLYSACCHARIDE formed by the action of an enzyme of the bacteria *Leuconostoc mesenteroides* on sucrose, was introduced into clinical praxis more than 30 years ago.[1] A number of alterations have been made in dextran since then. The most important concerns changes in the leuconostoc strain used for manufacturing of the dextran, a decrease in the average molecular weight as well as a narrowing of the molecular weight distribution.

Dextran was introduced as a plasma expander, and plasma expansion is its most important indication and effect. By increasing the blood volume dextran causes hemodilution, thereby decreasing blood viscosity, and increasing blood flow rate. This is obviously one way by which dextran counteracts thrombus formation. The antithrombotic effect of dextran is however also due to a specific and unique pharmacologic influence on the coagulation mechanism, different from that of anticoagulants. We now know that this is accomplished by an effect on the structure and function of factor VIII.[2]

Basic Pharmacology of Various Dextran Preparations

Pharmacologic effects of dextran depend on the following factors: average molecular weight, molecular weight distribution, molecular structure and concentration.

Considering the *average molecular weight*, two types of dextrans are commonly used: dextran 70, with an average molecular weight of 70,000, and dextran 40, with an average molecular weight of 40,000.

529

Molecular weight distribution is narrow; high molecular weight fractions must be eliminated since they cause aggregation of formed elements of blood and low molecular weight fractions must be eliminated since they are excreted rapidly. The *degree of branching* of the molecule should be as low as possible to avoid influence on blood coagulation and red cell aggregation. The *concentration* of the dextran 70 used is as a rule 6%. Since a 3.5% solution of this dextran preparation is iso-oncotic with plasma, the oncotic pressure of blood is increased after a rapid infusion of a 6% solution. A rapid infusion of a certain volume of this dextran results therefore in a more marked increase in blood volume than the volume infused. The dextran 40 used is available as a 10% solution. A 2.5% solution of dextran 40 is iso-oncotic with plasma. Therefore an infusion of this type of dextran increases the blood volume even more than dextran 70, though for a shorter period of time due to the more rapid elimination of the intravascular molecules. Since dextran has practically no osmotic effect it has to be infused in a solution of normal saline or 5% glucose.

Dextran is a reliable and predictable plasma expander compared to fresh blood or plasma, which sometimes is excreted quite rapidly from the blood stream.[3]

By the action of an enzyme present in the tissues dextran is completely broken down and metabolized as glucose.[1] In addition molecules with a molecular weight lower than about 50,000 are excreted in the urine. When this occurs a vacuolization of the cells in the renal tubuli can be seen, as after infusion of mannitol or glucose (osmotic nephrosis). These changes are transient, and there are no reasons to believe that dextran can damage the kidney function. It is, however, important to realize that dextran requires water. If the organism is dehydrated, the hyperoncotic dextran actually increased the dehydration. This may result, among other things, in a very pronounced water reabsorption in the tubuli. Since dextran has almost no osmotic effect it does not retain water in the tubuli. The water is readsorbed, but the dextran is not. The dextran concentration in the urine may increase tremendously, particularly after infusion of the more readily excreted low molecular weight dextran, resulting in an extremely thick and highly viscous urine, and a temporary oliguria. This is prevented by administration of water and/or mannitol.

Dextran has no antigenic properties. Shock-like side effects, so-called anaphylactoid reactions, do occur on rare occasions (see below). The mechanism behind these is still unknown.

Clinical Studies on Dextran in Postoperative Thromboembolism

Koekenberg[4] from Holland, interested to study whether avoidance of blood transfusion might decrease the incidence of thromboembolic complications following surgery, was the first to show that a group of patients given dextran instead of blood during surgery had a lower incidence of deep venous thrombosis (DVT). Following this investigation about 30 prospective randomized studies were published on the use of dextran on this indication. Most of the investigators used objective methods for diagnosing thrombosis, such as the ^{125}I-fibrinogen test and/or phlebography, but some used clinical methods on a double-blind basis. The great majority of investigators used dextran 70, a few used dextran 40. In practically all studies dextran was given during surgery; in most of them it was also continued for one or several days after surgery. In some series the control group did not receive any prophylaxis at all; in others dextran was compared to coumarin or heparin or antiplatelet drugs.

The studies found that dextran 70 decreases significantly the incidence of DVT following different kinds of surgery compared to controls and diagnosed with phlebography[5-14] or clinically.[4, 15] Generally the effect of dextran is most marked in surgery involving a major trauma, such as orthopedic surgery, particularly hip arthroplasty.

Comparing dextran to coumarin, Myhre and Holen,[8] Davidson et al.[16] and Bergqvist et al.[17, 18] found no difference in the incidence of DVT. Korvald and Støren[19] found a higher incidence and Lambie et al.[9] a lower incidence of DVT in patients treated with dextran compared to coumarin.

Comparing dextran to heparin, Myrvold et al.[20] and McCarthy et al.[21] found no difference in the incidence of DVT. Ruckley[22] found heparin to be more effective, and Hedlund[14] studying urologic patients found heparin to be slightly less effective than dextran.

When comparing dextran 40 with dextran 70 (giving equal volumes of 6% dextran 70 and 10% dextran 40, respectively) no significant difference was found.[15] Evarts and Feil[23] and Gruber et al.[24] found dextran 40 to significantly decrease the incidence of thrombosis compared to controls, using phlebography and radioactive fibrinogen, respectively, for diagnosis.

Dextran must be given *intraoperatively*. Jansen[15] and Stephenson et al.[25] found that dextran *not* given intraoperatively but for two consecutive days after surgery had no antithrombotic effect. It is unclear whether an additional prophylactic effect is achieved by continuing the dextran prophylaxis for one or several postoperative days. Jansen[15] gave the dextran only on the day of surgery; Bonnar and Walsh[10] also gave it on the first postoperative day. Other authors have continued the dextran administration for 3 or 4 postoperative days or even longer. It seems logical to continue the administration of dextran for a few days postoperatively if the patient is not mobilized, but there are no controlled studies confirming this assumption.

Regarding the *dosage*, most authors have used 500 ml during surgery. There is evidence to indicate that the effect of dextran is more marked if 1,000 ml is given.[10, 15, 22] This seems to be particularly important in major surgery requiring a long time on the operating table and several blood transfusions.[15] Postoperatively the dosage has as a rule been 500 ml per day or every second day.

Dextran appears to be about as effective when using phlebography for diagnosis as when the thrombosis is diagnosed clinically. On both occasions dextran decreases the incidence of thrombosis with 50-75%, depending on the type of surgery. Dextran seems to be less effective when using the iodine-labeled fibrinogen test, thereby diagnosing the thrombosis at an early, often reversible, stage. Daniel et al.,[26] using this test as the only diagnostic tool, found no effect of dextran compared to controls. Becker and Schampi,[27] using both the iodine fibrinogen test and phlebography, noticed that in the dextran-treated patients thrombi found with the iodine fibrinogen test were, in about one third of the cases, not detectable with the phlebography 4-14 days later. This discrepancy between the two diagnostic methods was not observed in the control groups. Becker and Schampi suggested that dextran might change the structure of the thrombi, making them more easily attacked by fibrinolysis. In a review of the literature Steinmann et al.[28] noticed that the prophylactive effect of dextran was more pronounced the longer postoperatively the phlebography was done.

With regard to the effect of dextran to counteract *pulmonary embolism* the diagnostic methods and criteria used by different authors are so variable that it is difficult to draw any conclusions. Regarding the incidence of *fatal pulmonary embolism*, verified at autopsy, there seems to be a significant decrease in dextran-treated patients as seen from Table 34-1, containing pooled data from the literature, and including only prospective randomized studies. It is of interest that while the incidence of DVT in treated versus untreated patients is 1:2 (general surgery, urology and gynecology) or 1:3 (orthopedic surgery), it is 1:6 (all specialties) for fatal pulmonary emboli.

In summary, dextran significantly decreases the incidence of thrombosis compared to controls, but there appears to be no difference

TABLE 34–1.—DATA FROM CONTROLLED STUDIES
ON THE VALUE OF DEXTRAN 70 IN THE
PREVENTION OF POSTOPERATIVE FATAL
PULMONARY EMBOLISM (FPE),
VERIFIED AT AUTOPSY

| | | NO. OF PATIENTS | | | |
| | | CONTROLS | | DEXTRAN° | |
AUTHOR	YEAR	TOTAL	FPE	TOTAL	FPE
Koekenberg	1962	105	1	94	0
Ahlberg	1968	47	2	39	0
Ahlberg	1969	52	2	32	1
Hartshorn	1969	104	2	99	0
Myhre	1969	55	2	55	0
Atik	1970	77	5	49	1
Stadil	1970	397	5	424	1
Huttunen	1971	100	4	100	1
Jansen	1972	301	4	304	1
Ruckley	1974	128	2	130	0
Kline	1975	435	7	396	1
Total		1801	36	1722	6

°The effect of dextran 70 is highly significant ($p < 0.001$).

when compared to coumarin or heparin. Six percent dextran 70 is about as effective as 10% dextran 40, given in the same volume. The dextran must be given during surgery; 1,000 ml may be more effective than 500 ml. In most studies dextran administration has been continued for one or several days postoperatively, but the additional effect of this regimen, as compared to the dextran given intraoperatively, is unclear.

The Mechanism of Action of Dextran on Coagulation, Hemostasis and Thrombus Formation

Dextran has been studied extensively with regard to its effect on hemostasis and coagulation since it was introduced. Most of the studies are, however, obsolete since they were done with dextran preparations containing high molecular weight fractions. By causing aggregation of red cells and platelets, these dextran fractions produce intravascular coagulation with consumption of clotting factors.[29]

Dextran is no anticoagulant. Modern dextran preparations do not cause any changes in the concentration of coagulation factors, except for those due to dilution. Dextran does, however, cause a decreased adhesivity of the platelets to a glass bead as demonstrated by Cronberg et al.[30] and Bygdeman et al.[31] In high concentrations in vitro it also causes a change in the fibrin morphology[32] and an increase in the

lysability of fibrin.[33] Dextran does not cause a measurable prolongation of the bleeding time if given in doses not exceeding 1.5 gm of
dextran 70, or 2 gm of dextran 40 per kilogram of body weight per 24
hr. A slight oozing from the capillaries may however occur, which
might be troublesome in surgery of parenchymatous organs (brain,
liver, etc.). This oozing may be related to the decreased platelet adhesivity and/or improved capillary circulation.

The antithrombotic effects of dextran are therefore *not* related to
any anticoagulant effects, but to the following two mechanisms.

1. *Hemodilution results in a decreased blood viscosity and increased blood flow rate.* — It is known that the blood flow rate in the
muscle veins in the lower leg approaches zero when the patient is
lying in anesthesia on the operating table, as demonstrated with
phlebography[34] or isotope technique.[35] These are the veins in which
postoperative thrombi are initiated. Hemodilution with dextran counteracts this decreased flow velocity.[35] It is also known that polycythemia increases the incidence of thrombosis, probably by increasing
blood viscosity and a decreasing blood flow rate. Hematocrit is the
most important factor in determining the blood viscosity, but after a
trauma the blood viscosity is increased even at unchanged hematocrit,
due to increased concentration of fibrinogen and globulin.[36] The
hematocrit should therefore be decreased after a trauma in order to
avoid a viscosity increase. This is actually what occurs in any traumatized or postoperative patient, even if there is no blood loss, or if the
blood loss is compensated for.[37] It is known[38] that the relative oxygen
transport capacity of blood, e.g., the oxygen concentration multiplied
by the cardiac output, reaches its peak at a hematocrit of about 30. A
higher hematocrit decreases the oxygen transport capacity because of
a decreased cardiac output. Also for this reason, lost blood should not
be substituted with blood until the hematocrit drops below 30. It is
however essential that the blood volume is not decreased
(normovolemic hemodilution). This is best accomplished by infusion
of a colloid. If a crystalloid solution is given, excessive amounts have
to be infused in order to avoid hypovolemia.[38]

2. *Dextran causes a change in the structure and function of factor
VIII, thereby impairing the function of the platelets and stability of a
thrombus.*[2, 39, 40] — The stability of thrombi formed ex vivo in Chandler
loops was tested by incubation with small amounts of plasmin, and
determination was made of the amount of fibrinolytic split products
released into the supernatant.[39] Infusion of 500 ml dextran 70 during 1
hr resulted in an increase in the lysability of the thrombi formed. This
increase was apparent already at the end of the infusion, but reached

its maximum after 4–5 hr, when the dextran concentration had decreased considerably. The increased lysability paralleled the decreased platelet adhesivity after dextran, and both were exclusively seen after infusion of dextran in vivo. This suggests a common mechanism for the two phenomena. This mechanism seems to be an effect on the structure and function of factor VIII, a coagulation factor known to be of importance both for the platelet function and for the stability of thrombi.[2, 40]

The temporary changes in the factor VIII structure after dextran can be demonstrated as a decrease in the concentration of factor VIII determined as an antigen, but not determined as factor VIII activity.[2] The explanation for this finding is probably that the large factor VIII molecule after dextran occurs in a less aggregated form and thus has a decreased stability to combine and precipitate visibly with rabbit antiserum. The changes can also be seen in gel filtration and increased immunoelectrophoresis. Furthermore dextran causes a decrease in the activity of the ristocetin cofactor for platelet-aggregation which is known to be a function of factor VIII. *All* of these effects of dextran are transient, but can be reversed immediately by infusion of a factor VIII concentrate.[2]

The changes in platelet function after dextran thus are due to the effect of dextran on factor VIII, in a similar way as the defect in platelet function in von Willebrand's disease is due to abnormalities in factor VIII.[2] Experimental studies have indicated that the increased lysability is secondary to a change in platelet function.[40] It is noteworthy that this increased lysability after dextran is not seen in clots, e.g., solidification of nonmoving blood, but only in thrombi, e.g., solidification of blood in a rotating Chandler loop.

Thus thrombi formed in the presence of dextran are more easily attacked by fibrinolysin. It is known that the most important fibrinolytic activators occur not in blood but in the vessel walls.[41] Individuals with low fibrinolytic activity in the vessel walls have an increased tendency to thrombus formation.[42] After surgery the incidence of subclinical "minithrombi," detectable early after surgery with the iodine-fibrinogen test, is very high. The majority of these thrombi disappear spontaneously within a few days, probably by the action of the fibrinolytic activity in the vessel walls. It is conceivable that by increasing the lysability of the thrombi by infusion of dextran, a larger number of these minithrombi will disappear. This is in agreement with the findings of Becker and Schampi,[27] of a lower incidence of thrombi detectable with phlebography 4–14 days after their detection by iodine-fibrinogen in dextran-treated patients but not in control patients, and with the observations of Steinmann et al.[28] that the reduction of the number of DVT in dextran prophylaxis is more evident the longer postoperatively the phlebography is carried out.

Side Effects and Contraindications

SIDE EFFECTS

There are three well known side effects of dextran infusion which can be avoided, and one which cannot be avoided at the present time.

Increased bleeding tendency is caused by modern dextran preparations only if the doses exceed 1.5 gm per kilogram of body weight per day for dextran 70, or 2 gm for dextran 40.

Oliguria or anuria occurs only if dextran is given in excessive amounts to a dehydrated organism, and is in any case only temporary.

Overexpansion of the blood volume and pulmonary edema is caused only if excessive amounts of dextran are given rapidly to elderly patients, to patients with imminent cardiac failure or patients with renal insufficiency without considering the fact that a rapid infusion of dextran, being a hyperoncotic solution, increases the circulating blood volume more than the volume infused.

The complication which at the present time cannot be avoided is an *anaphylactoid reaction* which occurs at an incidence of one in 3,000 to one in 40,000 infusions. This complication is not related to previous infusions of dextran, since dextran is not antigenic. It occurs immediately after the start of the infusion and is characterized by a drop in blood pressure, and occasionally cardiac arrest. Therapy consists of fluid administration rapidly, intravenous cortisone and adrenaline. A few deaths have been described, practically exclusively in elderly patients.

CONTRAINDICATIONS

Dextran should not be used in patients with a known bleeding disorder such as marked thrombocytopenia or defects in factor VIII (von Willebrand's disease or hemophilia). In patients with cardiac insufficiency dextran should be given slowly and under control of central venous pressure. In patients with renal insufficiency and uremia the doses of dextran should be decreased both because of the hemostatic defect, from which the uremic patients suffer, and because of a potential risk for retention of dextran and fluid. In complete anuria dextran should be avoided.

The Place of Dextran as an Antithrombotic Agent in Modern Surgery

An antithrombotic regimen has to be simple, safe and reasonably effective. Of these three requirements the first two are the most important, since "the net has to be cast widely" if the prophylaxis is going to be effective. It is true that we can define certain risk groups. These are patients with malignancy, patients with a previous history of thrombosis and patients undergoing extensive and prolonged surgical interventions with multiple blood transfusions. The most important risk factor is, however, high age. Ninety-seven percent of the fatal pulmonary emboli occur in patients above 50 years of age.[43] But all too often DVT and pulmonary emboli appear after operations on patients outside the risk groups. To improve the standard of the surgical care as many patients as possible should therefore be safeguarded.

The *advantage* with dextran as an antithrombotic agent is its simplicity, safety and low cost. It is given as an intravenous infusion during surgery, when the patients are going to have infusions anyway. By using dextran the number of blood transfusions can be decreased. Dextran does not cause bleeding, and other side effects are not of such a magnitude that the use of dextran is inhibited. The number of contraindications is low, and lower than for anticoagulants. For all these reasons dextran prophylaxis can be more universally applied than other types of prophylaxis.

The *disadvantage* with dextran is that it has to be given as an intravenous infusion. This makes it less suitable for prolonged therapy for instance in nonmobilized patients. In such cases coumarin is probably to be preferred.

At the present time there are three means available to decrease the incidence of postoperative DVT and pulmonary embolism: administration of coumarin, heparin or dextran. Mechanical methods may also prove effective, but no studies indicating the effectiveness of such methods to decrease the incidence of fatal pulmonary emboli are yet available.

Compared to both heparin and coumarin dextran is simpler to administer, it has fewer contraindications, and it can therefore be more universally applied. Strict comparisons between the three drugs from all the various aspects have as yet not been published. It appears that heparin is the most effective of the three drugs, particularly considering DVT diagnosed early with the iodine-fibrinogen method, and in general surgery. Heparin is definitely less effective, or ineffective, in orthopedic surgery and urologic surgery. If the thrombi are diagnosed with phlebography, dextran seems in general to be more effective. Dextran seems to be particularly valuable in extensive orthopedic surgery such as hip arthroplasty. Heparin and dextran should not be combined due to increasing hazard of bleeding. Coumarin, if started preoperatively and given with proper control, is as effective and safe as dextran and can be continued for a long time. It requires, however, laboratory control and should not be given to patients with severe hypertension, active ulcer or intracranial or visceral injury. Experience has shown that it is difficult to get this method applied in routine surgery in hospitals without special interest in the problem.

As the safety of surgery has increased, the relative importance of thromboembolism as a postoperative complication has increased. There are now several methods available to decrease the incidence of these complications. We cannot state at the present time that one is better than the other for all situations. Some kind of prophylaxis should, however, be used in order to improve the safety of surgery.

Summary

Dextran is a plasma expander with antithrombotic properties. Its effects are partly due to hemodilution, partly to a specific, transient effect on the structure and function of factor VIII, thereby influencing the platelet function and making the thrombi formed more easily attacked by the fibrinolysin released from the vein walls.

Dextran must be given intraoperatively; 1,000 ml seems to be more effective than 500 ml, and is definitely recommended in more extensive surgery. Continued administration of 500 ml a day (or every second day) for one or several days *may* add to the effectiveness. Dextran 70 is as effective as dextran 40.

Dextran is least effective against thrombi detected early postoperatively with the iodine-fibrinogen method. It is more effective against thrombi detected late with phlebography and against fatal pulmonary emboli.

REFERENCES

1. Grönwall, A., and Ingelman, B.: Untersuchungen über Dextran und sein Verhalten bei parenteraler Zufuhr, Acta Physiol. Scand. 7:97, 1944.
2. Åberg, M., Hedner, U., and Bergentz, S.-E.: The effect of dextran on factor VIII and platelet function, Ann. Surg. (in press).
3. Gruber, U. F., and Bergentz, S.-E.: Autologous and homologous fresh human plasma as a volume expander in hypovolemic subjects, Ann. Surg. 165:41, 1967.
4. Koekenberg, L. J. L.: Experimental use of Macrodex as a prophylaxis against postoperative thromboembolism, Bull. Soc. Int. Chir. 21:501, 1962.
5. Ahlberg, Å., Nylander, G., Robertson, B., Cronberg, S., and Nilsson, I.: Dextran in

prophylaxis of thrombosis in fractures of the hip, Acta Chir. Scand. [Suppl.] 387:83, 1968.

6. Johnson, S. R., Bygdeman, S., and Eliasson, R.: Effect of dextran on postoperative thrombosis, Acta Chir. Scand. [Suppl.] 387:80, 1968.

7. Ahlberg, Å.: *Tromboprofylax med macrodex i ett collumfrakturmaterial* (Lund, Sweden: Studentlitteratur, 1969), p. 89.

8. Myhre, H. O., and Holen, A.: Tromboseprofylakse. Dextran eller warfarin-natrium? Nord. Med. 82:1534, 1969.

9. Lambie, J. M., Barber, D. C., Dhall, D. P., and Matheson, N. A.: Dextran 70 in prophylaxis of postoperative venous thrombosis. A controlled trial, Br. Med. J. 2:144, 1970.

10. Bonnar, J., and Walsh, J.: Prevention of thrombosis after pelvic surgery by British dextran 70, Lancet 1:614, 1972.

11. Harper, D. R., Dhall, D. P., and Woodruff, P. W. H.: Prophylaxis in iliofemoral venous thrombosis. The major amputee as a clinical research model, Br. J. Surg. 60: 831, 1973.

12. Carter, A. E., and Eban, R.: The prevention of postoperative deep venous thrombosis with dextran 70, Br. J. Surg. 60:681, 1973.

13. Kline, A. L., Hughes, L. E., and Campbell, H.: Dextran prophylaxis of deep vein thrombosis. Organization of a clinical trial, Br. J. Surg. 61:332, 1974.

14. Hedlund, P. O.: Postoperative venous thrombosis in benign prostatic disease, Scand. J. Urol. Nephrol. [Suppl. 27]:1, 1975.

15. Jansen, H.: Postoperative thromboembolism and its prevention with 500 ml dextran given during operation, Acta Chir. Scand. [Suppl.] 427:1, 1972.

16. Davidson, A. I., Brunt, M. E. A., and Matheson, N. A.: A further trial comparing dextran 70 with warfarin in the prophylaxis of postoperative venous thrombosis, Br. J. Surg. 59:314, 1972.

17. Bergqvist, E., Bergqvist, D., Bronge, A., Dahlgren, S., and Lindqvist, B.: An evaluation of early thrombosis prophylaxis following fracture of the femoral neck. A comparison between dextran and dicoumarol, Acta Chir. Scand. 138:689, 1972.

18. Bergqvist, D., and Dahlgren, S.: Leg vein thrombosis diagnosed by ^{125}I-fibrinogen test in patients with fracture of the hip: A study of the effect of early prophylaxis with dicoumarol or dextran 70, Vasa 2:121, 1973.

19. Korvald, E., and Støren, E. J.: Deep venous thrombosis after major operations, J. Oslo City Hosp. 23:105, 1973.

20. Myrvold, H. E., Persson, J.-E., Svensson, B., Wallensten, S., and Vikterloef, K. J.: Prevention of thromboembolism with dextran 70 and heparin in patients with femoral neck fractures, Acta Chir. Scand. 139:609, 1973.

21. McCarthy, T. G., McQueen, J., Johnstone, F. D., Weston, J., and Campbell, S.: A comparison of low-dose subcutaneous heparin and intravenous dextran 70 in the prophylaxis of deep venous thrombosis after gynaecological surgery, J. Obstet. Gynaecol. Br. Commonw. 81:486, 1974.

22. Ruckley, C. V.: Heparin versus dextran in the prevention of deep-vein thrombosis. A multi-unit controlled trial, Lancet 2:118, 1974.

23. Evarts, C. M., and Feil, E. J.: Prevention of thromboembolic disease after elective surgery of the hip, J. Bone Joint Surg. [Am.] 53:1271, 1971.

24. Gruber, U. F., Rem, J., Altorfer, R., Schaub, N., Frede, K. E., Fridrich, R., and Duckert, F.: Efficacy of dextran 40 or heparin in prevention of deep vein thrombosis after major surgery, Eur. Surg. Res. 5:15, 1973.

25. Stephenson, C. B. S., Wallace, J. C., and Vaughan, J. V.: Dextran 70 in the prevention of post-operative deep-vein thrombosis with observations on pulmonary embolism: Report on a pilot study, N.Z. Med. J. 77:302, 1973.

26. Daniel, W. J., Moore, A. R., and Flanc, C.: Prophylaxis of deep vein thrombosis with dextran 70 in patients with a fractured neck of the femur, Aust. N.Z. J. Surg. 41:289, 1972.

27. Becker, J., and Schampi, B.: The incidence of postoperative venous thrombosis of

the legs. A comparative study on the prophylactic effect of dextran 70 and electrical calf muscle stimulation, Acta Chir. Scand. 139:357, 1973.

28. Steinmann, E., Duckert, F., and Gruber, U. F.: Wert von Dextran 70 zur Thrombo-embolie-prophylaxe in der allgemeinen Chirurgie Ortopädie, Urologie and Gynäkologie, Schweiz. Med. Wochenschr. 105:1637, 1975.

29. Bergentz, S.-E., Eiken, O., and Nilsson, I. M.: The effect of dextran of various molecular weight on the coagulation in dogs, Thromb. Diath. Haemorrh. 6:15, 1961.

30. Cronberg, S., Robertson, B., Nilsson, I. M., and Niléhn, J.-E.: Suppressive effect of dextran on platelet adhesiveness, Thromb. Diath. Haemorrh. 16:384, 1966.

31. Bygdeman, S., Eliasson, R., and Gullbring, B.: Effect of dextran infusion on the adenosine diphosphate-induced adhesiveness and the spreading capacity of human blood platelets, Thromb. Diath. Haemorrh. 15:451, 1966.

32. Muzaffar, T. Z., Stalker, A. L., Bryce, W. A. J., and Dhall, D. P.: Dextrans and fibrin morphology, Nature 238:288, 1972.

33. Tangen, O., Wikk, O., Almqvist, J. A. M., Arfors, K. E., and Hint, H. C.: Effects of dextran on the structure and plasmin-induced lysis of human fibrin, Thromb. Res. 1: 487, 1972.

34. McLachlin, A. D., McLachlin, J. A., Jory, T. A., and Rawling, E. G.: Venous stasis in the lower extremities, Ann. Surg. 152:678, 1960.

35. Jansen, H., and Lewis, D. H.: The effect of dextran 40 on the venous flow pattern in the lower extremity before and after operation, Acta Chir. Scand. [Suppl.] 427:48, 1972.

36. Bergentz, S.-E., Gelin, L.-E., Rudenstam, C.-M., and Zederfeldt, B.: The viscosity of whole blood in trauma, Bull. Soc. Int. Chir. 20:464, 1963.

37. Gelin, L.-E.: Studies in anemia of injury, Acta Chir. Scand. [Suppl.] 210, 1956.

38. Messmer, K., Görnandt, L., Jesch, F., Sinagowitz, E., Sunder-Plasmann, L., and Kassler, M.: Oxygen transport and tissue oxygenation during hemodilution with dextran, Adv. Exp. Med. Biol. 37B:669, 1973.

39. Åberg, M., Bergentz, S.-E., and Hedner, U.: The effect of dextran on the lysability of ex vivo thrombi, Ann. Surg. 181:342, 1975.

40. Åberg, M., Hedner, U., and Bergentz, S.-E.: Effect of dextran and induced thrombocytopenia on the lysability of thrombi in dogs, Acta Chir. Scand. (in press).

41. Pandolfi, M., Nilsson, I. M., Robertson, B., and Isacson, S.: Fibrinolytic activity of human veins, Lancet 2:127, 1967.

42. Isacson, S.: Low fibrinolytic activity of blood and vein walls in venous thrombosis, Scand. J. Haematol. [Suppl.] 16:1, 1971.

43. Sagar, S., Massey, J., and Sanderson, J. M.: Low-dose heparin prophylaxis against fatal pulmonary embolism, Br. Med. J. 4:257, 1975.

Discussion: Chapters 33 and 34

DR. NORMAN BROWSE: I think everybody here is interested in these problems, and has followed the many publications that have appeared over the last few years. I would like to make a few general points. First, we must appreciate that, when we decide to give or not to give a form of prophylaxis, we must be clear in our minds whether we are just making a decision on the basis of an opinion or a fact. The fact is, when one looks at all of the data, there is no evidence that using any means of prophylaxis increases the number of patients who leave the hospital alive.

What I am going to say about heparin, for example, applies to all of the other techniques. If you look at the data for the heparin trial, there were 16 people who died of fatal pulmonary embolism in the control group and two in the test group. This is highly significant. One then has to ask, how was that data achieved. One discovers that it was achieved using the assessment of a multitude of different pathologists who were each deciding that a particular patient died of pulmonary embolism. They were also excluding many others who had pulmonary embolism but in whom they thought that a particular embolus was not the prime cause of death.

If you look at the total mortality rate, 100 died in one group and 80 in the other. That isn't a significant difference. The same thoughts can be applied to the study of Kline, which is the other big prospective study of dextran. In terms of hard evidence, there isn't anything to say that, if you use these techniques, fewer patients are going to die.

If you are prepared to accept the presented evidence that fatal pulmonary embolism is reduced, then you make the judgment that there will be fewer fatal pulmonary emboli and that will justify using one of these methods.

Doctor Nicolaides may have said that perhaps it wasn't ethical not to give prophylaxis. I don't think I go along with that yet. I don't think the evidence is hard enough to say it is unethical not to give prophy-

541

laxis. I am sure that, in my opinion, it is better to use one or another of
these methods.

There is one other point to make. That is the noticeable difference
between dextran and heparin. Heparin reduces the incidence of calf
thrombosis and also pulmonary embolism. The evidence for dextran
suggests a much smaller effect on the calf vein thrombosis, but probably as good an effect on pulmonary embolism. This raises one or two
questions.

First, can we use the ^{125}I-fibrinogen test as a screen to determine
whether a particular technique is going to be a good prophylactic
agent? The answer is yes and no. If you reduce the incidence of peripheral thrombosis, you are likely to reduce the incidence of pulmonary embolism, but the opposite does not follow. There are techniques, perhaps, which won't affect the peripheral thrombosis, but
will affect pulmonary embolism. So one can't discard methods just
on the basis of a study with the fibrinogen test.

Finally, do we want to abolish all peripheral thrombi? Why are we
necessarily assuming that this is a bad thing? It has bad side effects,
yes, because people get pulmonary emboli. But calf thrombosis must
happen for some reason, and maybe this is part of the response to surgery. Perhaps we shouldn't be tinkering with it in such a massive way.

DR. ANDREW NICOLAIDES: I first would like to say that I agree with
all of the points Professor Browse has made. I would like to make two
points myself. One, like everybody else, I am very much aware that
dextran is far more effective in preventing pulmonary embolism than
the thrombi of the calf diagnosed by the radioactive fibrinogen test.
There is something missing here, and what we must look for is the
natural history of thrombi which form in the presence of dextran. We
have a very powerful tool in our hands, the radioactive fibrinogen test.
I suggest by scanning the legs of patients who receive dextran, that we
can find out what is happening to the thrombi—whether they last a
short time, lyse very quickly or propagate proximally. These answers
can be attained with the radioactive fibrinogen test, and that link is essential to our understanding of what is going on.

The second point I would like to make is that many people feel that
we are entering a period when we can be criticized if we have a study
with a control group receiving nothing. We are beginning to witness
many trials in which two methods of prophylaxis are compared. Now,
the more efficient these methods are, the lower the incidence of deep
vein thrombosis in the two groups is going to be, and the large number
required to show a difference between whatever is being compared.
Many of these studies, I predict, will be inconclusive. What we really

need is a method of predicting the risk for an individual patient, a means of saying that this particular method of prophylaxis will have this effect with this morbidity attached to it. We are not in a position to do this at the moment.

DR. EUGENE STRANDNESS: I really wanted to ask Doctor Nicolaides some questions and bring up some points that I would like to have clarified for my benefit. I think that a recent report in the *JAMA* on 820 randomized patients with low dose heparin has brought up some interesting points. First, I was surprised that 10% of the patients on the low-dose heparin regimens had dispensing errors during their hospitalization. Second, there were 8.6% bleeding complications. Third, the amount of blood required in the heparin group was on the average of 1 unit higher in the treated group than the nontreated group. Furthermore, most striking to me, was the very low incidence of femoropopliteal thrombosis in the control group, which was 2.9% as compared to 1 percent in the treated group. Also, in 820 patients, there were two pulmonary emboli, one in the control group and one in the treated group. The one in the treated group occurred after the heparin was discontinued on the 7th day.

Now, for those of us who are surgeons, some of these facts are important. We may think our patients are getting low-dose heparin but the nursing staff isn't giving the heparin on time. Second, a mean blood loss of 400 cc means that some patients required more blood than 400 cc when heparinized. I wondered in view of these statistics, are we justified in going ahead and recommending that all patients over 40 having major surgery receive low-dose heparin as a method of prophylaxis.

DR. ANDREW NICOLAIDES: These points are some of the things that worry many people. I don't think I can answer them completely. We are worried about the danger of an overdose, and it is a real possibility. I can't explain the 400-cc apparent increase in blood transfusion. However, blood loss studies at operation are extremely difficult because of the variation from patient to patient. It varies with surgical technique also and I am always skeptical about these studies. The point is that many surgeons who are going to do a major operation involving massive dissection do not want to use subcutaneous heparin. Also, the question arises: How long do we go on giving it? We always say until the patient is ambulatory. We are very much aware that no patient in the hospital is fully ambulatory. They have to spend quite a lot of time in bed. We would give heparin for about 10 days, until the patient is ready to go home. If he is going home earlier, we stop earlier.

Dr. Simon Sevitt: First, a word about dextran. We have a prophylactic program at our hospital. Sometimes we have patients in whom anticoagulants are contraindicated. Therefore, we have a few patients in whom dextran 70 was given intravenously. Among that group, we have three patients who died within a day or two. When we came to necropsy and examined the veins of the legs and the pulmonary arteries, all of these patients had a calf vein thrombus. Dextran does not stop calf vein thrombosis. Histologically, the thrombi were no different from those you would find in the patients without any prophylaxis. We did not find any pulmonary emboli. But, certainly, dextran does not stop deep vein thrombosis.

I would like to say a word, if I may, about miniheparin. It is certainly true that miniheparin, in my opinion, has been an effective agent in low-risk patients, the general surgical patients. But all of the evidence today indicates that it is of little or no value in the high-risk patients. The advantages claimed initially by the miniheparin protagonists were (1) it was sufficient, (2) no laboratory tests were needed and (3) there were few side effects. Now, we know that the laboratory tests may be needed to make sure that one is steering a course between effective therapy and bleeding. Second, apparently, we are now told that if we overstep some level of heparin in the blood, we get a high incidence of wound hematomas. This is in patients in whom the nurses have to go around three times a day to give subcutaneous injections. In warfarin therapy, all we have to do is give a pill once a day.

35 / Prevention of Venous Thromboembolism by Oral Anticoagulants and Drugs Affecting Platelet Function

EDWIN W. SALZMAN, M.D.

Dept. of Surgery, Harvard Medical School and Beth Israel Hospital, Boston, Massachusetts

Oral Anticoagulants

THE ADMINISTRATION of vitamin K antagonists to human subjects was first reported in 1941,[1] and within a year appeared the first description of their administration prophylactically to patients at high risk of venous thromboembolism.[2] Not until 10 years had passed, however, were the results of a controlled trial of their efficacy reported,[3] and almost another 10 years elapsed before the landmark account by Sevitt and Gallagher[4] of their experience with prophylactic administration of oral anticoagulants to patients with fractures of the hip. Over 40 reports of the prophylactic administration of coumarin derivatives have now appeared. Although the reported studies vary widely in adequacy of design and reliability of diagnostic criteria, the combined impact of the reported experience is overwhelming. The subject has been extensively reviewed,[5-8] and these papers should be consulted for a detailed listing of the available studies. The combined experience[5] in controlled clinical trials reports an incidence of venous thrombosis of 0–36% (average, 7.7%) in treated patients compared with 1.1–56% (average, 20.8%) among controls. Pulmonary embolism was encountered in 0–2.5% (average, 0.8%) of treated patients compared with 1.3–18% (average, 8.4%) of controls. A more meaningful tabulation,[5] considering specific diagnostic categories, reveals: in patients with congestive heart failure a ratio of treated to untreated patients of 1 :3.2 for venous thrombosis and 1 :5.3 for pulmonary embolism; in general and thoracic surgery, 1 :8.3 for venous thrombosis and 1 :4.6 for pulmonary embolism; among orthopedic patients with fractures of the hip or elective surgery of the hip a ratio of 1 :3.2 for venous thrombosis and 1 :4.2 for pulmonary embolism.

Many of the older studies of the efficacy of oral anticoagulants can be criticized, since by modern standards they are deficient in methodology, being based on clinical diagnostic criteria. The unreliability of clinical diagnosis of venous thromboembolism is well recognized today, in this era of phlebography, radioactive fibrinogen scanning and other sensitive objective diagnostic methods. However, even if one confines consideration to studies employing such "hard" criteria as those based on autopsy evidence, the impression is the same, and the effectiveness of vitamin K antagonists is beyond dispute.

Only two of the many studies examining this question have failed to show a clear advantage for the prophylactic administration of oral anticoagulants.[9, 10] Closer scrutiny of these reports reveals defects in design of the studies that in fact reinforce the conviction that oral anticoagulants are highly effective for prevention of venous thromboembolism, despite the apparent negative result. These papers report trials in which administration of the anticoagulant drug was not begun until the time of operation or later. Thrombi were detected by the sensitive radioactive fibrinogen uptake test, and most appeared within the first day or two postoperatively, too soon for the vitamin K antagonist to have become effective as an antithrombotic agent. These reports actually reinforce the conclusion that oral anticoagulants are beneficial, since in neither study did the patients with demonstrated thrombi go on to develop clinically significant consequences. Only one of the 75 anticoagulated patients had a pulmonary embolus. A major advantage of oral anticoagulants is the safety with which they can be administered in therapeutic or near therapeutic dosage in postoperative patients, so that the physician may achieve a therapeutic effect in patients with an already established venous thrombus, an advantage not shared by other prophylactic programs such as the use of low-dose heparin or antiplatelet agents.

Despite the well-established efficacy of oral anticoagulants, their use in the prevention of venous thromboembolism has not become a routine, even in very high-risk patients such as those undergoing surgery of the hip. A national survey of orthopedic surgeons[11] indicated that only 17% of those responding routinely employed prophylactic vitamin K antagonists in their practice, and only another 27% used

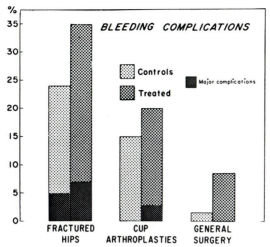

Fig 35–1.—Bleeding complications in prospective trials of prophylactic anticoagulation with warfarin in patients with fractures of the hip, elective cup arthroplasty of the hip or general surgical operations. (From Salzman et al.,[12] Harris et al.[13] and Skinner and Salzman.[14])

these drugs occasionally in selected high-risk patients, primarily because of concern about the hemorrhagic side effects of anticoagulation in surgical patients. A tabulation[5] of major bleeding complications reported in controlled trials with oral anticoagulants reveals a frequency of 0–7.2% (average, 2.0%) in patients receiving the drug compared with 0–4.8% (average, 0.9%) of controls. Our own experience (Fig 35–1) appears to be typical. Bleeding complications are more frequent in patients receiving warfarin than in a control group, but not much more frequent, and the occurrence of serious bleeding is not common, provided one is careful that the prothrombin time not exceed twice the control value at the time of operation and in the early postoperative period, and provided one observes certain important contraindications to prophylactic anticoagulation (Table 35–1).[5]

TABLE 35–1.—CONTRAINDICATIONS
TO PROPHYLACTIC ANTICOAGULATION*

Active peptic ulcer
Intracranial or visceral injury
Hemorrhagic diathesis
Gastrointestinal bleeding
Severe diastolic hypertension
Gross hematuria or hemoptysis

*From Clagett and Salzman.[5]

A substantial advance in practical therapeutics was obtained when O'Reilly and Aggeler[15] demonstrated that the use of a loading dose of oral anticoagulants offers no advantage and that the rate of disappearance of the vitamin K-dependent clotting factors after initiation of anticoagulation was the same when treatment was begun with a smaller daily dose. The latter practice appears to increase significantly the safety of anticoagulation by reducing the risk of early overdosage leading to a precipitous fall in factor VII. Despite the hemorrhagic complications of oral anticoagulants and the tedium of their administration and laboratory control, they remain the best established and probably most effective prophylactic drugs in high-risk patients and may well be the agents of choice in nonoperative patients. In surgical patients, the bleeding complications attending their use cause one to look further for a less hazardous mode of prophylaxis.

Drugs Affecting Platelet Function

Although the bulk of a venous thrombus consists of fibrin with enmeshed erythrocytes, anatomical studies provide evidence that platelet aggregation is a common feature in early lesions and may in fact be the initiating event in many, perhaps most, cases of peripheral venous thrombosis.[16-18] Accelerated platelet consumption has been reported in patients with clinically evident venous thrombi[19] and in those with recurrent venous thrombosis.[20] The technique of determining platelet survival is not sufficiently sensitive to detect platelet consumption in early thrombi recognizable only by radioactive fibrinogen scanning,[21] but it seems likely that this represents a limitation of the technique rather than evidence against their participation. Platelet hyperactivity has been described in cases of idiopathic recurrent deep vein thrombosis.[22] Excessive platelet coagulant activity was reported[23] in an interesting group of patients who subsequently developed postoperative deep vein thrombosis, a particularly interesting observation since it suggests that the assessment of platelet function may have predictive value. There is thus ample reason to suspect that agents inhibiting platelet function might have prophylactic value in patients with a high risk of venous thromboembolism.

The use of antiplatelet drugs to prevent venous thromboembolism is an attractive prospect because of the ease of their administration and their relative freedom from hemorrhagic side effects. Such drugs originally were hailed for their potential antithrombotic action in the arterial circulation because of the known contribution of platelets to arterial thrombosis. As it has turned out, these agents have actually been more widely evaluated for their influence on venous thrombosis, probably primarily because of the prevalence of venous thromboembolism and the relative convenience with which they can be tested in this regard, compared with the relative infrequency and difficulty of assessment of arterial thrombotic events.

Aside from investigations of the use of dextran as a prophylactic agent, discussed earlier in this Symposium, the first demonstration that platelet active agents might have preventive value was a report in 1971[24] of a group of patients undergoing vitallium mold arthroplasty of the hip who received either aspirin, dipyridamole, dextran or, for comparison, warfarin. Dipyridamole was not protective, but aspirin and dextran were as effective as warfarin in prevention of clinically apparent venous thromboembolism in these patients. There followed a series of clinical trials in a number of patient groups who received various platelet active drugs. The literature of the next several years was marked by conflicting claims of efficacy and of absence of an effect. Sufficient time has now elapsed to provide a somewhat clearer picture, and a tentative judgment seems permissible.

Several critical reviews have appeared.[25-27] There is substantial evidence for the effectiveness of drugs that alter platelet function as a result of their ability to inhibit the platelet synthesis of prostaglandins. These include aspirin, phenylbutazone and sulfinpyrazone. Well-designed studies employing objective criteria for diagnosis report the efficacy of these agents in patients undergoing elective surgery of the hip[28] or suffering from fractures of the hip[29] and in patients with recurrent deep vein thrombosis.[20, 30] In such patients, direct operative trauma to the peripheral veins or pathologic affections of the venous walls might be expected to exaggerate the role of platelets in the genesis of venous thromboembolism and provide a plausible explanation for the benefit of platelet active agents. A beneficial effect of aspirin in general surgical patients has also been observed,[21] but the results were less striking and the significance marginal. In such cases, with no particular injury to the veins, one might expect stasis of blood and postoperative hypercoagulability to be the predominant influences leading to venous thrombosis, and the role of platelets might be expected to be a secondary one. Other platelet active agents whose mode of action is less well established have also been examined for their prophylactic effect. Hydroxychloroquine has in two trials been reported to protect against venous thrombosis in the postoperative period.[31, 32] Dipyridamole has been found to be ineffective,[24, 33] but the combination of dipyridamole with aspirin was recently reported to be of value.[34] At present, it would be premature to recommend platelet inhibitors except in specific clinical situations in which they have been successfully tested by controlled trials. The ultimate role of platelet active drugs for prevention of venous thromboembolism will require many further contributions for a comprehensive assessment.

REFERENCES

1. Butt, H. R., Allen, E. V., and Bollman, J. L.: A preparation from spoiled sweet clover [3,3'-methylene-bis-(4-hydroxycoumarin)] which prolongs coagulation and pro-thrombin time of the blood: Preliminary report of experimental and clinical studies, Proc. Staff Meet. Mayo Clin. 16:388, 1941.
2. Allen, E. V., Barker, N. W., and Waugh, J. M.: A preparation from spoiled sweet clo-ver [3,3'-methylene-(4-hydroxycoumarin)] which prolongs coagulation and pro-thrombin time of the blood: A clinical study, JAMA 120:1009, 1942.
3. Anderson, G. M., and Hull, E.: Effect of dicumarol upon the mortality and inci-dence of thromboembolic complications in congestive heart failure, Am. Heart J. 39:697, 1950.
4. Sevitt, S., and Gallagher, N. G.: Prevention of venous thrombosis and pulmonary embolism in injured patients, Lancet 2:981, 1959.
5. Clagett, G. P., and Salzman, E. W.: Prevention of Venous Thromboembolism, in Sonnenblick, E. H., and Lesch, M. (eds.): *Progress in Cardiovascular Diseases*, Vol. XVII, no. 5 (New York: Grune & Stratton, 1975).
6. Hume, M., Sevitt, S., and Thomas, D. P.: *Venous Thrombosis and Pulmonary Em-bolism* (Cambridge, Mass.: Harvard University Press, 1970).
7. Aggeler, P. M., and Kosmin, M.: Anticoagulant Prophylaxis and Treatment of Ve-nous Thromboembolic Disease, in Sherry, S., Brinkhous, K. M., Genton, E., and Stengle, J. M. (eds.): *Thrombosis* (Washington, D.C.: National Academy of Sci-ences, 1969).
8. Salzman, E. W., and Harris, W. H.: Prevention of venous thromboembolism in or-thopaedic patients, J. Bone Joint Surg. [Am.] 58:903, 1976.
9. Pinto, D. J.: Controlled trial of an anticoagulant (warfarin sodium) in the prevention of venous thrombosis following hip surgery, Br. J. Surg. 57:349, 1970.
10. vanVroonhoven, T. J. M., vanZijl, J., and Muller, H.: Low-dose subcutaneous hepa-rin versus oral anticoagulants in the prevention of postoperative deep-venous thrombosis: A controlled clinical trial, Lancet 2:375, 1974.
11. Simon, T. L., and Stengle, J. M.: Antithrombotic practice in orthopedic surgery: Results of a survey, Clin. Orthop. 102, 1974.
12. Salzman, E. W., Harris, W. H., and DeSanctis, R. W.: Anticoagulation for prevention of thromboembolism following fractures of the hip, N. Engl. J. Med. 275:122, 1966.
13. Harris, W. H., Salzman, E. W., and DeSanctis, R. W.: The prevention of throm-boembolic disease by prophylactic anticoagulation: a controlled study in elective hip surgery, J. Bone Joint Surg. 49A:81, 1967.
14. Skinner, D. B., and Salzman, E. W.: Anticoagulant prophylaxis in surgical patients, Surg. Gynecol. Obstet. 125:741, 1967.
15. O'Reilly, R. A., and Aggeler, P. M.: Studies on coumarin anticoagulant drugs: initia-tion of warfarin therapy without a loading dose, Circulation 38:169, 1968.
16. Paterson, J. C.: The Pathology of Venous Thrombi, in Sherry, S., Brinkhous, K. M., Genton, E., and Stengle, J. M. (eds.): *Thrombosis* (Washington, D.C.: National Aca-demy of Sciences, 1969).
17. Sevitt, S.: Venous Thrombosis in Injured Patients (with Some Observations on Pathogenesis), in Sherry, S., Brinkhous, K. M., Genton, E., and Stengle, J. M. (eds): *Thrombosis* (Washington, D.C.: National Academy of Sciences, 1969).
18. Freiman, D. G.: The Pathology of Pulmonary Embolism and Venous Thrombosis,

in Fratantoni, J., and Wessler, S. (eds.): *Prophylactic Therapy of Deep Vein Thrombosis and Pulmonary Embolism*, publ. no. (NIH)76-866 (Washington, D.C.: Dept. Health, Education and Welfare, 1975).

19. Harker, L. A., and Slichter, S. J.: Platelet and fibrinogen consumption in man, N. Engl. J. Med. 287:999, 1972.

20. Steele, P. P., Weily, H. S., and Genton, E.: Platelet survival and adhesiveness in recurrent venous thrombosis, N. Engl. J. Med. 288:1145, 1973.

21. Clagett, G. P., Schneider, P., Rosoff, C. B., and Salzman, E. W.: The influence of aspirin on postoperative platelet kinetics and venous thrombosis, Surgery 77:61, 1975.

22. Wu, K. K., Barnes, R. W., and Hoak, J. C.: Platelet hyperaggregability in idiopathic recurrent deep vein thrombosis, Circulation 53:687, 1976.

23. Walsh, P. N., Rogers, P. H., Marder, V. J., Gagnatelli, G., Escovitz, E. S., and Sherry, S.: The relationship of platelet coagulant activities to venous thrombosis following hip surgery, Br. J. Haematol. 32:421, 1976.

24. Salzman, E. W., Harris, W. H., and DeSanctis, R. W.: Reduction in venous thromboembolism by agents affecting platelet function, N. Engl. J. Med. 284:1287, 1971.

25. Salzman, E. W.: Prevention of Venous Thromboembolism with Drugs that Alter Platelet Function, in Fratantoni, J., and Wessler, S. (eds.): *Prophylactic Therapy of Deep Vein Thrombosis and Pulmonary Embolism*, publ. no. (NIH)76-866 (Washington, D.C.: Dept. Health, Education and Welfare, 1975).

26. Genton, E., Gent, M., Hirsh, J., and Harker, L. A.: Platelet-inhibiting drugs in the prevention of clinical thrombotic disease: Part 1, N. Engl. J. Med. 293:1174, 1975.

27. Gallus, A. S., and Hirsh, J.: Prevention of venous thromboembolism, Semin. Thromb. Hemostasis 2:232, 1976.

28. Harris, W. H., Salzman, E. W., Athanasoulis, C., Waltman, A. C., Baum, S., and DeSanctis, R. W.: Comparison of warfarin, low molecular weight dextran, aspirin and subcutaneous heparin in prevention of venous thromboembolism following total hip replacement, J. Bone Joint Surg. 56A:1552, 1974.

29. Zekert, F.: *Thrombosen Embolien und Aggregationshemmer in der Chirurgie* (Stuttgart-New York: F. K. Schattauer Verlag, 1975).

30. Evans, G., and Gent, M.: Effect of Platelet Suppressive Drugs on Arterial and Venous Thromboembolism, in Hirsh, J. (ed.): *Platelets, Drugs and Thrombosis* (Basel: S. Karger Co., 1975).

31. Carter, A. E., Eban, R., and Perrett, R. D.: Prevention of postoperative deep venous thrombosis and pulmonary embolism, Br. Med. J. 1:312, 1971.

32. Carter, A. E., and Eban, R.: Prevention of postoperative deep venous thrombosis in legs by orally administered hydroxychloroquine sulphate, Br. Med. J. 3:64, 1974.

33. Browse, N. L., and Hall, J. H.: Effect of dipyridamole on the incidence of clinically detectable deep-vein thrombosis, Lancet 2:718, 1969.

34. Renney, J. T. G., O'Sullivan, E. F., and Burke, P. F.: Prevention of postoperative deep vein thrombosis with dipyridamole and aspirin, Br. Med. J. 1:992, 1976.

36 / The Prevention of Postoperative Deep Venous Thrombosis by Intermittent Compression of the Legs

LEONARD T. COTTON, M.CH., F.R.C.S.

Dean, King's College Hospital Medical School, London, England

AND

V. C. ROBERTS, PH.D., M.I.E.E.

Deputy Director, Department of Biomedical Engineering, King's College Hospital Medical School, London, England

SINCE THE DESCRIPTION of the ^{125}I-fibrinogen test by Atkins and Hawkins in 1965,[1] it has been possible to measure with great accuracy the effectiveness of methods that might decrease the incidence of postoperative deep vein thrombosis (DVT). It has proved to be the simplest method by which clinical trials can be conducted, simpler than routine phlebography. Some critics have claimed that the ^{125}I-fibrinogen test on which we have placed so much reliance is irrelevant to the problems of pulmonary embolism and fatal pulmonary embolism and suggest that finding "hot spots" in the calf muscles in no way reflects the incidence of thrombi in the femoral or iliac veins from which many pulmonary emboli arise.[2] MacIntyre has shown that in 2,029 patients pulmonary embolism occurred only in 24 and in all there were positive leg scans.[3] Kakkar has stated that the fibrinogen uptake test still provides the most dynamic and practical test for the detection of DVT.[4] This is potent evidence of the value of the ^{125}I-fibrinogen test in DVT prophylaxis. There is no doubt that patients who have positive leg scans do go on to develop signs of venous disease such as aching and swelling some years later.[5] Also we know

TABLE 36–1.—METHODS OF PROPHYLAXIS AGAINST DEEP
VENOUS THROMBOSIS (DVT)

METHOD	DVT DEPRESSION (%)*
Mechanical	
Elevation of legs on the operating table[6]	NS
Static compression of the legs[7]	NS
Static graduated compression of the legs[8]	47
Passive exercise of the legs[9]	77
Electrical stimulation of the calf muscles[10]	61
Intermittent compression of the arms[11]	60
Intermittent compression of the legs[12, 13, 17]	80, 75, 82
Intermittent compression of the legs in cases of	
malignancy[13]	89
Chemical	
Aspirin[14]	NS
Dextran	Variable
Warfarin	Variable
Dipyridamole[15]	NS
Dihydroergotamine[16]	74
Subcutaneous heparin[17]	77
Combinations	
Oxyphenbutazone and static compression[18]	69
Intermittent compression ± subcutaneous heparin[19]	No difference
Dihydroergotamine and subcutaneous heparin[20]	77
Aspirin and dipyridamole[21]	50

*NS, not significant.

many thousands of people suffer from leg ulceration and other post-phlebitic symptoms, the results of DVT after surgery, so anything that can depress the incidence of DVT must be a positive gain. One could even argue it would be as important to prevent the thousands of post-operative DVTs leading to life-long invalidism as to save a few lives from fatal pulmonary embolism.

Broadly two main groups of methods of prophylaxis against DVT can be defined, the mechanical and the chemical. We have prepared a list of many of the methods that have been tried, both successfully and unsuccessfully, and have tried to indicate their efficacy by their potential to depress the ^{125}I-fibrinogen test or less often by clinical tests of DVT (Table 36–1).

Our work on DVT prevention has been on mechanical methods of prophylaxis. The places in the veins of the leg where thrombosis begins are in the soleal sinuses[22] and in the deep valve pockets of the popliteal and femoral veins.[23] We were able to demonstrate how the induction of anesthesia more than halves the venous flow in the legs of patients.[24] Application of static compression achieved only a transient increase in flow and above 15 mm Hg there was a marked decrease in flow.[25] Passive exercise during surgery produced by a foot mover increased blood volume flow rate and flow pulsatility.[26] Intermittent compression of the legs increased blood flow pulsatility alone.[27]

Measurements of blood flow in the femoral veins of patients during varicose vein surgery showed that maximal pulsatility of flow was achieved by application of pressure to the leg at a rate of 8 mm Hg per second to a maximum of 45 mm Hg at an interval of 2 min. This interval is allowed so that the limb may fill with venous blood.[17] Cinephlebography shows that with each cycle of compression the entire deep venous system is emptied and the jet of blood from the limb is seen to flow well into the inferior vena cava.

The intermittent compression machine we have constructed is marketed as the British Oxygen Company's Roberts Venous Flow Stimulator which is comprised of two plastic boots that cover the legs to the knees and are inflated by a cylinder of oxygen or air to the limits described above. This machine can be used in any operation except obviously in those on the legs and has been in routine use in our theaters in all patients except children. It has been used without hazard in many hundreds of operations during the last 4 years. The method in no way interferes with the operation or embarrasses the surgeon.

Clinical trials using the ^{125}I-fibrinogen test to measure the incidence of DVT showed that passive exercise during surgery produced a depression of 77% and intermittent compression a depression of 80%.[12, 13, 17] Thus increasing pulsatility of blood flow in the leg veins during surgery was clearly more important than increasing mean blood flow. In cancer patients intermittent compression was even more efficient, depressing the DVT rate by 89%.[13] The reason for this was thought to be because DVT in cases of malignancy occurs more frequently in the first 24 hr after surgery than in nonmalignant cases and so methods which function only during the operation might therefore be more effective on thrombosis initiated during the early hours after surgery. It is remarkable that the effects of intermittent compression acting only during the operation should be so identically effective as subcutaneous heparin acting during the operation and in the subsequent 6 postoperative days.[17] It was a great disappointment that when intermittent compression and subcutaneous heparin were used together their combined action was no more effective than either method alone.[19]

It has been the purpose of this review to pause and survey progress that has been made in the prevention of DVT. We believe that the evidence produced in recent years pins the cause of DVT on *stasis* and *hypercoagulability.* Which is more important? We believe stasis is the more important if only because abolishing stasis by intermittent compression of the leg is just as effective as intermittent compression plus low-dose heparin which presumably reverses hypercoagulability. Subcutaneous heparin may also have an effect on blood flow by its effect of reducing blood viscosity. Dextran has a similar effect in lowering viscosity by diluting the blood. Dihydroergotamine seems to have an effect on DVT prevention by selective venoconstriction speeding deep venous flow.

The results of intermittent compression and low-dose heparin are equally effective in reducing DVT by about 80%. We have no idea of the quality of the 20% of cases which are resistant. There is no evidence that the resistant cases are more prone to pulmonary embolism. So far the evidence is that heparin and dextran dramatically reduce deaths from pulmonary embolism. We can only assume that intermittent compression does the same, though for financial reasons we cannot prove this.

Our thesis is that intermittent compression should be the preferred method of prevention of DVT because of its effectiveness, its cheapness, its freedom from side effects and the ease of application to all patients. In the future we hope to be able to use intermittent compression during operations for hip replacement which have so far proved resistant to DVT prophylaxis. We also intend to extend intermittent compression into the postoperative period for known high-risk cases such as hip operations and where there is a previous history of DVT and pulmonary embolism.

REFERENCES

1. Atkins, P., and Hawkins, L. A.: Detection of venous thrombosis in the legs, Lancet 2:1217, 1965.
2. Mavor, G. E., Mahaffy, R. G., Walker, M. G., Duthie, J. S., Dhall, D. P., Gaddie, J., and Reid, G. F.: Peripheral venous scanning with I-125-tagged fibrinogen, Lancet 1:661, 1972.
3. MacIntyre, I. M. C.: A Controlled Trial of Heparin and Dextran, in Ruckley, C. V., and MacIntyre, I. M. C. (eds.): *Venous Thromboembolic Disease* (London: Churchill Livingstone, 1975).
4. Kakkar, V. V.: Low-dose heparin in total hip replacement, Lancet 2:373, 1976.
5. Browse, N. L., and Clemenson, G.: Sequelae of an ^{125}I-fibrinogen detected thrombus, Br. Med. J. 2:468, 1974.
6. Rosengarten, D. S., and Laird, J.: The effect of leg elevation on the incidence of deep vein thrombosis after operation, Br. J. Surg. 58:182, 1971.
7. Rosengarten, D. S., Laird, J., Jeyasingh, K., and Martin, P. C.: The failure of compression stockings (Tubigrip) to prevent deep venous thrombosis after operation, Br. J. Surg. 57:296, 1970.
8. Holford, C. P.: The effect of graduated static compression on isotopically diagnosed deep vein thrombosis of the leg, Br. J. Surg. 63:157, 1976.

9. Sabri, S., Roberts, V. C., and Cotton, L. T.: Prevention of early postoperative deep vein thrombosis by passive exercise of the leg during surgery, Br. Med. J. 3:82, 1971.

10. Browse, N. L., and Negus, D.: Prevention of postoperative leg vein thrombosis by electrical muscle stimulation, Br. Med. J. 3:615, 1970.

11. Knight, M. T. N., and Dawson, R.: Reduction of the incidence of deep vein thrombosis (DVT) in the legs by intermittent compression of the arms, Br. J. Surg. 63:668, 1976.

12. Sabri, S., Roberts, V. C., and Cotton, L. T.: Prevention of early postoperative deep vein thrombosis by intermittent compression of the leg during surgery, Br. Med. J. 4:394, 1971.

13. Roberts, V. C., and Cotton, L. T.: Prevention of postoperative deep vein thrombosis in patients with malignant disease, Br. Med. J. 1:358, 1974.

14. O'Brien, J. R., Tulevski, V., and Ethrington, M.: Two in vitro studies comparing high and low aspirin dosage, Lancet 1:399, 1971.

15. Browse, N. L., and Hall, J. H.: Effect of dipyridamole on the incidence of clinically detectable deep vein thrombosis, Lancet 2:718, 1969.

16. Butterman, G., Theisinger, W., Oechsler, H., and Hör, G.: Untersuchung über die postoperative thromboembolic Prophylaxe nach einem neuen medikamentosen Behandlungsprinzip, Dtsch. Med. Wochensch. 100:2063, 1975.

17. Roberts, V. C., and Cotton, L. T.: Mechanical Methods for the Prevention of Venous Thromboembolism, in Ruckley, C. V., and MacIntyre, I. M. C. (eds.): *Venous Thromboembolic Disease* (London: Churchill Livingstone, 1975).

18. Tillberg, B.: Prevention of postoperative deep vein thrombosis by leg bandaging and oxyphenbutazone, Br. Med. J. 1:1256, 1976.

19. Roberts, V. C., and Cotton, L. T.: Failure of low dose heparin to improve efficacy of peroperative intermittent calf compression in preventing postoperative deep vein thrombosis, Br. Med. J. 3:458, 1975.

20. Sagar, S., Nairn, D., Stamatakis, J. D., Maffei, F. H., Higgins, A. F., Thomas, D. P., and Kakkar, V. V.: Efficacy of low dose heparin in prevention of extensive deep vein thrombosis in patients undergoing total hip replacement, Lancet 1:1151, 1976.

21. Renney, J. T. G., O'Sullivan, E. F., and Burke, P. F.: Prevention of postoperative deep vein thrombosis with dipyridamole and aspirin, Br. Med. J. 2:992, 1976.

22. Cotton, L. T., and Clark, C. C.: Anatomical localisation of venous thrombosis, Ann. R. Coll. Surg. Engl. 36:214, 1965.

23. McLachlin, J., and Paterson, G. L.: Some basic observations on venous thrombosis and pulmonary embolism, Surg. Gynecol. Obstet. 93:1, 1951.

24. Clark, C., and Cotton, L. T.: Blood flow in the deep veins of the leg, Br. J. Surg. 55:211, 1968.

25. Spiro, M., Roberts, V. C., and Richards, J. B.: Effects of externally applied pressure on femoral vein blood flow, Br. Med. J. 1:719, 1970.

26. Roberts, V. C., Sabri, S., Pietroni, M. C., Gurevich, V., and Cotton, L. T.: Passive flexion and femoral vein flow, a study using a motorised foot mover, Br. Med. J. 3:78, 1971.

27. Sabri, S., Roberts, V. C., and Cotton, L. T.: The effects of intermittently applied external pressure on the haemodynamics of the lower limb in man, Br. J. Surg. 59:223, 1972.

Discussion: Chapter 36

DR. ASCHER H. SHAPIRO: The review presented by Mr. Cotton presents convincing evidence that intermittent compression is a serious competitor to subcutaneous heparin as a prophylaxis against DVT. A remarkable feature is the high efficacy of the pneumomechanical device even though used solely during surgery. One cannot but wonder whether still further reduction of DVT might not be effected by application in the postoperative period.

It seems clear from the evidence at hand that we really do not know *why* intermittent compression is effective. Mr. Cotton mentions the common assumption that the important feature of the method is the elimination of stasis. But how can we be sure, for instance, that the important feature is not mere mechanical manipulation that dislodges small thrombi as they form? Alternatively, if elimination of stasis is indeed the significant feature of the method, how does this fit with the observation that the incidence of thrombi in the leg is reduced by intermittent compression of the arms? The thought has been expressed that either the hemodynamic effects or the mechanical manipulation produced by the device somehow leads to thrombolysis. If true, this might explain the experimental observations that (1) intermittent compression and subcutaneous heparin seem equally effective and (2) the two methods in combination produce no increase in protection over either.

Coupled with the hypothesis that the method works by elimination of stasis, Mr. Cotton suggests as the criterion of optimal performance the degree of flow pulsatility proximal to the compression boot. However, there are in fact several hemodynamic parameters of potential significance, and it is not clear which is the governing one tending to reduce DVT: (1) volume flow rate (ml/sec), (2) blood velocity (cm/sec) and (3) shear stress. Moreover, these must be considered not only proximally to the boot but at all sections under the boot.

It seems reasonable to hope that an understanding of the detailed mechanisms by which intermittent compression works against the formation of thrombi would lead to improvements in the method.

In our laboratory at M. I. T., my colleague Roger D. Kamm has been using hydraulic models and theoretical calculations to investigate the hemodynamic details of intermittent compression. Our aim is to understand, and to be able to predict, how the area, volume flow rate and fluid speed vary with time at each location along the venous return path, and, further, how the aforementioned curves depend upon the type of pressure cycle used.

The rapid application of external pressure does not produce uniform collapse of a long vessel. As shown schematically by Figure 1, the collapse starts at the knee end (that is, at the downstream end with regard to flow), and a "wave of collapse" proceeds distally toward the

Fig 1.—Mode of collapse due to rapid application of pressure. **a,** Before pressure is applied. **b, c** and **d,** Successive configurations after application of pressure.

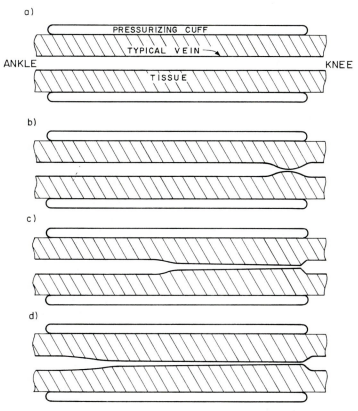

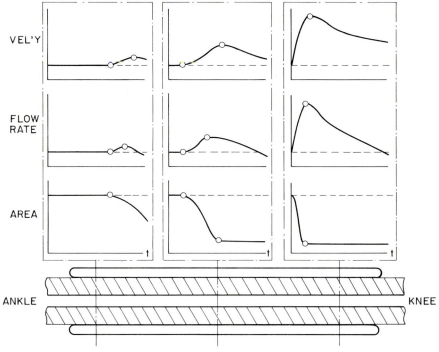

Fig 2. — Curves of area versus time, flow rate versus time and fluid velocity versus time, at three locations under the cuff.

ankle, but more and more slowly because of the flow-limiting resistance due to the small area downstream. The fluid dynamic reason for this mode of behavior, which we observe both experimentally and by theoretical calculation, is that the fluid can accelerate in the downstream direction only if the intraluminal pressure downstream is less than it is upstream. The consequences of this behavior on area, flow rate and velocity are shown schematically in Figure 2, where these variables are plotted versus time for three locations: near the knee end, near the ankle end and midway between. The area collapse is more and more delayed from downstream (knee) to upstream (ankle). Both the flow rate and velocity reach maximums and then decrease; however, the time of the maximum increases from knee to ankle, and the amount of the maximum is very much decreased. Naturally the shapes of all of the curves depend upon the type of pressure cycle used.

We believe that we shall soon have a quite good understanding of the hemodynamic details, but we stress that intelligent improvement of the intermittent compression method depends equally upon physiologic knowledge of how the hemodynamic details relate to the formation of thrombi.

37 / The Prevention of Venous Thromboembolism by Mechanical Methods

NORMAN L. BROWSE, M.D., F.R.C.S.
Professor of Vascular Surgery, St. Thomas' Hospital Medical School, London, England

SINCE VIRCHOW[1] POSTULATED that stasis was an important factor in the production of deep vein thrombosis, surgeons — being mechanically minded — have been particularly interested in mechanical methods of combating venous thromboembolism.

The theoretical justification of the hypothesis that the prevention of stasis will prevent thrombosis is not easy, for it has to embrace such opposite experimental observations as those of Hewson,[2] who showed that blood held in a horse's jugular vein would remain liquid for 6 hr, and Wessler[3] who showed that blood held in the jugular vein of a rabbit would clot within 2 min if the animal had been made hypercoagulable by pretreatment with an injection of an homologous serum. Nevertheless it is generally believed that the abolition of venous stasis should reduce the incidence of thrombosis.

The factors that influence venous blood flow are well established. The prime mover is the "vis a tergo" — the cardiac pump. The principal mover is the peripheral muscle pump. The intrathoracic negative pressure normally helps by sucking blood into the chest, but when this pressure is reversed during positive pressure ventilation it may impede venous return.

The velocity of blood flow depends not only upon the forces which actually move the blood and the quantity of blood being moved, but also upon the caliber of the vessels. The size of the veins can be altered by changes in venous tone and transmural pressure, the latter being accessible to control by direct external compression. Thus it should be possible to alter both the velocity and the volume of venous blood flow, but it is important to remember that such hemodynamic considerations treat the veins as smooth tubes; the way in which changes of blood flow affect the circulation of blood in and around the valve cusps has not been properly explored. It seems logical to assume that the only way to empty a valve cusp, the site of maximum stasis, is by direct compression of the segment of vein containing the cusp or by suddenly increasing the volume of flow so much that it flattens the valve flat against the vein wall. This is an important point to remember when predicting the possible effectiveness of a new method of prophylaxis.

The methods of changing venous blood flow can be divided into passive methods, which only change the velocity of flow, and active methods, which alter the volume and the velocity of flow.

Passive Methods

The two passive mechanical methods of prophylaxis that have been studied in detail are elevation of the legs and elastic bandages/stockings.

Elevation of the Legs

Elevation of the legs up to 15–20 degrees doubles the linear velocity of venous blood flow without reducing the arterial inflow,[4] but above this angle the arterial inflow becomes less.

There is no good evidence that elevation of the legs before, during or after operation reduces the incidence of deep vein thrombosis. In our own studies,[5] in which we compared the effect of elevating one leg to 20 degrees during operation against the other leg kept horizontal, the incidence of thrombosis in the elevated leg was 19% and in the horizontal leg 16%.

Elastic Bandages/Stockings

Any form of external compression which reduces the diameter of the veins will increase the linear velocity of blood flow, but there is no firm evidence to show that constant elastic compression of the limbs reduces the incidence of deep vein thrombosis. In our own study,[5] in which we used Tubigrip stockings, the incidence of thrombosis in the stockinged leg, worn from the day of entry into the hospital until the day of discharge, was 24% and in the control leg 29%.

The principal problem with any form of constant elastic compression is the control of the compressing force. Most experimental studies which have tried to assess the ideal external pressure to give the maximum increase of flow velocity conclude that it is about 15 mm Hg.[6] However, in those studies where different surgeons have applied the bandages, or different types of stocking have been compared, the applied pressure has been found to be extremely variable. Thus, any attempt to apply a uniform controlled pressure with stockings or bandages is likely to fail. Pressures above 15 mm Hg reduce arterial inflow and venous flow.

Although elastic stockings fail to alter the incidence of deep vein thrombosis, there is some evidence which suggests that they may reduce the incidence of pulmonary embolism. After a large study of 9,917 patients, partly randomly allocated and partly sequential and based on physical signs and postmortem evidence, Wilkins and Stanton claimed that the use of elastic stockings reduced the incidence of significant emboli from 0.4 to 0.15%, without changing the incidence of clinically detectable peripheral thrombosis.[7] This study has a number of defects, but it is probably worth repeating using better objective methods of assessment because it recently has been shown that intravenous dextran reduces the incidence of embolism without affecting the incidence of peripheral thrombosis and it would be extremely valuable to know if elastic compression has the same effect.

Active Methods

EARLY AMBULATION

It has been the fond belief of surgeons and physiotherapists for many years that rapid mobilization after an operation reduces the incidence of deep vein thrombosis. There is very little evidence to support this view. Two studies, one by Flanc et al.[8] and one by Tsapogas et al.[9] suggest that there is a slight reduction of the incidence of thrombosis in patients given intensive multifactorial postoperative physiotherapy (exercises, stockings and elevation), but the part played by early ambulation cannot be clearly isolated.

Early ambulation has many valuable effects and should be encouraged, but it is important that it be encouraged for the right reasons and not the unjustified belief that it prevents pulmonary embolism.

ELECTRICAL STIMULATION

The first clinical studies of the effect of electrical stimulation of the calf were by Doran et al. in 1964.[10] He showed that stimulating the calf muscles increased the linear velocity of venous blood flow and doubled the arterial inflow to the calf muscles, and claimed that this reduced the incidence of pulmonary embolism. In view of his findings we studied the incidence of thrombosis after operation using the fibrinogen uptake test for diagnosis[11] and found that the incidence of thrombosis in the stimulated leg was 9% and in the test leg 23%. Nicolaides et al[12] confirmed these results and also studied the frequency of stimulation required to produce the optimum change in blood flow. The best stimulus appears to be a square wave at 4-sec intervals (15/min), lasting 50 msec, using a voltage that produces a firm dorsiflexion of the foot—usually 35–45 v.

MECHANICAL FOOT PEDAL

Many surgeons have suggested that the blood flow from the leg could be increased during an operation by mechanically dorsiflexing and plantarflexing the foot. This method has been studied by Sabri et al.[13] at King's College Hospital, who showed that it does reduce the incidence of thrombosis but no other studies have been published on this method because the apparatus is cumbersome and not really suitable for intraoperative use.

PNEUMATIC COMPRESSION

The logical extension of passive compression of the veins with elastic bandages was to use pneumatic compression so that the pressure could be accurately controlled and applied intermittently to allow the veins to fill between compressions. This technique was first studied in the United Kingdom by two groups—Cotton at King's College Hospital[14] and Calnan at the Hammersmith Hospital.[15] Both have shown that it does reduce the incidence of deep vein thrombosis.

The Hammersmith device which produces a slow sine wave change in pressure does not appear to be as effective as the King's College device, which delivers a more frequent square wave pressure change, because in the Hammersmith study the incidence of thrombosis in patients with underlying malignant disease was not reduced.

Roberts et al.[16] made careful measurements of femoral vein blood flow to assess the optimum rate and degree of compression and found that a 40-mm Hg compression lasting 5 sec, applied every minute, gave the greatest increase of femoral vein velocity and peak volume flow. As there is no change in arterial inflow the minute volume flow from the leg does not change but a relatively steady flow is converted to a pulsatile flow.

No workers have confirmed the effectiveness of the Robert's pump, but Clark et al.[17] have had similar results to Hills et al.[15] with the sine wave pump.

My own unpublished studies suggest that pneumatic compression is not as effective in preventing calf thrombosis as electrical stimulation or subcutaneous heparin.

There have been no studies of the effect of pneumatic compression alone on the incidence of pulmonary embolism. We have studied a combination of pneumatic compression and intravenous dextran on the incidence of pulmonary embolism and found it to be effective.

Why do the passive methods, that increase the linear velocity of blood flow, fail to reduce the incidence of thrombosis when the active methods are effective? I would suggest that this is because the active methods directly compress the veins and so empty the valve cusps, as well as suddenly increasing the volume of venous blood flow; electrical stimulation has the additional advantage of increasing the arterial inflow because it causes active muscle contractions.

Discussion

The mechanical methods of prophylaxis are simple, safe and, consequently, very attractive. However, they must compete against the well-documented effectiveness against calf thrombosis of subcutaneous heparin and the less certain effectiveness against embolism of both subcutaneous heparin and intravenous dextran. Until acceptable trials have been performed with the mechanical methods it is not possible to be certain that they will reduce the incidence of embolism, but it is highly likely that they will be effective because there is a close correlation between thrombosis detected in the calf by the fibrinogen uptake test and the development of pulmonary embolism.[18]

If the mechanical methods are found to be as effective against embolism as systemically administered substances then I think most surgeons would prefer them, but on theoretical grounds such a finding is unlikely. It is well established that thrombosis can begin anywhere between the veins of the foot and the vena cava, and there is little doubt that the present mechanical methods affect only the blood flow in the veins of the calf and lower thigh. Blood flow in the tributaries of the profunda vein and in the pelvic veins is unaffected by any of the current mechanical techniques. These considerations make one suspect that a systemic agent is likely to be more effective than one locally applied, but many surgeons might be prepared to accept a slightly less effective technique if it were clearly much safer.

A new approach to the use of mechanical methods is being studied at the Hammersmith Hospital — the production of a systemic change in coagulation by mechanical means. It is well known that venous congestion stimulates the release of fibrinolytic activator from the vein wall and it has been postulated that the way in which pneumatic compression affects thrombosis is by enhancing fibrinolysis rather than by changing the blood flow. In a group of 28 patients who wore pneumatic leggings during their operation, we were unable to find any changes in blood fibrinolytic activity significantly different from untreated patients, but the Hammersmith group does claim to have observed such a change and has been studying the effect of applying small cuffs to the upper arms which are repeatedly inflated to produce mild venous congestion for a number of hours in the hope of increasing blood fibrinolytic activity. If this method does increase fibrinolysis, it may reduce the incidence of deep vein thrombosis, although I remain skeptical because we have not found any correlation between the development of deep vein thrombosis and the changes in fibrinolysis after surgery. Indeed we think that the fibrinolytic shut-down that follows surgery is either a response to the underlying disease or the development of a thrombosis and not a cause of thrombosis. Many patients have a profound fibrinolytic shut-down but do not get a thrombosis.[19]

Summary

In summary one must conclude that the currently available mechanical methods of prophylaxis have been overshadowed by the development of systemic methods, but I do not think that they should be discarded. Electrical stimulation and pneumatic compression are worthy of further study in large clinical trials to assess their effect on the incidence of pulmonary embolism and, remembering the hazards of the systemically administered agents, their effect on total mortality.

REFERENCES

1. Virchow, R. L. K.: *Thrombose and Emboli (1846–1856)* (Leipzig, J. A. Barth, 1910).
2. Hewson, W.: *Experimental Enquiries* (London: T. Caddell, 1771).
3. Wessler, S.: Thrombosis in the presence of vascular stasis, Am. J. Med. 33:648, 1962.
4. Wright, H. P., and Osborn, S. B.: Effect of posture on venous velocity, Br. Heart J. 14:325, 1952.
5. Browse, N. L., Jackson, B. T., Mayo, M. E., and Negus, D.: Value of mechanical methods of preventing post-operative calf vein thrombosis, Br. J. Surg. 61:219, 1974.
6. Sabri, S., Roberts, V. C., and Cotton, L. T.: Effect of externally applied pressure on the haemodynamics of the lower limb, Br. Med. J. 3:503, 1971.
7. Wilkins, R. W., and Stanton, J. R.: Elastic stockings in the prevention of pulmonary embolism, N. Engl. J. Med. 248:1087, 1953.

8. Flanc, C., Kakkar, V. V., and Clarke, M. D.: Post-operative deep vein thrombosis. Effect of intensive prophylaxis, Lancet 1:477, 1969.

9. Tsapogas, M. J., Gousous, H., and Peabody, R. A.: Postoperative venous thrombosis and the effectiveness of prophylactic measures, Arch. Surg. 197:561, 1971.

10. Doran, F. S. A., Drury, M., and Sivyer, A.: A simple way to combat the venous stasis which occurs in the lower limbs during surgical operations, Br. J. Surg. 51:486, 1964.

11. Browse, N. L., and Negus, D.: Prevention of post-operative leg vein thrombosis by electrical muscle stimulation, Br. Med. J. 3:615, 1970.

12. Nicolaides, A. N., Kakkar, V. V., Field, E. S., and Fish, P.: Optimal electrical stimulus for prevention of deep vein thrombosis, Br. Med. J. 4:756, 1972.

13. Sabri, S., Roberts, V. C., and Cotton, L. T.: Prevention of early postoperative deep vein thrombosis by passive exercise of leg during surgery, Br. Med. J. 3:82, 1971.

14. Sabri, S., Roberts, V. C., and Cotton, L. T.: Prevention of early postoperative deep vein thrombosis by intermittent compression of the leg during surgery, Br. Med. J. 4:394, 1971.

15. Hills, N. H., Pflug, J. J., Jeyasingh, K., Boardman, L., and Calnan, J. S.: Prevention of deep vein thrombosis by intermittent pneumatic compression of the calf, Br. Med. J. 1:131, 1972.

16. Roberts, V. C., Sabri, S., Beeley, A. H., and Cotton, L. T.: Effect of intermittently applied external pressure on the haemodynamics of the lower limb in man, Br. J. Surg. 59:223, 1972.

17. Clark, W. B., MacGregor, A. B., Prescott, R. J., and Ruckley, C. V.: Pneumatic compression of the calf and post-operative deep vein thrombosis, Lancet 2:5, 1974.

18. Browse, N. L., Clemenson, G., and Croft, D. N.: Fibrogen-detectable thrombosis in the legs and pulmonary embolism, Br. Med. J. 1:603, 1974.

19. Browse, N. L., Gray, L., and Morland, M.: Changes in blood fibrinolytic activity after surgery. Effect of thrombosis and malignant disease, Br. J. Surg. (in press).

38 / Postoperative Venous Thrombosis — The Dynamics of Propagation, Resolution and Embolism

MICHAEL HUME, M.D.

Professor of Surgery, Tufts University School of Medicine and Chief of the Surgical Services, Lemuel Shattuck Hospital, Boston, Massachusetts

AT ONE TIME the true scope of postoperative vein thrombosis was apparent only to the pathologist. Careful dissections of veins of the lower limb at autopsy[12] revealed that (1) thrombi may have multifocal origins with predilection to form at certain sites, (2) thrombi are found with increasing frequency as postoperative (or postinjury) immobilization is prolonged and (3) thrombi are "silent" more often than they are recognized by the clinican. By similarly detailed dissections the fate of thrombi has been demonstrated.[13, 14] Most venous thrombi are finally recanalized. While the picture so revealed seems rather complete, the time course of propagation, lysis and embolism has been assembled from single cases studied at one point in time — the point of autopsy. The dynamics of thrombus growth and resolution in any given patient could be demonstrated only with the advent of practical screening methods that allow repeated observations in postoperative patients. Admittedly, the contrast phlebogram allowed the same one-time perspective of the problem in living patients that the pathologist obtained at necropsy. However, by analogy, the phlebogram is to more recent screening techniques as the snapshot is to cinema. Contrast phlebography makes its most significant contribution to this moving picture by proving the accuracy of the screening methods which in turn reveal the dynamic view of postoperative thrombosis which is now emerging.

571

Besides revealing the fate of thrombi in postoperative subjects, screening methods seem to present some inconsistencies that need to be reconciled with the perceptions of the pathologist. Before the 4th postoperative day necropsy rarely reveals thrombi in leg veins. On the other hand, thrombosis revealed by isotope leg scan characteristically arises earlier, possibly during the day of operation, though there is active debate about this point.[3] Moreover thrombosis demonstrable by leg scan has an even higher incidence than thrombosis confirmed by phlebograms, and is many times more frequent than symptomatic embolism. To the pathologist, already aware of the silent aspect of postoperative thrombosis, this represents no surprise. To the clinician, into whose hands the tools for diagnosis have passed, this discrepancy has presented a challenge. Either it must be dismissed as overly sensitive diagnosis, which casts doubt on the credibility of the isotope leg scan method, or it requires a commitment to prevention which can no longer be ignored.

The results of monitoring postoperative patients at risk of thromboembolism following hip joint reconstruction seem to reconcile these apparent discrepancies, furnish the best evidence to date that acute postoperative thrombi often resolve spontaneously, justify renewed commitment to prevention and show that screening methods themselves may become a useful part of a plan for management of selected, complex cases. These conclusions derive from results of monitoring patients over a 5-year period during which time drug alternatives to warfarin prevention were sought.[5-7]

Methods

The development of ^{125}I-fibrinogen leg scan has been presented elsewhere.[1, 4, 9] The ^{125}I-fibrinogen leg scan is positive in more patients immediately postoperatively than it is on any subsequent day.[7] The number of patients in whom this test becomes abnormal for the first time declines progressively and almost smoothly during successive days. After hip joint reconstruction, some instances of thrombosis arise as late as the 3d postoperative week. Immediately after operation, these patients are encumbered by balanced suspension, and transport to the radiology department for contrast phlebography is a formidable undertaking. Nevertheless, an attempt was made to obtain ascending phlebography as early as possible after sustained significant isotope localization appeared. The extent of thrombosis demonstrated radiographically was less than anticipated from the leg scan results.[5] Of 47 phlebograms, only 11 showed extensive thrombosis, another 10 had moderately extensive thrombosis, 14 only showed minute thrombi and 12 were normal (no thrombosis). Thus 55%, or over half of those abnormal to leg scan, were subsequently shown by phlebography to represent insignificant extent of thrombosis or none at all. In terms of the efficacy of prevention, the leg scan seemed to be an unambiguous endpoint criterion, but it was disappointing to realize that at least half of those considered failures of prophylaxis did not suffer from any important extent of thrombosis. With or without whatever treatment was given, thrombosis in these might well have been on the way to resolution. The experimental data of Kerrigan et al.[11] was published at about this time revealing that thrombi incorporating ^{125}I-fibrinogen may lyse to the extent that patency can be demonstrated by phlebogram though local radioactivity is still present in significant concentration. This could well explain the occurrence of apparent false positives with the leg scan. A more specific screening technique than ^{125}I-fibrinogen was obviously needed which would discriminate between clinically important thrombosis and whatever thrombosis was insignificant or resolving.

The isotope leg scan data were searched for evidence that could provide such discrimination. It was learned that in the United Kingdom leg scan monitoring, if abnormal, did not lead to a decision for full-dose anticoagulant drug therapy unless it appeared to be extending proximally and involved portals above the knee.[10] Contrast phlebograms and ^{125}I-fibrinogen worksheets were reviewed. Overlay tracings were made of thrombi demonstrated in phlebograms, and their area was compared with the maximum accumulation of radioactivity in the abnormal limb prior to radiographic examination. A rough, but significant correlation appeared. Large thrombi are revealed by more isotope localization than small ones, not surprisingly.[16] The calculations were a bit cumbersome, however, and individual variation was large, so that clinical decisions could hardly be based on such calculations. It seemed that ^{125}I-fibrinogen leg scan did a better job of identifying patients with thrombosis than it did of sizing the thrombi. Others, too, noted disparity between the numbers of thrombi demonstrated by leg scan and the numbers of thrombi subsequently revealed by ascending phlebography[2]

Ultrasound and impedance plethysmography also were being used for monitoring the same postoperative patients. The Doppler probe was certainly specific, but not sufficiently sensitive. Only the most extensive thrombi were reliably detected. Impedance, by the original breath-held technique, was slightly better. By comparison with phlebograms it appeared that the more extensive was thrombosis, the more reliable was detection by impedance.[17]

The technique of venous occlusion by thigh cuff added to impedance a degree of sensitivity which soon was seen to approach the requirements of a noninvasive screening test capable of discriminating small thrombi from large. By the time 46 limbs had been studied by both techniques it was found that the only false negative results by cuff impedance (hereafter referred to as IPG) were in patients with minute thrombi which, except for the ^{125}I-fibrinogen leg scan abnormality, would have passed without notice. Extensive thrombi were all properly classified. Moderately extensive thrombi, even some in calf veins which did not block the popliteal vein itself, were also properly classified. The diagnostic accuracy of IPG with the cuff for monitoring asymptomatic patients at risk of thrombosis was evidently comparable to its accuracy for diagnosis of symptomatic patients as reported by its originator[15] and others.[8] Plethysmographic techniques, additionally, are most accurate for detection of thrombosis in the iliofemoral vein segments, an area not adequately revealed by ^{125}I-fibrinogen leg scan, particularly after hip surgery. It has been appreciated that thrombi in this segment, if detached as emboli, have the most serious implication, because of their large size.

With this new capability to discriminate large from small thrombi it was perceived that the combination of ^{125}I-fibrinogen leg scan and IPG was particularly appropriate for further clinical investigation of drugs for prevention after hip surgery. The combined techniques reveal the full scope of silent thrombosis, and so offer additional reassurance that patients at risk can safely be included in drug protocols requiring use of placebo. No patient had incurred an embolus while ^{125}I-fibrinogen surveillance was used, perhaps because when that test became positive, phlebography and appropriate treatment followed promptly. Such was the confidence in cuff-IPG that it was decided to postpone contrast phlebography until an abnormal result of *both* ^{125}I-fibrinogen leg scan and IPG occurred. Two objectives would thereby be served. The specificity of IPG and the safety of relying upon it as a major screening method would be tested critically. Moreover, evaluation of drug effectiveness could be judged not only by the criterion of ^{125}I-fibrinogen leg scan—which seemed overly sensitive, since some cases were included in whom no thrombi were seen by phlebography—but also by the criterion of both tests becoming positive, indicating that thrombosis had reached a clinically important extent.

Confidence in the safety of combined peripheral monitoring was generally upheld as subsequently shown. In the next 140 patients two drugs were evaluated which proved no better than placebo. Six subjects incurred minor embolism, and 35 had venous thrombosis requiring anticoagulant treatment. No major embolus occurred, no resuscitation was needed, and there was no fatality. There was no recurrent embolism after heparin was administered. At the same time, the evolution of thrombosis, its spontaneous resolution and the time course of these events was unambiguously revealed.

The schedule of monitoring was as follows. If either ^{125}I-fibrinogen leg scan or IPG was abnormal both tests were repeated daily and when both were abnormal a phlebogram was requested. As long as both were *normal* IPG was performed twice weekly and leg scan daily for 3 days postoperatively and on alternate days thereafter. If only the leg scan was abnormal phlebography was deferred, but was obtained just prior to discharge from the hospital. Monitoring techniques, the method of phlebography and classification of the extent of venous thrombosis found were as previously described.[7]

Results

Of the 140 patients, 78 (56%) were normal throughout by both techniques. This percentage of normal results might be expected to be higher after other operations which require less postoperative immobilization than hip reconstruction. One of these patients, nevertheless, had a symptomatic embolus. Lung scan showed a very small perfusion defect. This illustrated the possibility that thrombosis may arise in veins inaccessible to present monitoring techniques, and that embolism can occur from such sites. Evidently this is most unusual. In a total experience with more than 360 patients, only twice has embolism occurred while isotope leg scan was normal. Significantly, in both patients, the embolus was small as judged by lung scan, though sharp pain was present for a few days.

Thrombosis was demonstrated in the remaining 62. The extent of thrombosis and its evolution can be subdivided according to the IPG result. In one quarter (35 of 140) impedance became abnormal, and contrast phlebograms were requested. Extensive or moderately extensive thrombi were shown except as follows: in three, thrombi were minute; in two none were found; and in four others, unavoidably delayed 2 or more weeks, the phlebogram showed minute thrombi or none. In these latter cases lysis may have occurred between the time monitoring became abnormal and the phlebogram was done, thus accounting for the discrepancy. The possibility of a falsely positive

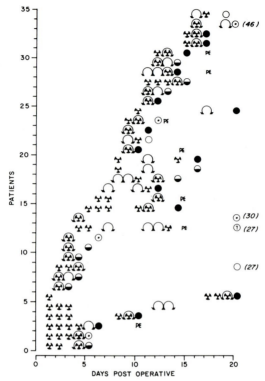

Fig 38–1.—Thirty-five patients (from group of 140) in whom venous thrombosis was demonstrated postoperatively by abnormal results of both impedance and leg scan. Where no symbol appears in the horizontal row corresponding to any patient, the monitoring techniques were either normal or were not scheduled to be done on that date. (See text for surveillance schedule.) Contrast phlebography was obtained in all but two, patients 5 and 16. *Numbers in parentheses* on the right refer to the date of phlebography if performed after the 20th day. ○, normal contrast phlebogram. ⊙, minute thrombus by phlebogram. ◑, moderately extensive thrombus. ●, extensive thrombosis. ☘, abnormal ¹²⁵I-fibrinogen leg scan. Ω, abnormal impedance plethysmography. *PE*, symptomatic pulmonary embolism confirmed by lung scan.

IPG is illustrated by the others. The importance of obtaining a phlebogram before or soon after beginning anticoagulant therapy is confirmed by the fact that "falsely positive" IPG results occur at times.

Reference to Figure 38 – 1 shows that during the first postoperative week phlebography demonstrated extensive thrombosis only once, but moderately extensive thrombosis five times and minute thrombi in two other subjects. Extensive thrombosis is proportionately more common if phlebograms are indicated and obtained during the 2d or 3d postoperative week. That thrombosis is more extensive after the 1st week corresponds to the time course of thrombosis revealed by autopsy dissections, which revealed few thrombi early, and to a progressive process — propagation of small thrombi to become large ones.

On the other hand, thrombus propagation may proceed quickly in some cases. In 18 of the 35, isotope leg scan was abnormal for 1 day or more before IPG became abnormal. However in five subjects both were abnormal on the same day and in an additional 12 the abnormal result of IPG preceded significant isotope localization. As evidence for propagation of small thrombi to become large thrombi, combined monitoring suggests that the process may be abrupt particularly after the 1st week. In these patients, appropriate treatment of venous thrombosis was recommended. In virtually all, anticoagulant drug

Fig 38–2.—Twenty-seven patients with abnormal leg scan but whose impedance plethysmogram remained normal. ○, normal contrast phlebogram. ◉, minute thrombus by phlebogram. ◐, moderately extensive thrombus. ●, extensive thrombus. ⚜, abnormal ¹²⁵I-fibrinogen leg scan. Ω, abnormal impedance plethysmography. *PE*, symptomatic pulmonary embolism confirmed by lung scan.

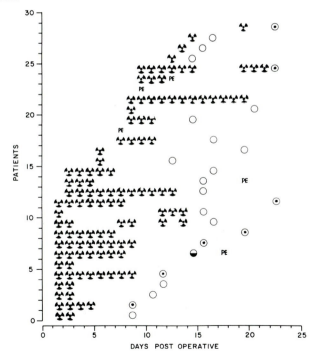

therapy was given. No residual edema persisted after hospital discharge except in those few with a history of prior thrombotic episodes. The follow-up period is necessarily too short to reveal whether any will develop chronic venous insufficiency. It is a reasonable speculation however that serious late sequelae will be fewer in monitored patients than in those who incur silent thrombosis, but because there was no leg monitoring, the process passed unnoticed.

The picture of spontaneous resolution is presented in Figure 38–2, summarizing those patients with abnormal leg scan postoperatively, but who were *normal* to IPG examination. There were 27 such, and in these, because IPG remained normal, contrast phlebograms were delayed until shortly before hospital discharge. During this interval, daily monitoring revealed that some "hot-spots" may "cool off." By the time that phlebography was performed, minute thrombi or none at all were shown, with a single exception. There can be little doubt that spontaneous thrombolysis was observed in these patients. It is seen in Figure 38–2 that symptomatic embolism can occur as part of the process of spontaneous resolution. In both instances the perfusion defect was small, smaller in fact than the defect revealed by lung scan in those three patients in Figure 38–1. This is consistent with the fact that the latter three patients had abnormal IPG results, such that leg vein thrombosis in them may have occurred in larger veins from which emboli, when detached, would be larger than those occurring in patients normal to IPG screening.

Discussion

As a practical matter the use of combined monitoring appears to compensate for any lack of sensitivity or specificity of either isotope leg scan or IPG if used separately. Large thrombi can be distinguished from small thrombi, evidently with sufficient accuracy to permit postponement of specific therapy in certain patients until it is clearly indicated on the basis of thrombus size. It would have been fortunate if the available screening techniques allowed treatment before any embolism occurred. This does not seem to be within present capability. The one thing worse than a small, symptomatic embolus, however, is a large, unheralded embolus. Since this did not occur, the prospective monitoring of patients appears to have practical implications for management besides adding to our knowledge of the evolution of fresh postoperative thrombosis. Until one universally effective and applicable drug treatment is available, a monitored patient may be better protected than an unmonitored patient, particularly if available drug prophylaxis is not completely effective, as is the case after hip reconstruction, or imposes unacceptable risk of hemorrhage. In some patients, perhaps almost half, fresh postoperative thrombi resolve spontaneously. The present experience suggests that postoperative monitoring can identify these patients with acceptable accuracy. For them, anticoagulant therapy could be withheld safely pending a change from normal to abnormal in IPG testing. If instituted thereafter, anticoagulant therapy would begin when hemostatic complications in fresh operative wounds are less likely. In the author's opinion, a phlebogram should be obtained before, or soon after, beginning anticoagulant drugs. Requiring positive proof by radiograph of thrombosis is justified by the duration and complexity of anticoagulant therapy. Postoperative monitoring can establish which circumstances require phlebographic examination and will reduce superfluous radiologic procedures to the few falsely positive cases that occasionally will be encountered. Finally, it is gratifying that as the dynamics of propagation and resolution of fresh postoperative venous thrombosis and of embolism are revealed by these techniques, broader opportunities for management of patients are served by the same diagnostic tools that illuminate our understanding of the pathogenesis of thromboembolism.

Summary

The results of monitoring postoperative patients at risk of thromboembolism following hip joint reconstruction furnish the best evidence to date that acute postoperative thrombi often resolve spontaneously. When the ^{125}I-fibrinogen lung scan was used, it was positive in more patients immediately postoperatively than on any subsequent day. Although transport to the radiology department was a formidable undertaking, an attempt was made to obtain ascending phlebography as early as possible after significant isotope localization appeared. Fifty-five per cent of abnormal leg scans were subsequently shown by phlebography to represent insignificant extent of thrombosis or none at all. The addition of the impedance plethysmograph to the fibrinogen scan technique was thought to be particularly appropriate for further clinical investigation. Ultimately, 56% of 140 patients were normal throughout by both techniques. One of these patients had a symptomatic pulmonary embolus. Thrombosis was demonstrated in 62 patients. In 35 of these, the impedance test became abnormal and contrast phlebograms were done. Extensive or moderately extensive thrombi were shown in nearly all patients. There were 27 patients with an abnormal leg scan but who were normal on IPG examination. By the time phlebography was done, minute thrombi or none at all were shown. There can be no doubt that spontaneous thrombolysis was observed in these patients. It appears that the use of combined monitoring may compensate for lack of sensitivity or specificity of either the isotope leg scan or the IPG if used separately.

REFERENCES

1. Atkins, P., and Hawkins, L. A.: Detection of venous thrombosis in the legs, Lancet 2:1217, 1965.
2. Harris, W. H., Salzman, E. W., Athanasoulis, C., Waltman, A., Baum, S., DeSanctis, R. W., Potsaid, M. S., and Sise, H.: Comparison of ^{125}I-fibrinogen count scanning with phlebography for detection of venous thrombi after elective hip surgery, N. Engl. J. Med. 292:665, 1975.
3. Heatley, R. V., Hughes, L. E., Morgan, A., and Okwonga, W.: Preoperative or postoperative deep-vein thrombosis? Lancet 1:437, 1976.
4. Hobbs, J. T.: External measurement of fibrinogen uptake in experimental venous thrombosis and other pathological states, Br. J. Exp. Pathol. 43:48, 1962.
5. Hume, M., Kuriakose, T. X., Zuch, L., and Turner, R. H.: ^{125}I-fibrinogen and the prevention of venous thrombosis, Arch. Surg. 107:803, 1973.
6. Hume, M., Kuriakose, T. X., Jamieson, J., and Turner, R. H.: Extent of leg vein thrombosis determined by impedance and ^{125}I-fibrinogen, Am. J. Surg. 129:455, 1975.
7. Hume, M., Turner, R. H., Kuriakose, T. X., and Surprenant, J.: Venous thrombosis after hip replacement—combined monitoring as a guide for prophylaxis and treatment, J. Bone Joint Surg. [Am.] 58:933, 1976.
8. Johnston, K. W., Kakkar, V. V., Spindler, J. J., Corrigan, T. P., and Fossard, D. P.: A simple method for detecting deep-vein thrombosis. An improved electrical impedance technique, Am. J. Surg. 127:349, 1974.
9. Kakkar, V. V.: The diagnosis of deep vein thrombosis using the ^{125}I-fibrinogen test, Arch. Surg. 104:152, 1972.
10. Kakkar, V. V.: Personal communication.
11. Kerrigan, G. N. W., Buchanan, M. R., Cade, J. F., Regoeczi, E., and Hirsh, J.: Investigation of the mechanism of false positive ^{125}I-labelled fibrinogen scans, Br. J. Haematol. 26:469, 1974.
12. Sevitt, S., and Gallagher, N. G.: Venous thrombosis and pulmonary embolism: A clinico-pathological study in injured and burned patients, Br. J. Surg. 48:475, 1961.
13. Sevitt, S.: The mechanisms of canalisation in deep vein thrombosis, J. Pathol. 110:153, 1973.
14. Sevitt, S.: The structure and growth of valve-pocket thrombi in femoral veins, J. Clin. Pathol. 27:517, 1974.
15. Wheeler, H. B., O'Donnell, J. A., Anderson, F. A., Penney, B. C., Peura, R. A., and Benedict, Jr., C.: Bedside screening for venous thrombosis using occlusive impedance phlebography, Angiology 26:199, 1975.
16. Wolfe, E., and Hume, M.: The semiquantitative classification of thrombus size by the ^{125}I-fibrinogen technique, Thrombos. Res. 4:757, 1974.
17. Zuch, L., and Hume, M.: Thrombus size and vein obstruction related to impedance phlebography, Surg. Gynecol. Obstet. 139:593, 1974.

Discussion: Chapters 35 through 38

DR. ROBERT KISTNER: Now we are presented with a plethora of information, a number of choices. Many of us are confused as to exactly where to go, but our choices are quite good. Some of the choices compare the mechanical and chemical means of prophylaxis. Doctor Cotton's approach allows us to prevent 80% of the thrombi that occur preoperatively and immediately postoperatively. This would seem to be the simplest and most practical method available. He also tells us that it is the cheapest. He only uses it during the operation, and this is an advantage. Certainly, it doesn't induce bleeding in the postoperative state. However, one wonders what happens to all of those clots that form after 1 week or after several days. How are they prevented by simply compressing the leg during surgery? Perhaps, as Doctor Hume suggested, these are two different groups and, perhaps, two different mechanisms. Perhaps the clots that we find after a week may be the ones that produce the more important emboli.

Doctor Salzman gave us a choice of chemical means. Perhaps this can be used selectively. Platelet inhibitors for hip operations and oral or intravenous anticoagulants for general surgical procedures. I would suggest that we have challenging, interesting and now objective ways to approach the entire problem.

The thought that I am left with is that we are neglecting the objective approach to the embolic aspect of thromboembolic disease, and I would like to see the same control studies performed on pulmonary embolism that we are performing on venous thrombosis.

DR. ELIAS HUSNI: Relative to the prophylaxis against thromboembolism by mechanical means, Doctor Cotton is quite convincing. While this method can be readily applied to some high-risk surgical patients, it is not feasible for the other hundreds of medical patients who make up the majority of hospital populations. As far as the elastic stockings are concerned, we are equally disappointed as Doctors Browse, Hobbs and others with the Tubigrip stockings, since they do

TABLE 1.–ELASTIC STOCKINGS–
THROMBOEMBOLISM

GROUP	NO. OF PATIENTS	THROMBOEMBOLISM		NO. OF FATALITIES
Stockings	7,115	11	0.077	1
Control	7,008	106	0.71	20
Total	14,123	117	0.81	21

not provide the physiologic environment for the significant reduction of venous stasis, the basic underlying cause for thromboembolism. On the other hand, graduated pressure stockings, applying a mean pressure of 22–26 mm Hg at the ankle and gradually reducing to a mean 12–16 mm Hg at the popliteal fossa, afford an excellent reduction in the venous pool of the leg. While this stocking may be uncomfortable, it was tolerated by some 7,000 of our patients in a just concluded 3-year study on 14,123 patients.

As can be seen in Table 1, and as confirmed by our statisticians, this type stocking does seem to be effective in reducing the incidence of thromboembolism in hospital patients.

DR. JOHN HOBBS: I think that I came here rather confused about the prophylaxis. Now, I think I understand the mechanisms because of the superb demonstrations of logic by Doctor Wessler and the scholarly approach of Professor Salzman. Now we have come to the question of prevention, much like the belt and braces story. It doesn't matter which way you do it and you don't have to do the two together. Regarding the question of elastic stockings, it hasn't been shown at all that the hemodynamic effect is consistent. In other words, stockings have to be well-fitted to produce an effect.

DR. GEZA DE TAKATS: This has been a marvelous symposium, of course. I can say that freely because I had nothing to do with the organization of it. But of course, without your attendance and participation, it really wouldn't have been anything like it is.

Now, as I look at this problem from the standpoint of a man who sat around and did, perhaps, a little thinking and had absolutely no evidence, one of the most exciting things is that so much of what we had been thinking about can now be proved. As you know, this is not a static problem, nor is anything static, and what we think has been proved and is straightforward today may be again found to be wrong tomorrow.

I would like to go back, in thinking about the homeostatic mechanisms. You may remember that we have talked about the thrombotic-fibrinolytic balance which appears to be present in the body. Under certain forms of stress such as surgery, trauma and a number of other things, the balance shifts toward the thrombotic or defibrinating side. I hope that some day there will be a test, where you can say, "Now, this patient's fibrinolytic activity is too high, it is too much, you have got to throttle it," or you may say, "This patient now is in an early phase of thrombosis."

Now, that would be Utopia. Maybe there is no such thing. Looking at patients over a period of years, you can see how a patient who has reacted to 10,000 units of heparin one day will react entirely different-ly the next day. I was tremendously impressed by the evidence that giving the same dose of heparin will result in different heparin levels in the blood. You may remember that, many years ago, the question arose whether or not the heparin we are giving to patients is standard-ized. As far as my biochemist friends tell me, we still don't have a stan-dard heparin. We are talking about units of heparin, but one manufac-turer's heparin is different from another. In fact, even the same manu-facturer's heparin isn't the same. When we talk about how many units to give, we are really giving an unknown quantity. This is one field in which we very urgently need standardization.

I am tremendously impressed by intermittent compression. Many years ago, we treated patients with peripheral arterial disease with a rhythmic compressor. We would have a little conference and ultimate-ly pumped the device up to 60 mm Hg, and then released it and pumped it up and released it. Some patients said they felt better. We thought it was a placebo. We had no idea we were really producing fibrinolysis. I am tremendously impressed by the work coming out of England, that you can get a change in the fibrinolytic mechanism by intermittent compression of the arm, rather than compressing the leg.

Well, I could go on about this for weeks. But now I just want to tell you how gratifying it is to see this tremendous audience and how many of the problems have actually been solved and how many prob-lems still remain to be solved.

EPILOGUE

Geza de Takats was honored by a banquet attended by many friends and by the participants in the Symposium. His longtime friend, Dr. Alton Ochsner, acted as toastmaster, Dr. John Reynolds told several "Gezadotes," J. Leonel Villavicencio presented a plaque from the Mexican Society of Angiology and Dr. W. Andrew Dale told about Dr. Geza de Takats, A Legend in His Own Time.

LADIES AND GENTLEMEN, it is indeed a privilege to participate in this splendid Symposium on Venous Disease with you in honor of Dr. Geza de Takats. It is a fitting tribute to a pioneer vascular surgeon who has been intimately involved with the development of this field nationally and internationally during a long and useful life which includes a distinguished surgical career of more than 50 years.

The accomplishments of Dr. Geza de Takats are far too numerous for me to recount all of them during the brief time available tonight. Indeed were I simply to read the list of offices to which he has been elected, the surgical honors bestowed upon him and the distinguished associations of which he is a member, the time allotted to me would be past. Perhaps, however, I may briefly note that he has been elected by his colleagues to serve as their leader in many groups including Chief of Surgical Staff at St. Luke's Hospital, President of the Chicago Heart Association, President of the Chicago Surgical Society, President of the North American Chapter of the International Cardiovascular Society from 1952 to 1954 and later International President of the same organization from 1965 to 1967. He served as President of the Society for Vascular Surgery in 1953.

May I briefly comment upon three aspects of his exceptional career which have left a significant mark upon the surgical scene in the United States.

First, he has continually exhibited an intellectual curiosity manifest by animal experimental research and clinical research in the field of vascular disease and its treatment. Thirty-seven years ago in 1939 we find his experimental and clinical report of pulmonary embolism which appeared as a now classic presentation in the journal *Surgery*. Further such studies continued and his Presidential address to the

585

Society for Vascular Surgery in 1953 was a remarkably advanced discussion of anticoagulation therapy and its closing line is quite significant when he stated that "heparin is regarded as the best anticoagulant; its adequate use by surgeons should be studied as carefully as a technique of vena caval ligation or thrombectomy." Shortly thereafter when he visited us at the University of Rochester as Visting Professor he discussed at a patient's bedside what today would be easily recognized as a prophylactic "miniheparin" program which 20 years later is widely recognized.

Secondly, Doctor de Takats has pursued his constant interest in teaching. He established the first Vascular Clinic at Northwestern University and later moved to the University of Illinois where his efforts continued as Clinical Professor of Surgery. In 1959 his text book *Vascular Surgery* was published and spurred a new interest in that field as well as establishing standards of excellence. This occurred prior to publication of any of the presently available similar books and added brilliance to his known reputation as a splendid teacher.

Finally, Doctor de Takats may be characterized as a splendid gentleman in the best sense of the word. In a field where fierce intellectual competition may lead to ill-advised criticism of others, he has regularly spoken only in praise. During a distinguished career when an older and established individual might easily bypass or overlook his younger colleagues, he has constantly demonstrated a concern and friendship for those to follow. In an era when rush and bustle were the order of the day, he has invariably exhibited charm, thoughtfulness and friendship for his colleagues.

I have long deemed it an honor to be reckoned as a friend by Doctor de Takats. This splendid Symposium and the enthusiasm of those in attendance tonight offer a small token of the sincere respect and regard in which he is held by his friends and colleagues throughout the United States as well as the world. Ladies and gentlemen, it is accurate to state that Dr. Geza de Takats has become a legend in his own time.

W. ANDREW DALE

APPENDIX

GEZA DE TAKATS: BIOGRAPHY AND BIBLIOGRAPHY

Geza de Takats

MORE THAN 50 YEARS AGO, Dr. Geza de Takats was well started on the fascinating career which was to extend to the present. At that time, he was Assistant Professor of Surgery at the University of Budapest. He had already been a Traveling Fellow for the Rockefeller Foundation and an Exchange Assistant in the Surgical Clinic at the University of Copenhagen. Earlier, he had been House Surgeon at the University of Budapest and a Resident Surgeon there after 1916. His career as a First Lieutenant in the Medical Corps on the Russian Front during World War I was behind (Fig 1). His short stories of this time, "The Miracle of Bochnia" and "The Maltese Knights," indicate his capacity as a decision maker and free thinker, characteristics which were to become evident in the long surgical career to follow.

Elsewhere in this volume, Doctor de Takats describes the founding of the Vein Clinic at Northwestern University under the encouragement of Dr. Allen Kanavel (Fig 2) and the founding of the Vascular Clinic at the University of Illinois in 1936. What is omitted is the profound influence which he was to have on vascular surgery as it developed and grew. In the next 25 years, he actively advanced vascular surgery, summarizing each year's achievements in articles for the *Archives of Internal Medicine*. He watched the growth of treatment of vascular disease from the vantage of one who was in the front ranks. He led investigations which were to change therapy. He stimulated others to think. As vascular surgery changed from purely venous surgery before 1945 to direct arterial reconstructive surgery after that time, he presided at the birth of the new specialty. He was instrumental in the development of the artery bank which flourished in Chicago under the aegis of the Chicago Heart Association through the mid-1950s. It was this bank which allowed arterial reconstruction to proceed in mid-America in that important time prior to development of fabric grafts.

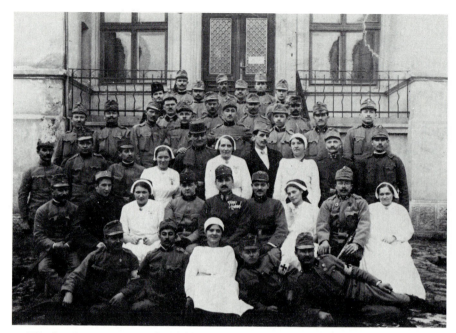

Fig 1.—In 1916, Geza de Takats was a lieutenant in the Medical Corps and served on the Eastern front. Here, he is seen, moustachioed (*right of center, second row*), in front of the surgical hospital headed by Soubbotich.

Eventually, Geza de Takats served as President of the Society for Vascular Surgery during 1953 and President of the North American Chapter of the International Cardiovascular Society in the years 1952 through 1954. Residents trained by him participated in the development of the new specialty. Interestingly, some of his earliest contributions to medical care were development and use of regional nerve blocks to determine functional versus organic components in vascular occlusion. These blocks were used to assess the effect of vasospasm, not only in the extremities but also in the brain, heart, kidney and pancreas. He described the effects of sympathetic blocks upon apoplexy, myocardial infarction and acute renal ischemia. His descriptions of reversal of perifocal edema and vasoparalysis surrounding an infarct recorded in the early 1930s sound remarkably modern when reread in the mid-1970s. It was in the mid-1930s that he suggested that there was a functional factor in the vascular tree in the lung during pulmonary embolization. This concept was mainly ignored but has been rediscovered recently.

Doctor de Takats felt that spontaneous thrombolysis occurred in

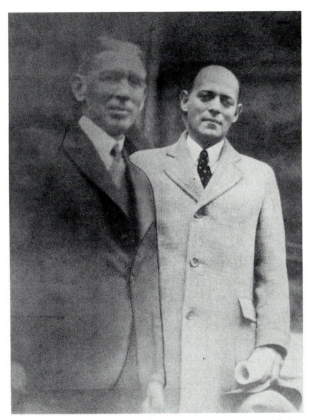

Fig 2.—Allen B. Kanavel, sixth Chairman, Department of Surgery, North-western University Medical School, and Geza de Takats *(right)*, Director, Vein Clinic at Northwestern (1930). In that year, de Takats published articles on barbiturate premedication for surgery, injection treatment of varicose veins, diabetic gangrene and ligation of the tail of the pancreas for juvenile diabetes.

pulmonary embolization and thought that he could demonstrate re-flexes from baroreceptors in the superior vena cava, right heart and pulmonary artery. He felt that these could be interrupted by pharma-cologic or autonomic nerve blockade. His experiments with atropine and papaverine mixtures to relieve pseudoangina and cor pulmonale in the acute phase of pulmonary embolism were quite convincing, even though more modern views of this subject implicate serotonin release mechanisms. His publications on pulmonary embolism in *Surgery* (6:339, 1939 and 7:819, 1940) are still fascinating examples of deductive reasoning which take experimental observations and give them important clinical relevance.

The subject of homeostatic balance between thrombosis and thrombolysis has always intrigued Doctor de Takats. His heparin tolerance test described in *Surgery, Gynecology and Obstetrics* (7:31, 1943) showed that no two people react exactly alike to heparin therapy. He was able to show quite clearly that the heparin response fluctuates within any individual as well as between individuals, and that complications of such therapy, including thrombosis and hemorrhage, are due to faulty or ill-regulated dosage. His investigations would lead to the very modern conclusion that continuous infusion pumps with accurate regulation of the thrombotic system is the only way to give heparin.

A subject of great interest to Doctor de Takats, the storage of heparin in tissue and release on stress, was the subject of the Presidential Address of one of his co-workers, J. Leonel Villavicencio, at the meeting of the Mexican Society of Angiology in Acapulco in 1976.

After numerous publications indicating profound interest in treatment of thromboembolic disease, causalgia, varicose veins and use of sympathectomy in the treatment of peripheral vascular disease, he turned to investigations concerning Buerger's disease, surgical treatment of aneurysms of the aorta and use of splanchnicectomy for treatment of pancreatic pain. After all of this, sufficient accomplishment for many when extended to an entire career, he returned to an interest in the thrombosis and lytic system. By 1950, he was suggesting that subcutaneous heparinization would be useful in preventing the venous thromboembolic events that attended surgery. At that time, he advocated the use of subcutaneous heparin 3 days prior to operation and suggested stopping this the night before surgery, having in mind that the majority of thromboses occurred during operation. This suggestion, made more than 25 years ago, is remarkably appropriate today.

Indicating a restless and constantly curious intellect, in the 1930s, Doctor de Takats and his co-workers became involved in the effect of adrenergic stimulation and blockade upon the islet cells in the pancreas. Their work included splanchnic nerve section in an effort to increase glucose tolerance and block glycogen release. Today, it has been shown that adrenergic stimulation does inhibit insulin release from the beta cells of the pancreas, and such stimulation also facilitates release of glucagon from the alpha cells.

In his investigations on causalgia, Doctor de Takats' observations have been particularly interesting. He has felt that a remarkable homeostatic mechanism obtains and that an adrenergic-cholinergic balance occurs. Sympathetic blockade sets up a cholinergic dominance, especially under stress. He has felt that, because of a causalgic state occurring not only in the extremities but also in partial nerve injury after amputation of a breast or even after myocardial infarction, emotional stress, which might decrease renal blood flow and induce hypertension, would have a reverse effect after sympathectomy, when terminal sensory nerve endings cannot release norepinephrine.

His literary style in scientific articles has always been distinctive. An example from a 1962 article on hand ischemia is illustrative. Describing episodic digital ischemia, he states, "Raynaud's phenomenon creates a feeling of uncertainty and apprehension in patient and physician alike. Is it a fleeting, harmless color change of anemic hypometabolic girls, occurring in cold, damp weather, or is it the forerunner of an ominous collagen disease?"

In commenting upon his contributions, Doctor de Takats has referred to the words of Alvin Feinstein in the August 22, 1972 issue of *Lancet,* saying that, "Our primary challenge is to assemble information which is meaningfully human, even if scientifically imperfect. We shall advance the progress of neither science nor humanity by obsequious adherence to scientific doctrines that provide quantitative glitter and 'statistical significance' while dehumanizing our data, confusing our sensibility, and diverting our attention from the people who are the only proper subjects for the study of mankind."

Which, of course, recalls the admonition of Aesculapius, that the true role of the physician is ". . . to observe and record for mankind."

In a prologue to his collection of short stories entitled *A Breach of Etiquette,* Doctor de Takats has said, ". . . it's fascinating to speculate what would have happened to this immigrant surgeon if he had gone into the diplomatic service in Austria-Hungary, if he had become an eye surgeon like his father was, if he had not accepted a Rockefeller Fellowship in the United States, and if he had done a number of things other than land in Chicago."

For our part, those of us who have shared his humor, admired his spirit and been touched by his humility in the face of greatness, we give thanks that he did indeed come to this land.

JOHN J. BERGAN
JAMES S. T. YAO

PUBLICATIONS OF GEZA DE TAKATS

IN HUNGARIAN

The Surgical Anatomy of the Mediastinum. Thesis, Master of Surgery degree, University of Budapest, 1918.

Causes and surgical treatment of exophthalmia (109 operated cases), Orvoskepzes 12:125, 1921.

Plastic of the orbit after exenteration, Orv. Hetil. 65:3, 1921.

Tumors of the optic nerve. Report on four cases, Trans. Hung. Surg. Soc., 1922.

Periarterial sympathectomy: Indications, results, Orvoskepzes 13:1, 1923.

A functional test of the bone marrow. Preliminary report, Trans. Hung. Surg. Soc., 1923.

Insufflation of air into the knee joint, Trans. Hung. Surg. Soc., 1923.

Letters to the Editors: Medical conditions in the U.S.A. (annual meeting of the AMA, Chicago, June 24, 1924; Mayo Clinic, July 1924), Orv. Hetil. 1924.

General anesthesia in the United States with a special regard to ethylene. Orv. Hetil. 68:1, 1925.

The functional tests of the liver with phenotetrachlorphthalein, Orv. Hetil. 68:4, 1925.

Surgical treatment of hyperfunction of the thyroid gland, Orv. Hetil. 71:1010, 1927.

Circulatory disturbances of the extremities, Orvoskepzes, 1934.

IN GERMAN

Plastic closure of the orbit after exenteration, Dtsche. Med. Wochenschr. 47:1132, 1921.

The clinical value of bilirubin determinations in the blood, Klin. Wochenschr. 1:1732, 1922.

Intravenous administration of urotropin, Arch. Klin. Chir. 125:544, 1923.

Prolongation of local anesthesia with cinchona alkaloid, Klin. Wochenschr. 5:1324, 1926 (with Paunz).

Surgical attempts at increasing sugar tolerance, Klin. Wochenschr. 12:623, 1933.

Surgery of juvenile diabetes, Arch. Klin. Chir. 177:242, 1933.

IN SPANISH

The role of surgery in arteriosclerosis, J. Bras. 3:1, 1946.

TRANSLATIONS INTO ENGLISH

Gatellier, J.: Internal drainage of the common bile duct. From the Clinic of Professor Pierre Duval, Surg. Gynecol. Obstet. 42:546, 1926.

Schmieden, V.: The technique of cardiolysis. From the Surgical Clinic of the University of Frankfurt am Main, Surg. Gynecol. Obstet. 43:89, 1926.

Franz, K.: The technique of abdominal hysterectomy for carcinoma of the uterus. From the University Clinic for Women's Diseases, Berlin, Surg. Gynecol. Obstet. 43:185, 1926.

Polya, E.: Technique of operation for carcinoma of the buccal mucous membrane, Surg. Gynecol. Obstet. 43:343, 1926.

IN ENGLISH

Some problems of jaundice and their significance in surgery, Ann. Surg. 79:669, 1924.

Latent jaundice as a symptom of biliary colic, Ann. Surg. 81:108, 1925.

Cholecystectomy for hyperacidity, Surg. Gynecol. Obstet. 40:221, 1925.

Chemotherapy with Rivanol, Surg. Gynecol. Obstet. 29:91, 1925.

The surgery of gastric and duodenal ulcers, Ann. Surg. 83:217, 1926.

Prolongation of local anesthesia, Surg. Gynecol. Obstet. 43:100, 1926.

Editorial: Local anesthesia, Surg. Gynecol. Obstet. 43:233, 1926.

The perverted physiology of the stomach after gastric operations, Am. J. Med. Sci. 172:45, 1926.

Splanchnic Anesthesia, in Piersol (ed.): *The Cyclopedia of Medicine* (Philadelphia: F. A. Davis Co., 1927).

Extraperitoneal hernia of the bladder, Ann. Surg. 85:156, 1927.

Indications for partial gastrectomy, M. J. Rec. 125:266, 1927.

Splanchnic anesthesia, Surg. Gynecol. Obstet. 44:501, 1927.

Indications for thyroidectomy, Ill. Med. J. 51:306, 1927.

The effect of jejunal mucosa on transplantation into the lesser curvature of the stomach, Ann. Surg. 85:698, 1927 (with Mann).

Subacute gastric phlegmon, Ann. Surg. 86:629, 1927.

Local Anesthesia. A Short Course for Students and Surgeons (Philadelphia: W. B. Saunders Co., 1928).

A goitre survey at Northwestern University, JAMA 90:1008, 1928 (with Grey).

Varicose veins and their sequelae, JAMA 92:775, 1929.

The impairment of circulation in the varicose extremity, Arch. Surg. 18:671, 1929 (with Crittendon, Tellotson and Quint).

The ligation of the popliteal vein for impending gangrene, JAMA 92:1264, 1929.

The treatment of varicose veins, Surg. Gynecol. Obstet. 49:114, 1929.

Problems in vascular surgery, Lancet 2:339, 1929.

The treatment of varicose veins and ulcers, Ill. Med. J. 56:114, 1929.

The injection of varicose veins: Indications, treatment and results. Int. J. Med. Surg. 42:475, 1929.

Hyperglycemia following head injuries: An experimental study, Ann. Surg. 90:190, 1929 (with Mock).

Correlations of external and internal pancreatic secretions, Arch. Surg. 19:771 and 20:866, 1929.

Isolation of the tail of the pancreas in a diabetic child, JAMA 93:606, 1929.

Premedication for local anesthesia with barbituric compounds, Surg. Gynecol. Obstet. 50:494, 1930.

Injection treatment of varicose veins, Surg. Gynecol. Obstet. 50:545, 1930.

Ambulatory ligation of the saphenous vein, JAMA 94:1194, 1930.

Diabetic gangrene, Int. J. Med. Surg. 43:415, 1930.

Ligation of the tail of the pancreas in juvenile diabetes, Endocrinology 14:255, 1930.

Push fluids, Am. J. Surg. 11:39, 1931.

The value of physical therapy in peripheral vascular disease, Physiotherapy Rev. 11:2, 1931.

Causes of failure in the treatment of varicose veins, JAMA 96:1111, 1931.

The indispensable use of narcotics in local anesthesia, JAMA 96:1228, 1931.

The effect of ligation of the tail of the pancreas in juvenile diabetes, Surg. Gynecol. Obstet. 53:45, 1931.

The differentiation of organic and spastic vascular occlusions, Ann. Surg. 94:321, 1931.

Postgraduate medical instruction in Hungary, J. Assoc. Am. Med. Coll. 6:290, 1931.

The cutaneous reactions to histamine as a test for collateral circulation in the extremities, Arch. Intern. Med. 48:769, 1931.

The effect of coeliac ganglionectomy on sugar tolerance of dogs, Proc. Soc. Biol. Med. 29:217, 1931 (with Cuthbert).

The mechanism of thrombophlebitic edema, Arch. Surg. 23:955, 1931 (with Zimmerman).

Management of chronic vascular occlusions in the extremities, Ill. Med. J. 61:79, 1932.

The "resting infection" in varicose veins, Am. J. Med. Sci. 134:57, 1932.

Vascular anomalies of the extremities, Surg. Gynecol. Obstet. 55:227, 1932.

Surgery of the orbit, Arch. Ophthalmol. 8:259, 1932.

Acute pancreatic necrosis and its sequelae, Ann. Surg. 96:418, 1932 (with MacKenzic).

Problems in the treatment of varicose veins, Am. J. Surg. 18:26, 1932.

The effect of coeliac ganglionectomy on the sugar tolerance of normal dogs, Am. J. Physiol. 102:614, 1932 (with Cuthbert).

Ligation of the saphenous vein, Arch. Surg. 26:72, 1933.

The management of acute thrombophlebitic edema, JAMA 100:34, 1933.

Splanchnic anesthesia, Sajous Encyc. Med. 1:549, 1933.

Surgical attempts to increase sugar tolerance, Arch. Surg. 26:750, 1933 (with Cuthbert).

Problems in the treatment of varicose veins, Int. J. Med. Surg. 46:269, 1933.

The effect of Salyrgan and x-ray on the rate of disappearance of thrombophlebitic edema, J. Lab. Clin. Med. 19:243, 1933 (with Zimmerman et al.).

Bilateral splanchnic nerve section in juvenile diabetes, Ann. Intern. Med. 7:422, 1933 (with Fenn).

The preparation of local anesthesia solutions. Bull. Am. Coll. Surg. 17:40, 1933.

Diagnosis and treatment of circulatory disturbances of the extremities, Surg. Gynecol. Obstet. 58:667, 1934.

Splanchnic nerve section in juvenile diabetes. I. Selection of cases for operation, Ann. Intern. Med. 7:1201, 1934 (with Fenn and Trump).

Diagnosis and treatment of peripheral vascular diseases of the extremities, J. Med. Surg. 47:180, 1934.

The effect of surgical procedures on sugar tolerance of diabetic patients, Med. Clin. North Am. 17:1507, 1934.

Diagnosis and treatment of peripheral vascular diseases of the extremities, J. Med. 15:512, 1934.

The determination of the proper level of amputation, Int. J. Med. Surg. 47:7, 1934.

Obliterative vascular disease. A preliminary report on treatment by alternating negative and positive pressure, JAMA 103:1920, 1934.

The effect of suprarenal denervation and splanchnic section on sugar tolerance of dogs, Arch. Surg. 3:151, 1935 (with Cuthbert).

Peripheral vascular disease, JAMA 104:1463, 1935.

Surgery in diabetes, J. Kans. Med. Soc. 36:177, 1935.

Splanchnic nerve section in juvenile diabetes. II. Technique and postoperative management, Ann. Surg. 102:22, 1935.

Peripheral vascular diseases, Arch. Intern. Med. 56:530, 1935 (with Scupham).

Cervical sympathectomy in retinitis pigmentosa, Arch. Ophthalmol. 14:441, 1935 (with Gifford).

The present status of the surgery of the sympathetic nervous system, Ill. Med. J. 68:512, 1935.

Gangrene, Surg. Clin. North Am. 16:317, 1936.

Varicose Veins; Thrombosis and Thrombophlebitis; and Embolism, in Christopher, F. (ed.): *Textbook of Surgery* (Philadelphia: W. B. Saunders Co., 1936), pp. 168, 175 and 180.

The use of papaverine in acute arterial occlusions, JAMA 106:1003, 1936.

Acute arterial occlusions of the extremities, Am. J. Surg. 33:61, 1936.

Obliterative vascular disease: Treatment by alternating negative and positive pressure, Am. J. Nurs. 36:763, 1936.

Peripheral vascular diseases, Arch. Intern. Med. 58:531, 1936 (with Scupham).

Surgical treatment of peripheral vascular disease, N. Y. State J. Med. 36:22, 1936.

Reflex dystrophy of the extremities, Arch. Surg. 34:939, 1937.

Intermittent venous hyperemia in the treatment of peripheral vascular disease, JAMA 108:1951, 1937 (with Hick and Coulter).

The effect of sympathectomy on peripheral vascular disease, Surgery 2:46, 1937.

Trauma and Peripheral Vascular Disease, in Brahdy and Kahn (eds.): *Trauma and Disease* (Philadelphia: Lea & Febiger, 1937).

Revision of Varicose Veins. Pamphlet prepared for the scientific exhibit of the AMA, September 1937.

Peripheral vascular diseases: A review, Arch. Intern. Med. 60:552, 1937.

Sympathectomy for peripheral vascular disease, Arch. Intern. Med. 60:990, 1937.

Intermittent venous hyperemia, Physiotherapy Rev. 18:7, 1938.

Management of peripheral vascular disease, Arch. Phys. Ther. 19:88, 1938.

The use of sodium nitrate for testing flexibility of the peripheral vascular bed, Am. Heart J. 15:158, 1938 (with Beck).

Diagnosis and management of peripheral vascular disease, Nebr. J. Med. 24:81, 1939.

The late effects of bilateral carotid sinus denervation in man, J. Clin. Invest. 17:385, 1938 (with Capps).

A case of arteriosclerotic gangrene, St. Luke's Hosp. Staff Bull. 1:19, 1937.

Observations on congenital megacolon, J. Pediatr. 13:819, 1938 (with Biggs).

Varicose Veins; Thrombosis and Thrombophlebitis; and Embolism, in Christopher, F. (ed.): *Textbook of Surgery* (Philadelphia: W. B. Saunders Co., 1939), pp. 190, 197 and 202.

The use of Neo-Synephrine in spinal anesthesia, Surg. Gynecol. Obstet. 68:1021, 1939 (with Brunner).

Pulmonary embolism, Surgery 6:339, 1939 (with Beck, Fenn, Roth and Schweitzer).

Peripheral vascular disease: A review, Arch. Intern. Med. 64:590, 1939 (with Scupham, Van Dellen and Beck).

Hernia, Hygeia 17:889, 1939.

Acetylcholine as a diagnostic test in cases of congenital megacolon, Surg. Gynecol. Obstet. 69:763, 1939.

The neurocirculatory clinic: A summary of its activities. I. Peripheral vascular disease, Ann. Intern. Med. 13:957, 1939.

Analysis of results following sympathectomy for peripheral vascular disease, Am. J. Surg. 47:78, 1940.

Amputation for peripheral vascular disease, Arch. Surg. 40:253, 1940 (with Reynolds).

Pulmonary embolism: Suggestions for the diagnosis, prevention and management, JAMA 114:1415, 1940 (with Jesser).

The meteorologic factor on pulmonary embolism, Surgery 7:819, 1940 (with Mayne and Peterson).

Vascular diseases: A review of some of the recent literature with a critical review of the surgical treatment, Arch. Intern. Med. 66:707, 1940 (with Scupham, Van Dellen and Beck).

Revascularization of ischemic kidney, Arch. Surg. 41:1394, 1940 (with Scupham).

Postoperative thrombosis and embolism, Ill. Med. J. 79:25, 1941.

We use flannel masks, Mod. Hosp. 55:61, 1941 (with Ante).

Postoperative infection: Measures of control, Surg. Gynecol. Obstet. 72:1028, 1941 (with Jesser).

Visualization of the pulmonary artery during its embolic obstruction, Arch. Surg. 42:1034, 1941 (with Jesser).

Sterility of the male after sympathectomy, JAMA 117:30, 1941 (with Helfrich).

Pulmonary embolism, Am. J. Nurs. 41:379, 1941.

Management of peripheral vascular disease, Ill. Med. J. 80:307, 1941.

Vascular diseases: 7th annual review of some of the recent literature, Arch. Intern. Med. 68:599, 1941 (with Scupham, Van Dellen and Jesser).

Surgical treatment of acute vascular occlusions, Surg. Clin. North Am. 22:199, 1942.

The surgical approach to hypertension, JAMA 118:501, 1942 (with Heyer and Keeton).

Use of direct heat and indirect heat to increase blood flow to the extremities, War Med. 2:429, 1942.

Obituary of Emile de Grosz, Am. J. Ophthalmol. 25:7, 1942.

Vascular diseases: 8th annual review, Arch. Intern. Med. 70:444, 1942.

The bronchial factor in pulmonary embolism, Surgery 12:541, 1942 (with Jesser).

Reflex pulmonary atelectasis, JAMA 120:686, 1942 (with Fenn and Jenkinson).

Post-traumatic dystrophy of the extremities: Sudeck's atrophy, Surg. Gynecol. Obstet. 75:558, 1942 (with Miller).

Vascular surgery in the war, War Med. 3:291, 1943.

Post-traumatic dystrophy of the extremities: A chronic vasodilator mechanism, Arch. Surg. 46:469, 1943 (with Miller).

Neurovascular lesions of the extremities, Bull. Am. Coll. Surg. 28:139, 1943.

Heparin tolerance: A test of the clotting mechanism, Surg. Gynecol. Obstet. 77:31, 1943.

Nature of painful vasodilation in causalgic states, Arch. Neurol. Psych. 50:318, 1943.

Vascular diseases: 9th annual review, Arch. Intern. Med. 72:518, 1943 (with Van Dellen and Scupham).

The effect of sulfur compounds on blood clotting, Surgery 14:661, 1943.

Causalgic states following injuries to the extremities, Arch. Phys. Ther. 24:647, 1943.

Sympathectomy in the treatment of peripheral vascular diseases, Ill. Med. J. 84:373, 1943.

The effect of digitalis on the clotting mechanism, JAMA 125:840, 1944 (with Trump and Gilbert).

The value of sympathectomy in the treatment of Buerger's disease, Surg. Gynecol. Obstet. 79:359, 1944.

Varicose Veins. Pamphlet prepared for the scientific exhibit of the AMA, October 1944.

The surgical treatment of thromboembolism and its sequelae, Bull. N. Y. Acad. Med. 20:623, 1944.

Nervous regulation of clotting mechanism, Arch. Surg. 48:105, 1944.

Causalgic States and Neurotrophic Lesions of the Extremities, Lectures on Reconstruction Surgery (Ann Arbor, Mich.: J. W. Edwards Publishers, Inc., 1944).

The problems of thromboembolism, Surgery 17:153, 1945 (with Fowler).

Vascular diseases: 10th annual review, Arch. Intern. Med. 75:125 and 197, 1945 (with Van Dellen, Scupham and Fowler).

Causalgic states in peace and war, JAMA 128:699, 1945.

Varicose Veins; Venous Thrombosis; and Embolism, in Christopher, F. (ed.): *A Textbook of Surgery* (4th ed.; Philadelphia: W. B. Saunders Co., 1945).

Peripheral vascular disease, J. Mich. Med. Soc. 44:477, 1945.

Venous thrombosis, Ky. Med. J. 43:130, 1945.

The technique of lumbar sympathectomy, Surg. Clin. North Am. 26:56, 1942.

The peripheral neurovascular lesions in diabetics, Proc. Am. Diabetes Assoc. 5:183, 1945.

Sympathectomy in the treatment of peripheral vascular sclerosis, JAMA 131:495, 1946 (with Fowler, Jordan and Risley).

Surgical approach to hypertension (second report), Arch. Surg. 53:111, 1946.

Peripheral vascular sclerosis, Am. Practitioner 1:251, 1947 (with Fowler).

Sympathectomy for peripheral vascular sclerosis, JAMA 133:441, 1947 (with Evoy).

The surgical treatment of aneurysms of the abdominal aorta, Surgery 214:443, 1947 (with Reynolds).

The surgical treatment of hypertension. III. The "neurogenic" versus renal hypertension from the standpoint of operability, Surgery 21:773, 1947 (with Fowler).

Indications for lumbar sympathectomy, Ill. Med. J. 92:6, 1947.

The treatment of pancreatic pain by splanchnic nerve section, Surg. Gynecol. Obstet. 85:742, 1947 (with Walter).

The immediate treatment of cerebrovascular accidents, Am. Practitioner 2:5, 1948 (with Gilbert).

Diagnosis and management of Buerger's disease, Postgrad. Med. 3:3, 1948.

The emergency treatment of apoplexy, JAMA 136:659, 1948 (with Gilbert).

The place of intermittent venous hyperemia in the treatment of obliterative vascular disease, Arch. Intern. Med. 81:3, 1948 (with Evoy).

The effect of penicillin upon the clotting activity of blood in normal human subjects. J. Pharmacol. Exp. Ther. 96:291, 1949 (with Dolkart, Halpern, Larkin and Dey).

The surgical treatment of essential hypertension. IV. Case selection and technique as influencing results, Surgery 24:469, 1948.

The surgical treatment of hypertension, Quart. Phi Beta Pi vol. 54 no. 3, November 1948.

The side effects and complications of sympathectomy for hypertension, Arch. Surg. 59:6, 1949 (with Fowler).

Emergency treatment of apoplexy, Postgrad. Med. 5:184, 1949.

The corticoadrenal factor in hypertension, Surgery 26:67, 1949.

The water tolerance of the hypertensive patient. Its relation to operability, Am. Heart J. 38:234, 1949.

Roentgen therapy of thrombophlebitis, JAMA 141:967, 1949 (with Snead, Lasner and Jenkinson).

Splanchnic nerve section for pancreatic pain (second report), Ann. Surg. 131:44, 1950 (with Walter and Lasner).

Editorial: Clinical research, Angiology 1:3, 1950.

Lymphedema, Angiology 1:73, 1950 (with Evoy).

Anticoagulant therapy in surgery, JAMA 142:527, 1950.

Sensitized clotting time, Angiology 1:317, 1950.

Causes of failure in the surgical treatment of hypertension, Angiology 1:457, 1950.

The subcutaneous use of heparin. A summary of observations, Circulation 2:837, 1950.

Care of the diabetic foot, ADA Forecast, September 1950.

Management of pulmonary embolism, Postgrad. Med. 8:506, 1950.

Recent advances in the surgical treatment of peripheral vascular disease, Med. Ann. D.C. 20:9, 1951.

Causes of failure in the surgical treatment of hypertension, Postgrad. Med. 9:128, 1951.

Selection of hypertensive patients for sympathectomy, Chicago Med. Soc. Bull. 53: 797, 1951.

Division of the popliteal vein in deep venous insufficiency of the lower extremities, Surgery 29:342, 1951 (with Groupner).

Periarteritis nodosa following thiouracil therapy of hyperthyroidism, resultant hypertension benefitted by sympathectomy, Angiology 2:4, 1951 (with Barnum and Dolkart).

Management of varicose veins of the lower extremities, Surg. Clin. North Am. 31: 1463, 1951 (with Fowler).

Sensitized clotting time, JAMA 146:1370, 1951.

The phenomenon of stress in relation to human essential hypertension, Angiology 2:461, 1951.

Diagnosis and management of peripheral vascular disease, Med. Clin. North Am. 36:141, 1952.

The response of the clotting equilibrium to postoperative stress, Surgery 31:13, 1952.

Surgical treatment of arteriosclerotic aneurysms of the abdominal aorta, AMA Arch. Surg. 64:307, 1952 (with Marshall).

Limitations of sympathectomy in treatment of diastolic hypertension, JAMA 148: 1382, 1952.

Segmental nature of peripheral arteriosclerosis: Special application, Angiology 4: 12, 1953 (with Julian and Dye).

The reactivity of the clotting mechanism, Proc. Inst. Med. Chicago 19:319, 1953.

Response of the clotting mechanism to ACTH, Angiology 4:283, 1953 (with Voight).

Peripheral Arterial Disease — Raynaud's Syndrome, in Conn, H. (ed.): *Current Therapy* (Philadelphia: W. B. Saunders Co., 1954), pp. 207–210.

Anticoagulant therapy, Surgery 34:971, 1953.

Peripheral arterial embolism after myocardial infarction, JAMA 155:10, 1954 (with Lary).

Vertebral vein thrombosis: A clinical syndrome, Gynaecologia 138:135, 1954 (with Coelho).

Aneurysms: General considerations, Angiology 5:173, 1954 (with Pirani).

Revascularization of the arteriosclerotic extremity, Surg. Gynecol. Obstet. 99:243, 1954.

Acute arterial occlusion, Surg. Clin. North Am. 35:265, 1955.

Revascularization of the arteriosclerotic extremity, AMA Arch. Surg. 70:5, 1955.

The controversial use of cervical sympathetic block in apoplexy, Ann. Intern. Med. 41:1196, 1954.

The management of venous thrombosis in the lower extremities, Surgery 37:507, 1955.

Arterial stenosis: A correlation of clinical and angiographic findings, Postgrad. Med. 17:286, 1955.

Traumatic axillary aneurysm of thirteen years' duration, AMA Arch. Surg. 70:390, 1955 (with Lary).

Clinical and angiographic correlations in arterial stenosis, JAMA 158:1502, 1955.

Sympathetic block in apoplexy, Surgery 38:915, 1955.

The experimental use of steel mesh tubes for the replacement of arterial segments, AMA Arch. Surg. 72:69, 1956 (with Lary and Meine).

Use of the cervical sympathetic block in the early treatment of apoplexy, Geriatrics 2:249, 1956 (with McDonald).

The Recognition and Management of Arterial Stenosis, vol. XIII, American Academy of Orthopedic Surgeons Instructional Course Lectures (Ann Arbor, Mich.: J. W. Edwards Publishers, Inc., 1956).

Fundamental factors affecting vascular surgery, Surgery 41:444, 1957.

Surgical treatment of hyperhidrosis, AMA Arch. Dermatol. 76:31, 1957.

Postphlebitic syndrome, JAMA 164:1861, 1957.

The vicious circle in hypertension, its surgical significance, Surgery 43:113, 1958 (with MacDonald and Harridge).

Mast cell activity under various forms of stress, Surgery 44:312, 1958 (with Villavincencio).

Place of sympathectomy in the treatment of occlusive arterial disease, AMA Arch. Surg. 77:655, 1958.

Ten-year follow-up study of surgically treated hypertensive patients, Geriatrics 14: 361, 1959.

Use of homografts dispensed by central artery bank of Chicago Heart Association, JAMA 178:2132, 1959 (with Weinberg, Fell and McElwaine).

Acute vascular occlusion of the extremities (summary of a talk given at the 119th annual meeting, Illinois Medical Society, Chicago, May 1959), Ill. Med. J. vol. 116, p. 254, 1959.

Bovine arterial grafts, Ann. Surg. 150:1017, 1959 (with Thompson and Dolowy).

Parkinson's law in medicine (special article), N. Engl. J. Med. 262:126, 1960.

Arterial inflammation, Surg. Clin. North Am. 40:45, 1960.

Injuries to Large Blood Vessels, in Cole, W. H., and Puestow, C. B. (eds.): *First Aid: Diagnosis and Management* (New York: Appleton-Century-Crofts, 1960).

Response of the arteriosclerotic limb to injury, Industrial Med. Surg. 29:192, 1960.

Treatment of Arterial Insufficiency of the Lower Extremities by Lumbar Sympathectomy, in Mulholland, Ellison, and Frieson (eds.): *Current Surgical Management II* (Philadelphia: W. B. Saunders Co., 1960).

Intermittent claudication studied by electromyography, AMA Arch. Surg. 81:94, 1960.

Intermittent Claudication, *Extrait du XVIII Congres de la Societe Internationale de Chirurgie,* Munich, September 13 – 20, 1959.

Bovine Arterial Grafts, *Extrait du XVIII Congres de la Societe Internationale de Chirurgie*, Munich, September 13 – 20, 1959 (with Thompson and Dolowy).

Intermittent claudication, J. Cardiovasc. Surg. 2:97, 1961 (with Griffiths, Thompson, and Frost).

The scrub nurse — a vanishing species, Surg. Gynecol. Obstet. 112:494, 1961.

Raynaud's phenomenon, JAMA 179:1, 1962 (with Fowler).

The neurogenic factor in Raynaud's phenomenon, Surgery 51:9, 1962 (with Fowler).

Surgical physiology of hypertension, Surg. Clin. North Am. 42:91, 1962.

Symptoms and signs of peripheral arterial disease, Med. Clin. North Am. 46:647, 1962.

The surgical treatment of diabetic vascular disease, Ill. Med. J. 121:627, 1962.

The three-legged stool, or, the patient's dilemma, JAMA 180:1145, 1962.

Experimental production of renal hypertension, Ann. Surg. 156:292, 1962 (with Lindstrom, Medgyesy and Wibin).

Bifurcational anastomosis of small arteries with pedicled grafts, Surgery 53:340, 1963 (with Lindstrom).

Trauma to the arteriosclerotic limb, Trauma, April 1963 (with Fowler).

Arterial emergencies, Med. Times 91:957, 1963.

Peripheral Arterial Disease, in *Current Therapy* (Philadelphia: W. B. Saunders Co., 1964), pp. 168–173.

Diabetic vascular disease, South. Med. J. 57:1143, 1964.

Sympathetic reflex dystrophy, Med. Clin. North Am. 49:117, 1965.

Smoking withdrawal: The physician's role, Ill. Med. J. 127:141, 1965.

The significance of intermittent claudication, South. Med. J. 58:50, 1965.

Vascular injuries associated with fractures, Chicago Med. 68:513, June 12, 1965.

Letter to the Editor: Fibrinolysis following surgery, JAMA 192:1105, 1965.

Microcirculation: The third force, JAMA 195:302, 1966.

Phlebitis, World-Wide Abstr. vol. 9, no. 3, March–April 1966.

The early fate of autogenous grafts in the canine femoral vein, J. Cardiovasc. Surg. 7:148, 1966 (with Eadie).

Peripheral Arterial Disease, in Conn, H. L., Clohecy, R. J., and Conn, E. B., Jr. (eds.) *Current Diagnosis* (Philadelphia: W. B. Saunders Co., 1966), pp. 226–237.

Diabetic vascular disease, Am. Surg. 32:355, 1966.

Frostbite, Presbyterian-St. Luke's Bull. 5:12, 1966.

Farewell to Ferdinand, Grant Gazette vol. 5 no. 2, September 1966.

Editorial: Scientism: A new blight, JAMA 180:155, 1962.

Letter to the Editor: Heparin treatment of thromboembolic disease, JAMA 199:862, 1967.

Microcirculation: The last frontier, J. Cardiovasc. Surg. (special no.) Philadelphia Congress, September 7, 1965.

Reverence review, Arch. Surg. 96:1015, 1968.

Letter to the Editor: Thromboembolic disease and oral contraceptives, JAMA 206:2792, 1968.

Pulmonary embolism: A second look, J. Cardiovasc. Surg. (special no.) Vienna Congress, September 1967.

The fibrinolytic potential, Rev. Surg. 25:453, 1968 (with Vaithianathan).

Editorial: Spontaneous fibrinolysis, Surgery 65:399, 1969.

Sympathetic reflex dystrophy following hand injury. Questions and answers, JAMA 208:872, 1969.

Pitfalls in the diagnosis of venous thrombosis, Ill. Med. J. 136:687, 1969.

Bodily defenses against thrombosis, Am. J. Surg. 120:73, 1970 (with Vaithianathan).

How to forecast and prevent thromboembolism, Med. Times 99:49, 1971.

Heparin tolerance — revisited, Surgery 70:318, 1971.

Defective thrombolysis, J. Cardiovasc. Surg. 12:323, 1971.

The surgical aspects of thromboembolic disease, Curr. Med. Dialogue 38:41, 1971.

Book review: *Arterial Surgery* by H. H. G. Eastcott, JAMA 211:2160.

Book review: *Peripheral Arterial Disease: A Physician's Approach* by Robert L. Richards, JAMA 215:801, 1971.

Letter to the Editor: Urokinase-heparin treatment of embolism, JAMA 215:1325, 1971.

The meaning of health and the nature of disease, Rush-Presbyterian-St. Luke's Med. Bull. 10:75, 1971.

Letter to the Editor: Palliation or cure in hypertension, JAMA 219:1477, 1972.

Book review: *Arterial Occlusive Disease* edited by W. A. Dale, JAMA 220:732, 1972.

Sympathectomy revisited, Rush-Presbyterian-St. Luke's Med. Bull. 12:188, 1973.

Editorial: Urokinase pulmonary embolism trial, Am. J. Surg. 126:311, 1973.

Sympathectomy for hypertension, Am. J. Surg. 127:521, 1974.

Local amputation: Feasible for diabetic foot lesions? Mod. Med. 33:35, 1974.

Book review: *Vascular Disorders of the Extremities* by David Abramson, JAMA 231:420, 1975.

Letter to the Editor, N. Engl. J. Med. 293:407, 1975.

Sympathectomy revisited: Phoenix or dodo? Surgery 78:644, 1975.

Adequate use of heparin, Ill. Med. J. 149:245, 1976.

Index